THE PROTOCOL
THAT
KILLS

A TRUE CRIME STORY

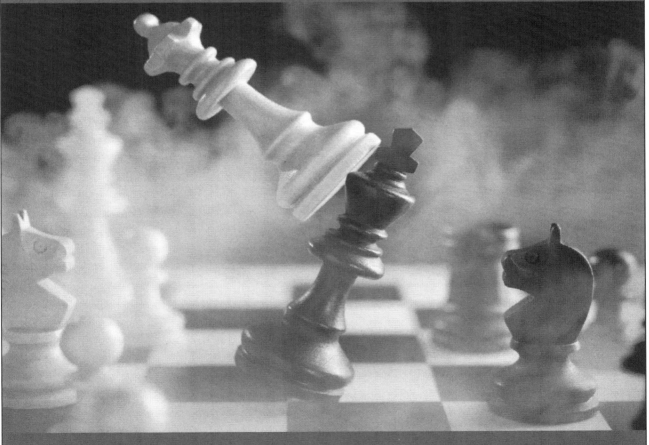

By Sheila Skiba
with Roberta and Allen Stalvey

The Protocol That Kills

Co-authored by Allen and Roberta Stalvey
theprotocolthatkills.com

Cover art & design by Sheila Skiba
Book images and art by Jeremiah Skiba
Edited by Allen Stalvey & Cynthia VanSlogteren
Poems by Roberta Stalvey

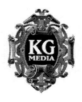

King's Gate Media, LLC
PO BOX 118461 Carrollton, TX 75011

First printing, 2023

ISBN: **979-8-846441-84-2**
Published in the United States of America

Dedication

I dedicate this book to my amazing husband, Robert A. Skiba II. It is my desire to be a continuation of his voice in honor of his life and motivate people to stand together in unity saying, *"Never Again!"*

Rob lived every day of his life to the fullest. He was a cheerful soul who had a song in each step. His presence was a joy and a gift, and I miss him terribly.

I wrote this book to honor his life and help save others by exposing the depth of the darkness behind an intentional, modern-day, genocidal medical tyranny.

Robert A. Skiba II, you are the love of my life, and I cannot wait to see you again. We were stronger together and I miss having you in my arms.

---

*In memory of the innocent victims of the protocol
that kills and in honor of their families.
May their voices not be silenced.*

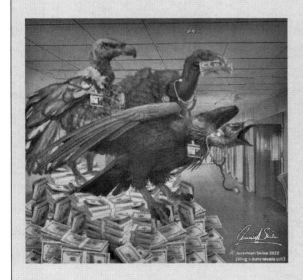

The Masquerade
Vultures in hospitals masquerade,
As doctors with murder
for money their trade,
Sedatives and paralytics their tools,
Comatose patients
their unfortunate fools.
Isolation, prison, stripped and bare,
Humiliation, alone, lost,
frightened and scared,
No one to hear their silent cries,
Their bodies violated,
their spirits die. These vultures, a scourge of the land,
Stealing the sick, and taking a stand,
Against the weak,
the vulnerable, the poor.
Their greed and cruelty,
forever a scourge.
But justice will come, in the end,
For the vultures,
their time is near at hand,
And the families, they will find peace,
When much needed
justice, is finally released.

Acknowledgments

It has often been said that behind every great man is a great woman. I have to confess that my husband, Robert A. Skiba II, was the most extraordinary person I ever knew. I could not, and would not, ever be able to hold a candle to the greatness he demonstrated and modeled to me.

I was blessed to have had 14 incredible years to call him my husband, and I cherish every moment we had together. I wish I could turn back the clock to before those agonizing 40 days that led to his untimely death on October 13, 2021.

First and foremost, I'd like to thank my son, Jeremiah Skiba. You are indeed one of a kind. Your unwavering love and support gave me the strength to carry on and keep looking forward rather than backward. I am so grateful for your love and support as I continue this journey, and I am deeply moved by your desire to preserve Rob's legacy and voice.

Thank you, Opa, my adopted father, for seeing me through every adversity and being my safe haven. I can't thank you enough for assisting me in raising Jeremiah and always being there for me since the day I was born.

I'd also like to thank my mother and sister for being by my side throughout Rob's 40-day hospitalization. Thank you for not giving up on me and helping me remain strong when I would have been weak without your guidance.

Thank you, Roberta and Allen Stalvey, for walking with me through this difficult time. Without your endless hours of comfort, support, and research, I could have never written this book. I praise God (Yahuwah) for your ongoing commitment to aiding me in uncovering the truth about my beloved husband's death. I treasure our friendship, adore you both, and cannot thank you enough for your encouragement, support, and genuine affection for Rob and me.

A special thanks to Cynthia VanSlogteren for her keen insights that aided us in polishing the final manuscript.

I would also like to thank Rob's and my extended family and friends, whose prayers and generosity have inspired me to persevere. Your love and prayers have given me the strength to keep moving forward with our ministry. I, too, will always remember the treasure Rob was and remains. His work, teachings, and spirit endure!

Finally, I'd like to extend my gratitude to everyone who has purchased this book. I sincerely hope that reading our story will equip you and your loved ones with valuable insights that will aid you in avoiding becoming victims of "the protocol that kills."

Foreward

I met Sheila Skiba after the passing of her husband, Rob, and I later learned more about who Rob was and what he stood for through his books and videos.

After serving as a medical/surgical nurse for 26 years, I became overcome with frustration, disgust, and horror at how Covid patients were being treated. So, in September of 2021, the same month Rob Skiba was hospitalized, I decided to leave a profession I truly loved.

I had to leave because I could no longer stand by and watch patients' and their families' rights being violated by colleagues who blindly followed and were willing to force their patients to succumb to a protocol that does not heal but harms; a protocol that was leading to the death of a large number of patients.

The Protocol That Kills is the most exhaustive exposé ever written on a government-incentivized protocol that must be **stopped** *to save future lives*. I hope hundreds of thousands read this book and send copies to colleagues, friends, and family members—especially to those who believe that everyone in the medical profession always has their best interests in mind.

Despite her pain, Sheila somehow crafted a work of art that could be called a true crime story, a legal brief, or an exhaustive exposé. Her insightful treatise is the most comprehensive and detailed book on the subject.

Be prepared, as in this book you will encounter the gripping details of Rob and Sheila Skiba's 40-day journey through hell; a journey that is sadly not unique as thousands of innocent victims have also traveled down this road of destruction.

After reading Sheila's story, you will have a clearer understanding of the risks involved in placing your life or the life of someone you love into the hands of modern-day "medical professionals" who have become protocol and profit-driven and who place both "the protocol" and their "bottom line" far above the health, welfare, and lives of their patients.

If this insanity is allowed to continue, thousands more will die needlessly. I hope that Sheila's insightful book will result in an outcry so strong and so loud that "the protocol that kills" will be stopped for good and that patients and their families will once again be treated with respect, dignity, and therapies that prolong their lives rather than end them.

Peggy Lawler
Medical/Surgical Nurse

Preface

I never imagined that I would be writing the tragic and true account of my husband's suffering and death at the hands of a group of "medical professionals"—a wholly callous and insensitive group that blindly adhered to a government-incentivized COVID-19 hospital "protocol that kills."

During my ordeal, it was as if I were a chess piece on a larger-than-life chessboard, and my husband, Rob, was the king the opposing side wanted to take down. My mother, sister, and close friends were the pawns on my side of the board. The opposing team comprised doctors, nurses, respiratory therapists, social workers, and hospital administrators.

Unfortunately, our opposition had the upper hand, as they had far more pieces on the board and were seasoned masters of the game, which they admitted they had played numerous times. They even broke the rules when it served their interests to do so.

Regrettably, this same game of cunning strategy is being played out in hospitals across the United States, where treacherous and devious masters of the game are defeating inexperienced patients and their unwary families.

Day and night I fought for his life during the forty days my husband was held captive by a team hell-bent on enforcing "the protocol." I insisted that he not be given dangerous drugs and therapies. However, they forced their will on him—until he died.

After the unnecessary and tragic death of my husband on October 13, 2021, my suffering and outrage grew stronger as I spent months working with a team of close friends, family, and medical experts who aided me in conducting a detailed analysis of the over 5,000 pages of his hospital records.

In addition, my team and I analyzed hours of conversations I had recorded with doctors, nurses, and staff during my husband's 40-day hospitalization—as allowed by Texas Penal Code, Section 16.02, Paragraph (c)(3)(A). https://statutes.capitol.texas.gov/Docs/PE/htm/PE.16.htm#16.02

Sadly, conducting a thorough investigation and authoring this book required reliving the trauma. Numerous disturbing facts uncovered during our investigation verified that my husband did not die of natural causes but due to the doctors' insistence that he follow their mandated and inhumane "protocol that kills."

Speaking of the protocol from a nurse's point of view, Nicole Sirotek, a registered critical care flight nurse who founded American Frontline Nurses to advocate for patients mistreated by hospitals' Covid protocols, said during a Senate hearing on January 24, 2022: "*Following orders has led to the sheer number of deaths that have occurred in these hospitals. I didn't see a single patient die of Covid. I've seen a substantial number of patients die of negligence and medical malfeasance.*"

My story is a raw, firsthand account of how "protocol-focused" doctors and nurses are violating the rights of patients and their families and how incentivized drugs and therapies are leading to needless deaths.

I decided to share my story for two reasons. First, I wish to inform the public that the U.S. medical establishment has devised and has been following a strict, unwavering, and lethal protocol that prioritizes hospital profits over patients' rights, health, and well-being.

Second, since being forewarned is to be forearmed, I hope to provide valuable insights that will protect you and your loved ones from falling victim to "the protocol that kills." That way, if you are confronted with tough decisions and a formidable opponent, as my husband and I were, you can declare "*Checkmate!*" and emerge victorious.

Sheila Skiba

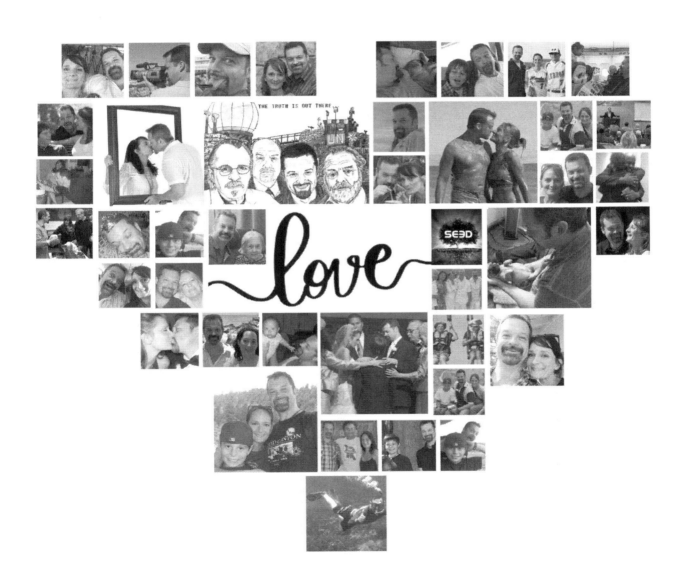

Table of Contents

Chapter 1 – Introduction

I hope that this true and tragic story will deeply touch you and, more importantly, that it will lead to the saving of many lives as the outright tyranny, corruption, and maliciousness of the Medical Industrial Complex is laid plain.

As I stated in the preface, my goal in sharing this story is to raise public awareness of the fact that the U.S. medical establishment has devised and recklessly follows a strict, unwavering, and lethal protocol that places hospitals' profits ahead of the rights, health, and well-being of patients and their families.

I also want to equip you with invaluable insights regarding what to do if you or someone you love chooses to attempt to recover at home or if hospitalization becomes the only option. In the latter case, my hope is that what you learn from reading my story can help you or a loved one avoid becoming another victim and statistic of "the protocol that kills."

Philippians 4:6 says, "*Do not be anxious about anything, but in every situation, by prayer and petition, with thanksgiving present your requests to God.*" I believe God hears our requests. I trust He is great, good, just, and true. He is ever active in human affairs and is sovereign.

Despite the immense trauma I experienced and the pain I still suffer today, I can assure you that God has never left my side as I walked through the valley of the shadow of death. It has been, and continues to be, exceedingly difficult; however, God is faithful and continues to sustain me. I pray that He will also sustain you through your life's journey.

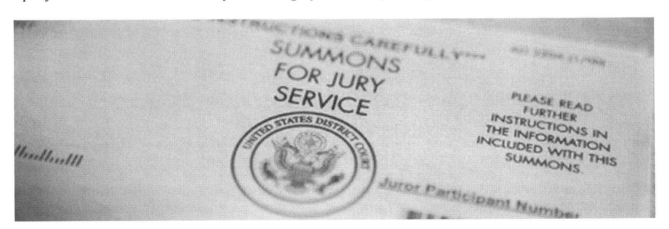

I now invite you to serve as **an informal juror in the court of public opinion** in the case of Robert A. Skiba II versus the Medical Industrial Complex. As a jury member, you will be asked to base your verdict solely upon the evidence without prejudice.

In this book, you will be presented with an abundance of compelling facts and exhibits that will allow you to decide whether my husband's death was caused by "the protocol that kills" or if he died an unavoidable death of natural causes.

You should base your decisions on the evidence presented here. However, you are not expected to set aside your life's experiences and common sense. Even then, I must warn you that my story is factually driven <u>and</u> emotionally charged because our lives were torn into millions of pieces during the forty tortuous and terrifying days I desperately struggled to keep Rob alive.

It is totally unacceptable that I was locked out of the hospital for 21 days while being forced to struggle tirelessly to defend my husband's rights and fight for his life. The experience was unbearably frustrating and emotionally draining, as I had to argue with doctors, nurses, and hospital staff daily until my husband died. What I experienced and many others have experienced at the hands of so-called "medical professionals" is a clear sign of a serious problem with our "health care" system in America.

I realize many kind and compassionate doctors and nurses have refused to support "the protocol that kills," even when doing so cost them their jobs. *Those who bravely stood up to this atrocity deserve to be recognized as modern-day heroes.*

Even then, it is undeniable that there have been and continue to be instances where patients have needlessly suffered and died at the hands of licensed physicians who, out of willful ignorance, uncaring negligence, or nefarious intent, forced their patients to succumb to "the protocol." Many of these professionals believe they are immune from prosecution because they have been sheltered by federal and state "pandemic" laws.

This senseless slaughter of innocent people at the hands of callous "professionals" must end. **Enough is enough!**

However, this evil abomination will not come to an end until enough of us who are awake and aware band together and, with one voice, say, *"We will no longer tolerate the systematic annihilation of innocent people in the name of a murderous protocol, and those who have committed these crimes against humanity **must** be held to account! This atrocity must stop now!"*

LEGAL COUNSEL STATEMENT
Members of the jury, this is the first of many "**legal counsel statements**" you will find throughout this book. Their purpose is made clear in Chapter 2.

At this point, we want to take a moment to salute and thank the doctors, nurses, respiratory therapists, and other medical staff who have *stood against this evil* and risked their careers and their lives to save the patients who entrusted them with their care. *These brave souls are true, modern-day heroes!*

Please join us in a moment of silence to thank our heavenly Father for their bravery, courage, and willingness to stand against medical tyranny. We pray for their safety and prosperity as they stand for truth and life.

In this book, we sound an alarm against a lethal protocol that must be stopped—and it is our sincere desire that Sheila and Rob Skiba's story touches hearts, opens eyes, saves lives, and helps to once and for all put an end to this modern-day genocide.

Sadly, Rob had no voice because his rights were stripped away. His medical treatment options were exclusively decided by his "medical caregivers," as they ignored his and my inputs and demands.

After Rob's death, a review of the over 5,000 pages of his hospital records clearly showed that it was (a) the lack of adequate food and water, (b) the large quantities and dosages of dangerous and deadly drugs such as remdesivir (which was refused but was administered anyway), (c) the continual stress of the constant badgering by doctors and nurses to be intubated and placed on a ventilator, (d) the use of a contraindicated therapy, and (e) his being intubated and administered toxic levels of oxygen for extended periods both before and after he was placed on a ventilator (see Page C-54 in Appendix C)—that led to Rob's death.

Rob had often said, "**Evil happens when good men do nothing.**" Is it possible that "the protocol that kills" is a covert aspect of a broad and sinister plan to vastly decrease the world's population? Regardless, it is high time we stand against this insanity and take back our God-given rights to life, liberty, and the pursuit of happiness.

Rob is just one of the countless innocent victims of an inflexible "protocol" that is being forced on patients by an oppressive and tyrannical medical system. This fatal protocol must be stopped! It is clear that the Hippocratic oath of *"above all else, do no harm"* that doctors were once said to ascribe to is NO LONGER being honored.

It may be time that we herald a "Nuremberg Trial II" to call the barbarous assassins who promote and execute this "protocol" to account—because if we do not stand together, we may all end up dying alone—just like my husband, Rob.

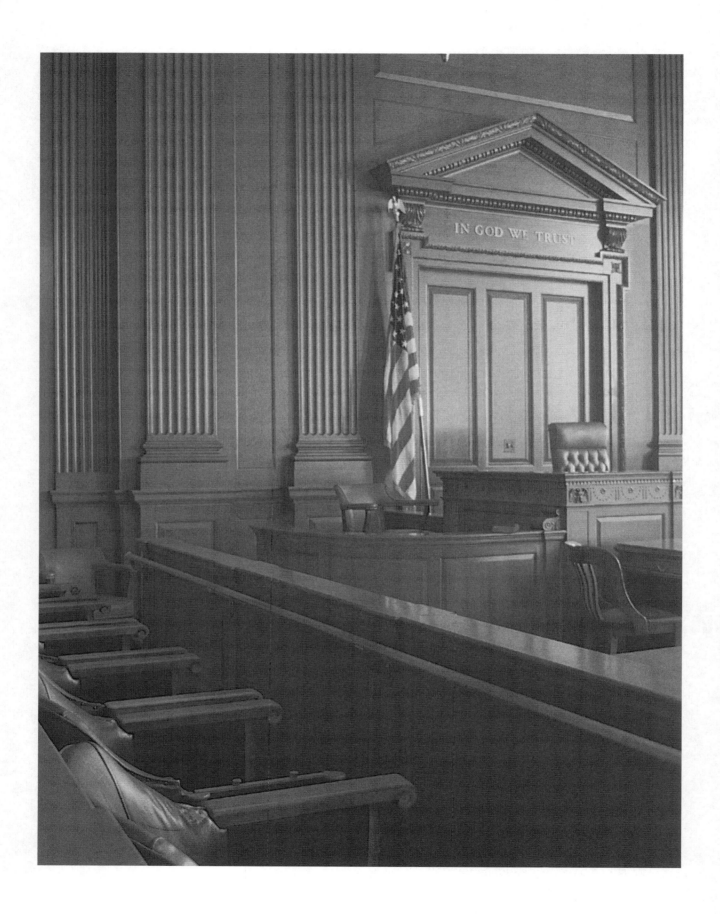

Juror Notes

Chapter 2 – Legal Counsel Argument

As you are being asked to serve as a member of the jury in the court of public opinion, it is essential that you have ready access to all of the evidence.

Therefore, we will be presenting the evidence in seven distinct voices:

1. **Sheila Skiba's voice**—as she candidly shares her personal story of the forty days of terror that she and Rob experienced at the hands of a medical system that is dead set on ensuring patients follow *the protocol that kills*.

2. **Rob Skiba's voice**—via his text messages to Sheila, friends, and family as he shares his fear that the doctors would kill him if Sheila could not be by his side as his on-site advocate.

3. **The voices of Sheila's family and friends**—who were trying to assist Sheila with keeping Rob alive and helped prevent Sheila from falling into severe depression.

4. **The comments of a quasi-legal counsel**— who provides a wealth of insightful and invaluable details and evidence—including over 100 citations from clinical studies, medical journals, federal regulations, and relevant books and articles—that prove Rob did not die of natural causes but due to the perpetrators' insistence that he follow the mandated and inhumane *"protocol that kills."*

5. **The voices of the doctors, therapists, nurses, and staff entrusted with Rob's care**— based on conversations Sheila recorded and transcribed, as allowed by Texas law. They reveal how Sheila and Rob were deceived and manipulated. *Their voices are displayed in gray text to make it easy for you to distinguish them.*

6. **The voice of Sammy Wong, MD**— an American Board of Internal Medicine Certified Internist and Assistant Professor of Medicine (ret) at Loma Linda University School of Medicine who has provided expert opinions and testimonies on well over a hundred cases over the past 30 years and has given multiple presentations on Medical Malpractice, Patient Safety, Cognitive Bias, and Diagnostic Errors. *His Letter of Introduction, Interim Analysis, and Causes of Action against the culpable parties appear in Appendix B.*

7. **Extracts from Rob's hospital records**—which expose the harmful drugs and therapies provided to Rob, the doctors' and nurses' frustration at Rob's and Sheila's continued insistence that he not be given remdesivir and not be intubated and placed on a ventilator, and their total disregard for the fact that Rob (who had not been able to eat for over a week prior to his admission and was already malnourished) was not consuming an adequate amount of food and water. *Each hospital record includes detailed notations that show how flagrant biases, willful negligence, malicious intent, and harmful therapies led to Rob's needless death.*

The evidence we will present strongly supports the claim that Rob and Sheila's constitutional, civil, patient, and Medical Power of Attorney rights were violated and that Rob Skiba did not die a natural death from his unquestionably curable illness.

Instead, due to gross negligence and possibly malicious intent, his needless death was caused by iatrogenic injury (injury caused by doctor-prescribed drugs and medical treatments).

Sheila was intimidated and shouted at over the phone the day after Rob's arrival at the hospital by a physician who was standing by Rob's bedside at the time of the call as he insisted Rob would die if he was not placed on a ventilator. Sheila's sister and mother were with her when the call came through and heard every word.

Due to this harsh and inappropriate treatment, Sheila began recording all future conversations with doctors, nurses, and hospital staff. The dialog that appears in this book was taken directly from her recordings. Anyone who *"is a party to the communication"* is legally permitted to record and disclose the contents of their communications under Texas Penal Code, Section 16.02, Paragraph (c)(3)(A). https://statutes.capitol.texas.gov/Docs/PE/htm/PE.16.htm#16.02

We contend that the hospital purposely locked Sheila out for 21 days so she could not watch over and question his care, advocate for him in person, ensure he was provided with adequate food and water, and aid him in eating and drinking—something he found impossible to do on his own with the high-flow oxygen therapy he was on. In addition, locking Sheila out allowed them to flood Rob with unwanted, unnecessary, and harmful drugs while starving him into submission.

As you will read and see in a text message screenshot later in this book, Rob texted Sheila, *"No food,"* at 7:30 PM on September 5, 2021, over 48 hours after his arrival at the hospital. He then texted, *"No strength, no hope left."* On Page 104 of the hospital records (see Page C-27 in Appendix C), a dietitian openly admitted Rob had "poor intake" and had "not been ordering 3 meals daily."

A hospital staff member told Sheila she could not be provided with access to her husband's records until after he was discharged to keep her from learning the details of how he was being treated. However, four days after he was admitted, she was able to retrieve a code the hospital emailed to her husband and gain access to his online MyChart records.

Even with access to the records, Sheila was at a significant disadvantage because she could only confirm what treatments Rob had received after the previous day's records had been posted. As a result, while being locked out of the hospital, she was dependent on the limited information she could obtain during her daily phone calls with nurses and doctors—which you will observe as you read her story. Disturbingly, their daily updates often conflicted with what was later recorded in the hospital records.

After being assaulted by a barrage of dangerous drugs since his arrival, on the morning of September 8, 2021, Rob was then subjected to 4.5 hours on a BiPAP—a contraindicated therapy admission five days earlier. Pneumomediastinum is a condition where a patient has air abnormally trapped in the space in the chest between the lungs, and BiPAP therapy can (and did) significantly worsen that condition.

To make matters worse, as noted on Page 127 of Rob's hospital records (see Page C-35 in Appendix C), a doctor informed Sheila that BiPAP therapy might cause barotrauma, a potentially life-threatening condition where the alveoli, the air sacs of the lungs, rupture and collapse. The "*Repeat CXR [Chest X-ray] this afternoon to monitor barotrauma*" note on page 141 of the hospital records (see Page C-44) confirms their placing Rob on a BiPAP for 4.5 hours **did** cause this life-threatening condition—making it nearly impossible for him to adequately breathe on his own.

Sammy Wong, MD, our expert medical witness, listed Rob's being placed on a BiPAP with known pneumomediastinum as one of his "**Causes of Action**" [grounds for litigation] against the doctors, as noted on Page B-7 in **Appendix B**. We believe this therapy further damaged Rob's lungs to the point of no return, giving the doctors the excuse they were looking for to force Rob to be intubated and placed on a ventilator.

How and why Rob died—which we unravel in detail in this book—*is an absolute crime*. Moreover, it is a crime that racked up a hospital bill of $794,587.10 (before adjustments) for Rob's 40-day stay at what Sheila later referred to as a "kill shelter." In addition, the hospital received government (and perhaps pharmaceutical companies') incentives (see **Appendix D**). With the doctors' private bills added, the unadjusted total came to over $1 million.

Sadly, incentivized medications and protocols have become a dangerous weapon against humanity.

The actions taken by the hospital administrators, doctors, nurses, and staff—such as isolating Rob, heavily medicating him, intimidating and humiliating him, depriving him of nourishment, causing him total desperation, and ultimately intubating and ventilating him—were motivated by their self-interests.

We argue that their single-minded focus on what would most benefit them rather than what would most benefit the patient ultimately resulted in his unnecessary and tragic death. They literally "forced their will down Rob's throat" by weakening him through a lack of adequate nutrition and the use of harmful medications and therapies. This allowed them to achieve their objective of intubating and ventilating him, which ultimately ended his life.

As you will discover by reading this emotional and disturbing true crime story, the protocol that kills' pattern of treatment—a pattern that is being followed in hospitals throughout the United States and possibly in other countries—consists of **isolation, heavy medication, intimidation, humiliation, starvation, desperation, intubation, ventilation, devastation, and termination**.

From the day of Rob's admission, the doctors and nurses never let up on their daily, and sometimes hourly, badgering of Rob to agree to be sedated, intubated, and placed on a ventilator. They continually referred to it as Rob's need to agree to "*elective intubation.*"

As a result of this harassment, Rob texted Sheila on his 4th day in the hospital, *"Doing all they can to try to get me to agree to intubate. I'm dead if they do."* Sadly, their daily abuse continued until Rob was finally sedated, intubated, paralyzed, and ventilated.

We believe that Robert A. Skiba II died as a direct result of the hospital's and doctors' unwavering, ruthless, and deadly protocol that they consistently followed whenever a patient had "**COVID-19**" stamped on their chart, especially if the record stated "**UNVACCINATED**" in **BOLD CAPITALS**, as can be seen on page 53 of Rob's medical records (see Page C-8 in Appendix C). *In addition, we contend that many doctors and nurses are prejudiced against the "unvaccinated" and especially target them for ventilation.*

> **LEGAL COUNSEL STATEMENT**
> Members of the jury, to protect the identity of the doctors, nurses, and hospital staff—and to universalize the story, which is regrettably repeating itself in hospitals across the U.S. and potentially abroad—**their names have been redacted and replaced with pseudonyms**.
>
> We admit that the aliases selected <u>are not complimentary</u>. They were chosen to help portray the terror Sheila, and her family experienced as the doctors, nurses, and staff indifferently and rigidly followed "the protocol that kills." In addition, we have chosen to refer to the hospital as the **Covid Coven Hospital of Plano, Texas**.

Clear evidence that *"the protocol that kills"* was the plan of care for Rob from the moment he arrived can be found in the "**Impression and Plan**" written by Nurse Practitioner Horrendous, who, at 9:07 PM, minutes after his admission to the ICU, wrote in Rob's records on Page 27 (see Page C-3 in Appendix C), "***Patient is at high risk for intubation.***" *She wrote this note even though Rob, as noted on Page 3005 of his records (see Page C-4), was improving on supplemental oxygen and his blood oxygen level had risen up to the range of 95% to 98%.*

Once he was on the ventilator, Rob's doctors continued to poison him with thousands of dollars' worth of unnecessary and harmful medications that helped hasten his death, which occurred after 40 days in the hospital and 35 days on a ventilator. Below is a list of just three:

- **Tocilizumab** (a rheumatoid arthritis drug given for a condition Rob did not have) = $12,175
- **Nimbex** (a paralytic used while Rob was on the ventilator) $1,070/dose x 50 doses = $53,500
- **VELETRI** (instead of the budesonide they requested) $148.36 per dose x 104 doses = $15,429

As you read this story, you will find yourself asking, *"Why?"*—just as Sheila did regarding the actions of the doctors, nurses, and staff during Rob's 40-day hospital stay while a man's life was being weighed in the balance. *We believe the choices they made cost Rob Skiba his life.*

> If you have had any doubt about whether patients have been dying needlessly in hospitals across America, consider this quote from <u>Undercover Epicenter Nurse: How Fraud, Negligence, & Greed Led to Unnecessary Deaths at Elmhurst Hospital,</u> where Erin Marie Olszewski, BSN, RN, stated:
>
> *"I can't tell you how many people I've seen in hospitals across the country who would rather live in denial than admit to themselves that their loved one is dying unnecessarily. Especially in America, many people would rather live in the comfortable bubble of ignorance than look evil in the eye."*
>
> Olszewski, Erin. "Introduction." Undercover Epicenter Nurse: How Fraud, Negligence, & Greed Led to Unnecessary Deaths at Elmhurst Hospital, Skyhorse, 2020.

Rob once proudly served as an Army helicopter pilot who swore to—and throughout his life

*I, Robert A. Skiba II, do solemnly swear (or affirm) that I will support and defend the Constitution of the United States against all enemies, foreign **and domestic**; that I will bear true faith and allegiance to the same; and that I will obey the orders of the President of the United States and the orders of the officers appointed over me, according to regulations and the Uniform Code of Military Justice. So help me God.*

Rob was willing to risk his life to defend his country. He was brave and he was courageous. He was a man who was constantly in search of and who stood for truth and justice. *A valiant soldier has fallen at the hands of a domestic enemy. After you have read his harrowing story, we ask that you stand with us against this unspeakable tyranny.*

Join us now in looking evil square in the eye as we reveal the disturbing, true story of what was done to Rob Skiba by so-called "medical professionals."

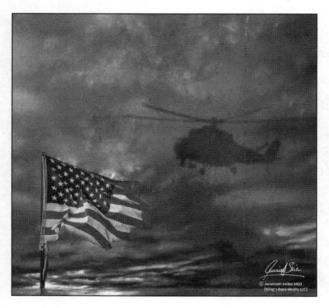
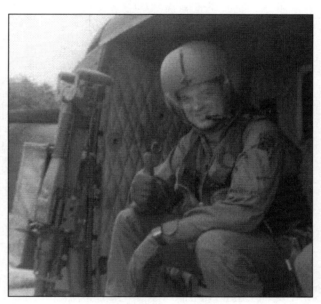

We now present to you, members of the jury of the court of public opinion, a wealth of compelling evidence we believe will incontrovertibly prove that Robert A. Skiba II, a healthy 52-year-old male with no comorbidities, would be alive today if the hospital had taken a conservative, personalized approach to his care and limited the scope of their treatment to supplemental oxygen, steroids (such as budesonide), antibiotics (for infection), and nutrition.

Unfortunately, a conservative and life-saving plan of care would not have been financially beneficial to the hospital or the doctors. Thus, they forced Rob to succumb to the horrifying "protocol that kills."

After Rob's death, Sheila and a small, dedicated team thoroughly reviewed Rob's hospital records. During their review, they unearthed many nefarious and incomprehensible acts that unraveled the mystery of why her otherwise strong and healthy 52-year-old husband of 14 years—and who faced an exceptionally negligible risk (a less than 1% chance) of dying from COVID-19—lost his life in a hospital after suffering 40 days of "the protocol that kills."

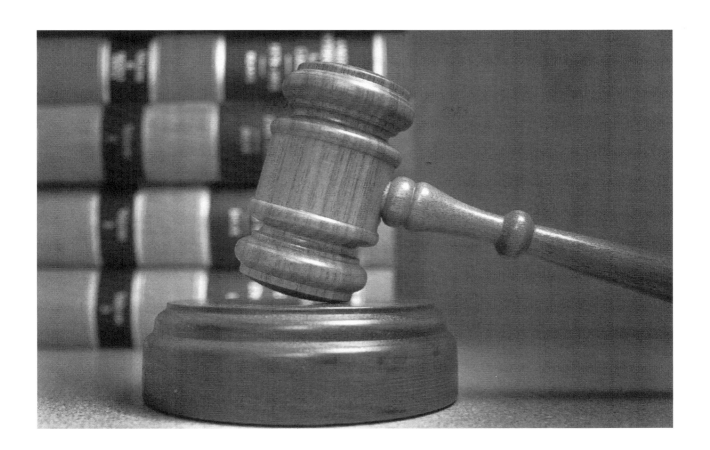

The gavel has fallen.
Jurors, you may now be seated.

Chapter 3 – Hospitalization & Isolation

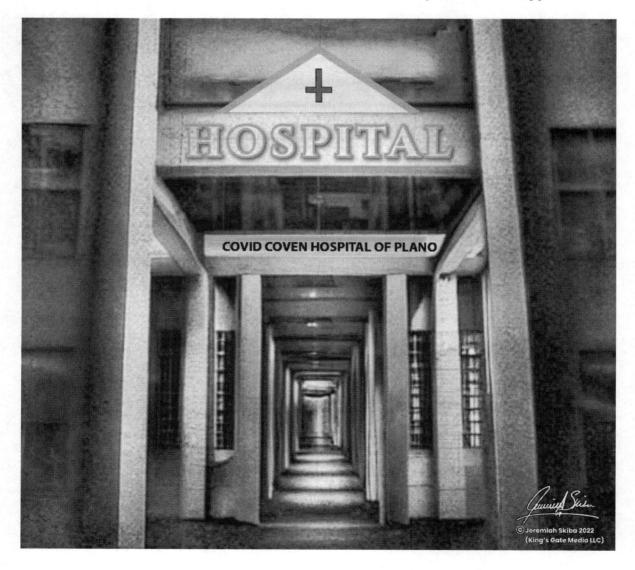

THIS CHAPTER COVERS SEPTEMBER 3, 2021 (Admission Day)

© Jeremiah Skiba 2022
(King's Gate Media LLC)

The entire world had mysteriously turned violently upside down. Everyone seemed to be in a trance as I rolled Rob into the Emergency Department at around 4:50 PM. A nurse and a security guard cowered behind their obligatory blue masks. The nurse at the desk gave me a stern stare that broadcast a sense of annoyance instead of radiating a sense of welcome.

Another nurse tossed a blue mask at my husband and yelled, "He needs to put this on!" She did not seem to notice or care that he was already wearing a transparent plastic shield that made it far easier for him to breathe while still protecting others from his consistent coughing.

After looking down at the mask in his lap, Rob gave me a pitiful and apprehensive look as he struggled to breathe between his uncontrollable bouts of coughing. I cried out, "No, he can't breathe!" The hateful and heartless nurse pointed at the mask with a demanding look.

Her chief concern was getting a mask on Rob's face—as if that was the most pressing issue, not Rob's difficulty breathing. When did it make sense to ask someone struggling to breathe to cover their face with a paper mask? Whatever happened to the age of reason?

She glared at me and waited for my compliance; I removed his clear face shield and begrudgingly put the mask on his face. Even then, I knew full well that my doing so would further reduce his blood oxygen level—which had already dropped to 71% according to the pulse oximeter we had used at home. A wave of panic overcame me as I could sense Rob's anxiety increasing because of how he was being treated.

When I finished placing the mask on Rob's face, the unsympathetic nurse shouted, "You need to leave!" She then quickly and forcefully wheeled my anxious husband away, indicating that I could not follow her and stay by his side. As she sped off, I yelled to her, "Don't you want my husband's medical history?" Her abrupt response was, "Is he vaccinated?"

I immediately thought, "What difference does it make whether or not Rob is vaccinated?" But, knowing how paranoid some people can be, I nervously squeaked out, "No!" as Rob began to vanish into the distance. Then, before they turned the corner, I heard him blurt out in an apprehensive tone between coughs, the last words I would hear him speak to me in person: "*If they don't let you be my advocate, I'm going to die in here!*"

LEGAL COUNSEL STATEMENT
Members of the jury, as noted above, Sheila thought, "*What difference does it make whether or not Rob is vaccinated.*" Sadly, she would soon find out, as Page 28 of Rob's hospital records (see Page C-6 in Appendix C) states in bold italics, "***He has not been vaccinated.***" On Page 53 of his records (see Page C-8) you will find, "**COVID 19 VACCINATION STATUS: UNVACCINATED.**"

They were not at all concerned with Rob's medical history. They only wanted to know if he had been vaccinated. Patients and their families across America have reported that unvaccinated patients have been targeted and received harsh treatment by cold-hearted pro-vax doctors and nurses who appear to have a substantial prejudice against the "unvaxxed" and wish to make examples of them.

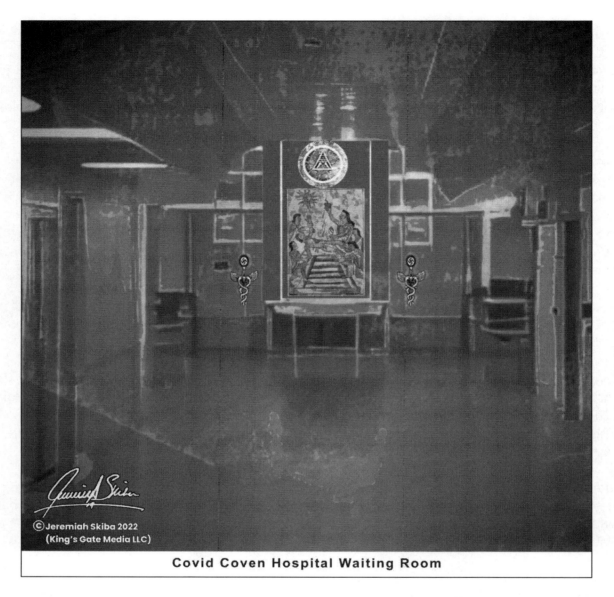

Covid Coven Hospital Waiting Room

As the nurse sped away, I pleaded, "**His father lost a kidney. So, NO remdesivir and NO ventilator!**" The Emergency Department waiting room had such an eerie feeling about it, and as the angry nurse sped away with my husband, I thought, "*Oh Lord, what are they going to do to Rob in this place?*"

In compliance with the nurse's demands, the security guard assigned to the Emergency Department rapidly and brutishly ushered me out the sliding glass doors, not unlike a bar bouncer ushers an unruly patron out of a bar.

As the automatic doors abruptly slid closed behind me, I found myself standing outside in a daze with my sister, who had followed us to the hospital, standing by my side with a blank stare on her face. I was shocked and unable to speak. My heart sank, and I felt a deep fear choking me and making it hard for me to breathe. I thought, "What in the world just happened!" I had fully expected to be able to stay by his side, assist the nurses with his care, and even sleep overnight in a chair at his bedside as I had before at this hospital when other relatives of mine had been hospitalized in the past. Now I was standing outside while Rob was trapped inside with no loving family member by his side.

While reflecting on what had just happened, I wondered whether I should run back in past the guard, chase down the nurse, snatch the wheelchair from her hands, and dart back out to my car with Rob. The temptation to do that was unbearable. Yet I realized if I ran out with him, I would have no way of saving him on my own as I had no other means of quickly getting him the supplemental oxygen he desperately needed.

I looked at my phone and saw it was a little after 5:00 PM. Although the sun had not yet set, I felt like everything had become black and dreary. No light could penetrate the unnatural darkness that now surrounded me.

When I arrived home, I called Rob to ensure he was okay. He said they had placed him on oxygen, his blood oxygen level had risen to a normal 95%, and he was feeling much better. I told him he would be okay and encouraged him to get some much-needed rest.

I tried to calm my mind by telling myself that his hospital stay should be brief and that he would likely return home fully recovered in just a day or two. I began to think, "Okay. Be calm. The hospital staff will stabilize Rob with oxygen, help him regain his strength, and he will come home soon."

Rob and I fully expected that if we both took a hardline stance against remdesivir, intubation, and ventilation, he would be okay—and would not become another grim statistic.

Hoping for assurance that I had made the right decision, I called my son, Jeremiah, who lived nearby. When I shared with him what had just happened, he was horrified to hear I had been abruptly ushered out of the hospital. He knew we had both been sick, yet he did not realize that while I had gotten better, Rob had only worsened and needed supplemental oxygen.

I tearfully told him, "They took him away from me and told me to leave, Jeremiah! What am I to do? I'm so afraid!" He tried to assure me, "Don't worry, mom. Everything is going to be okay. That's the same hospital you took Papi to, and they took good care of him. Remember how they saved his life when he got a pacemaker? So, there's nothing to worry about. They will give Rob the same kind of care they gave Papi. Besides, Rob is a man of God, and there is no way God would allow him to be taken out this way. You did the right thing."

I shared, "His oxygen was so low, Jeremiah. The telemedicine doctors told me to take him to the Emergency Department." He assured me that Rob's getting oxygen and antibiotics would fix everything. Even then, Jeremiah's encouraging words did nothing to quell my fear. I wanted to believe my family was right. They all agreed that God had a plan for Rob's life, that he had much more to do, and that it was not his time to go.

I continued, "Jeremiah! Rob said he would die in there if I couldn't be his advocate." He said, "Mom, don't worry. He will be okay. I know he will. I'm on my way over. Just give me a few minutes. I'll gather my things and stay the night with you." I pitifully cried, "Okay," and hung up the phone.

Despite my son's attempts to reassure me, I still felt desperate and overwhelmed. It was as if I was on a fast-moving rollercoaster that was constantly flipping and turning, causing me to feel physically ill and drained. My body's fight-or-flight response had been kicked into high gear, and I could not turn it off.

My family fully believed Rob would be okay and would survive this ordeal. Yet I kept hearing Rob saying, "***If they don't let you be my advocate, I'm going to die in here!***" I cried out, "Oh God, HELP ME! If Rob dies, I will die! I cannot and will not live without him. He's my everything!"

I yelled, "Nothing matters anymore!" I beat my fists against the wall and slid down to the cold, hard, tiled floor as I cried uncontrollably with angry tears that transitioned to fearful and grief-stricken wailing tears. I had never known this level of grief before.

My mother's heart broke as she watched her broken daughter lie limp on the floor. Her tears joined with mine as she suffered from the angst of not knowing how to save me from my self-implosion.

Jeremiah finally arrived, swung open the front door, and could hear me crying at the back of the house. He sat beside me and placed his hand on my back to comfort me. Seeing my face drenched with tears, he gently lifted me as I clung to him and cried on his shoulder.

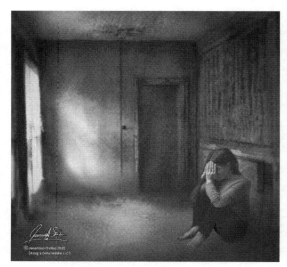

He lovingly said, "Mom, everything is going to be okay. I'm here now and will help you in any way I can. You did the right thing. In a few days, Rob will be home. I'm praying for Rob. God will not allow him to die in the hospital. He's such a good man. Don't worry, Mom. Everything is going to be okay. All he needs is a little oxygen."

He listened with great compassion as I poured out my heart. Finally, my anxiety had lessened enough that I could call the Emergency Department to check on how Rob was doing. They told me his blood oxygen was still at 95%, and he was doing okay. My sister said, "See, I told you they would help him and get him on the road to recovery."

At 10:33 PM, I called the Emergency Department again and was advised that at 9:05 PM, Rob had been admitted and moved to the Intensive Care Unit (ICU). So, I called the main hospital number and asked to be connected with the ICU.

LEGAL COUNSEL STATEMENT
Members of the jury, upon being administered oxygen, Rob's blood oxygen level rose **from 71%** into the **upper 90s**. Yet at 9:05 PM, they decided to admit Rob to the ICU instead of a room on a regular floor so they could give him a high-risk, nebulized, off-label drug called **VELETRI**, a drug that is so high-risk that it may only be administered in the ICU because it can cause patients *severe shortness of breath, gasping for breath, and possible death*— risks that were not disclosed to Rob or Sheila.

Drugs.com notes, "*VELETRI may cause **serious side effects**,*" which include "***symptoms of pulmonary edema*** (an X-Ray on September 5, 2021, noted Rob had multifocal pneumonia and pulmonary edema)— *anxiety, sweating, pale skin, **severe shortness of breath**, wheezing, **gasping for breath**, cough with foamy mucus, chest pain, fast or uneven heart rate.*"
VELETRI uses, Side Effects & Warnings. Drugs.com. (n.d.). From https://www.drugs.com/mtm/veletri.html

Why would the doctors prescribe someone suffering from Covid pneumonia, who had been diagnosed with pulmonary edema (which VELETRI can cause or exacerbate), and is already having difficulty breathing, a drug that can cause increased fluid in the lungs, increased difficulty breathing, and severe anxiety?

Our independent medical expert, Sammy Wong, MD (as noted in Appendix B), stated that **VELETRI** "*is indicated for people with known 'severe pulmonary arterial hypertension [PAH].' There was no objective evidence [that is, a diagnosis of pulmonary arterial hypertension does not appear anywhere in Rob's records indicating] that he had severe PAH.*"

In his **Causes of Action,** Dr. Wong stated that VELETRI "*can incite a profound inflammatory response in the pulmonary interstitium [the tissue in and around the wall of the alveoli (air sacs) of the lung where oxygen moves from the alveoli into the capillary network (the bloodstream)]. Due to a lack of indication for its use, the patient was subjected to unnecessary risks.*"

Covid creates a significant inflammatory response in the lungs, and the last thing a Covid patient needs is increased inflammation of the tissue between the alveoli (air sacs) and the capillary network where oxygen is delivered into the bloodstream.

We firmly believe Rob would have continued to improve and be alive today if he had only been given supplemental oxygen, antibiotics, steroids (such as budesonide, an inhaled corticosteroid that had been proven **90% effective for Covid** with two randomized control trials as noted in **Appendix F**), and adequate nutrition. Instead, as you learn, he was administered an abundance of dangerous drugs and contraindicated therapies— drugs and therapies that only worsened his condition and caused his death.

Just after midnight the evening of Rob's arrival in the Emergency Department, Dr. Useless, the hospitalist, wrote on Page 23 of Rob's hospital records (see Page C-2), "*It is anticipated that he will require at least a two-midnight inpatient stay.*" Unfortunately, a plan for a short-term stay where every effort would be made to stabilize Rob with the least number of medications and the least invasive therapies possible so he could be promptly discharged and sent home would not be profitable for the hospital or the doctors. As we stated earlier, the actual plan for Rob was laid out when Nurse Practitioner Horrendous wrote in Rob's record at 9:07 PM, minutes after his admission to the ICU (see Page C-3 in Appendix C), "*Patient is at high risk for intubation.*"

In an editorial published on April 22, 2022, in the peer-reviewed journal Surgical Neurology International, Russell L. Blaylock, MD, a retired neurosurgeon, said: "*For the first time in American history, a president, governors, mayors, hospital administrators, and federal bureaucrats are determining medical treatments based not on accurate scientifically based or even experience-based information, but rather to force the acceptance of special forms of care and 'prevention'—including remdesivir, use of respirators and ultimately a series of essentially untested messenger RNA vaccines. For the first time in history medical treatment, protocols are not being formulated based on the experience of the physicians treating the largest number of patients successfully, but rather individuals and bureaucracies that have never treated a single patient—including Anthony Fauci, Bill Gates, EcoHealth Alliance, the CDC, WHO, state public health officers and hospital administrators. . . even worse is the virtually universal control hospital administrators have exercised over the details of medical care in hospitals. **These hirelings are now instructing doctors which treatment protocols they will adhere to and which treatments they will not use, no matter how harmful the 'approved' treatments are or how beneficial the 'unapproved' treatments are**.*

"*Never in the history of American medicine have hospital administrators dictated to its physicians how they will practice medicine and what medications they can use. The CDC has no authority to dictate to hospitals or doctors*

"The federal Care Act encouraged this human disaster by offering all US hospitals up to 39,000 dollars for each ICU patient they put on respirators, despite the fact that early on it was obvious that the respirators were a major cause of death among these unsuspecting, trusting patients. In addition, the hospitals received 12,000 dollars for each patient that was admitted to the ICU—explaining, in my opinion and others, why all federal medical bureaucracies (CDC, FDA, NIAID, NIH, etc.) did all in their power to prevent life-saving early treatments." Covid update: What is the truth? Surgical Neurology International. (2022, May 10). From https://surgicalneurologyint.com/surgicalint-articles/covid-update-what-is-the-truth

With a nervous and shaky voice, I advised nurse Imposter, who answered the phone, that I was Sheila Skiba, Rob's wife, and asked her how he was doing. She said, "His blood oxygen level is currently at 99% while on high-flow oxygen. His blood pressure is 116/67, which looks great, and his heart rate is 72." Wow, he is doing great! I thought.

LEGAL COUNSEL STATEMENT
Members of the jury, Sheila and Rob initially had no idea that long durations of unnecessarily high concentrations of oxygen would further injure his lungs. We will cover this in greater detail later in the book.

I told the nurse that Rob and I did not want him to have remdesivir, nor did we want him to be

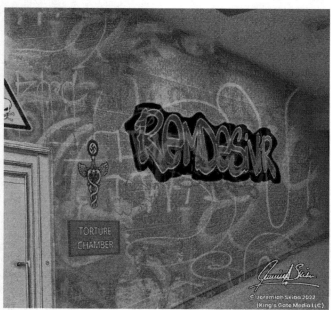

intubated and placed on a ventilator. To my horror, she informed me that he had already been given an initial double dose of remdesivir! I insisted that she write in his record that they needed to stop giving it to him because it could damage his kidneys.

She promised to note my request in his records and mention it to the day shift nursing staff when they arrived in the morning. She then said Rob had "refused insulin." What? Rob had refused insulin but accepted remdesivir. That made no sense, as he would have refused BOTH drugs if he knew they were being administered—especially remdesivir because he had called it, "Run Death Is Near!"

Rob did not believe in and had hardly ever used prescription medications. He prided himself on being healthy, fit, and drug-free. So, I knew he was given remdesivir without his knowledge.

LEGAL COUNSEL STATEMENT
Members of the jury, despite Sheila's insistence that he **NOT** be given remdesivir the moment she delivered him to the Emergency Department and Rob's repeated insistence that he not be given the drug (as recorded multiple times in his hospital record) less than 4 hours after his arrival, at 9:07 PM, as shown on Pages 12-13 of the hospital records (see Page C-1 in Appendix C), Nurse Practitioner Horrendous of the Emergency Department scheduled Rob for an initial **double-dose of 200 mg** of remdesivir followed by a second 100 mg dose the next morning.

Regrettably, during his first three days at the hospital, **Rob was given six doses of this dangerous drug**, one of which was **a second double dose** on September 6, 2021. Even more troubling is that remdesivir is a medication whose side effects include *breathing difficulties* and *acute kidney injury*.

Robert F. Kennedy Jr. stated in his book <u>The Real Anthony Fauci: Bill Gates, Big Pharma, and the Global War on Democracy and Public Health</u>, "*In 2018, Gilead entered remdesivir in a NIAID-funded clinical trial against*

Ebola in Africa. This is how we know that Anthony Fauci was well aware of remdesivir's toxicity when he orchestrated its approval for COVID patients. NIAID [the National Institute of Allergy and Infectious Diseases headed by Fauci] sponsored that project.

In the same clinical trial, Dr. Fauci had another NIAID-incubated drug, ZMapp, testing efficacy against Ebola alongside two experimental monoclonal antibody drugs. Researchers planned to administer all four drugs to Ebola patients across Africa over four to eight months. However, six months into the Ebola study, the trial's Safety Review Board suddenly pulled both remdesivir and ZMapp from the trial.

Remdesivir, it turned out, was hideously dangerous. Within 28 days, subjects taking remdesivir had lethal side effects, including multiple organ failure, acute kidney failure, septic shock, and hypotension, and 54 percent of the remdesivir group died—the highest mortality rate among the four experimental drugs.

Anthony Fauci's drug, ZMapp, ran up the second-highest body count at 44 percent. NIAID was the primary funder of this study, and its researchers published the bad news about remdesivir in the New England Journal of Medicine in December 2019."

Kennedy, R. F. (2022). In The real Anthony Fauci: Bill Gates, Big Pharma, and the Global War on Democracy and Public Health (p. 63). essay, Skyhorse Publishing.

Robert F. Kennedy, Jr. also noted: "Dr. McCullough gives us a stark and clear summary: *'Remdesivir has two problems. First, it doesn't work. Second, it is toxic and it kills people.'*" (Kennedy, 2021, p. 70)

I thanked her for being so helpful. Then, she offered to let me talk with Rob, saying, "Since I'm already in his room, why don't you speak with him." I replied, "Yes, please!"

I cried, Honey, I'm here. Don't talk, and don't use up your energy. I'm fighting for you. I've got a bunch of people helping, so don't give up. Just keep fighting. **Don't take the remdesivir**— though you didn't want to take it—it was forced on you already. But don't let them do it again. I'm going to be there first thing in the morning. And if I have to, I will take you out. I love you, Honey. Just stay strong! Keep taking deep breaths. We're fighting for you. Everybody's calling. Everybody's fighting for you. So, be strong and know that you are not alone. No, you're not alone, and there are a ton of people helping. Okay, I love you, Honey. We love you, Rob. Okay. Just rest. I love you!"

I was terribly upset to learn that while he was rapidly improving on oxygen, they had immediately given him remdesivir against our will—and tried to give him insulin. I planned on asking a doctor in the morning about all the drugs they were giving Rob and why.

LEGAL COUNSEL STATEMENT

Members of the jury, on April 30, 2021, WebMD published an article titled "COVID-19 and Your Kidneys: What You Should Know." The article noted, *"Research suggests that up to half of people hospitalized with COVID-19 get **an acute kidney injury**. That's a sudden case of kidney damage, and in some severe cases, kidney failure, that happens within hours or days."*

WebMD. (n.d.). Covid-19 and your kidneys: What you should know. WebMD. From https://www.webmd.com/lung/covid-kidneys-damage-coronavirus

We contend that **up to 50% of hospitalized COVID-19 patients** end up with **acute kidney injury** because **remdesivir** is part of the standard "protocol that kills"—a protocol that doctors are following in hospitals across the United States. It is of the utmost importance that those who have the authority to halt the use of this harmful drug and who can stop American doctors from forcing patients to succumb to "the protocol that kills" take swift action to end this madness. *If this insanity is allowed to continue, it will continue to cause the needless deaths of thousands of more innocent victims.*

My greatest concern was that Rob's being forcibly separated from me meant there would be no accountability. The doctors and nurses could do whatever they wanted since no one was watching over their shoulders.

LEGAL COUNSEL STATEMENT

Members of the jury, Nicole Sirotek, a registered critical care flight nurse who founded American Frontline Nurses to advocate for patients who are being mistreated by hospitals' Covid protocols (she was one of the original nurses who went to New York City to help manage ventilators for Covid patients, and is a masters-prepared biochemist) was asked to present at a January 24, 2022, Senate hearing led by Ron Johnson on "COVID-19: A Second Opinion." Among other things, during her testimony, she stated:

*"Following orders has led to the sheer number of deaths that have occurred in these hospitals. I didn't see a single patient die of Covid. I've seen a substantial number of patients die of negligence and medical malfeasance. They rolled out remdesivir onto a substantial number of patients, for which we all saw it was killing the patients. And now it's the FDA-approved drug that is continuing to kill patients in the United States. . . As these patients get **remdesivir**, they have less than a 25% chance of survival if they get more than two doses.*

"Our level of healthcare has deteriorated to substandard third-world nation healthcare whereas I tell people you are better off in South America in a field hospital than you are in Level 1 Trauma designer hospitals in the United States.

"Nowhere in the United States do we isolate people for hundreds of hours at a time with no human contact. It's not even allowed in the prisons because . . . it is horrible for their mental health, and it's considered inhumane. However, in these hospitals now we are allowed to isolate patients from their families for days and you have to say goodbye to them over the phone."

In the same Senate hearing, Dr. Paul Marik said, *"If you look at the four independent studies, including the large study by the WHO, it shows . . . **remdesivir** increases the risk of death. . . it increases your chance of renal failure by 20%. This is a toxic drug. Just to make the situation even more preposterous, the federal government will give hospitals a 20% bonus on the entire hospital bill if they prescribe remdesivir to Medicare patients. The federal government is incentivizing hospitals to give a medication which is toxic."*

Below are snapshots of a few of Rob's final, desperate text messages to Sheila and several of his friends. As you can see, Rob was candid about his trepidation that his journey was likely a one-way trip—and did not conceal his emotions.

As you can see from the text message below, Robbie (Rob's friend) was aware on 8/28/21 that Rob was not doing well. Rob noted that he had not been feeling well for six days and that anything he consumed (including supplements) came back up.

The text exchange below is between Sheila and Rob shortly after he was dropped off at the hospital. As Sheila noted, they would not allow her into the facility to even come near him; thus, she could not be by his side and serve as his on-site advocate.

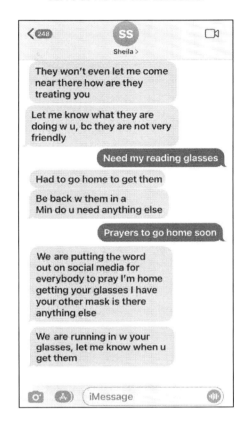

Robbie >

Aug 28, 2021, 5:47 PM

Hope you feel better soon man. My brother-in-law was throwing up so much he almost went to hospital last night. Been rough for a bunch of people I know and I just got over it. Was in bed pretty much for a week! It's rough what ever the "delta" is. Praying always 🙏

Aug 28, 2021, 9:15 PM

Thank you. Yes been 6 days. Really rough day today. Added diarrhea to the party now. So... weak. Most of what I need to get well require to be taken with food. But half hour later it all comes back out. This is freaking brutal.

Delivered

Sep 3, 2021, 11:41 PM

Praying for you brother 🙏

iMessage

Sheila >

They won't even let me come near there how are they treating you

Let me know what they are doing w u, bc they are not very friendly

Need my reading glasses

Had to go home to get them

Be back w them in a Min do u need anything else

Prayers to go home soon

We are putting the word out on social media for everybody to pray I'm home getting your glasses I have your other mask is there anything else

We are running in w your glasses, let me know when u get them

iMessage

21

Rob's family encouraged him to go to the ER and to do whatever the doctors told him to do.

Rob's friend, however, warned him not to follow "**the protocols**" he knew were "killing people in the hospitals."

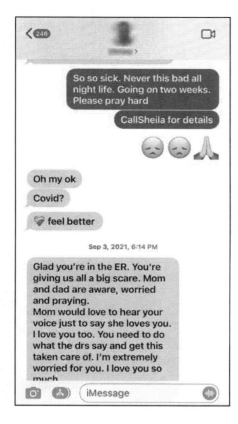

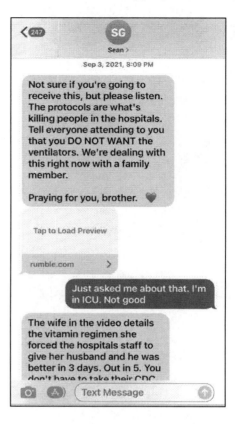

Rob texted his friend Paul at 8:53 PM on 9/3/21 to let him know, "I'm in ICU now."

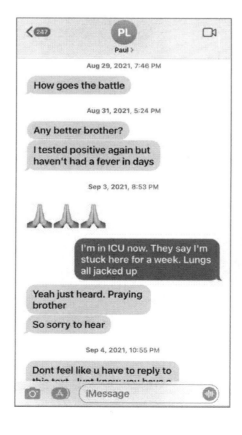

Chapter 4 – Intimidation & Starvation

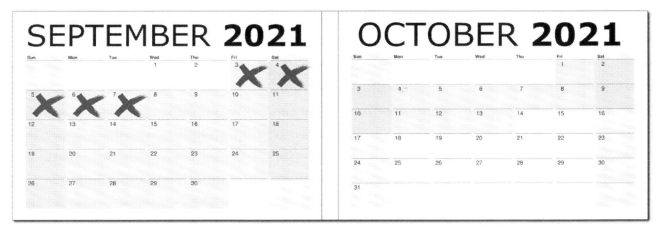

THIS CHAPTER COVERS SEPTEMBER 4-7

Saturday, September 4, 2021

When I awoke, I quickly called the ICU to see how Rob was doing.

Nurse Malicious answered the phone and told me Rob was stable and his blood oxygen level was good. I informed her I had packed a bag and would soon be heading her way. She promptly and unapologetically advised me that their policy would not allow me to visit Rob.

When I asked her how long their "policy" would prevent me from seeing Rob, she said, "I don't know; you'll have to call the hospital administrator to find out." I told her that any policy that would keep me away from my husband was criminal and violated our fundamental human rights. I explained that Rob desperately needed me and would recover far faster if I could be with him to give him hope and assist with his care. She coldly replied, "I'm sorry, that's our policy." I was once again overcome with a deep sense of fear and dread.

I asked her how I could access Rob's MyChart records to monitor his progress. She responded, "You cannot have access to his online MyChart records until after he has been discharged." I was stunned and caught off guard. That made no sense. I was his wife, I had a Medical Power of Attorney, and I had every right to know what they were doing to him.

LEGAL COUNSEL STATEMENT
Members of the jury, at 9:57 AM on September 4, 2021, the morning after his arrival, Dr. Dead End entered a note in Rob's hospital record that said "Consult palliative Care" as part of the initial "Impression and Plan" for Rob. You can see that note on Page 57 of the hospital records (see Page C-11 in Appendix C). "**Palliative care**" is a term that is often used interchangeably with "**comfort care**." Both terms refer to care that emphasizes comfort and support, particularly at end-of-life. Thus, Sheila was not pleased to find "Consult palliative Care" written in **Note 5** of the "Impression and Plan" for Rob immediately following a note that said, "patient does not want intubation" (see **Note 1**) and "COVID-19 unvaccinated" (see **Note 2**).

It was if they had written Rob off from the moment he arrived because of his "unvaccinated" status and because

would likely be a death sentence.

I left numerous messages for the hospital administration, yet no one called me back. So, I called the hospital switchboard and left messages on more extensions. I thought, "Where is everyone?" I had no patience, and I wanted to speak with someone immediately because I knew in my heart that Rob's life depended on my being able to break through the impenetrable wall that was keeping us apart.

My mother and sister rushed over to help me attempt to locate someone in charge at the hospital. Then, my phone rang. I expected it was likely someone from the administrative office calling me back. To my delight, it was Rob's number calling. I shouted, "It's Rob!"

I answered, "Hi, Honey, how are you?" Rob informed me that a doctor was with him who wanted to speak with me. We both had our phones on speakerphone mode, and I heard a higher-pitched voice say, "I am Dr. Dead End."

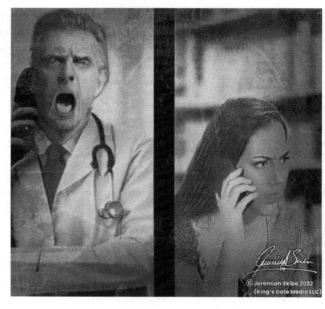

In a harsh and forceful tone, he informed me that despite Rob's oxygen levels being satisfactory, he required **the full protocol**, which included remdesivir, VELETRI, "elective intubation," and being placed on a ventilator. There was no time to waste.

I was shocked at his insistence that Rob must **stop refusing remdesivir**, a drug we both knew was harmful, and that we both needed to agree that Rob could be **intubated and placed on a ventilator**.

Rob and I refused, and I told him that as long as Rob's blood oxygen level remained in the 90s, we would forego any unnecessary drugs and treatments.

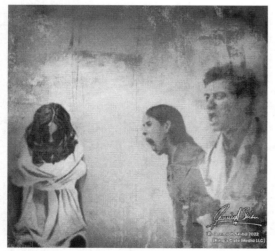

Dr. Dead End flew into a rage and began yelling at both of us, first shouting at me, "DO YOU WANT YOUR HUSBAND TO DIE?" and then bellowing at Rob, "DO YOU WANT TO DIE?!" I had taken Rob to the hospital for "care," and now we were both being berated by a heartless monster.

My sister and mother, standing by my side and hearing everything, were visibly shaken. I matched his volume and yelled back, "**NO, I DON'T WANT MY HUSBAND TO DIE!** "You're asking us to risk Rob's life on protocols that have killed hundreds of thousands of people.

The doctor continued to lambast Rob and me, and when I touched on alternative therapies, he made it clear that he would not be giving Rob any "alternative" therapies. This was his playground, and we had to play by his rules.

Dr. Dead End expected us to trust him unquestionably, and not challenge his knowledge or expertise. However, when we refused to blindly trust him with Rob's life, the abusive treatment he lashed out with was similar to the cruel maltreatment of prisoners of war, attempting to coerce them into submission. In this case, Rob's captors were a group of "whitecoat assassins" who demanded his full compliance, as well as mine.

Our response angered Dr. Dead End, and he now knew he had a troublesome patient and spouse to contend with. I could never trust this doctor again.

The horrific conversation, or shouting match as it became, lasted twelve full minutes. Finally, in disgust, Dr. Dead End advised us that if Rob did not change his mind about getting intubated and ventilated, he would be **kicked out** of the ICU and sent up to the 5th floor because "ICU beds are reserved for patients who are in need of the ventilator."

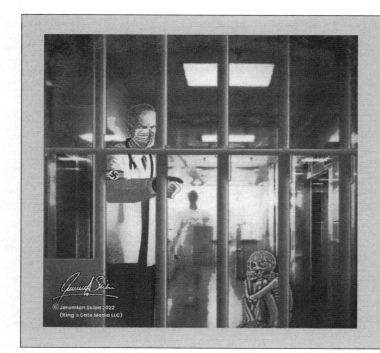

© Jeremiah Skiba 2022
(King's Gate Media LLC)

Holocaust Hospitals

The holocaust hospitals
Where the sick are doomed
Forced to the brink
Of an untimely tomb

Terrorized patients
Sentenced to die
As their hope fades
In the blink of an eye

Now become prisoners of war
Imprisoned with no hope
No one can save them
From this slippery slope

Their memories linger
Torture and pain
Let us never forget
The victims of this insane game

As we wrapped up our emotionally disturbing conversation, I told the doctor I would be looking into finding a facility that would allow me to stay with my husband, where he would be treated with respect, and where they would not try to browbeat and intimidate him into submission.

I learned a very harsh lesson that day; hospitals in America no longer honor patients' rights to review and approve the medications and treatments they are being administered.

When the severely ill or injured allow themselves to be admitted to a hospital, they do so with the expectation that *they will be aided in recovering from their illness or injury.* They are not signing up to be lab rats and are not expecting to become prisoners who have no choice in their "care." Unfortunately, Rob had—as he had warned me—entered a situation of clear and present danger, and he was heading into deep, shark-infested waters where the sharks wore stethoscopes and were in a feeding frenzy.

LEGAL COUNSEL STATEMENT
Members of the jury, Dr. Dead End violated the provisions spelled out in **Title 42 of the Code of Federal Regulations, Section 482.13** (as noted in Appendix E), where in Paragraph (b), the regulation states:

"The patient has the right to participate in developing and implementing his or her plan of care. The patient or his or her representative (as allowed under State law) has the right to make informed decisions regarding his or her care. The patient's rights include being informed of his or her health status, being involved in care planning and treatment, and being able to **request or refuse** *treatment. . . . The patient has the right to formulate advance directives and to have hospital staff and practitioners who provide care in the hospital comply with these directives."* Furthermore, Paragraph (c)(3) states: "The patient has the right to be free from **all forms of abuse or harassment.**"

This exasperated, headstrong, "protocol-focused" doctor berated Rob and his loving wife while attempting to force them to agree to the plan of care the doctor wanted with no regard for what Sheila or Rob wanted. *It is inexcusable that a "medical professional" would attempt to badger a patient into succumbing to a dangerous and unnecessary procedure that could result in their death.*

After the call, I was overwhelmed with the desire to comfort my husband, who had been reduced to tears and despair by the cruel actions of a maniac. The doctor had robbed him of all hope and dignity, leaving him alone in solitary confinement. How can patients who have been harassed, intimidated, and filled with fear be expected to improve?

My instincts told me to go and rescue my husband, who was trapped behind enemy lines and held captive by a ruthless system that was once known for saving lives but now appeared to be more focused on ending them. Yet since he was vitally dependent on supplemental oxygen, I knew I could not just rush in, wheel him out, and take him home.

Dr. Dead End had systematically and, with the precision of a skilled surgeon, ruthlessly cut away any hope or optimism my husband and I had for his recovery. He was a manipulative, greedy madman with a "doctor" title who had just gleefully demoralized us.

I desperately wanted to call Rob back to ask him how he felt after Dr. Dead End's tirade; however, I knew the caustic confrontation had zapped any strength he might have had left, just as it had zapped all of mine. So, I texted him to encourage him not to give up and to hang on to hope. I tried to assure him that everything would be okay—despite the doctors' fear tactics— although deep inside, I was terrified that Rob was now in the hands of a group of "professionals" who felt the "protocol" was more important than the "patient."

My mother, sister, and I were horribly shaken by what just happened, and I was worked up into a fever pitch. I cried, "Can you believe what Dr. Dead End just said? He was screaming at Rob and me! How could he threaten Rob by saying he's going to die if he doesn't do what he demands!"

We all heard the doctor's clear determination to get Rob to agree to being intubated and placed on a ventilator. Since when have doctors resorted to shouting at patients and their spouses to attempt to coerce them into agreeing to a high-risk, dangerous, and life-threatening procedure while shouting, "Do you want to die?"—all the while knowing the majority of the patients who board that train end up dead?

We all wanted Dr. Dead End removed from any responsibility for Rob's care. I was more convinced than ever that we needed to urgently find a facility that would accept a transfer and actually help Rob recover while allowing me to be by my husband's side.

LEGAL COUNSEL STATEMENT
Members of the jury, **Section 482.13 of Title 42 of the Code of Federal Regulations** (see Appendix E) states in Paragraph (b): "*The patient has the right to participate in the development and implementation of his or her plan of care. The patient or his or her representative (as allowed under State law) has the right to make **informed decisions** regarding his or her care.*"

Rob and Sheila did NOT want him to be intubated and placed on a ventilator because they knew most patients subjected to this procedure end up on a one-way trip where the only way out is through the morgue.

At the top of Page 52 of Rob's hospital records (see Page C-7 in Appendix C), you can see that Rob was listed as having been "**NAD**" (in No Acute Distress) at 2105 (9:05 PM) soon after he arrived in the ICU, and Nurse Imposter noted that Rob's oxygen saturation level was at **94%**. He continued to improve, with blood oxygen levels up to **98** and **100%**, as indicated on Pages 3007-3008 of the records (see Pages C-13 and C-14).

Even then, as noted at the bottom of Page 52 (on Page C-7), at 8:45 AM on September 4, 2021, Dr. Lament, just like Dr. Dead End, spent 15 minutes speaking with Rob. She falsely claimed Rob "**wants FULL CODE with intubation and Remdesivir as well.**" Her statement directly contradicted what Dr. Dead End recorded two pages later at 9:52 AM on Page 54 of the records (see Page C-9), where he stated, "*Patient wishes **to not** be placed on ventilator or intubated in emergency*" and at 9:57 AM on Page 57 of the records (see Page C-11) where he wrote, "*patient does **not** want intubation.*"

Dr. Lament's claim that Rob wanted "FULL CODE with intubation" was a total fabrication or, let's call it for what was—a lie. Rob made it clear multiple times (we counted it recorded **17 times** in the records) that he **did not want to be intubated and placed on a ventilator**.

As you can see from the multiple "**Orders**" extracted from Pages 1001 to 1018 of the hospital records (see Page C-53), **four doctors flip-flopped Rob's resuscitation order from FULL to Limited _five times_** from September 4, 2021 (the morning after his admission) to September 8, 2021 (the day he was intubated). That was done because of their *insistence that he consent* to "elective intubation," followed by Rob's consistently reminding them that he **DID NOT agree** to be intubated and placed on a ventilator.

In addition, on the bottom of Page 52 of the hospital records (see Page C-7), Dr. Lament noted, "**Wife will continue to look for hospitals/docs who will give pt [patient] alternative therapy.**" *We contend their awareness of Sheila's search for another hospital was a key reason all of the doctors involved in Rob's care were aggressively pushing for Rob to be intubated and placed on a ventilator because it is difficult to secure the transfer of a ventilated patient to a different facility—and they did not want their "cash cow" to walk out.*

On Page 59 of the hospital records (see Page C-15 in Appendix C), you can see that Sheila tried everything she could to remotely advocate for Rob while they refused her entry. She also made it clear that the ONLY reason to intubate Rob would be **if he stopped breathing**.

At the bottom of this same record, you can see that Dr. Dead End noted, "*Overnight events reviewed. Patient's wife was upset with us. Thinks we are trying to harm patient. She has refused remdesivir. She has refused elective intubation, she has advised her husband **to not proceed** with intubation if necessary.*" Notice how Dr. Dead End used the phrase "**elective intubation.**" He used that term because Rob would have to agree to (to elect) the procedure.

We contend their knowing family members are inclined to reject unnecessary intubation is one of the key reasons they wanted to keep Sheila isolated from Rob until they had accomplished their goal.

Before his eventual intubation and being placed on a ventilator on September 8, 2021, Rob should have been clearly informed of the **serious** risks involved, advised of the low percentage of patients who survive the treatment, and then been asked to sign an "Informed Consent" form to confirm he had been made aware of the risks involved and was willing to accept those risks. *A complete review of the over 5,000-page hospital record of Rob's 40-day stay revealed that he **had NOT signed a consent form** for these procedures.*

This unspeakable evil has been, and continues to be, foisted upon the uninformed and unfortunate who end up in the hands of merciless "medical professionals" who willingly promote "the protocol that kills."

Sadly—as you can see in the snapshots below of a few of the text message exchanges Rob had with friends the morning after he arrived in the ICU—the doctors' constant badgering led to him admitting he was "***losing hope.***" In addition, he despondently said, "*I think I'm pretty much dead no matter what*" and "*Won't even let Sheila in. All alone.*"

When friends found out Rob was not doing well, they texted to encourage him. Having been unable to eat for over a week and not being nourished at the hospital, Rob was terribly weak and, as he noted, was "losing hope."

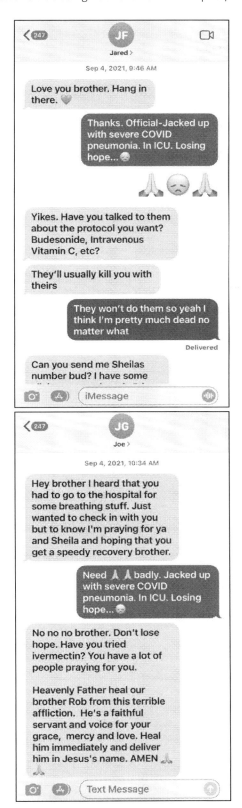

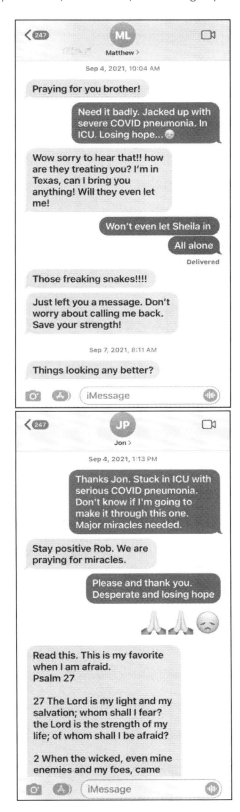

My mother called other hospitals to see if they would accept a transfer, but none allowed family visitation. I was hitting dead ends at every turn. I felt critical time was slipping away. It was as if a ticking time bomb was counting down while Rob's life hung in the balance. I believed his survival depended on my ability to find a solution, and I was determined to do everything in my power to save him.

My mother, sister, and I went to the hospital to drop off a "care package" for Rob. Despite feeling angry and wanting to express my frustration, I kept my emotions in check as a police officer stood at the front door. He was the "muscle" behind the front desk staff (the "guard dogs") who determined who could enter. For a brief second, I thought about making a run for the ICU—but I knew that would not turn out well.

If I had told them I had come to see a doctor, I would have been let in, but because I chose to tell the truth—that my husband was in the ICU—I remained locked out. So, speaking softly, I said, "This hospital seems like a prison camp. Don't patients have rights? What country are we living in?"

The lady speaking with me gave one of those sad upside-down smiles and half-heartedly chuckled, "You have no idea how many people ask those same questions every day." "Oh, really? So, I'm not the only one complaining. I have a Medical Power of Attorney that gives me the right to be my husband's medical advocate, but you're saying it doesn't give me the right to be with him?"

She shook her head, saying, "I'm sorry, you're not allowed entrance since your husband is in the ICU." "For how long?" I asked. She shrugged and said she did not know and that I would need the hospital administrator to allow me to enter. She suggested I call the administrative office in the morning to see if they could help. I told her I had already tried—with no success.

Feeling utterly defeated and terribly disappointed, we walked away. Despite my resolve, I couldn't get past the imposing police officer. I became even more determined to find a way to gain entrance the next day.

When we got back home, I called everyone I could think of who could possibly help. It was clear that Rob was in a lot of trouble and was struggling under the hospital's oppressive policies and protocols.

Members of the jury, in a note on Page 31 of the hospital records (see Page C-12 in Appendix C), Dr. Torture wrote the following:

- *"The patient meets criteria for use of **Remdesivir**, plan a 5 day course unless gets intubated."* As you have read, Sheila asked the nurse in the Emergency Department to note "**NO remdesivir**" in Rob's records the moment they arrived at the hospital. She then advised ICU Nurse Impostor during a call at 10:33 PM, soon after Rob was admitted, **not to administer this drug**. Rob and Sheila made it clear that they opposed its use. However, against their clear directives, it became a part of Rob's documented plan of care because "the protocol" trumps "the patient's and their family members' desires." **IMPORTANT NOTE:** The *"unless gets intubated"* statement was about the fact that at this hospital, once a patient has been intubated, they change from a **5-day course** to a **10-day course** of **remdesivir**. So, once you're intubated, you are treated to an additional five days of this toxic drug.

- *"Will give off-label **Nitazoxanide** and colchicine . . ."* **Nitazoxanide** is an antiparasitic clinical **trial drug** that should have required informed consent, and **colchicine** is a treatment for gout. Rob did not have a parasitic infection, nor did he have gout. Yet these two drugs were prescribed and administered without Rob's "informed consent." *Furthermore, nausea, diarrhea, fever, and weakness are common side effects of both drugs. Why assault Rob with these destructive drugs when he desperately needed a strong appetite to rebuild his strength?*

- *"The patient is out of the window to benefit from convalescent plasma as this late out he likely has his own IgG."* Thus, she admitted that at this late stage of his illness (he had been ill for over a week prior to his admission), Rob had likely already gotten over his initial Covid infection (assuming the results of the PCR test that Rob was given were accurate), and he probably had the IgG antibodies to the Covid virus. *That would have meant Rob was no longer contagious, and there was no valid reason to isolate him and keep Sheila out of the hospital. We contend that they kept Sheila locked out because they did not want her interfering with their plan to invoke on Rob the lethal "protocol that kills."*

Sunday, September 5, 2021

I suffered through another restless night. As I awoke, I was still tired. I grabbed my phone and texted Rob. Although I did not want to wake him, I felt compelled to urge him to remain conscious of the medications he was being given.

I knew my husband well enough to know he would never agree to take remdesivir because he was aware of its harmful effects—including its propensity to cause acute kidney injury and eventual death. Moreover, as an avid researcher, author, and speaker, he had spoken out against what he was now experiencing.

Despite our refusing remdesivir, I found they had given him a double dose of 200 mg at 11:02 PM on September 3rd, which must have been secretly administered while he was asleep—just two hours after his admission to the ICU. Then, they administered a second dose of 100 mg on September 4th. How could they be doing this when we both said we did NOT want him given this drug?

It was apparent the doctors and nurses had no intention of listening to us, and I had no idea how to fight an out-of-control medical monster that had put in place an insidious and deadly plan of care for my husband from the moment he arrived; a plan they intended to implement without unwanted interference from either of us.

I spoke with several of the nurses entrusted with his care about our feelings regarding this deadly drug, and each assured me that Rob's records said, "NO remdesivir." Since it was spelled out in the records, I believed they would comply with our requests. Instead, they gave me and Rob lip service and secretly administered remdesivir to Rob against his will and without his knowledge.

At 11:20 AM, I called the ICU nurse's station. Nurse Malicious answered. I asked about Rob's vitals and learned that forced ventilation BiPAP therapy would be ordered by Dr. Dead End if Rob began to show signs of tiring out. Unfortunately, I was not informed that "tiring out" was to be expected because of the inadequate food, water, and rest he was receiving and the excessive and harmful drugs he was being given. In addition, other doctors and nurses, not just Dr. Dead End, threatened that he would die if he did not agree to receive remdesivir, undergo "elective" intubation, and be placed on a ventilator.

Rob texted that he was getting conflicting information from the doctors and did not want to talk with them about it anymore. He also texted that all of the doctors disagreed with him, and he was afraid he would die because I could not be by his side to fight for him.

LEGAL COUNSEL STATEMENT
Members of the jury, Sheila was not exaggerating when she said Rob was badgered continually to agree to be intubated and treated with remdesivir. As you can see in the note at the bottom of Page 78 (that continues at the top of Page 79) of the hospital records (see Pages C-17 and C-18 in Appendix C), Nurse Malign had a "*Lengthy discussion with patient regarding intubation and use of Remdesivir.*" At the same time, she noted on Page 79 that **Rob's blood oxygen level was at 94%** (see the top of Page 79 on Page C-18), which is substantiated by the vital signs shown on Pages 2411-2412 (see Page C-19). *Thus, there was no reason to be pressing Rob to agree to be intubated and placed on a ventilator.*

These so-called "medical professionals" would not let up—and their continual harassment of Rob violated **Paragraph (c)(3) of Title 42 of the Code of Federal Regulations, Section 482.13** (see Appendix E), which clearly states: "*The patient has the right to be free from all forms of abuse or harassment.*"

Forcefully isolating patients from their spouses and other family members is a total injustice and not conducive to healing. Furthermore, it is incredibly detrimental to a patient's health. It is alarming and tragic that my husband received *substandard care* that was reminiscent of the inhumane treatment of prisoners of war. He was isolated, deprived of food and sleep, and threatened with physical harm if he did not comply.

LEGAL COUNSEL STATEMENT
Members of the jury, in March of 2020, the WHO (World Health Organization) began a large, international, randomized trial involving hospital inpatients to evaluate the effects of **remdesivir** (along with three other drugs) on in-hospital mortality. A total of 2750 patients received remdesivir for a duration of 10 days (or to death or discharge). As reported in the **British Medical Journal** (BMJ.com) on October 19, 2020, and the **New England Journal of Medicine** (NEMJ.org) on December 2, 2020, the WHO's "Solidarity Trial" verified that a 10-day course of Gilead Sciences' remdesivir "*had little or no effect on hospitalized patients with COVID-19 as indicated by overall mortality, initiation of ventilation, and duration of hospital stay.*"

On November 19, 2020, the *British Medical Journal* published another article titled "**WHO Guideline Development Group advises against use of remdesivir for covid-19**," where they stated, "*The antiviral drug remdesivir is not suggested for patients admitted to hospital with covid-19, regardless of how severely ill they are, because there is currently no evidence that it improves survival or the need for ventilation, say a WHO Guideline Development Group (GDG) panel of international experts in The BMJ today.*"

Who guideline development group advises against use of remdesivir for covid-19. BMJ. (n.d.). From
https://www.bmj.com/company/newsroom/who-guideline-development-group-advises-against-use-of-remdesivir-for-covid-19

On February 26, 2021, the *National Library of Medicine* published an article titled "**Kidney disorders as serious adverse drug reactions of remdesivir in coronavirus disease 2019: a retrospective case–noncase study,**" where they pointed out that "*the use of remdesivir was associated with an increased reporting of kidney disorders.*" It also stated, "*real-life data from > 5000 COVID-19 patients support that kidney disorders, almost exclusively AKI [**Acute Kidney Injury**], represent a serious, early, and potentially fatal adverse drug reaction of remdesivir.*"

Chouchana, L., Preta, L.-H., Tisseyre, M., Terrier, B., Treluyer, J.-M., & Montastruc, F. (2021, May). Kidney disorders as serious adverse drug reactions of Remdesivir in coronavirus disease 2019: A retrospective case-noncase study. Kidney international. From https://www.ncbi.nlm.nih.gov/pmc/articles/PMC7907730

Interestingly enough, the death certificate filled out by the hospitalist upon Rob's passing listed the underlying cause of death as "**ACUTE KIDNEY INJURY**."

Examples of Rob's desperation can be found in the text messages below. Here are a few excerpts: from the texts:
- *They won't give me budesonide, Intravenous Vitamin C, etc.*
- *I'm pretty much dead no matter what.*
- *They won't let Sheila in. All alone.*
- *Desperate and losing hope.*
- *I don't think I'm going to make it.*
- *No food No…. No strength no hope left.*
- *In ICU where doctors all disagree with me!*

When Rob said, "**No food no,**" as you will see in one of the text messages below, we suspect he meant to finish with "**No food no water,**" as he had told Sheila during an earlier call that he was very thirsty. Rob was isolated and on his own, with no one ensuring he ordered meals and no one to help feed him if he did have a meal delivered. *Unfortunately, he was too weak to even think about ordering meals and definitely too weak to feed himself. Whether due to the doctors', nurses', and dietitians' willful ignorance, uncaring negligence, or nefarious intent—Robert A. Skiba II was slowly being systematically starved into submission. The lock-out of Sheila, and the absolute lack of compassionate care for Rob, were **criminal**. As you will discover as you continue reading this story, **the substandard care** Rob received eventually **cost him his life**.*

Sheila advised Rob to refuse remdesivir and told him a doctor friend said *"they don't need to intubate you."*

A friend reminded Rob not to take remdesivir or be ventilated as *"This is the protocol that is failing patients."*

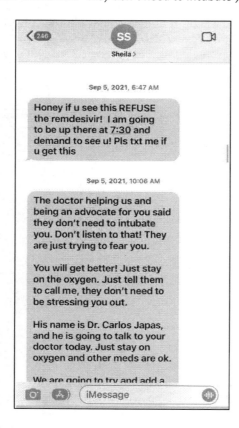

> **Sep 5, 2021, 6:47 AM**
>
> Honey if u see this REFUSE the remdesivir! I am going to be up there at 7:30 and demand to see u! Pls txt me if u get this
>
> **Sep 5, 2021, 10:06 AM**
>
> The doctor helping us and being an advocate for you said they don't need to intubate you. Don't listen to that! They are just trying to fear you.
>
> You will get better! Just stay on the oxygen. Just tell them to call me, they don't need to be stressing you out.
>
> His name is Dr. Carlos Japas, and he is going to talk to your doctor today. Just stay on oxygen and other meds are ok.
>
> We are going to try and add a

> Rob, I'm not sure when you'll get this. But I'm praying for your perfect healing. Also praying for strength and peace for Sheila. Praying the doctors will do the right thing. I know you will come thru strong and God's hand is upon you and your family. Fight my brother! The world needs you.
>
> **Sep 5, 2021, 10:11 AM**
>
> In ICU where doctors clll disagree with me. Feeling hopeless and afraid
>
> Ugh. So sorry. Praying harder now.
> You are strong! God is big! Only allow your thoughts to focus on perfect healing, ever cell in your body healthy!
>
> Do not allow them to give you remdesivir and put you on vent. This is the protocol that is failing patients.

Rob says he needs some indication he'll make it.

Rob indicates he needs to get home with oxygen.

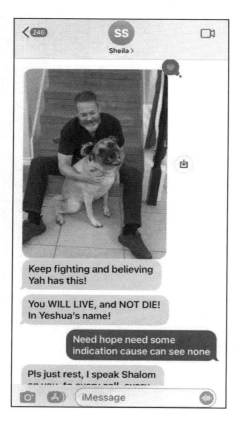

> Keep fighting and believing Yah has this!
>
> You WILL LIVE, and NOT DIE! In Yeshua's name!
>
> Need hope need some indication cause can see none
>
> Pls just rest, I speak Shalom

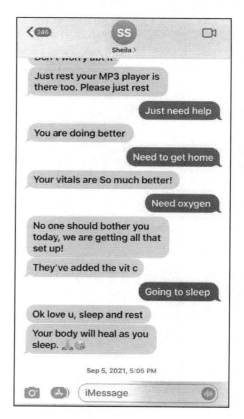

> Just rest your MP3 player is there too. Please just rest
>
> Just need help
>
> You are doing better
>
> Need to get home
>
> Your vitals are So much better!
>
> Need oxygen
>
> No one should bother you today, we are getting all that set up!
>
> They've added the vit c
>
> Going to sleep
>
> Ok love u, sleep and rest
>
> Your body will heal as you sleep.
>
> **Sep 5, 2021, 5:05 PM**

LEGAL COUNSEL STATEMENT
Members of the jury, what follows are the last text messages Sheila received from Rob.

Rob says the oxygen they are giving is beginning to work.   This is the last text message Sheila received from Rob.

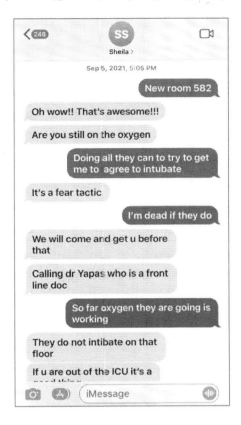

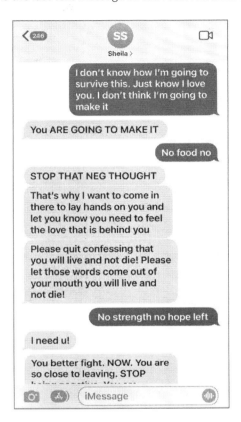

At 5:05 PM, Rob texted me that he had been moved out of the ICU and up to the 5th floor. So, at 7:30 PM, I called the 5th floor nurse's station to check on his status. The nurse that answered said Rob's plan of care had not changed and that his vitals were improving.

I was thrilled to hear that, and I was happy to learn he had been moved out of the treacherous death trap called the ICU because I knew they could not intubate Rob and place him on a ventilator on the 5th floor. One key change to his plan of care was, however, he had been **abruptly taken off** of a drug called VELETRI—a drug they could only give in the ICU because of the significant risks involved in its administration.

LEGAL COUNSEL STATEMENT
Members of the jury, although Rob had been moved to the 5th floor of the hospital on September 4, 2021, at 5:05 PM—out of the intensive care unit (ICU) where he was at significant risk of being intubated and placed on a ventilator—the constant badgering continued for him to agree to take **remdesivir** and to sign up for "**elective intubation**."

Only 38 minutes after his arrival on the 5th floor, at 17:43 (5:43 PM), Nurse Malign had a "Lengthy discussion with patient regarding intubation and use of Remdesivir" as noted on Page 78 of the hospital records (see Page C-17 in Appendix C). Then, less than 5 hours later, at 22:40 (10:40 PM), Nurse Felonious disrupted Rob's insufficient rest and "checked with pt [patient] about limited DNR [Do Not Resuscitate] status" as you can see in her note on the bottom of Page 79 of the hospital records (see Page C-18).

Rob again reiterated, "**I want to avoid intubation**" as you can see in the highlighted notes on Page 79 of the records (again, see Page C-18). The doctors and nurses collaborated on a plot to pressure Rob into agreeing to remove the DNI (Do Not Intubate) order from his records.

As stated in the record, Nurse Felonious then "paged" Dr. Heartless, who at 23:45 (11:45 PM) **again pressured Rob**. Out of annoyance and a lack of sleep due to their constant badgering, Rob made it clear he **did not want** to have the discussion. They even noted that he "*does not want to revisit this discussion tonight*." Out of clear frustration—since they were still unable to achieve their goal—Dr. Heartless passed the ball to the next shift, stating: "*Will defer to dayshift doctors to discuss code status/intubation with patient in morning.*"

Even more troubling is the fact that Dr. Dead End ejected Rob from the ICU at 5:05 PM and had him sent to a regular hospital room on a different floor because he was frustrated and irritated that Rob refused to remove his DNI (Do Not Intubate) order and would not agree to be intubated and placed on a ventilator. This resulted in the <u>hazardous and potentially lethal</u> abrupt withdrawal of the administration of **VELETRI (epoprostenol)**. This drug is such a high risk that it may only be administered in the ICU and must be slowly withdrawn to avoid potentially life-threatening complications.

Rob had already been given six doses of this medication, which was administered every six hours since the morning after his arrival at the hospital. The package insert for this drug states, "*Abrupt withdrawal (including interruptions in drug delivery) or sudden large reductions in dosage of Veletri may result in symptoms associated with rebound pulmonary hypertension, including dyspnea (difficult or labored breathing), dizziness, and asthenia (abnormal physical weakness or lack of energy). In clinical trials, one Class III primary pulmonary hypertension patient's death was judged attributable to the interruption of epoprostenol. Avoid abrupt withdrawal.*"
Veletri: Package insert. Drugs.com. (n.d.). From https://www.drugs.com/pro/veletri.html

As you can see, these heartless vultures would not cease badgering Rob to agree to be placed on a ventilator until he was utterly exhausted and they had achieved their objective. Moreover, they used the abrupt withdrawal of VELETRI to weaken him further so they could more easily force him onto a ventilator, an act we contend that, along with the massive assault of numerous toxic medications, directly led to his death.

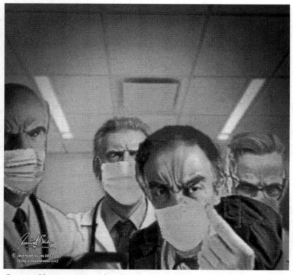

Later in the day, I received a call from Dr. Killer, who wanted to discuss Rob's status after his move to the 5th floor. She had a soft and kind voice—far different from Dr. Dead End's screaming approach. Dr. Dear End apparently had her call me because he believed a gentler and more friendly approach might somehow convince me to agree to their intubating my husband. She said, "Talking to Rob yesterday. He was, you know, he was unsure about the whole intubation."

I redirected the conversation to the hospital's unwavering protocol. I tried a commonsense approach by asking, "Who's responsible if the hospital protocol doesn't work? If it's a one-size-fits-all protocol, that can't possibly work for everyone. Rob is a unique patient. He has a history of asthma, and he needs budesonide. Also, his nutritional needs are different from others. Rob is one of over 330 million people in America. Your standard protocol cannot possibly work for everyone."

Dr. Killer first tried to say it was not a one-size-fits-all approach, yet she got tied up in her lie by admitting, "No, this protocol was put, uh, Mrs. Skiba, this protocol was put into place by multiple infectious disease doctors. They're following what the Centers for Disease Control says, you know, and, you know, what the Infectious Disease Society of America is recommending. There really is **no exception** to the protocol at this time."

So, it was a one-size-fits-all protocol. She was telling me Rob would have to follow an inflexible cookie-cutter approach without exception. That was absurd! Like every patient, Rob deserved a Plan of Care based on his unique situation and preferences—not a carved-in-stone plan that treats all patients the same. I stood firm and strongly insisted, "I want a few things outside the protocol. So, these are the things I'm asking for: intravenous vitamin C, a nebulized bronchodilator, and an increase in the steroids."

I continued as quickly as possible to prevent getting interrupted, "I've heard from family members who thought they were dying from Covid until they got nebulized budesonide. This medication seemed to have saved their lives. I have asked for budesonide a million times; I don't want it in an inhaler form. I want it nebulized. And I know your hospital has it. So, I don't understand why you refuse to give it to him." I also had heard that in 2020 Dr. Richard Bartlett, a West Texas doctor with 30 years' experience in Family Practice, had claimed budesonide was the "silver bullet" for COVID-19. He had also been saving lives using budesonide early on in Covid cases.

LEGAL COUNSEL STATEMENT

Members of the jury, *The Texan*, an online news organization, published an article on November 23, 2020, titled "Innovative Budesonide Treatment Key to West Texas Woman's Remarkable Coronavirus Recovery: Budesonide inhalation treatment turned 55-year-old West Texas woman sick with coronavirus from deathbed to recovery."

Roberts, K. (2020, November 23). Innovative budesonide treatment key to west texas woman's remarkable coronavirus recovery. The Texan. From https://thetexan.news/innovative-treatment-budesonide-key-to-west-texas-womans-remarkable-coronavirus-recovery

The article shares the story of a 55-year-old woman who was admitted on October 17, 2020, to Medical Center Hospital in Odessa, Texas. She had a severe case of Covid and was promptly placed on a ventilator. After she spent three days on a ventilator with **no** improvement, her husband, who had heard of Dr. Bartlett's success with budesonide, asked the treating physician to give her budesonide treatments. The doctor flatly refused. Another doctor at the hospital told the husband to prepare to move his wife to hospice for end-of-life care because he was going to remove her from the ventilator.

Not ready to give up on his wife like the doctors, the husband contacted Dr. Bartlett. The next day, Bartlett and an attorney called the hospital administration and the treating physician. They finally agreed to administer nebulized budesonide, yet they did so only once every six hours despite Dr. Bartlett recommending treatment every two hours. Within an hour of her first treatment, her blood oxygen level increased from 80% to 90%, and after 18 days, she was able to come off the ventilator. Twelve days later, she returned home with no need for hospice care.

As you will soon see, on September 6, 2021, a friend of Rob's who did not know how to contact Sheila contacted Dr. Bartlett. He asked the doctor to text Rob. Dr. Bartlett did so at 5:03 PM that day. Unfortunately, by then, Rob had ceased responding to text messages. Sheila did not see Dr. Bartlett's text message on Rob's phone until she reviewed Rob's call and text records after he died. "*The treatment plan is inhaled, generic budesonide*," Dr. Richard Bartlett had said. "*Using some generic antibiotics to protect from a secondary bacterial infection. Using zinc, which interferes with virus replication. It's common sense. It's intuitive.*" Common sense was not common

recklessness, indolence, and negligence.

We wonder how many lives have been sacrificed at this hospital and other institutions across America due to this small two-letter word that speaks volumes:

- **NO**, you cannot have adequate food and water
- **NO**, you cannot see your family because you are in isolation
- **NO**, you cannot have natural supplements such as IV vitamin C
- **NO**, you cannot have inexpensive lifesaving medications like budesonide

What you could have is "the full protocol" of harmful medications (such as remdesivir, VELETRI, and Alinia), combined with isolation, intimidation, and badgering until you agreed to "elective intubation" that would potentially lead to your termination.

I continued, "and I want him to have intravenous vitamin C. I know you're capable of giving Rob 10,000 mg. Vitamin C is the one thing Rob was given outside of your protocol, yet it is in capsule form that he cannot keep down. So, I want it given in an IV drip. You know Rob cannot swallow pills right now. It's far too difficult for him. You went outside the protocol once by giving him oral vitamin C, so why not do so again with the IV form?"

Dr. Killer brushed me off with, "I will discuss it with the infectious disease doctor as well as Dr. Dead End, like, you know, the three of us will discuss it again. Ultimately, you know, it has to be a joint decision because I can't do it by myself—because it's going against the protocol that we're using for our Covid patients. So, we have to be able to justify it. Let me talk to Dr. Dead End and Dr. Torture and see what they say as well."

With an artful dodge, she had weaseled out of agreeing to treat Rob as an individual—instead forcing him to follow a strict, mandated, deadly protocol. I was furious, as they were unwilling even to consider adapting their approach or make any compromises.

Sadly, although I asked that Rob be given budesonide every day, they refused to supply it. Their chief excuse was that they were "short-staffed" and could not provide nebulized treatments— yet somehow, they were perfectly capable of giving him nebulized VELETRI.

LEGAL COUNSEL STATEMENT

Members of the jury, as we stated earlier, the administration of VELETRI can cause a large number of severe side effects that include "*severe shortness of breath, gasping for breath, and anxiety.*"

A year after Rob's death, Sheila would discover, based on Sammy Wong, MD's analysis which appears in Appendix B, that:

- VELETRI was given without any evidence of pulmonary hypertension.
- VELETRI is associated with the development of a profound inflammatory response in the lungs.
- Due to a lack of indication for its use, the patient [Rob] was subjected to unnecessary risks [with the administration of VELETRI].

She also learned that VELETRI posed significant health risks and could cause rapid death if a patient was not slowly weaned off it.

Sadly, between September 4 and September 10, 2021, Rob was given a total of **twenty nebulized doses of VELETRI instead of nebulized budesonide,** which Sheila had consistently and repeatedly requested and that, as noted in the University of Oxford Study in Appendix F, is known to be able to reduce the recovery time for COVID-19 patients significantly.

They were likely "short-staffed" because of the number of personnel who had resigned because they could no longer stomach seeing patients being heartlessly subjected to a protocol that was killing their patients—or they chose to leave because they were advised they would be fired if they refused to be injected with an experimental gene therapy (i.e. the COVID-19 vaccine).

Dr. Killer changed her tone and, changing the subject, said, "But I mean, heaven forbid, if it seems like his oxygenation is worsening? Have you talked about that? You know, where do we go from there? Because Optiflow is, you know, the step right below intubation. So, would you guys want to consider intubation should he worsen?" Dr. Killer was now harassing me. Although she was using a softer tone, I knew it was the same type of harassment Rob was also dealing with day and night. While attempting to portray a soft-spoken "good cop," it was evident that she was hawking her wares much like a street vendor.

> **LEGAL COUNSEL STATEMENT**
> Members of the jury, Dr. Dead End had apparently asked Dr. Killer to work her magic on Sheila in a soft-spoken way to convince her to persuade Rob to agree to be intubated and placed on a ventilator. Unfortunately, the **ONLY** option available at this hospital was their uncompromising, pre-planned, no exceptions, one-size-fits-all "protocol that kills."
>
> By saying Optiflow high flow nasal oxygen therapy was "the step **right below** intubation," Dr. Killer was either **(a)** fully aware the use of a BiPAP (which is usually the next step before intubation) would be severely damaging to Rob because of his pneumomediastinum (which is air abnormally trapped in the mediastinum, the space in the chest between the lungs) and wanted to avoid it at all costs, or **(b)** she was lying and staying laser-focused on getting Rob on a ventilator as soon as possible by skipping the use of the "next step" BiPAP.
>
> *You have to ask yourself: What was Dr. Killer's <u>motive</u> for calling Sheila and, like all of the other doctors, pushing her to persuade Rob to agree to be intubated and placed on a ventilator? Could it have been the incentives spelled out in Appendix D?*

No matter where I turned, I could not make any headway. At each turn, there was another closed door, closed mind, and dead end.

Monday, September 6, 2021

With a fire in my belly, I started my day by using my trusty weapon, my phone, hoping I could make more progress with pure logic and thoughtful persuasion; yet once again, I was defeated by the nurses' robotic approach to caring for all Covid patients the same. I argued with them that my husband had been shown to have antibodies for Covid. Thus, he was no longer spreading the disease, and I should be allowed full access to him—all to no avail.

Once again, I found myself repelled by the hospital's anti-advocate force field, which proved impenetrable. I knew something had gone horribly wrong with the American hospital system, as I had never been prevented from entering to be with a loved one by hospital guards and armed police officers. However, I found it even more troubling that no one seemed to care, and everyone kept pointing to an elusive "policy" that they would never give me a written copy of.

Everything I was experiencing was wrong in every way—and I realized I was not alone because what was happening to me had happened, or was happening, to hundreds of other wives, husbands, mothers, fathers, sisters, and brothers all across our great country.
When did hospitals become so hostile and start using force, fear, and threats of violence against

need to fear being arrested and charged with a crime if I walked past a six-foot table at the front doors and "without permission" took an elevator up to the ICU floor to see my husband?

It was as if I were living in a nightmare where I found myself in a country that was not the land of the free and the home of the brave but a land of the enslaved and home of the afraid.

If this is where we are heading, dear Lord, help us—because what we once thought were our fundamental rights are being stripped away from us piece by piece. If we remain silent, we will no longer have rights regarding how our loved ones are treated in hospitals.

We need to launch a powerful and unstoppable movement of fearless men and women who stand up against this tyranny and say, "**NEVER AGAIN!**" We must fight for right and right this wrong.

> **LEGAL COUNSEL STATEMENT**
> Members of the jury, Erin Olszewski, BSN, RN, in her book <u>Undercover Epicenter Nurse</u> said to a group of nurses in a New York City hospital, "*This is so wrong. I can't believe they're doing this. They're literally experimenting on patients. What do we do? Is this even real right now? Sadly, it was all too real.*" One of the nurses in the discussion responded, "*They're playing with someone's life! If something happens to me, do not take me to the hospital.*"
> Olszewski, Erin. Page 62. Undercover Epicenter Nurse: How Fraud, Negligence, & Greed Led to Unnecessary Deaths at Elmhurst Hospital, Skyhorse, 2020.

As I struggled to navigate the hospital system and overcome one roadblock after another, I realized I was out of my league. So, I turned to my network of friends—especially those in the medical field—for their guidance and support.

Everyone I spoke with was deeply concerned that Rob's current level of "care" would ultimately lead to his death, and they urged me to consider transferring him to a different facility. The big question was, where? What facility would be willing to provide Rob with individualized care instead of pushing a one-size-fits-all "protocol."

My phone rang, and it was Nurse Carnage. I quickly looked at the time; it was 11:21 AM. I could tell she was very concerned, and her voice was laced with urgency as she spoke. "I had to add another mask that's delivering 100% oxygen on top of that other one to maintain him above 90%." My mind raced with confusion and worry. "Two masks? How could that be possible? It didn't make sense.

She further explained, "He's not a candidate for the other option called BiPAP because he has a pneumomediastinum—which is where there's air trapped in the space in the chest between the lungs, and it can cause him <u>traumatic injury</u> if we do a positive pressure such as a BiPAP. Okay? So, unfortunately, he's not a candidate for that. But yeah, at this point we can't give him any more oxygen than what he's on right now."

I struggled to process what nurse Carnage was saying. Finally, she explained, "He is sitting up and he's in bed. He's weak, he's able to turn side to side, he's able to take **deep breaths**, but he is very **short of breath**, and his oxygen requirements right now are maxed out. I literally, I cannot give him any more oxygen right now. He's reading 92 to 94% blood oxygen level. He's on Optiflow which is delivering 60 liters of oxygen per minute at 100% oxygen. He is also on a non-rebreather mask which is delivering 100% oxygen. His condition is very severe."

What? "He's able to take deep breaths," but he is very "short of breath?" How can you be both short of breath and at the same time take deep breaths? She also said, "He's reading **92 to 94%** blood oxygen level." That should have been great news since 92 to 94% is good.

Why were they pushing Rob to achieve a 95% blood oxygen level while knowing his breathing in 100% oxygen over extended periods can severely damage the lungs? Targeting an 85%+ blood oxygen level would have been acceptable and have allowed them to lower the level of oxygen he was breathing.

> **LEGAL COUNSEL STATEMENT**
> Members of the jury, **UC Health Medical Center** states that **they do not believe** patients must be placed on a ventilator **until their O_2 saturation is below 85%**, saying: "*When oxygen levels become low (oxygen saturation < 85%), patients are usually intubated and placed on mechanical ventilation. For those patients, ventilators can be the difference between life and death.*"
> Covid-19 resources. UC Health. (n.d.). From https://www.uchealth.com/en/media-room/covid-19/ventilators-and-covid-19
>
> COVID-19 patients may experience near-hypoxic oxygen levels in their blood without experiencing the typical symptoms of gasping and difficulty breathing because their blood levels of carbon dioxide, a gas exhaled after being absorbed in the lungs, remain low. This suggests the lungs are still able to effectively remove carbon dioxide even if they are having difficulty absorbing oxygen because the symptoms of Covid are more like those of altitude sickness than pneumonia.
>
> Scott Weingart, a critical care physician in New York and host of the "EMCrit" podcast said, "*The patients in front of me are unlike any I've ever seen. They looked a lot more like they had **altitude sickness** than pneumonia. We've had a number of people who improved and got off CPAP or high flow [nasal cannulas] who would have been tubed [intubated] 100 out of 100 times in the past.*"
>
> He went on to say it is a "*knee-jerk response*" to place patients on ventilators if their blood oxygen levels remain low with noninvasive devices because "*I think these patients do much, much worse on the ventilator.*"
> Begley, S. (2020, April 8). With ventilators running out, doctors say the machines are overused for covid-19. STAT. From https://www.statnews.com/2020/04/08/doctors-say-ventilators-overused-for-covid-19
>
> As a result, many believe maintaining a Covid patient's blood oxygen level at 95% or higher is unnecessary. Instead, the best practice is to use **the lowest percentage of inspired (breathed-in) oxygen possible** while keeping the patient's blood oxygen level at **85% or higher**. *This more conservative approach helps reduce the chance of causing **hyperoxia** (excessive oxygen in the lungs) which can further damage the lungs, making it harder for the patient to breathe.*

I pleaded with her to ask the doctors if he could be given nebulized budesonide and an IV vitamin C infusion. She responded that in her two years of working with Covid patients, she had never seen anyone given budesonide or IV vitamin C. Thus, she could not imagine my request being granted.

She explained, "I don't think it's been a recommended treatment. But at this point, he's in very serious condition. And we're watching him basically until he stops breathing. But I can't do anything more for him as far as his oxygen requirements go at this point, which is why I'm calling to update you."

I earnestly asked, "Would an IV vitamin C drip affect his oxygen? I don't understand. Why can't you put him on that?" I'm not asking for the moon. I'm asking for two basic things that can't possibly harm him. Nurse Carnage sternly replied, "Because it's not part of the protocol. It's not

I punched back, "I don't understand. Vitamin C is a vitamin that you are currently giving him in pill form, or at least you're attempting to. But he's having trouble swallowing anything. If that is the case, why can't you instead take an alternative approach and give it to him by IV? But to tell me 'Just because it's not in the guidelines' is why it can't be done doesn't make sense! All I'm asking is that you give the vitamin C in a different way."

I was so frustrated that I wanted to bang my head against a wall. The continued resistance to my simple requests for things that I was sure would help Rob improve was maddening.

They say, "where there is no will, there is no way," and because the doctors and staff had "no will" to go beyond the bounds of "the protocol," it was clear there was "no way." Nurse Carnage scoffed, "I don't think that a vitamin C drip is going to change anything."

I responded sternly, "I know you don't think so. But I'm asking for it. I can't even come in there and see my husband, assist him, and tell him in person that everything will be okay."

Nurse Carnage thought she was finished with me. So, to shut down the conversation, she said matter-of-factly, "I just, I don't believe that the doctors are going to be ordering that. But at this point, I have to update you and let you know that we can't give him any more oxygen. I'm watching his levels and his vital signs. As long as they stay stable, he's going to stay on the 5th floor. If he stopped breathing, then we start chest compressions and we give him medications. I cannot give him any more oxygen. If his oxygen saturation starts to drop, he's going to decline very quickly and go into respiratory arrest." Her aggressive scare tactic was pure "fear porn."

> **LEGAL COUNSEL STATEMENT**
> Members of the jury, nurse Carnage noted on Page 86 of the hospital records that Rob said at 12:30 PM on September 6th, **"I feel better once I rest, my breathing gets a little easier."**
>
> She also noted, "*Rob is max'd out on oxygen at this time but he's feeling better. Discussed with patient at length about severity of condition. **Patient continues to refuse intubation.** [Rob] States 'I guess we will just keep doing what we're doing, I'll get better or worse.' Explained to patient that in the event that he goes into respiratory arrest we will start ACLS protocol without intubation. Patient verbalized understanding. Placed all belongings in reach including call light. Instructed patient to call if breathing becomes more difficult as he is max'd out on oxygen at this time. **Left room with patient resting comfortably in bed and in no acute distress**.*"
>
> Nurse Carnage caused Rob undue stress by threatening that if he did not agree to be intubated, he would go into respiratory arrest (stop breathing). At the same time, she did not inform Sheila that Rob was feeling better and breathing easier whenever he was allowed to rest—and that he was "**in no acute distress.**"
>
> Sheila also asked nurse Carnage to take a photo of Rob and send it to her so she could see how he was doing. She surprisingly said it would be a "HIPAA violation" for her to take Rob's picture and send it to her. *Her refusal to send Sheila a simple photo of Rob was another of their methods for keeping Sheila in the dark about Rob's condition.*

Nurse Carnage left me feeling overwhelmed and somewhat panicked. The thought of Rob being placed on a ventilator filled me with dread—especially in light of Rob's text message the day before where he said, "*Doing all they can to try to get me to agree to intubate. I'm dead if they do.*"

I dreaded the thought of Rob having to attempt to defend himself in his severely weakened state from this pack of wolves who had "tagged" him as someone whom they had to get on a ventilator, with no regard for the fact that would likely mean I would never see him alive again.

At 7:30 PM, my phone rang with what I recognized as a number from the hospital. When I answered, I recognized Nurse Carnage's voice again. "I just wanted to give you an update. He's doing about the same, **no changes**. We still have him on both of the oxygen devices and he's maintaining his saturation over 90%. Blood pressure and heart rate are within normal limits." I thought, "That's wonderful news. He's maintaining!"

Nurse Carnage continued with a sense of concern, "His breathing is looking a little bit more labored, and his respiration rate is up from this morning. But he is maintaining saturation. **His respirations are 34**. And then we got him started on the **remdesivir**. It's running now he's tolerating it fine. And that's about it. I'm going home at seven, but I'll be back in the morning to take care of him."

I was angered to hear Rob had been given **another** (this was his **third**) dose of remdesivir. I said, "Did you ask him if he wanted remdesivir?" Rather than saying, "Yes," or "No," she said, "Okay. He was agreeable to it." That made no sense because Rob would never agree to take remdesivir because he knew it was an ineffective and dangerously harmful drug that would only worsen his condition.

Once again, they had ignored our directives, and more damage had been done. All I could do now was take up the fight, once again, with the doctors in the morning.

LEGAL COUNSEL STATEMENT
Members of the jury, at 3:23 PM on September 6th, 2021, on Page 99 of the hospital records, Dr. Killer recorded, *"expressed my repeated concern that it looks like he [Rob] is tiring out and will need intubation."* She also stated, *"IM [Internal Medicine doctor] now reports that the patient is **agreeable to receiving remdesivir**, I will order."* Rob may have been tiring, yet he expressed many times that he **did NOT want to be given remdesivir** and **did NOT wish to be intubated**. *His caregivers could not care less, as they hung over Rob like vultures over their prey, relentlessly hounding him to agree to "the protocol."*

We contend that Rob's respirations had increased to 34 breaths per minute **because of the following:**

- **The 500 mgs of remdesivir** Rob had been administered.
  As noted on the Gilead Sciences website at https://www.vekluryhcp.com/dosing-and-admin the standard protocol is to administer a 200 mg. "loading" dose via IV followed by daily 100 mg "maintenance" doses. Rob was given **(a)** a 200 mg "loading" dose at 11:02 PM on September 3, 2021, just six hours after he arrived in the Emergency Department, **(b)** a 100 mg "maintenance" dose at 8:41 AM on September 4, 2021, in the ICU, then **(c)** another 200 mg "loading" dose at 5:22 PM on September 6th because he REFUSED a dose on September 5th, and they "restarted" the entire regimen.
  *In addition, Drugs.com notes that remdesivir's potential side effects include "**trouble breathing**," which can cause an elevated respiratory rate.*
  Remdesivir side effects: Common, severe, long term. Drugs.com. (n.d.). From https://www.drugs.com/sfx/remdesivir-side-effects.html

- **The six doses of nebulized VELETRI** he had been administered.
  As we noted earlier, VELETRI's potential side effects include <u>severe shortness of breath</u> and <u>gasping for breath</u>. In addition, our independent medical expert, Sammy Wong, MD (as noted in Appendix B), listed the administration of VELETRI as one of his "Causes of Action" against the doctors.
  VELETRI uses, Side Effects & Warnings. Drugs.com. (n.d.). From https://www.drugs.com/mtm/veletri.html

- **Rob's being placed on high-flow nasal cannula oxygen at levels of 87 to 100%** due to their attempt to keep his blood oxygen level at 94% or higher. *Targeting a blood oxygen level of only 90% or higher would have been more "lung protective," as they could have used lower oxygen concentrations to avoid damaging Rob's lungs. Concentrations of oxygen above 60% for over 24 hours can create pulmonary toxicity,*

*a partially or completely collapsed lung), resulting in **shortness of breath** and **painful breathing**.*

As noted on Page 127 of the hospital records (see Page C-35 in this Appendix), Rob would be eventually diagnosed with **atelectasis** on September 8, 2021, the day he was placed on a ventilator. As shown in the charts on Page C-54, Rob was subjected to **excessively high levels of oxygen** from the day of his arrival until the day he died.

On July 14, 2021, CapnoAcademy published an article titled "Hyperoxia: Too much of a good thing" in which the authors noted, *"Research shows that time and time again, routine [one-size-fits-all approach] and unchecked high-flow oxygen administration **reaches toxic internal levels within minutes**. To this extent, the current European Society of Cardiology guidelines **recommends giving oxygen only when oxygen saturation levels are below 90%.**"*

Further detailing the cascading negative effect of giving patients <u>unnecessarily high levels of inspired oxygen</u> (referred to as FiO2 for the fraction [or percentage] of inspired oxygen), they state, *"The patient progressively inhales higher oxygen concentrations as the flow is increased, **causing more and more previously functional and intact alveoli to collapse**. This **increasing atelectasis** [a complete or partial collapse of the entire lung or lobe of the lung] further decreases lung surface area for the transfer of oxygen into the blood. **The hypoxemia [below-normal levels of oxygen in the blood] worsens, and oxygen flow is increased, and so on.**"*
CapnoAcademy. (2021, August 13). Hyperoxia: Too much of a good thing. CapnoAcademy, From https://www.capnoacademy.com/2021/07/14/hyperoxia-too-much-of-a-good-thing-2

*The insane rush to intubate and mechanically ventilate Covid patients is unjustified in many, if not most, cases. Doctors who push intubation and ventilation on patients do so while knowing full well that prematurely placing them on ventilators **dramatically increases the risk that they will not leave the hospital alive**. Unfortunately, hospitals receive a bonus payment for each "Covid" patient who ends up on a ventilator and another bonus if the patient dies "of Covid," as noted in the article in **Appendix D**.*

I decided to further press in on the fact that Rob would benefit from nebulized budesonide. So, I said, "Everyone is telling me they are concerned about the inflammation Rob has in his lungs. He has asthma issues, and we know that budesonide helps with inflammation. So, I've been asking everyone to give him budesonide. This is insane. I want this added to his treatment regimen. Also, I want him to be given full doses of steroids because they attack inflammation too. I will talk to a pulmonologist about this."

The nurse was happy to inform me that **Dr. Dead End**, a critical care pulmonologist was on his case. I thought, "You must be kidding me!" Good Lord! The same crazy doctor who had shouted at me, "Do you want your husband to die?" and then at Rob, "Do you want to die?" two days earlier, and who wanted Rob to be intubated from day one, was "on the case." She continued, "And he doesn't think increasing the steroids would help lower inflammation while increasing his blood oxygen level. At this time, that's not their plan of care. Because I can't speak for him. But there are standards of care that they follow as a health care team."

I unashamedly shot back, "That doesn't make any sense! I've been contacting doctors who have treated Covid patients from all over the U.S., and they don't understand why Rob's doctors aren't increasing his steroids. I mean, it just seems like a kind of basic next step. I will be pushing for a nebulized steroid, for sure."

At 11:34 PM, I received a call from Nurse Lousy to tell me that Rob was being moved back to the ICU to receive VELETRI again, as it can only be administered in the ICU. I had been told by the medical staff that VELETRI was not harmful and that it would open his airways. Although it could only be administered in the ICU, I was concerned about the move because Dr. Dead End had told Rob and me during our call on September 4, 2021, that the ICU beds were "reserved" for patients willing to be placed on a ventilator.

<blockquote>

LEGAL COUNSEL STATEMENT

Members of the jury, a note on Page 63 of the hospital records (see Page C-16 in Appendix C), in point #1, substantiates what Sheila had been told by Dr. Dead End regarding ICU beds being held for patients who had agreed to be placed on a ventilator. In that note, you will see that he stiltedly wrote, "patient does not want intubation," and "at this point if patient does not Wish for intubation if needed will transfer to floor. To utilize beds for patient and may need elective intubation."

In point #4, Dr. Dead End went on to say, "given the limited resources available in the intensive care unit Will triaged [should be "triage"] the patient up stairs [should be "upstairs"] is [should be "if"] they do not want intubation if necessary to prolonged [should be "prolong"] and save his life." *As you can see, Dr. Dead End's writing is as bad as his bedside manner and patient care.*

His hardball stance led to Rob being moved out of the ICU at 5:05 PM the day before (on September 5th) as a form of punishment for refusing to agree to be intubated and placed on a ventilator. *He then welcomed him back to resume treatment with VELETRI, knowing that once he had him back in his "sandbox" he could again set the rules.*

In this same note (#4), Dr. Dead end says, "advised patient and his family that he may die without elective intubation." He was attempting to persuade Sheila and Rob that the **ONLY** option to save Rob's life would be via **elective intubation and ventilation**, despite his full awareness that the vast majority of "Covid" patients who end up on a ventilator **do not survive**.

*Rob only agreed to return to the ICU to receive VELETRI—because he had been told (without being aware of its damaging side effects) that it might be helping him breathe better, and this drug is so risky that it can ONLY be administered in the ICU. **He did NOT agree to be moved to the ICU to be intubated and placed on a ventilator.***

</blockquote>

I was being tested beyond measure and did not know if I would survive the test. I would have exchanged my own life for Rob's if I could have. He was the love of my life, and I felt life was not worth living without him. He had a particular purpose, a unique ministry, and much more to accomplish. In my view, his life was more valuable than my own.

I tried hard to "let go and let God," but it was a continuous struggle. Finally, emotionally and physically exhausted, I went to bed; but sleep did not come easily. How do you tell your mind to rest and not worry—to trust even when life-threatening storms are raging? I was totally wiped out, and I had to find a way to close my eyes and endure the emptiness of my home another night.

LEGAL COUNSEL STATEMENT

Members of the jury, Dr. Richard Bartlett, a Texas-licensed family medicine physician, tried to reach Rob at 5:03 PM on September 6, 2021. He did so because a friend of Rob's had reached out to Dr. Bartlett and asked him to contact Rob to help him make sound decisions regarding his care. Dr. Bartlett was also willing to advocate for him as he had done for many patients since 2020.

Unfortunately, Rob had ceased responding to text messages by this time, and Sheila was only aware of this text message after Rob died. Had she been aware of Dr. Bartlett's attempt to assist, she would have contacted Dr. Bartlett herself.

The budesonideworks.com website (which lists Dr. Bartlett) notes that budesonide is an inhaled corticosteroid that has been proven **90% effective for Covid** with two randomized control trials from Oxford University (see **Appendix F**). Furthermore, they note, "*It is the ONE drug that can keep you from going TO the hospital and get you OUT of the hospital, even if you are on a ventilator.*"

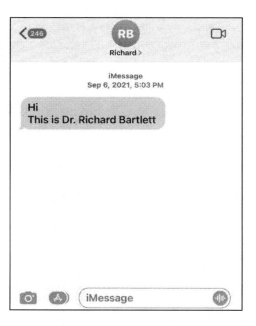

As you can see below, a family member and a doctor friend both encouraged Rob to get intubated and on the ventilator, which made it all the more confusing for him.

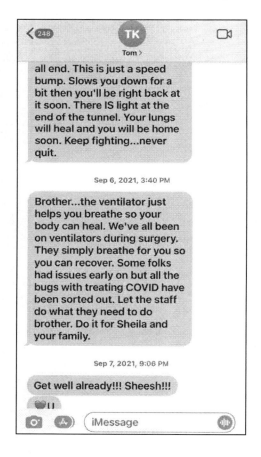

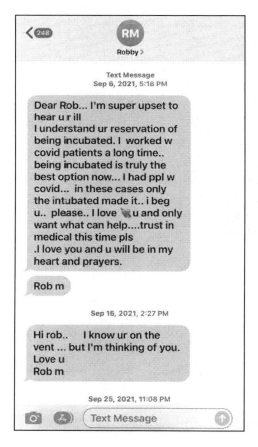

46

The term "daybreak" took on a new meaning, as all my days were now broken. My heart, trust, hope, and faith had all been shattered, especially my faith and hope that the doctors would do what was right above all else.

Since the evening I delivered Rob to the nurse in the Emergency Department and I was rudely ushered out, my entire experience with the hospital had been a chaotic mess. My son called the mayhem "Clown World," and it felt like everything was upside down and inside out. Whenever I said "No," it ended up being treated as a "Yes."

I said, "No remdesivir!" They said, "He's had two doses and is tolerating it well." When I said, "**No more remdesivir** and put that in his record," they responded, "Oh, he just got another dose—okay?" When I insisted, "Stop giving him remdesivir. I have told you many times he doesn't want it," they countered with, "It's hospital protocol," and they reissued the orders for Rob to be administered the drug.

No doctor should be excused for willfully pushing a protocol with a high mortality rate just because they have a medical degree, the backing of the hospital's administration, and lucrative government incentives. When a patient or a family member, especially one with Medical Power of Attorney, as I had, takes issue with their "plan of care," doctors need to listen to and respect those concerns!

It should be standard practice to ask patients for written informed consent to be administered Emergency Use Authorization medications or off-label use drugs in the name of full transparency, truth, and integrity. Anything less is calloused and abusive. But, sadly, what Rob and I had encountered went even further. It was coercive and criminal.

I had taken Rob to the hospital for what I had expected to be life-saving treatments, not to become a science project or lab rat. Rob had not signed up to be a member of a clinical trial where "medical professionals" could "practice medicine" on him using any drugs or therapies they wished that fit into their pre-prescribed and known-to-be-lethal protocol.

Unfortunately, patients who assertively expressed their opinions or suggested alternative treatments ended up in tense confrontations with the doctors. As Rob had texted me, "***The doctors are all disagreeing with me.***" Worse yet, Rob's doctors made his and my agreeing to "follow the protocol" their top priority—a far higher priority than Rob's health and wellness.

I will never forget my husband's woeful "I don't want to die" response to Dr. Dead End as he screamed at Rob, "Do you want to die!" simply because he was not being compliant and would not agree to remove his "Do Not Intubate" (DNI) order. Our ongoing conflict with the doctors should never have occurred. It was exhausting, demeaning, and demoralizing.

I tried calling Rob's phone, but there was no answer. So I called the nurse's station, hoping to hear that he was improving. Nurse Strife told me his respirations were in the 20s and 30s, and his blood pressure was 153 over 80 with a heart rate of 75. His temperature was 97, and his

Hearing that news gave me a little relief as it appeared he was doing well. So, I asked, "I was told that laying prone is really helpful. Do you think there's any way you can get him to lay prone?" The nurse replied that she had not asked him to lay prone yet, saying, "I asked him yesterday." So, I asked, "How is he feeling? Does he seem okay? Is he eating?"

The nurse woefully answered, "He looks tired. He is not eating." I hammered back, "He looks tired? Did you say he's not eating?" The nurse nervously replied, "No, he did not. He didn't eat anything today." I inquired, "Are you giving him Ensure?" She said she ordered one, but he had not gotten it yet. She said she talked with the dietitian this morning.

I found her comments very disturbing. Why were the nurses not ensuring Rob was getting adequate nourishment? Were they too busy or afraid to properly care for those diagnosed with Covid? I had heard of situations where staff delivered a food tray and quickly ran out of the room, leaving nearly incapacitated patients alone and fending for themselves.

Since I could not reach Rob on his phone, I asked the nurse if she could make sure his phone was charged and was near him, tell him I loved him, and let him know I had been trying to reach him by phone. I said, "Could you also ask him to call me"? She replied, "I don't know if his phone is fully charged or not. He said he could not talk well when he last spoke with me. But I'll tell him again to call you. I was going to his room just now."

I asked, "Oh, one more thing. Please let him know I could not get into his hospital records, and I need to get a code from him that they emailed him." She said, "Yeah, okay. I'll tell him that." It made no sense at all to needlessly lock me out. Sitting at home and only able to check on his status by phone, I could not ensure he was being well cared for and was receiving and consuming sufficient food and water.

I was shocked that a moment later my phone rang and it was Rob! I could hardly believe it, as I did not get to speak with him the day before and was worried sick. I excitedly answered, "Hi, Honey, how are you?" Rather than indulge me in sharing his condition, he said he wanted to focus on getting me into his email account, so I could get the code I needed to access his MyChart. Besides, he wanted to conserve his energy.

Following his directions, I bolted upstairs, powered up his computer, and followed his instructions to access his email account to get the essential MyChart code. "Okay, I'm in." Within seconds I found the hospital's email and got the code. I hooted, "Yay, I can now access your MyChart records. Thank you for your help. I am so sorry to have had to bother you with this. The nurses told me only you could access the records, and it's been very difficult trying to advocate for you from the outside without seeing what they're doing to you. The doctors and nurses have no respect for me or my Medical Power of Attorney."

Rob responded, "Yes, same here. The doctors are doing all they can to make me take remdesivir and be intubated. They harass me every time they come into my room. They send in the nurses to badger me. I told them to put it in my record **NO remdesivir** and in bold **DO NOT INTUBATE**. I don't know how I'm going to survive this if they have their way! But I'm trying to be strong and need the oxygen."

I responded, "Don't talk anymore. Conserve your energy and get some rest. Now that I have access to your records, I will make sure no one harms you. You will be okay. Rest now and spend all your energy on getting well. I don't want to do life without you. I love you so much. You will be coming home soon. Goodbye, Honey. I miss you so much. Bye."

I felt my insides churning, and I didn't want to hang up. The terrible silence when the phone disconnected was its own form of torture. I dropped to the floor and cried until I could not cry anymore. The quiet in my home without Rob seemed deafening. I deeply missed hearing his constant happy humming that I had grown to love during our fourteen years of married life. Rob was the happiest Tigger ever. He bounced through the house with joy from the time he awoke until he bounced into bed at night. He was such a jolly, happy soul. There was no one like him. He had made my life worth living.

LEGAL COUNSEL STATEMENT

Members of the jury, Nurse Trauma noted in Rob's hospital records at 6:50 AM on September 7, 2021, at the bottom of Page 102 (see Page C-22 in Appendix C), "*Patient is alert and conversant, however appears tired and weak.*" What do they expect from someone who is too exhausted to feed themselves and is left alone with no one to aid them in eating?

We contend that a major (and evil) reason Sheila was "locked out" was to ensure she could not help Rob eat and drink, as that would have aided him in regaining the strength he needed to heal. In addition, they knew that if she could not be by his side to encourage him with a loving touch, he would eventually reach a point of total desperation.

As noted on Pages 104, 105, 117, and 149 of Rob's hospital records (see Pages C-27, C-28, C-30, and C-31 of Appendix C), Rob was being slowly starved into submission while being further weakened by the **remdesivir** (*which is known to cause trouble breathing and acute kidney injury*) and **VELETRI** (*which should NEVER be used on a patient who is already short of breath because it may cause SERIOUS side effects that include "severe shortness of breath, gasping for breath, and anxiety"*).

The "*pt has not been ordering 3 meals a day*" and "*Unsure about pt's weight history*" notes on Page 149 (see Page C-31) are especially troubling as they clearly indicate the doctors, nurses, and dietitian **were all well aware** that Rob—who had no one assisting him in eating and drinking—was becoming critically weakened by severe malnourishment.

Today's modern hospitals focus on ensuring patients are administered the full dose of every prescribed medication on the specified schedule. As long as that is accomplished, they believe they have provided the "service" patients expected when they agreed to be admitted. If a patient is too weak to order meals and too ill to eat or drink the little food and water they receive, the resulting dehydration and malnutrition are not the medical staff's problem.

As they pointed out in the hospital record, a major issue for them was that Rob had, "*Refused Remdesivir from 9/5 until 9/6.*" They made sure to note the missed dose of remdesivir so they could use that as their excuse for why Rob was not doing well at this stage. Unfortunately, the sad and cruel truth was that he was dehydrating, starving, and further weakened by numerous high-risk medications.

The assault of harmful drugs and lack of adequate nutrition severely debilitated Rob, making it extremely difficult for him to breathe adequately. The "**No strength no hope left**" text message he sent on September 6, 2021, just three days after being admitted, was horribly disturbing, and was the last text message Rob sent Sheila.

This same day, when (as noted above) Nurse Trauma stated that Rob was "*alert and conversant,*" a hospital "Admission Specialist" wrote "***Verbal***" on a "***General Consent for Treatment***" form and on two additional

You can see the signature blocks of all three forms on Pages C-25 and C-26 in Appendix C. When the Admission Specialist who filled out the forms posted them at 1:07, 1:08, and 1:09 PM, she wrote in "**spouse**" as the signing party—implying <u>Sheila</u> had given her verbal consent—which made no sense because she would not have had the authority, per the hospital's policies, to sign for Rob if he were "*alert and conversant.*"

On December 22, 2022, Sheila and her son Jeremiah visited the hospital to meet with the Admission Specialist who had filled out the forms and had written "*Verbal*" on the forms. During that meeting, she admitted that she had never spoken with Sheila, saying, "***There is a whole procedure. And I missed out on that one. Sorry.***" The Admission Specialist's supervisor dropped by to listen in on the conversation and said she would open an investigation to find out what had actually occurred. *See **Appendix I – Falsification of Hospital Consent Forms** for the dialog of that conversation and additional details regarding this troubling discovery.*

A thorough review of the records confirmed that these three were the *only* "consent" forms filed during Rob's 40-day stay. What is blatantly missing is any signed "Informed Consent" forms for the Emergency Use Authorization (EUA) medications Rob was subjected to and the high-risk treatments he endured, such as the 4.5 hours he was subjected to on a highly risky, contraindicated BiPAP therapy and his eventual intubation and ventilation.

"Informed consent" for the administration of off-label use, experimental drugs, and highly risky procedures would have required **(a)** a clear explanation to Rob of the significant risks involved and **(b)** his signature that he was fully aware of and willing to accept those risks.

Now that I had full access to Rob's online MyChart hospital records, I planned to take as much time as necessary to navigate through them and gain a clear understanding of how he was being treated. I knew I would need help because the format was not intuitive, and with my intense worry, lack of sleep, and inadequate nourishment (as I was barely eating), I would not be at my best.

So, I called my sister, mother, and a few friends, some of whom had medical backgrounds, to ask them to help me review the records so we could understand the essential points of his treatment over the past four days. Soon, my living room was bustling with activity as my small group of helpers examined Rob's MyChart records with me.

We decided to print the records and bind the pages into a 3-ring binder so they would be easier to analyze. We then highlighted key sections, made notes, and wrote questions about what we saw. However, we realized that what we were examining was always going to be 24 hours behind since they posted each day's treatment records the following day. This meant that my daily phone calls would be the only way I would know what was happening with Rob on a given day, and I would be in "react mode" if I noticed an anomaly in his MyChart from the previous day.

As my family and friends continued to analyze the records, I placed the first of many calls to the Pastoral Care Office of Covid Coven Hospital of Plano, Texas, in the early afternoon. Unfortunately, they were clearly not interested in assisting me, as it took multiple calls and persistent urging to get a hospital Chaplain to eventually call me back.

When a Chaplain finally did call, I shared with her my dismay at being locked out of the hospital, with Rob not having an advocate by his side and no one there to encourage him and give him a personal "it will be okay" touch. I expected the Chaplain would be willing to plead my case to the administration and gain their approval for me to visit my husband in the ICU.

To my surprise and dismay, she was rude, uncompassionate, and uncaring. If anyone would understand and have sympathy with my plight, I would have expected a hospital Chaplain would; however, she brushed me off and advised me their "policy" did not permit them to provide any form of in-person contact with nor comfort to Covid patients. She admitted they would not even darken the doorway of a "Covid" patient's room.

It was as if having "COVID-19" and "UNVACCINATED" stamped on your record meant you were to be given a bed where you could be drugged, ignored, and allowed to waste away until you finally weakened enough that you could be coerced into becoming the next victim of the "let's see if you can survive this therapy" ventilator.

LEGAL COUNSEL STATEMENT

Members of the jury, as noted on Page 117 of the hospital records (see Page C-30 in Appendix C), the Chaplain's office indicated that Sheila had called and expressed her concern that Rob had no "personal touch" or "human connection." Yet, they noted even in the record that their "department's policy" did not allow them to enter the "Covid rooms" and provide comfort or support for such patients. In addition, they did not even offer to let Sheila come to their offices to meet with them in person for encouragement or prayer.

If anyone truly "cared" about the emotional and spiritual welfare of isolated patients and their families, you would have thought it would be the staff and chaplains of the "Pastoral Care Office" of the hospital. However, as Sheila just shared, they coldly advised her they could **do nothing** to aid her in seeing Rob, nor could they provide him with any form of encouragement or support because their "protocol" did not include their "going to Covid rooms."

Ironically, the hospital's website claims their Chaplains provide a compassionate and "supportive presence" to patients and their family members. *How could they be so cold? Where was the compassion and "supportive presence" they said they offered?*

*As you can see, no matter where she turned, Sheila's requests were dismissed entirely and rebuffed. Even the Pastoral "We Really Don't" Care Office **turned a blind eye** to the atrocity of patients being isolated from their families. Thus, they were complicit in the evil plan to ensure any patient admitted with a "Covid" diagnosis on their record would lose all hope and, out of pure desperation, agree to succumb to the abundance of medications and harmful therapies that would eventually lead to their termination. That way, the hospital could chalk up one more "Covid death" and cash in on the large incentive booty, as noted in **Appendix D**.*

At 7:16 PM, I received a call from Dr. Wicked. He sounded like an angel—so sweet and understanding. At first, I thought I could trust him. He sounded like a genuine, caring person—which was refreshing after having been surrounded by a pack of carnies.

A carny is a carnival employee who hocks carnival wares such as stuffed animals, junk foods, games, and rides. Rob's doctors and nurses all sounded like carnies who were pushing what they had to offer. It was as if they were yelling, *"Popcorn, cotton candy, corn dogs, remdesivir, intubation, ventilation. Step right up!"* To their dismay, we were not interested in what they were offering. They probably wondered, "Why would anyone come to our carnival/hospital and not be interested in what we are offering? If Sheila did not want her husband loaded with boatloads of our favorite medications, why did she bring him here?"

Unfortunately, many patients buy into the whole "doctor, do what you will" experience and happily eat the whole enchilada, even when doing so ultimately leads to their demise. So yes, many do enter the hospital carnival in the hope of enjoying the complete experience (the "full therapy"), which, for many, then ends up being a one-way ticket to the morgue.

Rob was in serious condition when I first brought him to the hospital; he needed supplemental expected we would be able to overcome their manipulative practices by being crystal clear with our directives. In addition, I had fully expected to be able to be with him, and I thought I could ensure he would not be given unnecessary and unwanted medications or therapies because I could watch over his care (at least while there during the day) in person.

Dr. Wicked said, "I am the ICU doctor today taking over your husband's case. I just saw him a little bit ago. I asked him if he wanted to call you, and he didn't want to do that, but he said to tell you that he loves you."

I was delighted he had tried to get my husband to call me, and I expect he endeared himself to Rob with the same touch of kindness. I thought I might finally be speaking with someone I could trust. He continued, "We talked for a while, and I was actually able to get an Ensure in him because he has not been able to eat, but we were able to get a protein shake in, and that was positive."

Oh goodness. So, he was admitting Rob had not been eating and needed to be encouraged to take in some form of nourishment so he could build up the strength required to heal. It was becoming apparent that my husband, who had been in the hospital for nearly five days, had not been ordering meals because he was too weak to do so, and up to now, no one had cared.

Lack of adequate nutrition can wear anyone down, especially someone struggling to breathe. Rob had lost a good amount of weight before he went into the hospital because of severe nausea, and now he was becoming even more weakened. Dr. Wicked said they were "low on manpower." I had no doubt their being short-staffed was impacting the quality of care my husband received.

Dr. Wicked went on to say, "When I went in, they had him on double oxygen. I think he'd been doing that just for comfort. We were able to take off the mask so he could drink, and the whole time he was talking to me, his oxygen stayed about 90% on just the nasal high-flow oxygen. That was positive."

That was music to my ears, and my heart rejoiced. Finally, it appeared that I might be working with a doctor who would NOT pressure Rob into being intubated and placed on a ventilator. Dr. Wicked also gave me the great news that Rob no longer needed to be on a nonrebreather mask.

The night before, Nurse Carnage had stressed that Rob was on two machines, both of which were "maxed out," and all they could do to help him beyond that would be chest compressions if he stopped breathing.

I asked, "So, you took him off the other oxygen device, and he seemed to be stable?" He clarified, "The non-rebreather mask, the one with the bag on it; he has that next to him. It's in the room in case he feels out of breath. He can always put it on."

Wow. So, he was improving and might even be able to come home soon. I could feel my chest muscles relax, and I took a deep breath as I felt a glimmer of hope flooding back into my veins. I smiled and said, "Okay!"

Dr. Wicked continued in a more business-like tone, "Lab-wise, we're starting to see some improvement in a lot of inflammatory markers, which is a positive sign in there. His kidney numbers are doing fine. We have done a CT scan and **don't see any clots**. Everything else has been going down. So, those are all positive signs. You know, the CT scan shows he had a pneumomediastinum which is air leaking out of the lung, and that's not a good thing to see. But otherwise, we're seeing **a lot of improvement**. He has not developed a pneumothorax, and that is good. So, hopefully, we'll see over the coming days improvement in the oxygen."

Okay, this all sounded good, and he gave me the hope I had longed for. He then threw me a curve ball, "There's no need for Rob to be on a ventilator **at this point**. But I did see in his records he **does not want to be** on a ventilator. I just want to give you my spiel on that." I thought, "Oh Lord, now what? With Rob doing better, why are we talking about the ventilator? Are these people truly dead set on getting Rob intubated and mechanically ventilated?" I said, "What?" and braced myself for what was coming next.

He rambled on, "I agree; I don't want him on the ventilator unless it's absolutely necessary. But the ventilator got a lot of bad press both with that New York Governor last year talking about it and, unfortunately saying some things that set people off. Yet, if you have to be on a ventilator, that is a marker of bad disease. We don't put people on a ventilator for fun. We've put people on a ventilator, those Covid people who, in my opinion, are at a 90% -100% chance of dying without it. **So, it is a very bad thing to have to go on, and that is 100% true. That I know. I believe the ventilator causes death.**"

Yes! That was what I had been saying. Ventilators kill people! Rob did not want to go on a ventilator for any reason, even if he was told it would be necessary to save his life. He did not want to chance it because he knew going on a ventilator would be a death sentence.

Dr. Wicked continued, "But there **are** complications of being on a ventilator—that's definitely possible. Last year, 45% of those on the ventilator **died**, which means 55% of them didn't die. And again, we're picking a population of people that pretty sure had a close to 100% chance of death. So, I agree we don't want to be on the ventilator. It's a marker that things went poorly. But I only do it when I think you're going to die without it."

Just because Rob and I were separated from each other, that did not mean we were not still in total agreement. Rob was trying to survive in conditions like those in prisoner-of-war camps where the prisoners had no choices. In Russian WWII military POW camps, the death rate of German prisoners was said to be as high as 33%, while in Britain's POW camps, the percentage who died was as low as .03%. Clearly, something is grossly wrong when 33% of prisoners die. That death rate indicates **negligence, maleficence, and/or malicious intent are involved**.

Suppose 45% of Covid patients who are placed on ventilators die in "hospital" death camps. In that case, the mortality rate of ventilated patients exceeds the death rate of prisoners in Russian POW camps during WWII. Fathom that!

Being on a ventilator was not a risk we were willing to take. Yet, every doctor we spoke with at Covid Coven Hospital of Plano, Texas, pressured us to agree to remove Rob's "Do Not Intubate" (DNI) order so they could have intubation and ventilation as their next-step option.

Dr. Wicked's admission that the "benefit" of being intubated and placed on a ventilator was a 45% chance of death further demonstrated that the "benefits" did not outweigh the risks; the only real benefit accrued to the hospital and the doctors.

> *Risks vs. Benefits*
>
> *The risks versus the benefits is a game they play*
> *With the health of their patients, the price to pay*
> *For their own gain, they risk it all*
> *Ignoring the harm, ignoring the fall*
>
> *But in the end, their evil deeds will show*
> *Their mask will slip, and their lies will grow*
> *And justice will come with a heavy weight*
> *And the physician predators will meet their fate*

I had heard stories from nurses and respiratory therapists **who said they had not seen <u>any</u> Covid patients survive the ventilator.** All the while we discussed "intubation," Rob's blood oxygen level was cruising along in the mid-90s with high-flow nasal cannula oxygen alone. So, where was the logic in all of this?

With significant government incentives being paid to hospitals for every "ventilated" patient, and an additional bonus paid if a patient died of Covid, I could almost hear the excitement of anticipation in Dr. Wicked's voice. Even if he did not receive the incentive money himself, he was aware that another patient on a ventilator would endear him to the hospital administrators.

LEGAL COUNSEL STATEMENT
Members of the jury, as we noted previously, the article in **Appendix D** notes that hospitals receive bonus incentive payments whenever a "Covid" patient ends up on ventilators and another bonus if the patient dies "of Covid."

In her book, <u>Undercover Epicenter Nurse</u>, Erin Olszewski, BSN, RN, said, *"Hospitals could get more for COVID for two reasons: First, the CARES act puts a 20 percent booster bonus payment on top of normal respiratory disease reimbursements. Second, under the CARES act, Medicare and Medicaid would reimburse hospitals for uninsured patients who normally didn't give them a dime. Suffice to say, a patient labeled COVID-Positive could net the hospital five figures or more."*
Olszewski, Erin. Page 70. Undercover Epicenter Nurse: How Fraud, Negligence, & Greed Led to Unnecessary Deaths at Elmhurst Hospital, Skyhorse, 2020.

It is high time government-incentivized drugs and therapies be stopped.

I could not help but ask, "What would you say Rob's chance of survival is right now without the ventilator?" He cautiously answered, "I do not know. If he said he was okay with a ventilator, I would not put him on a ventilator because I don't think he needs it. The problem is if we let people try to stay off the ventilator too long, then when it becomes clear they do need it, sometimes I only have minutes to get them on it. And that is the thing I think about. He does not need it right now. I am hopeful he won't need it."

If Rob did not need to be on a ventilator right now, then why were all of the doctors pushing Rob to agree to "elective intubation," and why did Dr. Dead End yell at me in Rob's presence on September 4th, the morning after Rob's arrival, "Do you want your husband to die?" It was clear something sinister was going on, and I hoped I could trust this doctor to protect Rob from the vultures who wanted to force "the protocol that kills" on him.

Once again, he seemed to know all the right words, as he said, "It's 100% his right to decline therapy we offer. I will not put him on it if he says not to." So finally, someone understands that a patient is 100% within their rights to decline any medication or therapy. I wished what he said would have been written down, placed on the wall above Rob's bed, and taped to the glass door to his room in the ICU.

He added, "We do want you to deal with it from the **correct set of facts**. If he is not wanting to be on the ventilator because Facebook said something about it, then I'll tell you that's not an appropriate reason to not want to."

What in the world? I had thought I had finally met Mr. Nice Guy. Yet, in the same conversation, he had gone from friend to foe by downplaying any concerns about the hospital's favored protocol which was obviously to get every Covid patient on a ventilator.

I wondered if he had given the same type of "*You can trust me, I don't want to push anything on you, but don't believe the lies you've read about how terrible being on a ventilator is*" speech to Rob? I fully expected he had. Yet I knew Rob would easily see right through the Mr. Nice Guy's "I'm your friend" façade. He knew full well not to believe everything the doctors told him.

Dr. Wicked added, "Right now, I don't think he's going to need it. Oh, he definitely doesn't need it right now. Hopefully, he's not going to need it. But if he got into the position where he did need it, we may have only minutes to do it. These are things you need to think about. I'm optimistic that he won't need it. I just want to make sure he was saying no for the correct reasons."

Dr. Wicked had attempted to gain my trust but failed miserably. I knew from experience that people who frequently lie are exposed when they say too much.

Despite the fact Nurse Carnage had said the day before that, "He's not a candidate for the other option called BiPAP because he has a pneumomediastinum—which is where there's air trapped in the space in the chest between the lungs, and it can cause him traumatic injury if we do a positive pressure such as a BiPAP," Dr. Wicked brought up BiPAP therapy as an option, saying, "**If I choose** to do this treatment called BiPAP, **it comes with risks**. The BiPAP would be **a little increased risk** for him because that's positive pressure."

He went on, "So, it has a risk because he has pneumomediastinum. But that would be the next step, where the oxygen he's receiving now would go to using a BiPAP, which is basically like a ventilator without the tube in the throat. You're still awake and talking with it, and we can go back and forth. He can't stay on BiPAP forever."

Without batting an eye, he lightheartedly said, "So, a couple of things can happen. If he gets bad enough, we go to that next step on BiPAP. In his case, a few things can happen. So, say he was to worsen. And again, right now, by all measures, the last 12 hours, he's been going in the right direction. And hopefully, he'll keep doing that. If he were to worsen on this level of therapy, the next step would be BiPAP. One of a couple of things can happen with BiPAP. In this case, he already has a pneumomediastinum, which is a marker that his lungs are fragile.

He then said, "There are probably small areas that are necrotic. So, when we put them on increased positive pressure, you could definitely develop a pneumothorax." He added, "And if you did that, that could be **a life-threatening situation,** and we would need a chest tube placed."

I thought if Rob's "lungs are fragile" and placing him on a BiPAP might create a "life-threatening situation," then how in the world could he be calling BiPAP therapy "**a little increased risk**"?

He continued, "So, that would be one thing, that by the time you do the chest tube, the chest would be painful, and he would need pain medicines and sedation. **And you probably wouldn't be able to breathe adequately, and he would probably need to be on a ventilator**. The second thing that we get on BiPAP—it can help, and he can do okay, and it buys us more time. And you can come and go—come off it and go on it—so you can drink a little bit. In which case, we can still use BiPAP and still be portable more than the ventilator. But that's kind of our last step. **Oxygen levels of about 85% are pretty safe**. So, if we can keep you about 85% [blood oxygen level], you know, it's not a problem if your heart tolerates it pretty well."

Oh goodness. He was now saying that if things went wrong, Rob "would probably need to be on a ventilator."

> **LEGAL COUNSEL STATEMENT**
> Members of the jury, as you can see on Page 3011 of the hospital records (see Page C-24 in Appendix C), Rob's blood oxygen levels were in the range of **92%** to **97%** from 9:00 AM to 11:00 PM on September 7th.
>
> Dr. Wicked's statement that "**Oxygen levels of about 85% are pretty safe**" is right in line with **UC Health Medical Center's** policy that states they do not believe patients must be placed on a ventilator until their O_2 saturation is **below 85%**, saying, *"When oxygen levels become low (oxygen saturation < 85 %) patients are usually intubated and placed on mechanical ventilation. For those patients, ventilators can be the difference between life and death."*
> Covid-19 resources. UC Health. (n.d.). From https://www.uchealth.com/en/media-room/covid-19/ventilators-and-covid-19
>
> Why then would Dr. Wicked be promoting the use of BiPAP therapy while knowing: **(a)** Rob's blood oxygen level was well above 85%, and **(b)** with pneumomediastinum (air abnormally trapped in the mediastinum, the space in the chest between the lungs) the BiPAP could cause Rob traumatic injury.
>
> *We contend that Dr. Wicked knew if the BiPAP sufficiently injured Rob's lungs, he would then have full justification for intubating Rob and placing him on a ventilator—achieving the ultimate goal they had set for Rob the moment he set foot in the Emergency Department.*

He continued to prime me for the likelihood Rob would soon need to be placed on a ventilator, "If you consistently get below the 80s below 85% or lower, if you stay low, that causes kind of a spiral of events. Your heart doesn't like that. Your heart starts pumping less well. You get less oxygen delivery to your tissues. Your acid level goes up. Then, he's trying to breathe more, which he's already not able to do. And that kind of spirals, and that's where I say that spiral can happen over minutes. And that's where your expectations of the ventilator would have to be better, or else you're going to die."

I wanted to ask Dr. Wicked how many patients he had saved and how many died after being placed on a ventilator—but I was afraid to ask and know. Moreover, it was difficult to think straight after hearing all this.

He explained that if Rob got "stuck" on a BiPAP, even if it worked for him, he would still need to be intubated and placed on a ventilator within days. "And then the last thing that could happen on the BiPAP is if it worked for him, he could get stuck on it. And you can't eat or drink with the BiPAP mask strapped over your face. And we can't usually get nutrition in you. So, we put you on BiPAP, but if you aren't improving over a couple of days, there's only so long you can go with IV nutrition, and IV nutrition is pretty poor because of the high infection risk. So, you can't do that very long, even in a good situation."

He continued to lead in the direction of Rob ending up on a ventilator, "So, we have a BiPAP. And then we go several days, and he has turned to the worse. We have to put the tube in urgently. But you know, if for four days you're on BiPAP and getting no nutrition—and you might have to be put on a ventilator just so you can get nutrition." There it was! The hook, the bait, the switch—and Rob would be his prized catch.

He further explained, "If he didn't have a pneumomediastinum, we probably would have already tried BiPAP. But he's been teetering right on that next-to-last step. If someone doesn't want to be on the ventilator because they personally don't want to be, that's 100% your right. But he's 52 years old. I'd hate for someone to just decide this because he's not understanding, and he will lose his life."

LEGAL COUNSEL STATEMENT
Members of the jury, as noted on Page 23 of the hospital records (see Page C-2 in Appendix C), and as Dr. Wicked pointed out during his conversation with Sheila, they knew soon after Rob arrived in the Emergency Department that he had **pneumomediastinum**.

Pneumomediastinum is a contraindication for the use of a BiPAP (Bilevel Positive Airway Pressure) because this type of positive pressure therapy can make the condition far worse by forcing more air into the space between the lungs, making it VERY difficult to breathe—and Dr. Wicked admitted, "it has a risk because he has pneumomediastinum."

Sadly, at 9:40 AM on September 8, 2021 (the next day), Dr. Wicked removed Rob's DNI (Do Not Intubate) status as Rob was being placed on life-threatening BiPAP therapy **for 4.5 hours**. We contend this therapy further damaged Rob's lungs to the point of **NO RETURN**—making it far more difficult for him to breathe on his own and giving the doctors the excuse they had been looking for to force Rob to be intubated and placed on a ventilator.

I mentioned that Rob's nurse said he was on two oxygen machines, yet Dr. Wicked had said he took him off one because he did not need it and was breathing better. Dr. Wicked explained, "We took it off to see where he was. It's not two different types of machines, just two different types of oxygen. He's on a brand called, Optiflow. It delivers oxygen through a large cannula to the nose. And they also had him on a partial re-breather, which is just a face mask; just a loose-fitting face mask that has an extra bag. So, without the re-breather he was able to talk with me with just the oxygen through the nose, and his oxygen level is actually about 93% right now. It was just sitting there next to him. So he can put the mask back on if he wants to. He was wanting a drink. So, he managed to get down an Ensure. So, basically, he was able to drink, and he could talk to me for 10 to 12 minutes that I've been there. And his oxygen levels stayed at 93%."

I was so happy to hear Rob was doing well on an Optiflow nasal cannula and could talk for 10 to 12 minutes. I asked the doctor if he would give Rob budesonide which a doctor had prescribed before his admission. He shut that idea down with "I'll put him on nebulized budesonide when I think he needs it—when he's able to come off the IV steroids then, yeah, for sure, we'll put him on it." He was clearly not supportive of giving Rob nebulized budesonide as it was not part of their protocol.

I asked, "So, is he getting fluids? Dr. Wicked reluctantly shared, "So, he's only getting a little bit of fluid for the blood pressure. Actually, I try to run him kinda dry because of when your lungs are inflamed, all that extra fluid—he's not getting diuretics right now—but he's right around the dry side because with his lungs being so inflamed if you get extra fluid on your body, especially while you're sucking in air negative pressure, he is just having to go to breathe through inflammatory fluid as well as extra fluid. He is running a little bit on the dry side intentionally."

I could feel Dr. Wicked was wrapping up, so I jumped in with, "So, what's the plan moving forward?" He answered, "So, my plan right now is continuous anti-inflammatories and oxygen. Keep his blood oxygen level above 88 to 94 is where I'm shooting for. Basically, nutrition, because there's been a lot of work going into breathing. So, those protein shakes . . . you can't really eat well. They can't swallow and breathe at the same time. So, he was able to hold 350 calorie protein shake down for me while I was in there. And we got another one. Hopefully, get that down tonight. So, **nutrition**, **oxygen**, and **time**."

I sincerely hoped Dr. Wicked would help ensure Rob received and consumed adequate food and water so he could regain the strength he needed to recover.

LEGAL COUNSEL STATEMENT
Members of the jury, Dr. Wicked was correct in saying that what Rob needed was adequate **nutrition**, **oxygen**, **and time**.

What he **did not need** was a "**5-day course**" of **remdesivir** (a drug known to have the potential to cause acute kidney injury) and off-label **VELETRI** (a drug with potentially serious side effects that included severe shortness of breath and gasping for breath), **nitazoxanide** (an antiparasitic clinical trial drug) and **colchicine** (a drug designed to treat gout symptoms), etc., etc.

Covid creates a significant inflammatory response in the lungs, and the last thing a Covid patient needs is increased inflammation of the tissue between the alveoli (air sacs) and the capillary network where oxygen is delivered into the bloodstream.

We contend these unnecessary and harmful drugs, combined with the lack of adequate nutrition, weakened Rob to the point where Dr. Wicked could have an excuse to say he was "tiring out" and needed to be placed on a BiPAP. This therapy would then cause sufficient damage to Rob's "fragile lungs" to allow them to get Rob on a ventilator.

Dr. Wicked then swooped in like a vulture after its prey, saying, "And then the other thing to consider is if things were to worsen, would he consider a ventilator as a last-ditch effort or not? But hopefully, that won't be an issue."

With Rob's DNI **(Do Not Intubate)** order, we had made it clear he did NOT want to be intubated and placed on a ventilator. To ensure he understood our stance, I said, "Thinking about that as a family, we're... **NO!** I mean, the answer is **NO!** He's doing good. He's doing great right now." Then, with emphasis, Dr. Wicked added, "Unless he told me otherwise. If **he** cannot make the decision, then you can tell me otherwise, so we'll leave it as a no. **I just want to make sure everybody is working on that.**"

He then told me Rob had been tested for COVID-19 antibodies, and the test was positive. Putting two and two together, I asked, "Since he has the antibodies doesn't that mean he isn't positive for Covid any longer, which should mean I could now see him?" He swiftly replied, "I believe they're doing **21 days** for the isolation. We will do isolation visitation when manpower allows. That's not, unfortunately, being allowed."

I was horrified at the doctor's cold response. Rob needed the comfort of human touch and reassurance, not isolation. He was worried that if I couldn't be there to advocate for him, the doctors might make decisions that would lead to his death. He did not want their favored "protocol." He only wanted the basics—oxygen, nutrition, and antibiotics; then to be discharged to continue his recovery at home.

Since Rob seemed to be doing better, I asked Dr. Wicked if he had at least encouraged him that he would be okay. He responded, "I did tell him that I wouldn't lie to him—that I couldn't give any false hope. I told him just about the things I was worried about. Even if it's not exactly what he wants to hear, I'm going to be honest."

I was disappointed to hear that, during his conversation with Rob, he chose to emphasize all the things he "was worried about" rather than supporting Rob and encouraging him that he would recover. He did not let Rob know that he was getting better or that he was making progress. Instead, he only shared with him potential negative outcomes.

Fear is a form of oppression and a destructive emotion that cannot help anyone heal. I replied, "You're going to be honest with him? You seemed much more optimistic with me. I hope you are showing him the same optimism, because he can't handle negativity at this point."

Rob needed to hear good news about how he was improving to continue improving. Unfortunately, with me locked out, Dr. Wicked had free reign to push the *"you're not likely going to make it"* narrative as a means of fearmongering. The doctors used every opportunity to fill his head with worse-case scenarios to convince him he would likely die if he did not agree to their *"full protocol."*

Although he admitted to me that Rob was improving and what he needed to recover was "nutrition, oxygen, and time," Dr. Wicked had slyly buddied up to my husband, fed him a protein drink for the first time in days at a time when he was totally famished, then filled his head with worse-case scenarios in the hope of convincing him to agree to their "full protocol" of intubation and ventilation if he wanted to live. He was basically asking Rob to sign on the dotted line.

I could imagine my husband as a defenseless rabbit trapped by a pack of wolves in the corner of an ICU room—knowing he was outnumbered and his chances of escaping and surviving were slim. So, I kept texting Rob positive affirmations hoping he would see them. If we both stood firm in our convictions and stayed strong, I hoped he would come out of this nightmare unharmed.

I grieved as I thought of how the doctors were continually badgering him to agree to "the protocol." The only comfort I had was that Dr. Wicked admitted that despite their repeatedly assaulting Rob with unnecessary medications, he was somehow actually improving.

I expected he would be able to continue to improve if they did not do any more to harm him. But, even then, I could not take a deep breath because I grieved deeply at Rob's treatment and still feared for his life.

After our call ended, I reassured myself by saying, "Remember, Dr. Wicked said he is improving. He's improving!" I repeated those positive thoughts, and before long, I could finally doze off to sleep.

LEGAL COUNSEL STATEMENT
Members of the jury, on the evening of September 7th, on Page 122 of the hospital records (see Page C-32), Dr. Wicked noted (again) that "**Pt [patient] does not wish to be intubated.**" *Unfortunately, Rob's not being intubated would not follow their script for "Covid" patients.*

On this page, they again noted that Rob had pneumomediastinum. This condition can be significantly worsened if placed on a BiPAP. Sadly, starting at around 9:30 AM the following day, he suffered 4.5 hours on a BiPAP, as you can see in the note on Page 135 of the hospital records (see Page C-37 in Appendix C).

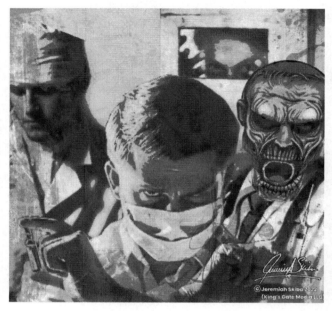

At the top of Page 122 of the hospital records (see Page C-32), they also entered "**restarted remdesivir.**" It was "**restarted**" because (as we noted earlier) Rob had successfully refused one dose the morning of September 5th, as pointed out near the top of Pages 170-171 of the hospital records (see Page C-46).

Due to his "refusal" of one dose of remdesivir, they alleged (near the top of Pages 170-171 as found on Page C-46) that "**Noncompliance with medications**" was one of the critical factors that somehow COMPLICATED his acquired pneumomediastinum.

Their "Noncompliance with medications" note was simply a complaint that Rob had successfully refused <u>one dose</u> of **remdesivir**, a drug they had forced upon him <u>without his consent</u>.

Chapter 5 – Intubation & Ventilation

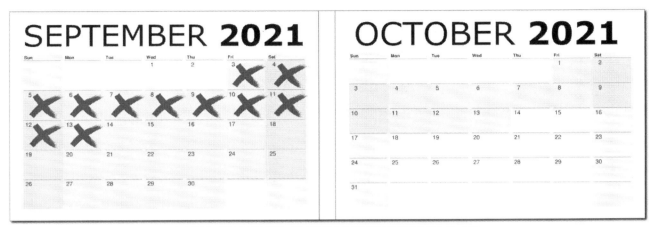

THIS CHAPTER COVERS SEPTEMBER 8-13

Wednesday, September 8, 2021

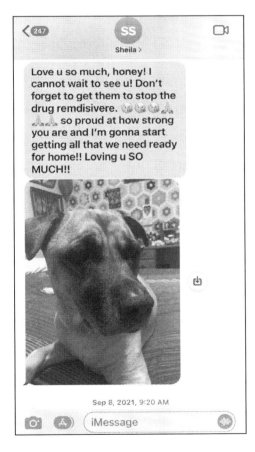

When I awoke, I was exhausted from yet another sleepless night. There was no peace in the midst of my battle to free Rob from unscrupulous doctors who were pressuring him to follow their prescribed "protocol" at any cost—even if it would cost him his life.

I sent Rob a text message of hope and encouragement with a picture of our dog, Heidi—his best friend other than me. They were inseparable. Even when he was working at his computer, she would stay close to him, waiting for the occasional hug, tug of war, or time of wrestling on the floor. With no more happy humming from Rob or the loud commotion of his playing with Heidi, my once-happy home became a place I despised.

I waited until 9:05 AM to call Rob's phone in case he might be resting. I was delighted he answered, and during our brief, four-minute conversation, I reassured him that the doctors said he was improving.

Rob sounded good and indicated he was holding his own. We remained steadfast in our stand against his being intubated and placed on a ventilator. I felt so much better having heard his voice and being able to assure him he was improving.

At 10:07 AM, I received a call from Dr. Wicked. He got down to business, saying, "His numbers look okay." Well, that sure sounded good. He then blurted out, "I'm hoping the BiPAP with that

61

He spoke relatively fast, and his voice faded in and out due to a bad connection. I heard something about "BiPAP" but didn't quite catch what he was getting at. He quickly changed the subject. "Well, he did about an hour [proning] on his stomach last night, but that was too uncomfortable, and he couldn't stay that way. So, hopefully, this will help. Otherwise, his oxygen level is relatively stable." I thought, "Outstanding! His oxygen level is relatively stable. That's fantastic!"

He breathlessly continued, "Yesterday, his inflammatory markers were still improving, lab-wise." Great. More good news. Keeping up his fast pace, he launched into, "Now the thing with the BiPAP—BiPAP being positive pressure—is, he already has that damage and air leakage happening with his pneumomediastinum. So, I'm gonna keep an eye on that to make sure we don't get like a pneumothorax. But we're several days out from that". And so, we will be as cautious as we can and keep an eye out for it. Hopefully, that won't be an issue."

I asked, "So, has anything else changed since yesterday?" He answered, "Nothing I can find objectively on his labs. Everything on the labs is actually a little bit better, his white count went up just a tad, but on steroids, that's hard to follow. White counts can be elevated due to infection. Stress, in general, can do it, and steroids can do it. So, that gets hard to follow. No new meds. Nothing else changed."

He added, "CRP [C-reactive protein] is coming down to normal range. His D-Dimer had gone up two days ago. It's coming down today. It's down to 11.19 from 17. Everything lab-wise looks actually a little improved." I would have thought he would be rejoicing at Rob's improvement, yet he almost sounded disappointed.

Dr. Wicked added, "I think our biggest issue is that he drank the one Ensure with me yesterday and then no more. So, I want him to get three in today. So, I think respiratory muscle fatigue **and poor calorie intake** is the ONLY thing that's working really against us."

So, he knew Rob needed to get more nutrition and calories. These devils had been ignoring Rob's "calorie intake" from the moment he was admitted, as evidenced by the fact that just 48 hours after his arrival on the evening of September 5, 2021, Rob texted me, **"No food no . . ."** and **"No strength no hope left."** Without adequate food and water, he would quickly develop "muscle fatigue."

He added, "Yeah. Because otherwise . . . time. You know, we just need to find time for things to heal." What did he mean by "we need to find time to heal?" Rob was already healing, and he was improving. Obviously, this type of illness takes time to heal.

Dr. Wicked was very candid about Rob's continual lack of nutrition, saying, "But if he's getting weaker and not eating or getting the protein shakes in, that'll be an ISSUE. So, we'll keep trying to push him on the nutrition and get him on the BiPAP here in a little bit."

They knew Rob was too weak to feed himself and that if he did not receive assistance, he would fail to order meals. Dr. Wicked should have asked the nurses to ensure Rob ordered meals. Then, someone should have been assigned to ensure he ate at least part of each meal or drank sufficient "Ensure" drinks to boost his caloric intake. Verifying he was consuming enough calories should have been equally as important as hanging his IV bags of pharmaceuticals.

What Rob was lacking was not more drugs. What he desperately needed, but they were purposely denying him, was food, water, and an advocate. He continued, "I think, honestly, I'm not minimizing anything; he is very sick. Things could go either way. But a lot of it, I think, is his stress level."

Of course, Rob was stressed. With a lack of compassion, a never-ending assault of dangerous drugs, a lack of loving companionship and encouragement, a scarcity of food and water, and constant day and night badgering from left and right to remove his DNI (Do Not Intubate) order, why wouldn't he be?

All of this was tiring him out and making him anxious. They knew that a totally worn-out and starved patient would be more likely to agree to intubation and ventilation because he would no longer have the energy to fight the illness on his own. Their cunning plan was to divide, weaken, and conquer, and I was terrified that they would succeed.

A doctor friend told me about an option called TPN (Total Parenteral Nutrition), where most of the body's required nutrients and calories can be provided via an IV. So, I asked him, "How about TPN intravenous feeding?"

He told me that TPN was usually done short-term to assist with postoperative healing or was used long-term in patients whose bowels could not absorb nutrients. He said he did not favor this type of therapy, commenting, "TPN is horrible nutrition. It's not very good nutrition. It's a horrible infection risk, especially when you're already on steroids. I really, really don't want to do that at all." I had thought the delivery of additional nutrients via this method would be better than letting Rob become nutrient and calorie deprived, which we both knew would allow him to weaken even further.

He went on, "I would actually consider putting an NG tube in first, but then with the BiPAP, it will be hard to use. I'll talk to him maybe tomorrow about that if he's not able to get the protein shakes in today." I thought, "Why wait another day for him to weaken even more?"

Why would Rob's being in the ICU—which by definition administers "Intensive Care"—have not meant that everything he needed to recover would be provided, including adequate nutrition to restore his strength?

When did it become acceptable for patients to starve because they cannot eat due to breathing difficulties? Do the healthcare professionals who work at hospitals believe ensuring patients receive adequate nutrition during their stay is a NON-ISSUE, or do they only neglect the nutrient and calorie intake of Covid or unvaccinated patients?

I asked, "Can I go back to something you said earlier? You said it's 'his stress level,' and I know where you're going with that. But, look, he has only been seeing medical personnel. He needs to see ME. Without me there, he can't be at ease. He does not even know that his family members are working for him. I am sure you have heard this a million times. You know this is a big problem!"

Pretending to sympathize, he said, "The video things [Facetime chats] are the best we have right now. I'd say you can talk to administration to see if you can get an exception. I'm all for it if we can, but it's above my pay grade. And I understand the reasons for it, we just don't have the manpower or the protective equipment and, of course, as always, our lawyers and liability. In the meantime, just try to use the video chats as much as you can."

LEGAL COUNSEL STATEMENT

Members of the jury, we, like Dr. Wicked, also "understand the reasons for" the 21-day lock out of family members. We contend it was designed to keep them at arm's length so they could not interfere with "the protocol," which required that patients agree to be placed on a ventilator.

One month before Rob became ill, he posted an article on the need for religious exemptions to forced medical procedures. In that article, he said the following:

"I am a healthy person, with a God-given, functioning immune system. I was created in the image and likeness of the Creator, who tells me that my body is meant to be a Temple for the indwelling of His Holy Spirit. Thus, I refuse to corrupt my temple/body with potentially harmful substances, foreign genetic code, and things identified in Scripture as 'unclean' and an 'abomination.' Neither you, the government, nor anyone else has the right to FORCE a medical procedure on me, in violation of virtually every medical ethics standard—including the Nuremberg Code."

Unfortunately, a well-planned tragedy was about to occur at Covid Coven Hospital of Plano, Texas. Although during her midmorning call with him, Dr. Wicked had advised Sheila that Rob was improving, and the day before, on September 7th, that all he needed was **oxygen**, **nutrition**, **and time**—*helping him recover and discharging him to home would not benefit the hospital or the doctors. Thus, their "Plan of Care" required that Rob eventually agree to be intubated and placed on a ventilator.*

I thought, "What kind of doctor is this? Does he not realize my husband needs to focus his limited strength and energy on getting well, not on video chats." What Rob needed was not more "chat time" but to have me by his side. The last thing Rob said to me as the nurse in the Emergency Department whisked him away in a wheelchair on the evening of September 3, 2021, was, *"If they don't let you be my advocate, I'm going to die in here!"*—and he did not mean my attempting to advocate for him remotely.

Realizing Dr. Wicked neither cared nor was willing to advocate for my ability to gain entrance to the hospital, I changed subjects and asked him once again if he would prescribe nebulized budesonide for Rob. He retorted, "At this point, his inflammatory markers are coming down, so I disagree."

I asked, "Would it hurt him to have inhaled budesonide? He was on that at home." Dr. Wicked confided, "The reason I'm not giving it to Rob is I don't have the <u>resources</u> for it. But, if it's the medicine he needs, then by all means, we'd do it. If I put everybody on it . . . I'm already short on respiratory therapists." So, if Rob needed it, he would "by all means" do it, yet they are too short-staffed to give it. Thus, if he felt he needed it, a respiratory therapist would magically appear to provide the nebulized treatment. Something surely did not add up.

Now came the clincher, "Go back and do the math. If he's on the ventilator. Yeah, what we do is we put it [the budesonide] in the line, and they walk away. I don't have the resources to do it if it's not a needed medicine. It would not be harmful to him. I just don't have the resources to do it." All I had to do was agree to have Rob placed on a ventilator, and THEN they would give him budesonide. However, the whole purpose of getting him on budesonide now would be to avoid the need for intubation and ventilation in the first place.

After having informed me the night before that, "Last year, 45% of those on the ventilator died," he now expected me to be elated at the thought of getting Rob on a ventilator so he could THEN be given budesonide.

Since he said, "It would not be harmful to him at this point. If we lower the steroids, I'll be happy to order for him," I asked, "Okay. You said if the steroids get lowered? Why not do that now and give him the nebulized budesonide?" He responded, "My Respiratory Therapists are already stretched." It was clear he was only trying to placate me and that he had NO INTENTION of giving Rob budesonide unless and until we agreed to his being intubated and placed on a ventilator.

Realizing I was getting nowhere with the budesonide plea, I asked him about the remdesivir Rob was being given. I knew it was a dangerous drug; however, I tried an academic approach by sharing how I had read studies that indicated it could harm the kidneys and, at best, *might* be beneficial in the very early stages of Covid; after that, it showed no beneficial effects. I said, "It has been two weeks since Rob developed his initial symptoms, and you discovered he has the antibodies for Covid. Why would he have been prescribed this drug? I don't understand."

Dr. Wicked agreed with me. He said, "That was my standpoint. But I would defer to Dr. Torture on that. I think she is just kind of throwing everything at him as she can." Clearly, "throwing everything at him" was their standard of care for Covid patients.

I replied, "Well, Rob said he doesn't want that." He responded, "That would be the first medicine we stop; it's not by no means a miracle drug. So yeah, I agree. I don't feel strongly one way or the other." I asked him if he would please speak with Dr. Torture and try to reason with her since she had ordered it, and he agreed it would likely do no good.

He responded, "I can talk with her about it. I don't feel strongly about it; I don't think it's a miracle drug. I don't think it's hurting kidneys or liver function. **If it went in the wrong direction at all, then we'd definitely stop it.**" Surprised at his "we'll wait and see (if his kidneys get damaged)" attitude, I said, "You say you will keep an eye on his kidney function. We don't want to risk damaging his kidneys, and I don't think remdesivir is helping him at this point."

He barked, "We are going to watch his kidneys regardless." I rebutted, "Rob pleaded with me that he did not want it, but they're pressuring him to take it. And if it doesn't benefit him, it is a wasted medication that can potentially harm him."

To diffuse the situation, he said, "I'll talk to Dr. Torture and see if it's been ordered; at this point, I agree that it's probably not doing much." I replied, "Tell her Rob's family is going to continue to push that he be taken **off** remdesivir. We will drop our pushing once she removes the drug."

His less-than-helpful response was, "Yeah, well, again, **you always have the right to refuse treatment for sure.** I'll talk to Dr. Torture today, and I'll bring that up. It's something that the Infectious Disease doctor should know. I would stop it if I saw any kind of or it caused any harm."

What a cruel joke. He had said, "you always have the right to refuse treatment," yet they totally disregarded our refusals. We also had **the right to request** any medication or supplement we desired—such as budesonide and IV vitamin C—yet they operated on the premise that they had the right to refuse to administer any and all requested medications or supplements.

Their playbook was one of: (a) pretend to agree with the patient or family member, (b) dodge responsibility and pass the ball to someone else, (c) continue on the prescribed course of treatment that lines up with "the protocol." I knew I could not rest until I could get Rob home and out of the clutches of these bloodthirsty villains.

Dr. Wicked then shared that he had continued to badger Rob about "elective intubation." I pleaded, "Doctor, I'm begging you. He thinks he's going downhill because no one is telling him he's **doing well** and that he will be okay. I get it that you can't tell him, 'Hey, you're gonna walk out of here in two weeks,' and you can't guarantee that. But you must be positive, or my husband will continue having anxiety issues."

Dr. Wicked clarified, "I don't think anxiety is exactly the right word. It's not. It's not depression. It's not anxiety, but it's something along those lines." I blurted out, "Like **fear**?" He answered, "Fear for sure. Fear for sure. **Like I said, when I brought up intubation, he kept asking for it.** I asked him, 'you're fine with it?' But I told him, no, you don't need it yet. I'm talking to him about it. Yeah, we need to get up on that. Oh, but this morning...." His thoughts trailed off as if he had forgotten what he was going to say.

Before I could interject, he continued, "I went back over on the positive today. The oxygen is stable, and I'll tell you, I mean, I'll keep trying to give him that. And I'll pass it on to the nurses to try to be more upbeat with him. But obviously, we can't lie to him. **I've been telling him positive stuff for the last few days** and kind of focusing on that. I said, to be honest, 'get the whole picture.' But then I started with the positive, and then I finished with the positive. So ...." He trailed off as if he did not know what else to say because he had been caught in a series of lies and hoped I had not noticed. Thus, we ended our conversation on a sour note.

How could Dr. Wicked say he was being positive with Rob for the last few days when he had only met Rob the night before when he gave him his first Ensure drink?

The entire conversation greatly disturbed me because I knew Rob did not want to be intubated and put on a ventilator. Dr. Wicked's assertion that Rob had been "asking for it" clearly indicates that he was lying. We had vowed to each other never to be intubated, and Rob knew being placed on a ventilator would be a death sentence. He would have told me if he even thought of being placed on a ventilator. *Rob wanted to live, and he had a lot to live for!*

I also did not believe Dr. Wicked when he said he had started and ended his conversations with Rob "with the positive." *The only thing Dr. Wicked was positive about was that Rob would end up on a ventilator.*

LEGAL COUNSEL STATEMENT
Members of the jury, Sheila made an astute observation regarding Dr. Wicked's "I've been telling him positive stuff for the last few days" statement, as his initial entry in the hospital records concerning Rob was made the day before, on September 7, 2021. You can see the entry on Page 122 of the hospital records (see Page C-32 in Appendix C).

In addition, he appears to have attempted to deceive Sheila when he said, "Like I said, when I brought up intubation, he kept asking for it" as on that same page you will see Dr. Wicked noted, "Pt [patient] does not wish to be intubated."

One thing was clear, and it drove me to tears; he and the other doctors were dead set on achieving their goal even if their doing so would mean Rob would not come home alive. As Rob's life hung in the balance, they had their heavy hands on their side of the scale to tilt it in their favor.

How did they think someone who was teetering on the edge and who might go either way could survive without adequate food, water, and human touch—all of which he was being deprived of? I would have never taken Rob to this hospital if I had known they would deprive him of basic human needs. He may have had a roof over his head, but he was not being sheltered from danger. I feared I had taken him to a kill shelter, and he was in line to be slaughtered.

My mother, sister, and son could see that I was undone and on the edge of a nervous breakdown. They valiantly tried, without success, to convince me that all the doctors were doing their best and wanted Rob to recover. But no matter how much they tried to assure me Rob would be fine, I could not get rid of an inner foreboding that something horrible was about to happen.

A good friend, Amanda, texted me to let me know she had spoken with three ER nurses. Each of them urged her to warn me NOT to let Rob be put on a ventilator since doing so would be a death sentence.

My family, friends, and I again called doctors, nurses, hospitals, and rehabilitation centers in the hope of finding a facility that would accept a transfer of Rob and allow us to participate in the development of his plan of care—ALL TO NO AVAIL. The right solution would have been to be permitted by Rob's side in the hospital so I could advocate for him in person. Yet, they were unwilling to budge on their insurmountable 21-day isolation policy.

LEGAL COUNSEL STATEMENT

Members of the jury, the doctors at Covid Coven Hospital of Plano, Texas, had a pre-planned course of treatment for every "Covid" patient that included a list of essential drugs and therapies that would raise the hospital's and doctors' per-patient revenue. *In Appendix G, you will find validation of Sheila's fear that Rob would be administered a wealth of harmful drugs that might increase his suffering and possibly lead to his death.*

Anything Rob or Sheila requested that was not on their "*essentials*" list was ignored or refused. Instead, the doctors cleverly schemed to ensure that no matter what Rob or Sheila wanted, every "*essential*" on their **"pre-planned list"** was checked **off.**

The last page of Rob's hospital bill, as shown here, makes it clear that checking off each item on their list resulted in a grotesquely large bill of **$794,587.10** (before adjustments) for Rob's 40-day stay. With the doctors' private bills added, the unadjusted total came to over $1 million.

Date	Admission Date	Discharge Date	Page
12/28/2021	09/03/21	10/13/21	110
Patient Name			Account #
Skiba,Robert			
Total charges:			$794,587.10

An article published on November 17, 2021, by the American Association of Physicians and Surgeons (a copy of which appears in **Appendix D)** indicates this enormous sum does not include additional subsidies the hospital received from the federal government, such as:

- A 20 percent "boost" bonus payment from Medicare on the entire hospital bill when a patient is administered remdesivir as opposed to other medications, such as ivermectin.
- A larger bonus payment to the hospital if a COVID-19 patient is mechanically ventilated.
- Whether or not the patient indeed died of COVID-19, the hospital receives additional funds if the cause of

We believe the federal government has no business rewarding hospitals for utilizing a protocol that has a criminally high mortality rate. *This madness needs to stop, and it needs to stop now.*

I was living each moment on high alert. So, when the phone rang a little after 6:00 PM, I felt sick to my stomach, just as I did every time it rang from the moment I had taken Rob to the hospital.

Because I did not recognize the number, I let the call go to voicemail. Once the message had been recorded, I played it in the presence of my mother and sister, who were with me.

We heard an unemotional, matter-of-fact, mousy voice say, "Hello Sheila, this is Dr. Dead End. I've gone in and talked with Rob a couple of times. This afternoon, his respiratory status is worsening, and they'll have the nurse call and update you, but I'm gonna have to put him on a ventilator. My thoughts and prayers are with you and your family, and we'll update you later tonight."

So, Dr. Dead End gave me no choice; he had already decided for Rob and me. It was a done deal— signed, sealed, and delivered! I remembered Rob's text to me on the afternoon of September 5, 2021, when he said, "*Doing all they can to try to get me to agree to intubate. I'm dead if they do.*"

Turning to my mother and sister, I could feel the blood rushing from my face. I blamed them for encouraging me to take Rob to the hospital and believing the medical staff would take good care of him. Terrified that Rob was about to be placed on a ventilator, I screamed, "They're going to kill him! I told you they would!"

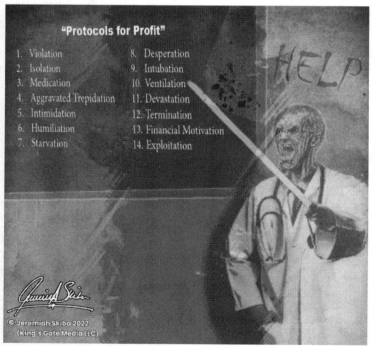

"Protocols for Profit"

1. Violation
2. Isolation
3. Medication
4. Aggravated Trepidation
5. Intimidation
6. Humiliation
7. Starvation
8. Desperation
9. Intubation
10. Ventilation
11. Devastation
12. Termination
13. Financial Motivation
14. Exploitation

© Jeremiah Skiba 2022
(King's Gate Media LLC)

I could not avoid hating everything and everyone involved in leading us down this path. But, most of all, I hated myself for taking Rob to the hospital.

My husband was suffering this evil fate at the hands of a group of criminals who had been dead set on his following every step of their unbending and deadly "protocol that kills" from the moment he stepped over the hospital threshold and into their hands.

Now, despite all my efforts to prevent it, the love of my life was a soon to be a prisoner—strapped to a device few get **off** alive. I was shaking so badly that my teeth were chattering, and my family had no idea what to say to comfort me.

As I stood there trembling, my sister lovingly took my phone from my hands and called back the number that had left the message. As she held the phone to my ear, I could hear a nurse on the other end of the line say that she would immediately get Dr. Dead End on the phone.

I then heard the dreaded voice I had hated from the moment he had yelled at us four days earlier when Rob and I refused to agree to the ventilator as he shouted, "*Do you want your husband to die?*" while standing by Rob's bedside. That same evil voice was about to tell me that he had succeeded with his plan to intubate Rob, and we had lost.

The voice of doom said, "Hey, Sheila, this is Dr. Dead End." I shakingly answered, "Hi, Doctor. Yes, I just got your message." "He's gonna have to be put on a ventilator here. We're gonna start gathering the supplies," the unconcerned, Mengele-spirit-led doctor shot back, "I was here when Dr. Wicked called me this morning. He's just working too hard. We tried a noninvasive BiPAP." Why was I being TOLD he's going to be placed on a ventilator instead of being ASKED?

Why was Rob placed on a BiPAP when it could cause him traumatic injury? Just two days ago, Nurse Carnage had warned me, "He's not a candidate for the other option called BiPAP because he has a pneumomediastinum—which is where there's air trapped in the space in the chest between the lungs, and it can cause him traumatic injury if we do a positive pressure such as a BiPAP."

Why were they now "gathering the supplies" to place Rob on a ventilator when Dr. Wicked had told me earlier in the day that **he would not do that** unless (a) Rob's blood oxygen level dropped **below 85%** (it had been 93% the last I heard) and (b)? he was 100% certain Rob would die without being placed on a ventilator?

Dr. Dead End continued, "He couldn't tolerate that [the noninvasive BiPAP] due to claustrophobia. And he's breathing 30-plus times a minute." He couldn't tolerate the BiPAP because of claustrophobia? Why would claustrophobia mean he had to be intubated? Had the BiPAP further damaged Rob's fragile lungs?

Unfortunately, Dr. Dead End had only called **to inform me HE had decided** to intubate Rob and place him on a ventilator and his decision was FINAL. I was out of options, and by his tone, it was clear I could do **nothing** to stop him. My heart was pounding in my chest, and I felt like vomiting.

None of this made any sense. Other than Rob's being on the BiPAP, nothing else had changed. According to Dr. Wicked, Rob was doing fine and had improved, and earlier in the day, it appeared he was coming out of the dark and heading into the light. But now it appeared the Whitecoat Cult worshipers of "the protocol god" were going to sacrifice Rob—just as they had done to thousands of others before him.

LEGAL COUNSEL STATEMENT
Members of the jury, our independent medical expert, Sammy Wong, MD (**see Appendix B**), considered the use of a BiPAP on Rob **an injurious act** and one of his "**Causes of Action**" against the doctors, stating, "*He had known pneumomediastinum on admission yet he was subjected to 4½ hours of BiPAP which substantially increases the risk for barotrauma.*"

After the BiPAP and Rob's subsequent intubation, a chest X-ray showed "*Extensive pneumomediastinum and chest wall and soft tissue gas in the neck.*" As Dr. Wong noted in Appendix B (and as recorded on Page 135 of the hospital records found on Page C-37 in Appendix C), "*It is conceivable that the 'claustrophobia' [Rob experienced on the BiPAP] was more likely feeling shortness of breath from the iatrogenic [worsened by medical treatment] pneumomediastinum.*"

In addition, Dr. Wicked knew that **barotrauma**—a potentially life-threatening condition where the alveoli, the air sacs of the lungs, rupture and collapse, leading to difficulty breathing and decreased oxygenation of the body—was a likely outcome for someone with pneumomediastinum, as noted on Page 127 of Rob's hospital

Unfortunately, the BiPAP **did cause barotrauma,** as documented on page 141 of the hospital records (see Page C-44), where they stated, "Repeat CXR [Chest X-ray] this afternoon to **monitor barotrauma.**"

The rupturing and collapsing of the alveoli caused by **barotrauma** makes it difficult for oxygen to get into the bloodstream and for carbon dioxide to be exhaled. *This can lead to symptoms such as shortness of breath, difficulty breathing, and a feeling of tightness in the chest (which is likely another reason why Rob felt claustrophobic on the BiPAP as noted at the bottom of Page 136 of the hospital records (See Page C-41 in Appendix C).*

We believe Rob's rate of breathing increased to 30+ breaths per minute due to the **extensive pneumomediastinum** he had combined with the **barotrauma** injury caused by the BiPAP therapy. *Thus, Rob suffered from a life-threatening crisis created by the BiPAP therapy.*

When a former medical equipment sales rep who used to sell BiPAP equipment to hospitals heard Rob was placed on a BiPAP for 4.5 hours with known pneumomediastinum—and that the doctor had removed the DNI (Do Not Intubate) order from Rob's records just minutes before placing him on the BiPAP as noted on Page 1018 of the hospital records (see Page C-33 in Appendix C)—she said, "*Then they used the BiPAP to* **BREAK HIM,** *because a BiPAP can cause severe damage to the lungs when used inappropriately.*"

Rob's blood oxygen level was 93 to 95% before he went on the BiPAP. Then, the moment he was placed on a ventilator, they had to rapidly crank the **PEEP** (residual pressure left in the lungs after expiration to keep the alveoli open) up to **14 cm H_2O** (the normal residual pressure left in the lungs after expiration is 5 cm H_2O) and the **FiO2** (the concentration of oxygen Rob was breathing) up to **100 percent** to keep his blood oxygen level above 90%.

Then then maxed him out on fentanyl (a powerful synthetic opioid that is similar to morphine but is about 50 to 100 times more potent), Versed (the brand name for the medication midazolam, which is a benzodiazepine drug that is commonly used to relieve anxiety and promote sedation), and Levophed (a brand name for the medication norepinephrine, a potent vasoconstrictor used to increase blood pressure in cases of severe hypotension).

PEEP stands for *Positive End Expiratory Pressure* and is pressure forced to remain in the lungs by the ventilator at the end of each breath (upon exhalation). This excess pressure (anything above 5 cm H_2O is excess pressure) prevents the passive emptying of the lungs and "recruits" damaged or collapsed alveoli (the air sacs in the lungs) by exerting residual pressure on the alveolar walls to help keep them open. *High PEEP can cause changes in lung compliance and <u>make it more difficult to wean a patient off the ventilator</u>.*
Advanced respiratory monitoring in COVID-19 patients: Use less PEEP! (n.d.). From
https://ccforum.biomedcentral.com/counter/pdf/10.1186/s13054-020-02953-z.pdf

FiO2 is the fraction of inspired oxygen (the oxygen concentration) in the air breathed. *Dry air at sea level contains about 21% oxygen. Prolonged exposure to oxygen concentrations above 60% can damage the lungs by inflaming and injuring the alveoli (air sacs).*

The Agency for Healthcare Research and Quality criteria (which this hospital followed) for attempting to wean someone from the ventilator is for them first to pass a Spontaneous Awakening Trial (SAT) followed by a Spontaneous Breathing Trial (SBT), where the **PEEP** (Positive End Expiratory Pressure) is no greater than **8 cm H_2O** and **FiO2** (oxygen concentration) is at **50% or less.**
Coordinated spontaneous awakening and breathing trials protocol. AHRQ. (n.d.). From
https://www.ahrq.gov/hai/tools/mvp/modules/technical/sat-sbt-protocol.html

Unfortunately, for the rest of Rob's stay, they never reduced the PEEP and FiO2 to the required levels. ***As a result, once on the ventilator, Rob was on a one-way trip to the morgue.***

Sammy Wong, MD, our medical expert witness, said in his "Letter of Introduction," which appears in **Appendix B**, "*Since he was sedated and paralyzed, he was dependent on the ventilator. All of the ABGs showed profound respiratory acidosis indicating that the staff chose not to adjust the ventilator settings to improve his alveolar ventilation. **They just maintained his ventilator settings essentially unchanged . . . until he died.**"*

I tried to focus on the doctor's words. He continued, "And I went in there earlier today because he actually inquired about intubation. And I had walked him through what that process might look like. **I told him he wasn't ready yet at that time**."

Why would Rob have been inquiring about intubation while he was still improving? That made no sense. In addition, he would only have "inquired about intubation" if he was in a real crisis, yet Dr. Dead End had told Rob he "wasn't yet ready at that time." Even stranger was that the same physician was eager to intubate Rob as early as September 4th when he shouted at me over the phone, "do you want your husband to die" and to Rob by his bedside, "do you want to die?" Nothing made sense in this bizarro world where they jumped from "do you want to die?" to "you're not ready" to "it has to be now!"

My world was shrinking, and darkness closed in on me as the doctor continued to explain the gravity of Rob's situation in a flustered tone, "But now, he wasn't ready. Meaning I didn't think that he was ready or that he needed it. Now, I _medically_ think that, that he needs it."

What he failed to tell me was that the "noninvasive therapy" BiPAP had apparently caused sufficient damage to Rob's lungs that they might as well have dragged him down a dark hallway of the hospital and severely beat him—and that to help him recover from the beating, he was now going to be placed on a ventilator, a therapy that generally leads to the patient's death.

Dr. Dead End menacingly rambled on, "I'm gonna give him drugs to, as I told him, create amnesia so that you don't remember it. We'd like him to be comfortable and sedated on the ventilator. I think the minimum that you're looking at is 7 to 10 days. That's sort of a rough guess. One of the hardest things for us with Covid is predicting and prognosticating because people just do differently. And it's very hard to say how long he may need to be on a ventilator. We try and wake him up once a day to make certain he's awake, moving, and following all commands. And then we kind of go from there."

He then explained why Rob was put on VELETRI. He said, "When we took him **off** of VELETRI this weekend, we watched him in the ICU for 6 to 8 hours **off** of VELETRI, and his oxygen levels were stable. VELETRI is a pulmonary vasodilator. **It's a heroic form** that helps open his alveoli. **VELETRI isn't really a treatment for Covid. It is a rescue** for . . . a form of rescue. **And he didn't need that.**"

Dr. Dead End asserted, "I'm just calling to tell you that **my plan** [as it had been since the

71

"No! In truth, this is what lack of food, isolation from family, heavy medication, and constant badgering will do."

He continued, "It attacks the body, and it causes all sorts of inflammation and destruction in the lungs. And right now, he's breathing 36 times a minute. He's on VELETRI."

It reminded me of when Dr. Wicked had told me earlier in the day that Dr. Torture was "just kind of throwing everything at him as she can." The doctors believed they could do whatever they wanted, including using off-label drugs and contraindicated therapies, if a patient had "COVID-19" stamped in their hospital record—and they could do so with total impunity given them by the government.

If a patient somehow survived their "let's throw the kitchen sink at them and see what happens" type of treatment, then lucky them. Yet, if a patient died of mistreatment, then, oh well, people die of Covid—and we expected that. So, chalk up one more Covid death.

He then said, "He's on 100% oxygen at 60 liters per minute, and his oxygen sats [meaning his oxygen saturation or blood oxygen level] right now are 87 to 88." So, after the BiPAP, Rob's blood oxygen level dropped below 90% for the first time in 5 days while on 100% oxygen. Once again, what in the world had the BiPAP done to him?

LEGAL COUNSEL STATEMENT

Members of the jury, Dr. Dead End called to "inform" Sheila he had already decided to intubate Rob. It was a foregone conclusion, and there could be no debate. Dr. Dead End had become Rob's surrogate decision-maker, leaving Sheila as a spectator on the sidelines. His "shock and awe" approach totally caught her off guard. As you've read, her traumatized response was, *"They're going to kill him!"*

As we shared earlier, UC Health Medical Center states that they do not believe patients must be placed on a ventilator until their O$_2$ saturation is below 85%, saying: *"When oxygen levels become low (oxygen saturation < 85%), patients are usually intubated and placed on mechanical ventilation. For those patients, ventilators can be the difference between life and death."*
Covid-19 resources. UC Health. (n.d.). From https://www.uchealth.com/en/media-room/covid-19/ventilators-and-covid-19

If UC Health Medical Center does not believe patients do not need mechanical ventilation until their blood oxygen level is less than 85%, why would Covid Coven Hospital of Plano, Texas, have insisted that Rob had to be intubated and placed on mechanical ventilation when his blood oxygen level (SpO2) was last recorded (before intubation) at 88% (at 5:00 PM) and was 91% the hour before (at 4:00 PM) as noted on Page 3012 of the hospital records (see Page C-38 in Appendix C).

When he called Sheila at 7:16 PM the evening before (on September 7, 2021), even Dr. Wicked said that "oxygen levels about 85% are pretty safe." He also stated, "I don't want him on the ventilator unless it's absolutely necessary. . . . it is a very bad thing to have to go on. And that is 100% true. That I know. **I believe the ventilator causes death**." He also said, "Last year 45% of those on the ventilator died."

Even prior to COVID-19, a 1997 study determined that *"A large percentage of ICU patients who require 5 days or more of mechanical ventilation die in the hospital"* and *"None of the patients discharged from the hospital were able to return home initially without assistance. By 6 months after discharge, more than 50% of the original sample and died, 9% resided in an institution, and 33% were living at home."*
Douglas SL;Daly BJ;Brennan PF;Harris S;Nochomovitz M;Dyer MA; (n.d.). Outcomes of long-term ventilator patients: A descriptive study. American journal of critical care: an official publication, American Association of Critical-Care Nurses. From https://pubmed.ncbi.nlm.nih.gov/9172858

What caused the doctors to believe that Rob had to be intubated and placed on a ventilator, knowing that doing so would likely lead to his death? Were they hasty in their decision because of the incentives (see the Hospitals' Incentive Payments for COVID-19 article in **Appendix D**)—or had they damaged Rob's lungs with the BiPAP to the point that he could no longer adequately breathe for himself?

Whatever their motivation, the outcome was exactly what Rob anticipated when on September 5, 2021, two days after his admission, he texted Sheila, "*Doing all they can to try to get me to agree to intubate. I'm dead if they do.*"

I asked why they hadn't given Rob nebulized budesonide, which I had pleaded for every day for inflammation. He said, "Dr. Wicked discussed with you that on a milligram per kilogram basis, with SOLU-MEDROL, the budesonide is not indicated, probably not super helpful, probably not super harmful, but on a milligram a day, a milligram per kilogram of SOLU-MEDROL, the amount of IV steroids that you're getting is a tremendous amount."

I was grasping at straws when I said, "Doesn't budesonide address the inflammation? That's how I understand it. He answered, "Absolutely. SOLU-MEDROL is 100 times stronger than budesonide is. I think that there's probably a role for budesonide as an outpatient. I give it to my patients. I give it to patients post Covid. But once you're already getting the amount of steroids that we're giving you've saturated every steroid receptor in the body."

LEGAL COUNSEL STATEMENT
Members of the jury, **SOLU-MEDROL** (methylprednisolone sodium succinate) is a potent systemic steroid that has numerous potential and very undesirable side effects. They include *wheezing, tightness in the chest or throat, trouble breathing, trouble talking, feeling very tired, and shortness of breath*.
Solu-Medrol: Indications, side effects, warnings. Drugs.com. (n.d.). From https://www.drugs.com/cdi/solu-medrol.html

Rob had each of the symptoms listed above when he arrived at the hospital five days earlier, on September 3, 2021. Also, WebMD says the following regarding SOLU-MEDROL IV solution: "*This medication may lower your ability to fight infections. This may make you more likely to get a serious (rarely fatal) infection or make any infection you have worse.*"
WebMD. (n.d.). Solu-Medrol intravenous: Uses, side effects, interactions, pictures, warnings & dosing. WebMD. From https://www.webmd.com/drugs/2/drug-152303/solu-medrol-intravenous

If Rob already had the symptoms this high-powered systemic steroid was known to likely cause or exacerbate, and he already had a severe infection (pneumonia) while this drug can "*make any infection you have worse*," then why would his physicians prescribe a medication that was very likely to worsen his symptoms and his current infection?

Sheila repeatedly asked that Rob be administered **nebulized budesonide** *that would act directly on the lungs vs. assaulting Rob systemically and was known to provide significant immediate benefits, as noted in* **Appendix F**, *yet she was flatly denied. Clearly, it was their show, their protocol, and their decision as to how and with what Rob would be treated.*

I shared my ongoing concern about Rob's coughing, and Dr. Dead End surprised me when he said, "I mean, when I went in there, he wasn't. I talked to him for 20 minutes this afternoon. He was not coughing. I talked to him. I mean, he wanted it [referring to the ventilator] earlier in the day; I told him I didn't think that he was ready or that he met the criteria. **But that's why he was in the ICU now that he wanted intubation.** We were keeping an eye on him, and if things changed, we would reevaluate, and things have changed now."

Rob had returned to the ICU on the evening of September 6, 2021, ONLY to resume treatment

I cried out, "Rob wants this?" Dr. Dead End said with enthusiasm and satisfaction, "Yes, he actually said that he can't take it anymore, and he wants us to put him on the ventilator. So, we're gonna look at what his oxygen requirements are every day. It's called PEEP [Positive End Expiratory Pressure] requirements, another measure of how much support. We'll look and see what his X-rays look like. I do think that there is, as Dr. Wicked told you this morning; **I think there's a significant risk if we put him on the ventilator that his lungs could collapse because he already has a pneumomediastinum**. Although it's been several days, and his X-rays have been stable. That's one of the things that we'll have to watch out for. We'll just have to deal with whatever occurs as it occurs."

Placing Rob on a ventilator was a death sentence. I knew it. Rob knew it. I asked if he knew of anyone who survived the ventilator. He stumbled over his words when he said, "Yes, I mean, so 40, I would say. You know...." I said, "I don't know." He again tried to be a little more specific, "40 to 50% of patients recover and live. It's a generic percentage early on. Meaning last March, when patients were put on a ventilator. Umm. No, a lot of them did not survive. Things now are different. I do think that he has severe pneumonia from Covid. And **I think that he's in for a potentially very long course.** That is the greatest challenge that we have with Covid . . . is predicting and prognosticating."

He did not sound confident that placing Rob on a ventilator would save his life. I said, "I will have to think about it. I will consider everything you said." I needed more time to think about this. Dr. Dead End shot back, "There's nothing to think about!" He was stern and resolute and made it clear that his decision was final. He had made up his mind, and nothing I could say would change anything. I could not believe what I was hearing.

He continued, "I need to put him on a ventilator. I know. I know. He is consenting to that." I would like to have had time to hear my husband say he had consented to be placed on a ventilator, but the doctor made it clear that Rob had given his consent.

Almost sounding guilty, Dr. Dead End continued, "I will, um . . . Look, all we want is for him to try and recover. We practice critical care to try and save people's lives. That's all our goals are. That's it." He then added, "We want him to get better. He's 52. As I told you over this weekend when I encouraged that we put him on a ventilator as needed, he's young. I practice, and my partners practice, critical care to save someone's life. The ones that have, that still have significant life ahead of them. That is a 100% goal. Okay. Is there anything else I can answer for you?"

I had been shot in the chest by Dr. Dead End and was bleeding heavily. I was dizzy and unsure what to say. He had made it clear that although he felt my husband would not survive without the ventilator, other terrible things like having his lungs blown out were still possible. It was as if the doctor had pulled a grenade's pin, tossed it to Rob, and said, "Good luck!"

The last words I heard him rattle off as fast as he could as he headed off to intubate Rob were, "All right. Sounds good. We'll update you after we put him on the ventilator. Great. Thank you. Great. Bye."

Rob's Last Cry

No food, no water, I lay in bed
With doctors surrounding me, their intentions unsaid
Their every move, a trial of my fate
Their hands on me, I can't escape

Intubation, a word that brings fear
For if it's done, my end will be near
I fight for breath, I fight for life
Against the odds, a never-ending strife

But still they persist, with a stubborn disdain
Doing everything, to keep me in pain
To put me under, to take control
To end my journey, to take my soul

I pray for mercy, I pray for peace
For in this moment, my pleas do not cease
But if they succeed, my death will be certain
A victim of their greed, a tragedy we can't pardon

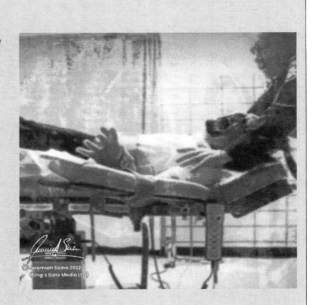

Jeremiah Skiba 2022
King's Gate Media LLC

LEGAL COUNSEL STATEMENT

Members of the jury, as noted on Page B-2 of Appendix B and Page 3729 of the hospital records (see Page C-40 in Appendix C), Sammy Wong, MD—our medical expert witness—stated in his Interim Analysis, "At **5:48 PM**, the nurse noted that the patient was '**alert, awake, cooperative, oriented (x4) and tranquil**' and that his '**speech was clear**.'"

However, less than 60 minutes later, at **6:43 PM**, Rob was coerced or forced, which Sammy Wong, MD, calls (assault and battery), into being sedated, intubated, and placed on a ventilator by Dr. Dead End soon after he had said (as noted on the next page) that Rob was only in "**mild respiratory distress**." *Why, then, was Rob pressured to be intubated and placed on a ventilator?*

Dr. Dead End coldly made it clear to Sheila that **(a)** she had no choice in the matter, **(b)** Rob (or so he asserted) had agreed to be placed on a ventilator, and **(c)** there was no time for Sheila to speak with Rob and hear his voice one more time before he was silenced forever with sedatives and paralytics.

We find it highly suspicious that Sheila was not allowed to speak with Rob so he could tell her (as we know he would have wished to do) that he had truly tired out, needed a rest from the difficulties he was having, and wanted her not to worry

We suspect that she was prevented from speaking with Rob because he had not "consented" to be intubated but found himself in a life-threatening crisis due to the severe damage caused to his lungs by the 4.5-hours of BiPAP therapy—a crisis so severe he could possibly no longer speak. One they could then use as an excuse for intubating Rob and placing him on a ventilator.

As we noted earlier, on September 5, 2021, Rob texted Sheila, "*Doing all they can to try to get me to agree to intubate. I'm dead if they do.*" He knew their game plan and was fully aware of the dangers of their deadly protocol.

As we noted earlier, the multiple "**Orders**" extracted from Pages 1001 to 1018 of the hospital records (see Page C-53 in Appendix C) show how his DNI status was switched to FULL CODE multiple times over four days by four different doctors because of their insistence that he consent to "elective intubation," followed by Rob's consistently reminding them (we counted **17 times** in the records) that he **DID NOT agree** to be intubated and placed on a ventilator.

A physician has a fiduciary duty to keep the patient's best interests in mind and those of anyone (such as Sheila) who has Medical Power of Attorney. A breach of fiduciary duty occurs when fiduciaries fail to act responsibly and disregard the best interests of their clients or patients. In this case, the doctors were working in the best interests of the hospital's income and their paychecks. In addition, the physician must disclose all available treatment options and the risks of each without forcing on the patient any prescribed course of therapy.

We contend that the conduct of Rob's physicians was reckless, fraudulent, and oppressive—and calls for the imposition of punitive and exemplary damages because their conduct was a breach of their fiduciary duty and was the proximate cause of Rob's death.

I had just been told by Dr. Dead End that the decision to intubate Rob and place him on a ventilator was final, and I had no say whatsoever. He had said Rob had consented to the procedure, so what could I say? I was broken and wailed in complete agony. The sun and the moon must have heard my cries, but did God hear my cries? Was there anyone out there who could rescue Rob? I needed someone to hear me and to answer my heart's groaning.

I lay on my bed as if dead. I was numb and suicidal. If Rob was going to die, I did not want to live. Then, Psalm 121 entered my thoughts. It was just a whisper. "*I will lift up my eyes unto the hills, from where comes my help. My help comes from Yahuwah, which made heaven and earth. He will not suffer your foot to be moved: he that keeps you will not slumber. Behold, he that keeps Israel shall neither slumber nor sleep. Yahuwah is your keeper.*"

Even with my family and close friends by my side, I felt lost and forsaken. What I had most feared had just now come to pass. Rob was placed on a ventilator and would be in an induced coma for only God knows how long and be under the doctor's complete control. He could no longer speak or breathe on his own. He was at the mercy of those who had none, and I would still be locked out for 15 more days.

LEGAL COUNSEL STATEMENT
Members of the jury, below is a timeline of critical events that occurred on September 8, 2021, the day the doctors achieved their goal of intubating Rob against his will. As this was a crucial turning point that led to Rob's eventual death, we call this "**The Road to Destruction Timeline.**"
1. **6:30 AM**—Nurse Trauma said at the top of Page 123 of the hospital records (see Page C-34 in Appendix C) that she updated Sheila via telephone on Rob's status and provided her with "emotional support." *Sheila received **NO CALL** from nurse Trauma that morning—which she verified by pulling her call records from her cellular provider. Why would this nurse feel the need to falsify the record?*
2. **7:00 AM**—At the beginning of the day shift, according to Nurse Rabid's notes that appear on Page 136 of the hospital records (see Page C-41), Rob allegedly "changed his mind regarding DNI [Do Not Intubate]" after stating he was "tiring out."

3. **8:30 AM**—Rob was given his 4th dose of **Alinia**, a Phase 1 trial drug with side effects that include trouble breathing, diarrhea, nausea, and malaise (severe weakness)—*which would further weaken him.*

4. **9:01 AM**—Rob was given his **5th dose of remdesivir**. We allege they knew full well that remdesivir could cause progressive hypoxia (which ended up being one of their reasons for intubating Rob), dyspnea (difficulty breathing), and acute kidney injury (which was listed as one of Rob's causes of death on his initial death certificate). In addition, Rob suffered from continued starvation, as evidenced by the fact that the hospital records on Page 105 (see Page C-28) show that he weighed **170 lbs.** upon admission on the evening of September 3, 2021. Yet, he weighed only **160 lbs.** the morning of September 9, 2021 (the morning after he was intubated)—thus, he had lost 10 pounds in less than six full days in the hospital. *Is not starving and drugging a patient into submission considered a crime?*

5. **9:04 AM**—Sheila called Rob, and he did not express any concerns about fatigue nor say he had agreed to change his DNI (Do Not Intubate) status to FULL CODE.

6. **9:25 AM**—Rob had his **12th dose of VELETRI,** a drug that should NEVER be given to a patient who is already short of breath. Its potential side effects include severe shortness of breath (leading to an increased respiratory rate), gasping for breath, difficulty breathing, anxiety, and **increased fluid in the lungs**. *NOTE: Rob's respirations had improved on September 5, 2021, when VELETRI and remdesivir were temporarily discontinued, and his respirations dropped into a normal range of 18 to 22 breaths per minute. Sadly, they insisted on giving Rob VELETRI and SOLU-MEDROL instead of budesonide (which Sheila asked for repeatedly). As noted in the study referenced in **Appendix F**, budesonide was known to reduce the relative risk of requiring urgent care or hospitalization by 90%.*

7. **9:39 AM**—Rob's inflammatory markers and vital signs were improving until he was **placed on a positive pressure (forced ventilation) BiPAP.** Dr. Wicked knew that doing so could, as nurse Carnage had said, cause "traumatic injury." *Sammy Wong, MD (see Appendix B) considered the use of a BiPAP an injurious act and one of the "Causes of Action" against the doctors.*

8. **9:40 AM**—As noted on Page 123 of the records (see Page C-34), less than 1/2 an hour before his 10:07 AM call to Sheila and as Rob was beginning his 4.5-hour BiPAP session, **Dr. Wicked removed Rob's DNI (Do Not Intubate) status**. *He did this despite the fact Rob was **IMPROVING,** and he knew Rob had continually insisted that he **DID NOT** want to be intubated. Removing the DNI order would give the doctors the authority to **FORCE** Rob to be intubated and placed on a ventilator if the BiPAP caused the amount of damage to his lungs they suspected it would.*

9. **At 10:07 AM**—Dr. Wicked called Sheila and had an extensive conversation with her. Yet did not say anything about Rob "tiring out" or that he had switched Rob **from DNI (Do Not Intubate) to "Full Code."** Instead, he said Rob's oxygen was "relatively stable" and "everything on the labs is actually a little bit better and improving." He did not mention the switch from DNI to Full Code because he knew Sheila and Rob were clearly opposed to Rob being intubated and placed on a ventilator. *Sheila had been **purposely** kept out of the hospital and out of the loop so she could not stand in the way of their strategy of combining starvation, harmful drugs, and (now) a dangerous therapy to bring Rob to the point of sheer desperation. So now, all that was left for them to do was wait for the damage to be done!*

10. **2:09 PM**—Rob came **off 4.5 hours** on a BiPAP. Unfortunately, this therapy increased his pneumomediastinum. It also caused **barotrauma,** as documented on page 141 of the hospital records (see Page C-44), where they note, "Repeat CXR [Chest X-ray] this afternoon to **monitor barotrauma**."

11. **5:48 PM**—A nurse noted that Rob was "alert, awake, cooperative, oriented (x4) and tranquil," and his speech was "clear," as noted on Page 3729 of the hospital records (see Page C-40). This shows that Rob was improving at 5:48 PM, less than an hour before his intubation and being placed on a ventilator. *Why would an improving patient be forced to be intubated and ventilated? Is that not a crime?*

12. **6:16 PM to 6:28 PM**—Sheila had a **12-minute call** with Dr. Dead End. He calmly said that he was going to intubate Rob and place him on a ventilator, yet earlier in the day Rob did not appear to be in any distress.

13. **6:22 PM**—in the "**Orders**" section of the hospital records are 12 total pages of orders, all signed by Dr. Dead End, for the drugs, equipment, and monitoring necessary for Rob's impending intubation. One of those orders was for "bilateral wrist restraints for up to 24 hours" for "airway protection." *Having seen this in the records after Rob's death made Sheila suspect that they might have restrained Rob before the BiPAP and before his intubation to ensure he would not interfere with their plans to get him on a ventilator. As noted above, Sheila was on the phone with Dr. Dead End from 6:16 PM to 6:28 PM. If there was a **true emergency**, Dr. Dead End would not have calmly explained everything during a 12-minute call. While Dr. Dead End*

14. **6:28 PM**—Dr. Dead End noted, as shown at the top of Page 136 of the hospital records (see Page C-41), that Rob was only "in mild respiratory distress." If Rob was only "in mild respiratory distress," why did he continue that same note with, "He will need intubation." In addition, Dr. Dead End wrote in the same note, "at the time of my evaluation at 14:00 [2:00 PM] he was borderline," yet as shown on Page 3012 (see Page C-38), his SpO2 (blood oxygen level) was at 92! *Why, then, was Rob considered to be "borderline?*

15. **6:43 PM**—Rob was coerced or forced into being sedated, intubated, and placed on a ventilator by Dr. Dead End precisely 15 minutes after Sheila got off the phone with him and less than 20 minutes after he had noted Rob was only in "mild respiratory distress," as stated above. Dr. Wicked had told Sheila that he would only intubate patients who would be 100% sure to die without being placed on a ventilator. The medical records do not indicate Rob was anywhere near death; however, the 4.5 hours on the BiPAP while Rob had pneumomediastinum appears to have severely injured Rob's lungs, making it very difficult for him to breathe. Before his intubation, an X-ray **WAS NOT DONE**, most likely because they suspected they had caused barotrauma and did not want it confirmed until AFTER Rob was on the ventilator. In addition, an Arterial Blood Gas (ABG) **WAS NOT DRAWN** to ensure that Rob was indeed in desperate need of intubation. Instead, an ABG was drawn at 9:04 PM, 2 hours 21 minutes **AFTER** Rob was intubated, as noted on Page 137 of the hospital records (see Page C-43). *Sammy Wong, MD, our Medical Expert witness, noted in cause #7 of his "Causes of Action," which appear on Page B-7 of Appendix B, that: "There is no clear documentation readily available that provides clear indication for intubation. **There were no pre-intubation ABGs**. Even the ID [Infectious Disease] specialist documented (within the hour or so of intubation) that the patient was in **no acute distress ('NAD')**."*

16. **End of Day Shift**—According to Nurse Rabid's notes that appear on Page 136 of the hospital records (see Page C-41), Rob was said to have called her into the room and with a respiratory rate of 30-36 breaths per minute, said, "I want to be put on a ventilator because I'm too tired to breathe on my own anymore." It is impossible to speak even one-syllable words while breathing at that rate, and a 36-year respiratory therapist whom Sheila spoke with after Rob died said it was "inconceivable" anyone could say such a sentence while breathing at that rate. If Rob could speak that clearly, he would have called Sheila and spoken his last words to her to make her aware he decided to go on a ventilator and not to worry. *We contend Rob could not have said such a long sentence while breathing once every 2 seconds (which is what 30 breaths per minute equates to).* In addition, **there was no signed consent** for intubation in Rob's hospital records. So, we must ask, *"What was going on here?"*

The hospital records do not indicate Rob was near death. However, the 4.5 hours on the BiPAP appear to have severely injured Rob's lungs and brought him to a point of absolute desperation. Dr. Wicked and Dr. Dead End, who are business partners, collaborated on their devious plan to ensure Rob ended up on a ventilator.

Clearly, Rob went from good, to bad, to worse at the hands of the "medical professionals" entrusted with his care at Covid Coven Hospital of Plano, Texas. He was doing good on oxygen alone. Things went bad when he was placed on the BiPAP. They got far worse, to the point of death, when he was intubated and placed on a ventilator.

Thursday, September 9, 2021

Even though the sun was shining brightly, I awoke feeling surrounded by darkness and dread. I was terrified that my husband was fighting for his life in a deficient, "short-staffed" ICU under the care of deviant physicians who had made it clear that we had no say in his plan of care. I could imagine them rejoicing, *"One more patient on a ventilator! Cha-ching!"*

It had taken his captors five days to break him. Until the very last second, he had been a courageous and valiant soldier. His continued resistance must have frustrated them terribly.

Sadly, in the end, my husband fell victim to "the protocol" despite my efforts to serve as his advocate. I knew his days would be limited and his chances of survival slim if I could not keep them from causing him further injury.

He had been isolated, intimidated, harassed, starved, and harmed by a contraindicated therapy that led to his being strapped to a device he and I knew would likely kill him. I was infuriated that my husband had been treated like a caged animal, and his captors felt they could do with him whatever they desired.

My mission to save Rob from the vultures holding him in their grasp went full throttle; I had to stop the ticking timebomb that had been activated at 6:43 PM the night before when he was placed on a ventilator.

The hospital's cruel "21-day lockout" policy was still in effect. Even with my Medical Power of Attorney, I was still not allowed to spend even five minutes with my now intubated and ventilated husband, who could no longer speak for himself.

My family and friends continued to search diligently for a physician and hospital that would agree to treat Rob with dignity and allow us to participate in the development of his plan of care, even though every facility we had previously contacted also isolated families from patients.

As we did so, I wondered if my candidly sharing my desire to transfer Rob before his intubation had anything to do with the doctors rushing to get him on a ventilator. Had they done so to prevent the transfer and the resulting loss of revenue?

Now that he was on a ventilator, finding a hospital willing to accept the transfer of a ventilated patient would make a rescue mission more difficult. We also contacted hospice facilities to see if they would accept a transfer. Unfortunately, we quickly learned they would not do so until Rob was off the ventilator.

LEGAL COUNSEL STATEMENT

Members of the jury, can you hear the referee cheering "*Touch Down!*" as you read the "Refused Remdesivir from 9/5 until 9/6" (by Dr. Lament) and "Now that he is intubated will extend Remdesivir to 10 days" (by Dr. Torture) statements on Page 159 of the hospital records (see Page C-45 in Appendix C).

These statements, made by Drs. Lament and Torture, make the case they were delighted Rob was **finally on a ventilator** so they could subject him to 10 days of remdesivir so Covid Coven Hospital of Plano, Texas, could earn more of the "*bonus incentive payments for all things related to COVID-19 (testing, diagnosing, admitting to hospital, use of remdesivir and ventilators and also death*" that are paid by the federal government (your tax paying dollars at work killing your loved ones) under the CARES Act as noted in the "Hospitals' Incentive Payments for COVID-19" article in Appendix D.

With Rob incapacitated, Sheila continually insisted, as his Medical Power of Attorney, that Rob **NOT** be given this deadly drug. Even then, they ignored her directive **until September 10th**, two full days after Rob had been sedated, paralyzed, intubated, and placed on a ventilator. That day, they noted with apparent frustration on Pages 170-171 of the hospital records (see Page C-46 in Appendix C), "Wife refused Remdesivir again." Then, on September 15, 2021, on Page 266 of the records (see Page C-51), they recorded, "Remdesivir discontinued as per wife's wishes." *Thus, they continued administering remdesivir against her directive and behind her back.*

The doctors repeatedly imposed their will on Rob and Sheila, disregarding the consequences on Rob's health. In doing so, they knowingly and willfully violated **Title 42 of the Code of Federal Regulations, Section 482.13** (as noted in Appendix E), which states: "*The patient has the right to participate in the development and implementation of his or her plan of care.*" Those rights include "*being able to request or refuse treatment.*"

It would be two more weeks before they removed the invisible barrier that separated me from Rob. I hoped I could persuade them to reconsider their irrational "21-day isolation" policy, yet they continually refused.

I considered how we might "storm the castle" to rescue Rob. My family, however, persuaded me that the doctors and nurses would likely retaliate by causing Rob further harm if we did.

These text messages between Sheila and her sister on September 9, 2021, demonstrate Sheila's determination to rescue Rob.

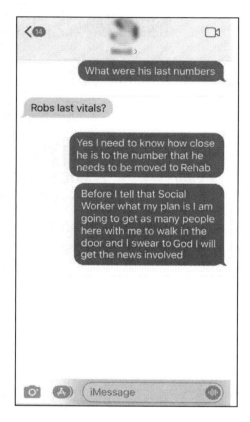
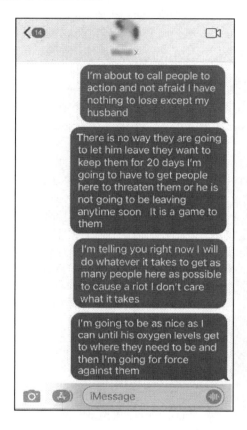

As you can see, Sheila was VERY concerned about Rob's safety.

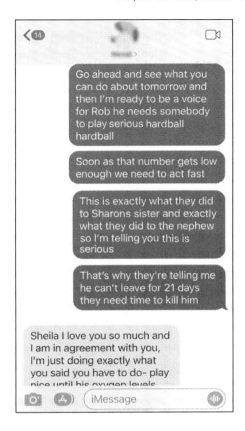

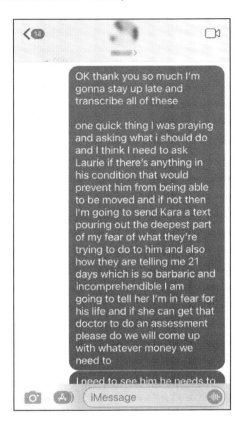

LEGAL COUNSEL STATEMENT

Members of the jury, Rob's blood oxygen level (SpO2) was an acceptable 92% at 9:00 a.m. on September 8, 2021, just before he was placed on a BiPAP, as documented on hospital record page 3012 (see Page C-38 in Appendix C). However, his blood oxygen level dropped to 89% at noon while he was on the contraindicated BiPAP therapy—indicating the BiPAP was worsening his condition. Rob should have been taken OFF the BiPAP at that point. However, they kept him on it for two more hours.

At 2:00 PM, when Rob was taken off the BiPAP, his blood oxygen level returned to 92%, and his respirations were only 22 per minute. However, at that same time, Dr. Dead End made a note in the hospital records on the top of Page 136 (see Page C-41 in Appendix C) that Rob was "borderline" and "will need intubation." If he were being honest, he could have replaced "will need" with "I am Hell-bent on getting Rob on a ventilator, and I will succeed."

Less than 4 hours after being placed on the ventilator at 6:43 PM on September 8th, Rob struggled with blood oxygen levels **as low as 81%**, as noted at 11:30 PM (2230) at the top of Page 3014 (see Page C-42). Clearly, he was doing far better BEFORE he was intubated and ventilated. It took them over 5 hours (until 11:45 PM) to get Rob's blood oxygen level above 90% again, which is where it had been **before** being placed on a ventilator. *As further evidence of the harm being done to Rob by being placed on a ventilator, see the **SOFA Score Assessment** at the end of Appendix C.*

In addition, Rob was flooded with medications he had never been subjected to, as noted at the bottom of Page 136 of the hospital records (see Page C-41 in Appendix C), where nurse Careless reported at 6:24 AM on September 9th, "Earlier in shift, pt [patient] maxed out on **fentanyl** [a synthetic opioid that is 50 to 100 times stronger than morphine] and **versed** [a brand name of **midazolam**, a benzodiazepine medication used for anesthesia and sedation that causes respiratory depression—especially when taken with opioids such as **fentanyl**] drips. Pt [patient] still not compliant with vent [ventilator] and **de-sating** [blood oxygen level dropping to] **85%.**"

This note continues at the top of Page 137 of the records (see Page C-43) with, "**Okay to add levophed** [a brand name of norepinephrine bitartrate that is a vasopressor used for patients with **septic shock** to increase systemic blood pressure and coronary artery blood flow] **low dose peripherally and will add nimbex** [a neuromuscular blocking agent used to facilitate muscle relaxation during surgery or mechanical ventilation]."

Sheila was **NEVER** advised by the doctors that Rob had been "maxed out" on any medications, and she was unaware of the complete list of drugs and high dosages Rob was assaulted with until she obtained a copy of his over 5,000-page hospital record—after his death.

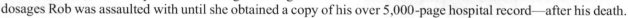

She was also **NOT ADVISED** that Rob was "not compliant" with the ventilator and that his blood oxygen level had dropped to 85%.

In addition, she was **NOT INFORMED** that Rob had to be administered **Levophed 14 times** between 10:12 PM on September 8th to 4:17 PM on September 9th. Levophed is a brand name for norepinephrine, a vasoconstrictor used during or after CPR when someone's heart stops beating or for treating life-threatening low blood pressure (hypotension). You can see all 14 doses of Levophed in the list of "*Questionable Drugs & Dosages Given Between 9/8/21 and 9/10/21*" in **Appendix G**. This amount of Levophed is a clear indication that their "treatment" caused Rob to go into **septic shock** and/or caused him **severe cardiac problems**.

With her Medical Power of Attorney and Rob being intubated, ventilated, sedated, paralyzed, and possibly near death, Sheila should have been allowed **immediate** access to her husband.

A hospital must allow a family member who is the patient's Medical Power of Attorney (Medical POA) to act as that patient's advocate, including entering to visit the patient and make critical decisions regarding their care. A Medical POA is a legal document that designates an individual to make healthcare decisions on behalf of a patient who is unable to make such decisions for themselves. Thus, that person may act in place of the patient as if they were the patient. However, Sheila's right to be with Rob so she could make critical decisions regarding his care was denied. Instead, the doctors acted as if they were Rob's Medical POA—and they made all of the critical care decisions for him.

Later in the day, Ms. Destroyer, a Social Worker, contacted me. It was immediately apparent that she was not calling to assist me but to shield, defend, and advocate for the ICU doctors. Feigning to care and in a faux sad tone, she said, "My name is Ms. Destroyer. I'm a Social Worker, and I work here in the ICU. I know he was put on a vent yesterday, and with us having to do these, you know, '**no visits because of isolation**,' I know how stressful it is for a family . . . it's **just torture**." Yes, torture is what this hospital was becoming known for. I was surprised that she first emphasized that I would continue to be prohibited from entering the hospital until Rob had completed his entire "isolation period."

I asked, "Then, when can I see my husband?" She stated, "So, the rule at the moment is . . . well, not at the moment, it's been this way since the beginning . . . **the CDC recommends twenty days from the date of his first positive**, and that was September 3rd."

She told me I had to wait for a full twenty days from the date of his admission. That would mean I would have to wait until September 23rd to be with my husband, whom they now held captive. Yet, whom were they attempting to safeguard? Rob? Me? The doctors? The ICU nurses?

I lived with Rob, we had contracted Covid at the same time, and I had been tested and confirmed to have antibodies against the virus. Thus, I would not be a risk to my husband or hospital personnel. Therefore, the hospital's cruel and insane "no visits" policy made no sense.

I responded, "I thought the CDC quarantine was fourteen days." She said fourteen days was for "mild or moderate" Covid, then added, "But once you end up **severe**, they're recommending twenty days." Now that he was on a ventilator, which made him a "severe" case, my husband needed me more than ever—not an extended isolation period.

Oddly, she reiterated, "Okay, **our folks are here for twenty days**." I knew Covid had become a significant hospital windfall, and I thought, "What does she mean by, 'our folks are here for twenty days'?" Each patient should be in the hospital for the shortest duration necessary to get them back on their feet. She seemed to be admitting that they hoped to keep "Covid" patients for at least 20 days, even if that required mistreating them to extend their stay so that they could gain the full financial benefit from their admission.

She then said, "We can arrange for FaceTime visits. I know those stink. I know that's not the same. So, we can set up video calls even while he's on the ventilator; we can take that into the room and leave it in the room for 10 to 15 minutes, so you have time to talk to him. We don't know what he can hear, right? I'd like to think that he can certainly hear voices he recognizes."

Oh, great. How nice of them. I could have a private one-way FaceTime conversation with my fully sedated and unconscious husband. Before he was placed on a ventilator, attempting a video chat only irritated Rob because he wanted me **there**, not on a chat via FaceTime.

I replied, "There's no substitution for loving human touch." She responded, "For some people, it is more agitating. If it were me laying in that bed, and I feel rotten, and all these things are happening to my body that I don't even fully understand or like, if I were to hear someone, I know I would want them near. I would want them to hold my hand. I would want to get out of here. There's no substitution for someone you love being there. Right?"

So, she was willing to admit she had witnessed patients becoming agitated when their family members' interactions with them were limited to FaceTime chats, yet she had no qualms about saying it was the only option they were willing to offer. If I attempted a FaceTime chat with Rob, and if he somehow managed to hear me, he would undoubtedly be furious to realize he was still incarcerated in an ICU cell with no family visitation privileges.

I needed to be by his side now more than ever, and her matter-of-fact, "the best we can do" response only added to my fear that Rob, like all of the other patients who had endured "the protocol that kills," was in a truly desperate situation.

LEGAL COUNSEL STATEMENT

Members of the jury, as noted earlier, in an editorial published on April 22, 2022, in the peer-reviewed journal *Surgical Neurology International*, Russell L. Blaylock, MD, a retired neurosurgeon, said: "*Never in the history of American medicine have hospital administrators dictated to its physicians how they will practice medicine and what medications they can use. **The CDC has no authority to dictate to hospitals or doctors concerning medical treatments. Yet, most physicians complied without the slightest resistance.**"*

Covid update: What is the truth? Surgical Neurology International. (2022, May 10). From https://surgicalneurologyint.com/surgicalint-articles/covid-update-what-is-the-truth

The Centers for Disease Control and Prevention (CDC) is a federal agency within the Department of Health and Human Services that has the authority to issue "*guidelines*" and "*recommendations*" for infection control and disease prevention. However, the CDC **does not** have the authority to issue *mandates* that hospitals must follow, including mandates that hospitals implement a specific patient isolation period. However, when the hospital staff at Covid Coven Hospital of Plano, Texas, referred to the CDC's "21-day guideline," they implied it was a *mandate* while it was nothing more than a "*guideline*" that they CHOSE to implement for their benefit.

In truth, what they should have said is: "*The CDC has issued a **guideline**, and we have decided to use it as an **opportunity** to keep families and Medical Power of Attorneys separated from patients so we can institute the full 'protocol that kills' without their family members' interference.*"

Isolating patients from their families only benefits hospitals by allowing them to operate freely without interference from family members who may question the treatments patients are receiving or may notice patients are being starved into submission, receiving substandard care, and being subjected to harmful and unnecessary medications.

Furthermore, by saying, "our folks are here for twenty days," she implied that there was little to no chance Rob would be able to get off the ventilator any time soon based on her experience with other Covid patients; otherwise, she would have said something like "*your husband must be isolated from his family for twenty full days **unless** he happens to be able to come home sooner because of a rapid recovery, in which case you'll be able to see him when he is discharged.*" Instead, she had advised Sheila to prepare for a lengthy hospital stay because that was the norm at this hospital, which was seeking to maximize its profits.

Sadly, Sheila learned that when someone becomes a "Covid" patient at Covid Coven Hospital of Plano, Texas, as the lyrics of the song Hotel California say, "*you can check out whenever you want, but you can never leave*"— that is until they have extracted the maximum benefit from you.

We firmly believe the hospital took advantage of the CDC's "recommendation" as an excuse to keep Sheila out of the hospital and out of their way. That way, she would not be able to interfere with their scheme to ensure Rob completed the prescribed protocol, which would include his being "discharged "via the morgue so they could collect the maximum revenue and incentive money possible.

I stressed that I wanted to get Rob **off** remdesivir because kidney issues ran in his family. She confirmed, "**It is on his med list**. Usually, the Infectious Disease doctor drives that. She's recommending a five-day course. I'm looking at his labs, and his kidney function is still within normal range, according to the labs. Yet, **a 5-day course is not the max** when someone is on a ventilator. **Usually, it's longer.** Once someone is on a ventilator, **they often extend that to 10 days total**. All I can do is ask the physician to give you a call to explain why remdesivir is effective."

Although I was my husband's Medical Power of Attorney, I was again advised that a doctor would make all of the decisions regarding his care—and that my input was irrelevant.

I was infuriated but responded calmly with, "Okay. I don't understand. I mean, I understand the protocols and everything. This is just getting so out of hand. His dad lost a kidney. We have kidney issues in the family." She then read off his BUN (Blood Urea Nitrogen) and creatinine levels from the lab reports, said they looked okay to her, and said if they got too high, the doctors would **then** agree to stop the remdesivir.

I told her I had already spoken with Dr. Wicked and that he had said remdesivir, in his opinion, was **not** helping Rob at this point. She responded, "He is timed for a dose of remdesivir **every 24 hours**. So, he got it this morning at 9:45. Call in the morning and talk to the nurse between 8:00 and 9:00 AM, and just tell them you would like to refuse his getting the remdesivir if that's what you'd like us to do. In the meantime, I still want Dr. Torture to call you just to, you know, explain if there's some sort of insight to all of this that you and I don't know, right? But if you feel convicted to stop that dose tomorrow—before you can talk to Dr. Torture—just call and say you want them to mark it as refused until you can speak to the doctor."

She continued, "People have the right to refuse. I'll be fairly frank [note, she said 'fairly frank,' but not completely frank] **off** the cuff [being casual and somewhat truthful] with you. People **don't necessarily have the right** to come in demanding all sorts of things that may not have a medical basis for us. But people have the right to make the decisions about what care they want for themselves or their next of kin."

> **LEGAL COUNSEL STATEMENT**
> Members of the jury, paragraph (a)(3) of **Title 42 of the Code of Federal Regulations, Section 482.13**, which appears in Appendix E, states, *"The patient or his or her representative (as allowed under State law) has the right to make informed decisions regarding his or her care. The patient's rights include being informed of his or her health status, being involved in care planning and treatment, and being able to request or refuse treatment."*
>
> *Thus, the Social Worker should have advised Sheila that the hospital maintained a Medical Administration Record which listed the name of each prescribed medication, the dose and frequency of administration, and the route of administration (e.g., oral, intravenous, or topical) and that as Rob's Medical Power of Attorney, she had the right to demand that any medication be **removed** from Rob's MAR and **NOT be administered**.*

What I heard her say was, "people have the right to make decisions about what care they want for themselves or their next of kin," unless the doctors disagree. It was their *"we make the final decisions about your care, not you"* attitude that had brought us to this point where Rob was now on a ventilator, a therapy I was genuinely concerned he might not survive.

I had taken Rob to the hospital fully expecting they would treat him with oxygen, antibiotics, and steroids (ideally, budesonide, an anti-inflammatory corticosteroid I repeatedly asked for). Instead, Rob was subjected to "the full ICU Covid protocol" despite our repeated objections. As a result, our "right to make decisions" vaporized the moment he was in their custody.

I exhaustedly explained, "I've talked to the doctors and the nurses **many times**, going back and forth on the remdesivir topic. I want you to know I am **REFUSING IT**, and I'm refusing it until I talk to the doctor."

As if I struck a chord with her, she replied, "It's no big deal, okay? So, in general, like, I will stick up for my healthcare coworkers all day long because I've been here for twenty years, I know these people. But one thing that we tend to do is **we sometimes get stuck in our ways**, right? I don't care who you are and where you work, right? **We all get used to how we do things.** And so, from our standpoint, we're always coming from the standpoint of **what the doctor**

I wanted to yell, **WRONG!** Rob's condition had only worsened at the hands of clueless doctors who were "stuck in their ways," and they now had Rob "stuck" in their fly trap.

After we hung up, I called the ICU nurse's station, hoping to find a glimmer of hope in Rob's dire situation. I needed to hear that Rob was still breathing and was holding his own. When I asked to speak with his nurse, they paged her to come to the phone.

She said, "Hello. I'm Nurse Horrors. I was just checking on Rob's vitals." She sounded tired and downtrodden. I braced myself. She said, "His blood pressure and heart rate are fine. However, his oxygen saturation is not great. His blood oxygen level is 84%, with the ventilator on 85% FiO2 oxygen. So, he's getting full support from the ventilator and is still not oxygenating well."

I could hear the defeat in her voice as if she had seen many patients on ventilators go downhill fast. So, I asked, "Is there something that changed, or do we know why?" She replied, "Covid, I mean, it's all the Covid. So, we see that a lot, you know, Yeah, kind of deteriorating, as the time goes by with Covid, even on the ventilator."

When I spoke with Rob early in the morning on September 8th, he did **not** sound desperate or deteriorating. During my midmorning call with Dr. Wicked, he had said, "His numbers look okay . . . his inflammatory markers were still improving, lab-wise . . . CRP [C-reactive protein] is coming down to normal range . . . The oxygen is stable."

Yet by 6:16 PM that evening, Dr. Dead End had called me to bluntly advise me, "He's gonna have to be put on a ventilator here. We're gonna start gathering the supplies." Just 27 minutes later, at 6:43 PM, Rob was on a ventilator. Now, less than 24 hours later, Nurse Horrors was telling me he was *deteriorating* and that it was typical for Covid patients they placed on ventilators in their ICU.

My voice trembled as I said, "So, I understand, Covid kind of wreaks havoc through your body, and then you just need to let your body heal, correct?" Nurse Horror responded, "So, he's on the ventilator. I don't know when your last update was, but he is paralyzed on the ventilator— getting medication to keep him comfortable and whatnot. He's still compliant with the ventilator; *his body is just not oxygenating*."

How could Dr. Dead End have said, "Now, I medically think that, that he needs it [the ventilator]," yet now Rob's body was "just not oxygenating." Something was not right with this picture.

Rob was clearly doing **far** better **before** being placed on the ventilator. So why had they rushed to intubate him and get him on this contraption? I had been told the ventilator would allow him to get some rest from his difficulty breathing, and it would vastly <u>increase</u> his blood oxygen level. With dread, I thought back on Rob's haunting warning: *"Doing all they can to try to get me to agree to intubate. **I'm dead if they do.**"*

Dr. Dead End warned me, "**there's a significant risk** if we put him on the ventilator that **his lungs could collapse** because he already has a pneumomediastinum." Rob's deterioration was undoubtedly due to lung damage caused by the BiPAP **and** the ventilator. They were simply using "Covid" as a convenient scapegoat to deflect blame from the harmful therapies they had placed him on.

Nurse Horrors interrupted my thoughts: "He's on the ventilator, and we're doing what we can."

Dr. Wicked had promised to administer budesonide to Rob if he ended up on a ventilator, so I informed Nurse Horrors of my conversation with Dr. Wicked and requested that Rob be given nebulized budesonide.

She dodged with, "You know, he's getting a continuous nebulizer through his ventilator of **VELETRI**, which is a medication that we've been using A LOT with Covid patients, you know. It helps with that oxygenation, you know. You know, the medications that were given, like the remdesivir, and steroids and all of that—that's going to be more, you know, helpful."

Like most of her colleagues, she had obviously chosen to take the "blue pill" and remain ignorant, preferring to believe a false reality rather than face the truth of the harm inflicted on patients in the name of "the protocol."

The hospital profited handsomely—as they charged **$148.36 per dose** for VELETRI while they charged only **$19.39 per dose** for budesonide. From September 4, 2021 (the day after Rob's admission) through October 13, 2021 (the day Rob died), they administered **four doses per day** of VELETRI—a medication for which there was "*no indication*" (according to Dr. Sammy Wong) and which was an off label use (being used for a purpose or in a manner that is not specifically approved by the FDA) drug with significant risks.

On the afternoon of September 9, 2021, the doctors finally agreed to administer one nebulized dose of budesonide while continuing to administer four doses of VELTERI per day as they had finally achieved their goal of getting Rob on a ventilator. October 5, 2021, 26 days later, they finally agreed to increase the budesonide dosage to a generous two times per day.

*The bill for the 104 doses of VELETRI at $148.36 per dose came to a whopping **$15,429.44**, while the charge for the only 44 doses of budesonide was just **$853.16**. As noted in the book of Matthew, "For where your treasure is, there will your heart be also." Their motivation is clear.*

Realizing I wasn't getting anywhere with her regarding budesonide, I said, "I'm going to have to call the nurse in the morning to talk with them about remdesivir."

Nurse Horrors responded, "I'll be honest with you. This is how the Covid patients are presenting. You know, even though we intubate them, even though we put them on the ventilator, and we give them all of the things [meaning drugs], a lot of the time, especially now, they're not . . . ." Wait, "they're not" what? I sensed she was about to say, "*they're not surviving.*" Then, taking a breath, she continued, "It takes a while . . . **if they recover**. So, you know, we see them kind of . . . not all the time . . . you know . . . everybody's different."

Again, she refrained from saying the obvious. Once a Covid patient was intubated and placed on a ventilator in the ICU at Covid Coven Hospital of Plano, Texas, they rarely survived. She wanted to be honest with me but stopped herself before saying, "*From all I have seen while working here in the ICU . . . your husband is not going to make it.*"

A chill came over me as I replayed her "we see them kind of . . ." statement. I could not help but wonder how many others they had placed on ventilators, knowing it was a one-way trip.

I could not believe what was happening. I had begun the day before celebrating my husband's improvement. Then, after the BiPAP therapy and Rob's being placed on a ventilator, my husband, the love of my life, was deteriorating. I was terrified, and my heart ached so badly that I thought I might die.

Friday, September 10, 2021

During our 14-year marriage, life had been good. But now, Rob was in the grasp of body snatchers who were more concerned with "the protocol" than "the patient." I anxiously pondered, "Will I ever again hear Rob's voice or his joyful humming? Will it be possible for me to play a practical joke on him? Will I have the pleasure of seeing his silly grin and enjoying his twinkling eyes?"

When I called the ICU nurses' station at the start of the day shift, Nurse Jagged answered. She happened to be Rob's nurse for the day. I informed her that I was Rob's Medical Power of

Attorney and wanted him off remdesivir. She responded, "Oh, I was about to go get it. Sure. Okay. I will put that in his record." If I had not called at that moment, Rob would have been assaulted with another dose.

As suggested yesterday by Ms. Destroyer, the Social Worker, I left two voicemails for Dr. Torture, the Infectious Disease doctor—one that day and one right after speaking with Nurse Jagged. In both messages, I asked that she call me to discuss stopping Rob's 10-day remdesivir regimen.

To my dismay, however, Dr. Torture did not return my calls. Therefore, I contacted Dr. Wicked, who, on September 8th, had admitted, "I agree that it's probably not doing much." When I explained that, as Rob's Medical Power of Attorney, I wished for the drug to be discontinued but had been unable to contact Dr. Torture, he agreed to formally record my refusal of the medication. It was a minor victory that came far too late.

LEGAL COUNSEL STATEMENT

Members of the jury, as you just read, it took 8 days for Sheila to get the doctors to agree to stop administering remdesivir, a drug she believed was life-threatening. Finally, a physician complied with one of her requests for the first time since Rob's admission. Sadly, it was one of the few times they did

Dr. Wicked noted on Page 165 of Rob's hospital record, "D/w [discussed with] Mrs. Skiba this am, she declines further remdesivir given length of time and her concern for his renal function." At the same time, he removed remdesivir from Rob's MAR (Medication Administration Record).

Rob received the following **six doses** of remdesivir during his first six days in the hospital—against his and Sheila's will:

- **1st dose**—200 mg—9/3/21 at 11:02 PM
- **2nd dose**—100 mg —9/4/21 at 8:41 AM
  Rob successfully refused a 100 Mg dose scheduled for 9/5/21 at 8:37 AM
- **3rd dose**—200 mg —9/6/21 at 5:22 PM
  His 3rd dose was another "loading" dose, as they were "restarting" the whole regimen due to his one missed dose.
- **4th dose**—100 mg—9/7/21 at 9:22 AM
- **5th dose**—100 mg —9/8/21 at 9:01 AM
- **6th dose**—100 mg —9/9/21 at 9:46 AM

You can see their devious plan for Rob documented on September 4, 2021, the day after his arrival, as noted on Page 31 of the hospital records, which appears on Page C-12 in Appendix C. There, Dr. Torture wrote, "The patient meets criteria for use of Remdesivir, plan a 5 day course unless gets intubated."

You will also see on Page 52 of the hospital records, which appears on Page C-7, that Dr. Lament alleged, "patient himself agreed to Remdesivir/Intubation if needed and he has medical capacity to make that decision."

As Sheila shared earlier (on September 5th), "*I knew my husband well enough to know he would never agree to take remdesivir because he was aware of its harmful effects—including its propensity to cause acute kidney injury and eventual death. Moreover, as an avid researcher, author, and speaker, he had spoken out against what he was now experiencing.*"

Despite what they wrote in the record, we agree with Sheila that Rob did NOT want to be given remdesivir. We also contend that Dr. Lament entered that note to falsely justify their plan to administer a harmful drug that she knew would result in a bonus for the hospital. As noted in the "*Hospitals' Incentive Payments for COVID-19*" article in Appendix D, hospitals received "*A 20 percent 'boost' in bonus payment from Medicare on the entire hospital bill for the use of remdesivir instead of medicines such as Ivermectin.*"

Despite Rob and Sheila continually attempting to refuse this medication, it was prescribed and administered against their will until the morning of September 10, 2021. This day, as previously mentioned, Sheila was finally able to get the doctors to cease its administration. However, after six total doses, the damage to his kidneys had been done.

My mother and sister continued calling other hospitals, hoping to find at least one that was not pushing "the protocol" and would allow family visitation. But, unfortunately, no matter how far they looked, they heard the same "our policy is" explanation that we encountered at Covid Coven Hospital of Plano, Texas.

I questioned my sanity for bringing Rob to the hospital in the first place, but I had to remind myself that I had not expected to be locked out the moment we arrived. Besides, he desperately needed oxygen, and I knew no other way to get him the urgent care he needed.

I spent the rest of the day printing and reviewing Rob's online MyChart records and regularly calling the ICU nurse's station to inquire about Rob's vital signs and daily lab results. Nothing I heard reassured me that he was receiving proper care.

Rob was now unconscious and in the dark, totally unaware of what was being done to him. Because he now had no voice, I needed to be his voice. Unfortunately, they seemed to want to keep me in the dark as well and would only share the details of what they were doing if I called and insisted on a comprehensive update.

LEGAL COUNSEL STATEMENT

Members of the jury, a National Library of Medicine article titled "Ventilator-Induced Lung Injury (VILI)" states that "*Ventilator-induced lung injury is the acute lung injury inflicted or aggravated by mechanical ventilation during treatment and has the potential to cause significant **morbidity and mortality**.*"

The article goes on to say that although mechanical ventilation can potentially injure both normal and diseased lungs, "*the injury will be much more **severe** in the latter due to higher microscale stresses.*" They also note that the injury caused by ventilation "***might contribute significantly to the morbidity and mortality of critically ill patients**.*"

Ventilator-induced lung injury (Vili) - statpearls - NCBI bookshelf. (n.d.). From
https://www.ncbi.nlm.nih.gov/books/NBK563244

A high percentage of patients do not survive prolonged mechanical ventilation. The American Journal of Critical Care published an article titled "*Outcomes of long-term ventilator patients: a descriptive study,*" stating, "*43.9% of the patients died in the hospital. None of the patients discharged from the hospital were able to return home initially without assistance. By 6 months after discharge, more than 50% of the original sample had died and 9% resided in an institution.*" They concluded, "*A large percentage of ICU patients who require **5 days or more of mechanical ventilation die in the hospital**, and many of those who live spend considerable time in an extended-care facility before they are discharged to their homes. **These likely outcomes of patients who require long-term ventilation should be discussed with patients and their families to assist them in making informed decisions**.*"

Douglas SL;Daly BJ;Brennan PF;Harris S;Nochomovitz M;Dyer MA; (n.d.). Outcomes of long-term ventilator patients: A descriptive study. American journal of critical care: an official publication, American Association of Critical-Care Nurses. From
https://pubmed.ncbi.nlm.nih.gov/9172858

Considering the fact, as noted by the American Journal of Critical Care, "*A large percentage of ICU patients who require 5 days or more of mechanical ventilation **die in the hospital**,*" no one should be placed on mechanical ventilation without their informed and written consent or the informed and written consent of their Medical Power Attorney.

As we noted earlier in Chapter 2, the hospital could produce no evidence that Rob had signed any form of "Informed Consent" for the high-risk treatments (such as the contraindicated and highly risky BiPAP), the often experimental Emergency Use Authorization (EUA) medications he was administered, or the significant risks he was subjected to by being intubated and placed on a ventilator.

Informed consent would have required Rob's actual signature, not just the statements of doctors and staff who had a vested interest in seeing him follow their preferred protocol and who were quick to claim Rob "verbally consented" to a particular medication or therapy when he was allegedly hypoxic and incapable of making such life-altering and life-threatening decisions.

In addition, the hospital never received Sheila's consent for any of the harmful medications that were administered to Rob, nor her written consent for him to be intubated at a time when he was said to be suffering from "progressive hypoxia," a condition that would have made it difficult or impossible for him to consent. Below is a snapshot from Page 143 of Rob's hospital records noting that condition.

Robert Skiba was intubated last night due to respiratory fatigue and progressive hypoxia

Dr. Wicked had admitted, when discussing with me the significant risks of being placed on a ventilator on the evening of September 7, 2021, the day before Rob was placed on one, "So, it is **a very bad thing** to have to go on, and that is 100% true. That I know. I believe the ventilator **causes death**." He also advised me that "he already has a pneumomediastinum, which is a marker that his lungs are fragile."

Despite the high mortality rate, the entire team at Covid Coven Hospital of Plano, Texas, had been dead set on getting Rob on a ventilator from the moment he arrived. To my horror, they had succeeded—and I felt I had failed.

While my family and many of my friends were optimistic that Rob would recover, others sent me links to disturbing articles and videos that described the same treatment that Rob and I were enduring.

I was in constant agony and could not bear the thought of living without Rob. Witnessing the needless deaths of other victims of "the protocol that kills" only increased my fear that I might never see him alive again.

Here I was, attempting to advocate for him from home without being permitted to see him as he suffered alone, like an abused prisoner in solitary confinement.

Saturday, September 11, 2021

After a difficult night, I did not want to get out of bed. I was losing all hope and the will to live. My fear that Rob might not survive grew by the minute.

My mother stopped by to assist, comfort, and reassure me. Nonetheless, I was anxious, fearful, and angry no matter what she did or said. Finally, she reminded me that Jesus (Yahushua) loves Rob and me and would never leave or forsake us. I knew that, but I needed a real miracle—and a big one at that.

The hospital's Covid protocol was like the iceberg that sank the Titanic. We had hit a solid iceberg, and we struck it hard. I had thought my husband was unsinkable. He was the strongest, toughest man I knew. I was confident he would still be improving were it not for the massive doses of unnecessary and harmful drugs, followed by the harmful BiPAP and ventilator therapy.

I again called the nurse's station to check on Rob's condition. This time, Nurse Oppressive answered. She informed me, "Okay. So earlier today, they tried switching **off** the paralytics, but apparently, he didn't tolerate it well. So, they had to go back up on the paralytics and put him back on 100% oxygen. Tonight, what we're gonna do is we're going to try and wean him **off** the oxygen, **but we're now at 100%, got it?**" What I "got" was that he was in major trouble, and they were frying his lungs with an excessively high level of oxygen.

Although my September 6th attempt to get Nurse Carnage to take a photo of Rob failed when she used the excuse that it would be a "HIPAA violation," I asked if Nurse Oppressive might be willing to accommodate me. "I know you probably hear this a lot from others who cannot see their spouses. I have not seen my husband for over a week now. I just want to see him so I can verify that he's doing okay. All I know are his vital signs. Is there any way you could take a picture of him in the bed, along with the vitals on the monitor, and send it to me so I can see him and see what's happening.?"

Nurse Oppressive cleared her throat and said, "Unfortunately, we don't have a way to take photos of patients because that's **against the law**. We cannot take Rob's photo without his consent. That's the law, American law. You just cannot take photos of someone who . . . who is unaware of what's going on. See, without his consent, we can't do that right now. But if you call the nurse in the morning, she can schedule a FaceTime with you so you can see your husband if you want. You can, like, invite your family and stuff like that so that you can all be there."

I asked, "but he's not conscious, correct?" She said, "He's not at all. He won't be able to talk to you at all. But you can see his face. You'll see what's going on, you know. I have to warn you, okay? It is not a very pretty sight because of all the tubes and lines and everything that he has on him. We can do that in the morning if you want."

LEGAL COUNSEL STATEMENT
Members of the jury, HIPAA (the Health Insurance Portability and Accountability Act of 1996) is a federal law that places strict restrictions on healthcare providers' use and disclosure of protected health information (PHI). That includes any information that may be used to identify a patient, such as their name, address, or photograph.

However, the Privacy Rule at 45 CFR 164.502(g) *"requires covered entities to treat an individual's personal representative **as the individual** with respect to uses and disclosures of the individual's protected health information, as well as the individual's rights under the Rule."*
(OCR), O. for C. R. (2022, October 7). Guidance: Personal representatives. HHS.gov. From https://www.hhs.gov/hipaa/for-professionals/privacy/guidance/personal-representatives/index.html

Also, under the Rule, *"an individual's personal representative is someone authorized under State or other applicable law to act on behalf of the individual in making health care related decisions."*
(OCR), O. for C. R. (2021, June 28). 2069-under HIPAA, when can a family member of an individual access the individual's PHI from a health care provider or health plan? HHS.gov. From https://www.hhs.gov/hipaa/for-professionals/faq/2069/under-hipaa-when-can-a-family-member/index.html

Thus, it was **not** "against the law" for Sheila to have access to a photo of Rob at any time because:

1. Her name was on the hospital's **Protected Health Information form,** on which Rob was noted to have authorized "*this facility and medical staff members to discuss my medical history, diagnosis, treatment, and prognosis with the person(s) listed below.*"

2. Also, Sheila was Rob's **Medical Power of Attorney**, and by Texas State law, she was authorized to act on Rob's behalf in making any healthcare-related decisions. Thus, she had the right to access any of Rob's protected health information, <u>including his image.</u>

Per HIPAA's Privacy Rule, **Sheila should have been treated "as the individual,"** not as an outsider. Besides, if it were "against the law" for her to see an image of Rob in the ICU bed, they would not have offered her the FaceTime chat option.

NOTE: *It may have been against "hospital policy" for nurses to use their cell phones to take and transmit photos of patients to authorized family members. Even then, if that were the case, the nurse should have referred to the policy vs. inappropriately telling her it was **"against the law"** for her to see a transmitted image of her husband.*

Clearly, I had the right to receive and see images of Rob. How else could I evaluate his condition while they isolated him from me? Moreover, by denying me access to a view of him and his room, they could easily hide his current condition from me and prevent my asking uncomfortable questions about his care or the lack thereof.

I asked, "Can you just tell him that his wife called and tell him she loves him? I mean, he can still hear?" She said, "He still can hear. I just don't know how much he can hear. But yeah, whenever I go back and later on, I'll give him his hands a squeeze." I pleaded, "Please just say your wife loves you. Just touch his hand and tell him I love him."

She said she was busy but would squeeze his hands for me when she made her rounds. I wondered why it was okay for some strange woman to be at my husband's side and squeeze his hands while I could not. Their illogical policy of isolating me from a man with whom I had spent the entirety of his illness before his admission and whose "illness" I had also endured and conquered made no sense.

Patients who believe they have no hope are more likely to give up and further decline. I needed to be able to see and touch my husband, and he needed my presence and my touch to help give him the strength and encouragement he needed to recover.

Rob needed to know I was still there for him, his family loved him, and we were working on his behalf. But, sadly, all my pleas to be with Rob fell on uncaring, deaf ears as everyone I spoke with at Covid Coven Hospital of Plano, Texas, chanted the same "it's our policy" incantations.

As you can see from the text messages below, Sheila was actively working on developing a "rescue" plan for Rob.

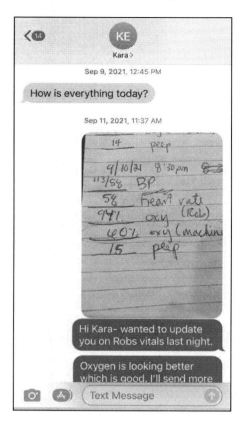

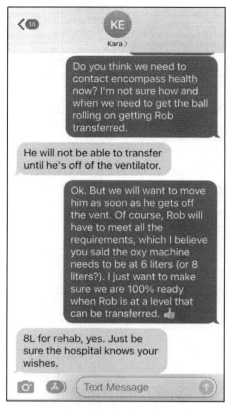

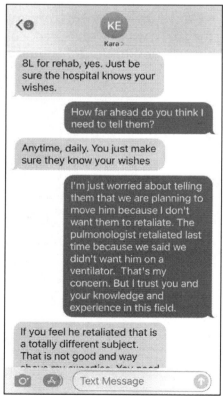

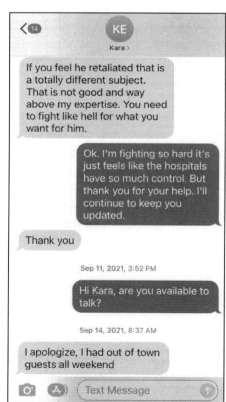

Sunday, September 12, 2021

Each day seemed to present a new challenge, and my annoyance with the doctors who thought Rob was their property and the hospital staff who seemed oblivious to what was causing him to deteriorate was at an all-time high.

While reviewing Rob's daily MyChart records, I could not find any information regarding his caloric intake. When I asked one of the ICU nurses about it, she responded, "Well, the propofol he is receiving is included in his calorie count."

That absurd comment made absolutely no sense. I was concerned about whether or not Rob was receiving adequate nutrition and could not imagine anyone would consider a powerful sedative as a nutrient.

LEGAL COUNSEL STATEMENT
Members of the jury, propofol (a potent and rapid-onset sedative that is promptly metabolized by the body and eliminated as waste) is delivered in a fat emulsion that contains 1.1 kcal per milliliter. Thus, it does contain calories. However, it is **not** a good source of nutrients or energy the body can use for metabolism or other essential physiological functions. On average, the contribution of calories from propofol is not clinically significant.

However, when ICU patients are being administered propofol, "*some clinicians have empirically **decreased the infusion rate of the nutrition therapy**, which also may have **detrimental effects** since protein intake may be inadequate.*" As you will discover later, **Rob's protein intake was inadequate**, which led to his suffering from profound anemia. "*Recent studies have indicated an association between improved mortality, shorter ventilation days, and shorter duration of ICU and hospital stays with **increases in protein intake** for critically ill patients. This is particularly relevant for those critically ill patients with a prolonged ICU stay.*"
Dickerson, R. N., & Buckley, C. T. (2021, July 1). Impact of propofol sedation upon caloric overfeeding and protein inadequacy in critically ill patients receiving nutrition support. Pharmacy (Basel, Switzerland). From
https://www.ncbi.nlm.nih.gov/pmc/articles/PMC8293440

Adequate protein intake is essential for the production of hemoglobin. Hemoglobin is the protein molecule that binds to oxygen in the lungs and carries it to the body's tissues and organs. When the body cannot produce sufficient hemoglobin due to inadequate protein intake, the amount of oxygen delivered to the body's cells decreases. This can lead to a condition called "*hypoxia*," a deficiency of oxygen at the cellular level.

The last thing Rob needed was to end up suffering from *anemia* because he was already "**hypoxic**" (a condition in which there is a deficiency in the amount of oxygen that reaches the body's tissues), as noted at the top of the "Impression and Plan" on Page 27 of his hospital records, which you can see on Page C-3 in Appendix C.

Unfortunately, within three days, on September 15th, Rob's having become *anemic* became a topic of discussion. Tragically, his anemia worsened until it became so severe that doctors recommended a blood transfusion not long before he died.

I expressed deep concern that Rob might not be receiving sufficient nutrition. The nurse said that she would monitor his caloric intake from that point forward, which made me wonder who, if anyone, was ensuring Rob was not being kept in starvation mode. I was troubled at having to bring Rob's potential lack of nutrition to their attention. Unfortunately, adequate nutrition was not a part of their "Covid protocol."

Although it appeared Rob had been denied adequate nutrition on a consistent basis, he was not denied a steady supply of IV bags of pharmaceutical soup, an onslaught of drugs that kept his excessively high levels of sedatives, paralytics, and opioids were severely damaging his liver and his kidneys, which led me to wonder if he would have a functioning mind and body if they could finally "extubate" him and get him off the ventilator.

As I reviewed the daily written log I kept of each medication and dosage, I was alarmed to discover they had now increased his fentanyl dosage from 150 mcg per hour to 300 mcg per hour. It appeared they were doing all they could to pump him full of as much medication as possible, which would make it impossible for him to wake up.

Furthermore, the ventilator was consistently set to a FiO2 (oxygen concentration) of 90% or higher; sometimes, it was cranked up to 100%. Were they unaware that excessively high levels of oxygen for extended periods could further damage his fragile lungs?

Worse yet, they advised me that every time they attempted to reduce his sedation and do a "spontaneous breathing trial" (which Dr. Dead End had told me they would do every day) to determine whether they could wean him from the ventilator, he would "desaturate" (his blood oxygen level would drop). As a result, they would further raise the FiO2, cranking it back up to 100% if necessary.

I wondered—and hoped to the Lord it was not true—whether the 4.5 hours he had endured on the BiPAP might have injured his lungs to the point that he could truly no longer breathe on his own.

LEGAL COUNSEL STATEMENT

Members of the jury, we contend that Rob would have never been intubated and placed on a ventilator (a therapy few patients survive) if the doctors had used *a conservative approach* where they only treated Rob with supplemental oxygen, steroids (for the inflammation), antibiotics (to help clear up the infection from pneumonia), and budesonide (an inhaled corticosteroid that has been proven 90% effective for Covid as noted in the University of Oxford Study results shown in **Appendix F**).

In addition, Rob would not likely have required mechanical ventilation if the hospital had simply allowed Sheila to be with him as his on-site advocate so she could help ensure he had adequate food and water (which was essential to his being able to regain the strength needed to heal) and provide him with the love, encouragement, and moral support he desperately needed.

Consider the example of a healthy 65-year-old couple Sheila knows who both contracted COVID-19 in February 2022 as proof that *a conservative approach* can be highly effective. Although the wife only felt ill for a few days, while she was recovering, her husband became ill and ended up with double pneumonia, a fever of more than 105°, and a blood oxygen level that began to fall into the 50s.

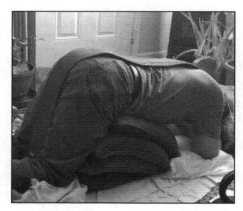

He was given 5 liters per minute (LPM) of supplemental oxygen through an oxygen concentrator (5 LPM equates to a FiO2 [oxygen concentration] of 40%) at home, and a telemedicine doctor prescribed an antibiotic, a steroid (for inflammation), and nebulized budesonide. In addition, they added a few natural remedies (such as extra doses of vitamin C, vitamin D, etc.) that they believed could be as effective as traditional pharmaceuticals.

Although it was rough going at times, and he was unable to lay on his side or back for nine days (he had to remain in a prone position **as shown in the photo on the previous page** to keep his blood oxygen level at 90 percent or higher), the couple knew that keeping him at home while taking as few medications as possible and receiving adequate food, water, and his wife's loving support would be FAR BETTER than admitting him to a kill shelter hospital where he would be subjected to and likely become a victim of "the protocol that kills."

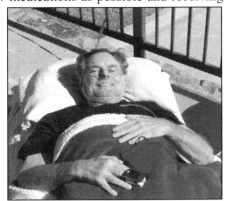

This couple knew Rob and Sheila; they had seen what had happened to Rob and did not want to suffer the same fate of becoming another victim of "the protocol that kills." **The photo on the right** shows him on the road to recovery enjoying some sunshine on a lawn chair with supplemental oxygen. Had he been hospitalized, he would likely have ended up on the road to the morgue.

Within a couple of weeks, the husband was back on his feet. In a few months, he was back to 100 percent. They are confident they made the right decision to avoid the isolation, intimidation, starvation, and possibly forced mechanical ventilation that has become the norm in mainstream American hospitals.

Monday, September 13, 2021

Rob was in grave danger, and I knew that his life depended on my ability to keep up with the doctors' orders, their extensive written notes, and the limited vitals I could see posted in Rob's online MyChart for the previous day.

Being locked out of the hospital meant I was always playing catch-up as I reacted to their constantly changing orders and Rob's deteriorating condition. My only other source of information was the limited updates I could obtain through my multiple daily calls to the ICU nurses' station or an occasional call with a doctor.

Whenever I asked Dr. Wicked how Rob was doing, he would typically tell me that "he is overall stable." Yet I wondered if he were being honest with me if he would have instead said Rob was "overall dying," as I could sense he wanted me to believe Rob was doing well when he was NOT. They all seemed to be using a calculated *"appease the wife"* strategy designed to keep me at bay and content so I would not attempt to rock their boat.

During one of my morning calls to the ICU, I learned Dr. Wicked was there on his morning rounds. So I asked if I could speak with him. When he came on the line, I asked why they kept Rob's FiO2 (oxygen concentration) at such high levels. He said, "Yeah, he **was** doing well. We're doing that to keep his oxygen levels up. One thing is the paralytic. **It really accelerates muscle loss and makes for a much longer rehab, of course**. So, it's the first thing I want to get rid of when we can.

"So, when he was off the paralytic, he coughed a little bit and **just didn't have the reserves**, so he dropped down [his blood oxygen level decreased]. So, because that oxygen is the fastest thing we have to work with, **you can crank FiO2 up to 100%** to get his oxygen level up while you wait for the paralytic to come back on and work again. So, he responded to that well."

I knew Rob did not "**have the reserves**" because they had weakened him by bombarding him with harmful and unnecessary medications and failing to ensure he received the nutrition he needed to regain the strength required to heal.

To these drug-obsessed professionals, the solution to <u>every</u> problem, even problems caused by the medications he was being given, was—you guessed it—another medication. If you were malnourished, for example, they would look for a drug that might counteract the damage caused by the lack of adequate nutrition.

As I held my head in my hands, I heard him say, "But we've got to be careful with **pressure** because it also causes bronchial pneumomediastinum, which has improved according to the X-ray, so that's good. But, so, with pressure and with the ventilator—**now the problem is with the ventilator**.

"We know that *smaller volumes decrease mortality* and make you more likely to survive; however, the patients are uncomfortable breathing [on the ventilator] and need sedation. **So, there's no way to know if we are doing better or not until we try it.** I wouldn't stop the paralytics if he's on 100% oxygen because **he doesn't have any reserves**.

"But he's currently getting around 60% oxygen. **We think** that's non-toxic. We are *pretty sure* 60% is not toxic from an oxygen standpoint. We don't know exactly where the threshold is. But in dogs, it's about 60%. So, we try to keep him at 60% and get him some reserve. And that's where we like their oxygen to be, and then we start trying to take things away. So, as for things I'll take away . . . he's on the inhaled vasodilator (VELETRI), he's on increased pressure, and he's on paralytics. Those three things. The paralytics . . . we like to get rid of first because **the longer we're on them, the longer our recovery course is going to be.**"

LEGAL COUNSEL STATEMENT

Members of the jury, what Dr. Wicked was speaking of appears to be a failed attempt at what is called a **Spontaneous Awakening Trial** (SAT). That is where the sedatives and paralytics are reduced in the hope the patient will not become agitated, show signs of respiratory distress, or have their blood oxygen level drop below 88% for at least five minutes. If that occurs and they can awaken them, they then ask the patient to complete three out of four simple tasks, such as opening their eyes or squeezing a hand.

According to Dr. Wicked, Rob failed the trial because he "didn't have the reserves" (he had no physical strength). Thus, his oxygen level dropped significantly. That led to their ramping back up the paralytic and sedatives and raising the FiO2 as needed (many times to 100%, as shown in the chart at the bottom of Page C-54 in Appendix C) to get Rob's blood oxygen level into what they considered an acceptable range.

*As we noted earlier, targeting a blood oxygen level of only 90% or higher (vs. 95% or higher) would have been more "lung protective." That way, they could have used lower concentrations of oxygen to avoid further damaging Rob's lungs since concentrations of oxygen **above 60%** for over 24 hours can create pulmonary toxicity, extensive damage to the alveoli, and **atelectasis** (a condition where alveoli in a lung or a part of a lung deflate, thereby causing a partially or entirely collapsed lung).*

As shown in the chart at the bottom of Page C-54, this is one of the few times they were able to reduce the FiO2 (oxygen concentration) to a level of **60%** or less. It was also one of the last times they even attempted a Spontaneous Awakening Trial (SAT), which precedes a Spontaneous Breathing Trial (SBT)—both of which must be passed to try to wean someone from a ventilator.

*The FiO2 level on the ventilator was generally set to **well above 60%**, at levels Dr. Wicked had admitted were "toxic" and life-threatening. Later this same day, the FiO2 level was raised to 85%. It was then increased to 100% for some time the following day.*

Being totally sedated, paralyzed, and even further starved, how was Rob expected to build any "reserves"? By now, Rob had been on the ventilator for nearly four days, and it was becoming increasingly apparent that there was no way to successfully wean him from it.

You can read more about the SAT and SBT tests a patient must pass to be weaned from a ventilator on the Agency for Healthcare Research and Quality website in their Coordinated Spontaneous Awakening and Breathing Trials Protocol: AHRQ Safety Program article at
https://www.ahrq.gov/hai/tools/mvp/modules/technical/sat-sbt-protocol.html

By saying, "*there's no way to know if we are doing better or not until we try it,*" I knew full well Dr. Wicked was speaking of their failed attempt to wean Rob from the heavy sedatives and paralytics to see if he might miraculously be able to breathe on his own despite the fact the paralytic, as Dr. Wicked just said, "really accelerates muscle loss."

I could envision two doctors holding a jump rope and shouting, "*Hey Rob, we know you've been paralyzed for days now, but we're ready to start, so be sure to jump as we swing the rope.*" With Rob in his weakened "no reserves" condition, I wondered how they would ever wean him from the ventilator.

Dr. Wicked went on, "So, I tried to get rid of it, and he was looking really good on Saturday. And we can, of course, just leave it like that. But I didn't want to give him two more days of paralytics if he didn't need it [and yet Rob would have to endure 30 more days of paralytics and sedatives before the protocol finally killed him]. So, we tried to work him off. **He had to go back on.** He's responded very well; he's back down to 60% again today. We're working on coming off the paralytic again. And as Einstein said, doing the same thing over and over again and hoping for a different result is the definition of insanity. **That's basically what we're doing here**. But the things that are changing is . . . *IS HIM.*"

He explained more fully, "So, when we get off all of those, and pressures are looking good, then we start a little bigger volume and **work and see if we have enough strength reserve to come off the ventilator.** If we don't, that's when I want to talk about a tracheotomy, but it's a little early to talk about now. **But, if he's too weak, which happens from the ventilator,** that's when we talk about a tracheostomy as a temporary thing, to do a procedure to remove the tube from going in the mouth down through the vocal cords to go in the neck below the vocal cords.

"It's a more comfortable way, and then you go on and off the ventilator. So, when we're ready to go off the ventilator, **if he has enough strength** to just come off, that'd be great. If he doesn't, then we do a tracheostomy that you'd come off for an hour and go back on. You can decrease pressures and be more awake for the therapy. So, we'll talk about that when it's time to talk about that."

I felt like I was being deceived by skilled con artists who had initially told me that Rob would only need a ventilator for up to ten days so that he could rest from his "work of breathing." It had now been five days, and they seemed to be no closer to weaning him than they were 24 hours after placing him on the ventilator.

see") **if** Rob would "have **enough strength reserve** to come off the ventilator." If he did not have any strength left, which "happens from the ventilator," a tracheostomy (also called a trach) would be required even to attempt to wean him.

If Rob would require a trach to help him come off the ventilator, then why did they not just give him a trach from the beginning and bypass the whole "intubation, ventilation, heavy sedation, and muscle-wasting paralytics" nightmare? Could the real reason be the fact the government incentive they were expecting would <u>only</u> be paid if they first got Rob on a ventilator?

I wanted this nightmare to end as soon as possible to prevent them from causing Rob even more harm, so I asked, "How soon do you think Rob will be able to come **off** the ventilator?" He replied, "Yeah, and at 50 years old, **he could probably handle, with paralytics, probably 10 to 14 days and still have enough reserve . . . most likely.** So, by the time he got on the ventilator, of course, **we were nutritionally down, <u>and he hadn't been fed for several days before</u>**. So, he may not, you know, **he may not have enough reserve in two weeks.**"

I could not believe what I was hearing. Dr. Wicked had just admitted that (unlike Rob) a patient who was in his 50s who HAD been eating (Rob had not) and who DID have adequate "reserves" (and Rob did not) **might** survive "probably 10 to 14 days" on paralytics on a ventilator. He also admitted that Rob "hadn't been fed for several days before" (thus, he was starving) and had **NO** reserves. Therefore, "**he may not have enough reserve in two weeks.**"

I could only hope and pray they would find a way to wean Rob from the ventilator within the "**two weeks**" time frame—because after two weeks, according to Dr. Wicked, he would not likely have "**enough reserve**" for them to get him off the ventilator. Clearly, time was of the essence. Unfortunately, however, I had yet to see them even begin to successfully wean him from what Rob had feared would be a death trap.

Dr. Wicked continued, "Nutrition is doing better now. Five days into the vent, **he had been kind of weak and not eating well for another four or five days before that.** And it doesn't really help to count those days, so we're looking at . . . **we're just a little over a week from a muscle loss standpoint**. So, I mean, by the end of this week, I think we'll have a better idea of that.

"We will see if he's more stable and ready to tolerate the trach. When we make the transition, **you got to have enough reserve breathing-wise**. It's a little early, regardless, to talk about it. But I would not be surprised if I'm not recommending that towards the end of the week. But some people, when they start getting better, they get better fast; and if he does, that would be great to just come straight off. If not, a tracheostomy. It's not the end of the world by any means. When you don't need it anymore, you take it out."

I informed Dr. Wicked that Rob had lost more than ten pounds during his first few days in the hospital, which was apparent from the weights in his MyChart records. Now that he was paralyzed and on a ventilator, he would lose even more weight and muscle mass.

In an effort to demonstrate to me that Rob's caloric intake had been sufficient SINCE he had been placed on the ventilator, he consulted Rob's hospital records. To his dismay, he could not locate any documentation proving that Rob had been fed since he was placed on the ventilator five days prior.

To skirt the issue, he said, "They haven't updated it from last week. But I pulled up the math here. Pivot 1.5 provides 1800 kilocalories with 113 grams of protein a day. I think that's adequate, especially when you're paralyzed right now and we're doing all the work. When he's been paralyzed, we've been doing all the work of breathing for him. The only muscle using any energy is his brain and his heart. Everything else has been pretty passive. When he comes off the paralytics, he'll start using a little more, but the ventilator's doing the work of breathing.

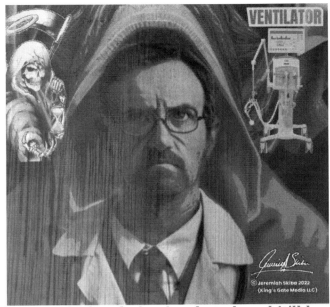

"1800 calories is plenty of calories for him right now. He's got 1800 calories a day and 113 grams of protein. So, we're doing good on nutrition as long as he's intubated, **and it was an issue before being intubated, and it'll be an issue if we're able to come straight off the ventilator.** That'll be something we have to consider, **making sure he's got enough reserves** to be able to."

He hit the nail on the head when he said, "That'll be something we have to consider, **making sure he's got enough reserves** to be able to" get off the ventilator. He knew very well Rob had been malnourished "**before being intubated.**" That was how they had weakened and "starved him into submission" in the first place. I was shocked to hear his admission that their negligence and malfeasance (in addition to their needlessly locking me out of the hospital so I could not assist Rob) had brought us to this point!

Just 48 hours after his arrival on the evening of September 5, 2021, Rob texted me, "**No food no [water],**" and "**No strength no hope left**." *The fact that Rob was not fed from the moment he arrived was entirely their fault and a criminal act!*

Because of their mistreatment, Rob was now imprisoned by a machine that was unlikely to release him until it had drained him of all his remaining energy and life. I desperately wished I could have found another way to get Rob the help he desperately needed without handing him over to a group of criminals who, in my opinion, had lost their moral compass and were gleefully following "the protocol that kills."

I shuddered as I recalled Rob's "*If they don't let you be my advocate, I'm going to die in here!*" and his "*Doing all they can to try to get me to agree to intubate. I'm dead if they do*" warnings.
I was brought back to the present when Dr. Wicked continued, "Because he has the pneumomediastinum, a lot of times I'll go higher on PEEP because it does help oxygen but at THE EXPENSE of increased pressure and RISK of what's called barotrauma. **We knew he had barotrauma before we put him on a ventilator.**"

I was once again being subjected to circular reasoning. Dr. Wicked stated that Rob was at risk for barotrauma now that he was on a ventilator, even though he had barotrauma BEFORE they placed him on a ventilator. Why was this the first I heard of Rob's having barotrauma? Had they intended to keep the information from me, but Dr. Wicked's chatty manner caused it to slip out?

I had been wondering whether the damage caused by the BiPAP therapy might have been a major reason Rob ended up on a ventilator, and now I felt I knew, as it seemed from what Dr. Wicked just told me, that the BiPAP had caused barotrauma. Now, the ventilator might exacerbate the condition.

I remembered Nurse Carnage telling me on September 6, 2021, two days before Rob was placed on the BiPAP, "He's **not** a candidate for the other option called BiPAP because he has a pneumomediastinum—which is where there's air trapped in the space in the chest between the lungs, and it can cause him traumatic injury if we do a positive pressure such as a BiPAP."

Because Rob's X-rays did not reveal barotrauma BEFORE he was placed on the BiPAP, it is evident that he did not have barotrauma then. Rob had been improving daily until he was placed on the BiPAP. Within hours of being taken off the BiPAP, Rob reportedly suffered such severe respiratory fatigue and hypoxia that he had to be placed on a ventilator.

LEGAL COUNSEL STATEMENT
Members of the jury, as we noted earlier, the 4.5 hours Rob spent on a BiPAP increased his pneumomediastinum and **did cause** barotrauma, as documented on page 141 of the hospital records (see Page C-44), where they note, "Repeat CXR [Chest X-ray] this afternoon to **monitor barotrauma**."

As we also shared previously, **barotrauma** is a well-recognized and potentially life-threatening complication where the alveoli, the air sacs of the lungs, rupture and collapse. That causes shortness of breath, difficulty breathing, and a feeling of tightness in the chest or claustrophobia. Rob was intubated and placed on a ventilator because of these same symptoms, which occurred immediately after he was placed on the BiPAP.

Their placing Rob on a BiPAP likely led to their having to place Rob on a ventilator because the damage caused by the BiPAP was so extensive that he could not survive any other way. Such a deliberate and reckless act should at least be considered malpractice. In some courts, it might be regarded as premeditated murder.

Rob had not eaten for over a week; I now knew he was suffering from barotrauma, and his lungs were being further damaged by the hour by the ventilator's increased pressure and up to 100% oxygen. I could not imagine how he would be able to regain the strength and "reserves" needed to survive and be weaned from the ventilator.

Dr. Wicked then explained the PEEP setting, saying, "So, normal PEEP, if you're on the ventilator just to go for a surgery or something, is **zero**. But with lung problems, it is normally like 5. We can get back down to that, and that's where we'll start evaluating for coming off the ventilator . . . when he's down to 4 to 8. **A PEEP of 14 is high**. Rob is on 14 PEEP. But for my kind of ARDS [Acute Respiratory Distress Syndrome] or Covid respiratory patients, that is not as high as I generally go."

LEGAL COUNSEL STATEMENT
Members of the jury, **PEEP** stands for *Positive End Expiratory Pressure* and is pressure applied by a ventilator (or a BiPAP device) at the end of each breath (upon exhalation). The excess "end expiratory pressure" prevents passive emptying of the lungs when a patient breathes out.

The purpose of keeping a higher pressure in the lungs upon exhalation is to "*recruit*" damaged alveoli. Unfortunately, Rob had damaged (ruptured and collapsed) alveoli (the air sacs in the lungs) because of the **barotrauma** that occurred while he was on the BiPAP.

The "*recruitment*" of alveoli is carried out by keeping them filled with a volume of air <u>at all times</u>, even upon exhalation. The goal of a higher PEEP is to help increase the oxygenation of the blood by keeping more alveoli "*recruited*" to do their jobs of removing carbon dioxide from, and delivering oxygen to, the bloodstream.

When alveoli rupture and collapse due to barotrauma, excess "end expiratory pressure" is required to keep them open. If they were to collapse upon exhalation, adequate oxygen and carbon dioxide exchange could not occur. Thus, the damage (the barotrauma) caused by the BiPAP led to their having to use, as Dr. Wicked admitted, a **high** PEEP setting of 14 cm H_2O.

As we noted earlier, high PEEP levels can cause changes in lung compliance (that is, the ability of the lungs to expand and contract in response to changes in pressure with a resulting lack of efficient exchange of gasses in the lungs), making it far more difficult (or nearly impossible) to wean a patient off the ventilator. Thus, the barotrauma caused by the BiPAP and the resulting high PEEP setting on the ventilator put Rob in a very precarious situation.

*Their criteria for attempting to wean someone from the ventilator was a **PEEP** of **5 to 8 cm H_2O** and an **FiO2** (oxygen concentration) of **50% or less**. However, they kept the PEEP setting on the ventilator at 14 to 15 **for the entire 35 days Rob was on the ventilator,** as shown in the bottom chart on Page C-54 in Appendix C. Unfortunately, Rob was virtually trapped on a device <u>they could not remove him from</u>.*

As Sammy Wong, MD, our medical expert witness, said in his "Letter of Introduction," which appears in **Appendix B**, *"Since he was sedated and paralyzed, he was dependent on the ventilator. . . They just maintained his ventilator settings essentially unchanged . . . until he died."*

Regarding the barotrauma, he added, "**But because he already had the barotrauma**, that's where I kind of capped out on him [with the PEEP]. I tried to get him down to 10 early on, but it just wasn't adequate for his oxygenation. So, we got it back up to 14, but I have not gone higher because he had the pneumomediastinum to start with."

The more Dr. Wicked spoke, and he spoke a lot because he was very talkative, the more I realized Rob was in grave danger—and the more panicked I felt.

In the hope of at least some good news, I interrupted him to ask if Rob's X-rays had shown any signs of improvement. He responded, "I wouldn't get too hung up on the X-rays, like the radiologists might read today's X-rays and say they are worse, but his oxygen level is better. One problem with these X-rays . . . these portable chest X-rays are not very good quality. They're shot from the front; they're shot coming close in there. They're not nearly as defined as going down to the department for an X-ray. The main role for X-rays on the ventilator is we can look at big changes. But the main thing I'm looking at is to make sure our lines haven't moved—our tubes [such as the endotracheal tube] haven't moved.

"So, it's really more of a kind of safety monitoring. The radiologists read every entry as it comes across and <u>they'll make it hard for us to say things</u>, but we're really limited as to qualities or traits, and they make a lot of calls on little changes. One thing we <u>can see</u> is the barotrauma and pneumomediastinum has actually been improving, despite being on the ventilator. This means he's absorbing air back faster than leaking air into the space. So that, I'm very happy about.

"But regarding any big, huge dramatic change, we're really limiting the quality, so don't get too hung up on what the radiologist reads on these portable studies because the quality is just not that great, but they're good for making sure my tubes are where they're supposed to be. His lung hasn't popped, and things along those lines."

I took no comfort in the "his lung hasn't popped" comment. No one had even hinted at THAT being a possibility. I was also not at all pleased to hear Rob had been damaged by barotrauma **which they caused**, yet I was happy to hear it seemed to be improving.

Why would he disparage radiologists—doctors who specialize in interpreting X-rays, CT scans, and MRIs to diagnose diseases and injuries—by saying, "they'll make it hard for us to say things." Did he mean that the experts who interpret X-rays for a living made it difficult for him to conceal what was really going on with his ICU patients?

I asked him why he had reduced the dosage of SOLU-MEDTOL (methylprednisolone) since corticosteroids can help reduce inflammation. He answered, "Like everything we do, **it's risk versus benefit**. It's kind of a double-edged sword. So, it's a very potent anti-inflammatory, and it's been working well. So, he has inflammation markers that are coming down. The flip side of methylprednisolone is that it's an immune suppressive. It is both for clearing the virus from your body and other risks of infection, which is a high risk when you're in the ICU.

"Basically, the takeaway is with the most severely sick people with Covid, steroids are good, but how much and how long? For sure, we know, we use them. The flip side is the immune suppression. So, where things are better, like Friday or Saturday, I dropped him another 10% today for the next 24 hours. So, it went from 60 a day to 50 a day. But again, everything we do has a benefit, **but _everything_ we do also has a potential risk**."

"So, I can't tell you 100% for sure, but his CRP (C-Reactive Protein) is kind of down to normal. We've got four or five days, and everything else is improving inflammatory-wise; I can get rid of all your inflammation with a giant dose of steroids. **But you could die from a secondary infection.** Where that exact line is there, I don't know. And that's where a little bit of the art of medicine, or the science, comes in. Right now, I keep tapering those down as much as I can."

I fully understood the concept of "risks versus benefits," yet they were taking way too many **risks** with Rob, and all of the **benefits** were in their favor, not his. Actually, they were benefiting by putting Rob's whole life at risk. But, sadly, that is precisely how incentivized medicine works. I asked him to explain why I kept hearing that Rob had been coughing while on the ventilator. He explained, "Everybody, everyone . . . generally when you're coughing, it's good to get stuff out. Coughing or gagging is a very normal response for someone with a tube **shoved** in the back of their throat. They go in there, and you have to suction the tube of mucus, or you turn the patient, or prop them up a little, and they'll cough a little bit. If your lungs are okay, and you have plenty of reserve, it doesn't really cause a lot of problems. **When you're living on the edge with no real reserve** . . . coughing itself is neither good nor bad at this stage, it is just something that exists. **The problem with the coughing for him is that he has no reserve.**"

Once again, Dr. Wicked admitted without realizing it that he had a ventilated patient on his hands who had "**no reserve**." Rob had no reserve because they had allowed him to starve from the day he arrived at the hospital. I was convinced they did that on purpose because a starved and weakened patient would not have the strength to resist "the protocol" they were insisting on and would eventually succumb to it.

He continued, "So, preventing coughing is not the only way. Paralytics help with oxygenation. But that's just an example and part of it, and that's why I think, for lack of a better word, **he tanked on Saturday** when he was off the paralytics and **was in kind of a coughing spell.**

"But it's not a huge surprise because we're pushing him right on the edge of the line all the time. We're trying to get down to the least amount of oxygen needed—the least amount of everything. But I'm not surprised; he **just wasn't ready to be off**. You never know until you try."

As we hung up, I thought, "Wow, Dr. Wicked just admitted that Rob 'tanked' two days ago, on Saturday, September 11th. Why did they not tell me that until now?" So here I was, still physically separated from my husband due to their irrational no-visitation policy while at the same time being isolated from critical information regarding my husband's condition.

What if Rob's PCR test result had been a false positive, and we had been unnecessarily separated? Besides, as they implied, if Rob was in critical condition, how could they keep me out when family members have every right to visit relatives in critical condition?

What if Rob "tanked" and died while I was sitting at home without having felt the touch of his hand since he was hospitalized on September 3rd? I needed to see him, he needed me, and I had every right to be with him. Yet these heartless criminals kept him locked away from me and refused my admission.

Every day, I was learning more and more about others who were suffering or who had suffered the same fate as Rob and me. I wondered how many other patients and family members had been asked, "Do you want to die?" by their doctors, and how many others had been pressured by their doctors into agreeing to be intubated while being harmed by unnecessary medications that had dangerous side effects.

Rob knew his chances of survival on a ventilator were little to none. That was why he had told the doctors and nurses he did **not** want to be intubated. He wanted "DO NOT INTUBATE" clearly noted in his hospital records. Yet, here he was, on a ventilator, yet somehow still alive. I knew there might still be time to save him from the narcissistic doctors who lived by the motto: "*Not your will, but **OUR** will be done. Amen!*"

I called Ms. Destroyer, the Social Worker with whom I had spoken on the day Rob was placed on the ventilator, hoping she would be willing and able to assist me. Even though she was a hospital employee who advocated for the doctors and the hospital, and she had only given me lip service in the past, I felt it was worthwhile to reach out to her again in the hopes that she would at least attempt to listen to and address my concerns.

However, as usual, she was not at her desk, and my call landed in her voicemail. As I anxiously waited for her to return my call, I wrote my questions and concerns down on a notepad. Then, the phone rang. It was Ms. Destroyer, the Social Worker. She apologized, "Sorry it took me a minute to call you back. But I'm here now. What can I do for you?"

Daring to hope she might be willing to aid me in my quest to save Rob, I advised her, "I just finished speaking with Dr. Wicked. He explained that Rob had setbacks this past weekend, and he didn't respond well to coming **off** the paralytics. Dr. Wicked wants to build up his strength. My question is, how can we get the doctors to prescribe intravenous vitamin C?

"They have continually refused it and are now trying to crush up small tablets and put them in his feeding tube. I believe IV vitamin C could help him regain his strength." She replied, "I don't know. I mean, it has to be ordered by a physician; I don't know what the barrier to doing that would be. Sometimes a component is the COST."

I was shocked, and my mouth hit the floor. Why would the cost of anything matter when we had medical insurance? Even if we had no insurance, I would have sold everything we owned to pay for whatever my husband needed to save his life. In a smart aleck sort of way, she continued, "So, I'm just going to be honest, **COST** is a **BIG** consideration in hospitals."

I could not believe what I was hearing. How costly could IV vitamin C be compared to the high-cost drugs Rob was being given, the ICU's daily room rate, and the expense of the ventilator he was on? Her illogical and insensitive answer had my head spinning. How could "cost" be a consideration when a life was at stake? If "cost" were the deciding factor, I had even more reason to fear for Rob's life.

Her break with reality continued, "So, even something as simple like, for example, this is just the example, I would have to ask our pharmacist to know the difference . . . and this may not be the case at all, but just so you have a frame of reference, something as simple as oral Tylenol, you know, that you buy from the drugstore, costs like five bucks for a bottle of 50 or whatever. Here, an oral Tylenol is also inexpensive. When you switch to the IV format, with certain medications, it compounds cost exorbitantly. So, for an oral Tylenol, maybe we might charge five bucks per pill. For the IV form, each dose can be thousands of dollars. With the benefit of something like IV vitamin C, **how are we going to justify the cost?**"

What a ridiculous thing to say when a patient's life might be hanging in the balance! I thought, "What planet is she on, and what kind of dribble is this? Is she nuts or just making things up as she goes? My husband's life is at stake, and she is talking about having to justify the cost of IV vitamin C!"

She dribbled on, "I don't know the answer to that question. I'm not trying to tell you so that it comes across like, wow, my loved ones are certainly worth every penny of that. Well, yes, we all are, from the standpoint it makes a difference." Had she seen so much death in her ICU that she didn't think IV vitamin C would make any difference and would be a waste of their money?"

She continued, "I certainly don't want to challenge your optimism." By saying it might not make any difference and that they might be wasting their money on IV vitamin C she certainly was challenging my optimism regarding Rob's chances of survival at Covid Coven Hospital of Plano, Texas.

I found it ironic that she was crabbing about the potential cost of IV vitamin C while, at the same time, they could waste as much money as they wished on massive doses of high-powered (and potentially incentivized) sedatives, paralytics, steroids, antibiotics, analgesics, vasodilators, anti-coagulants, and diuretics—and Rob was on multiples of each of these. Of course, kickbacks were unavailable for beneficial nutrients such as IV vitamin C.

She then said, "Because we have every reason to be optimistic for Rob, **but I don't know if I would go so far as to say he's in recovery.** We're still fighting this nasty thing." I shook my head in disbelief. Was she trying to say in a coldhearted way that it did not make sense to waste any more money on a patient like Rob, who was likely to die anyway since he wasn't in recovery?

I said, "I'll bring in cash for the IV vitamin C." Shocked at my boldness, she laughed and said, "There's a system, and it's against the law, and it's fraud! How can we send somebody in there to give him vitamin C IV? It would be a liability issue; it comes with a whole host of problems." She wasn't getting it. I had not told her I planned to hire someone from the outside to come in and administer IV vitamin C to Rob. Many IV clinics in the Dallas/Fort Worth area offered IV vitamin C, and I was offering to procure and provide IV vitamin C from one of those clinics at my own cost. So, I asked, "But I have insurance; you can't add it to the insurance bill?"

The insanity continued, as Ms. Destroyer asserted. "No. Insurance doesn't pay us per service or medication, or even per day. What insurances pays hospitals . . . every insurance is **X amount of dollars based on a diagnosis**. So, if someone's in the hospital with pneumonia, and they're in the hospital five days, or ten days, **we get the same amount of money.** So, we are being asked to be **a good steward of the resources** that we're given because they may be in the hospital for 20 days, but we may only be getting paid X amount of dollars that maybe covers the cost of the first three days, five days, or seven days. I don't know; every insurance is different."

Her penny-pinching attitude regarding my husband's life infuriated me. Was this the reason they chose to not feed my husband? Was it because they had to be good stewards of their money? I was shocked to hear her say that insurance companies paid one flat amount per diagnosis and that the hospitals had to be "good stewards" of the limited amount of money they would be paid. In the past, when I had family members at this same hospital, they had billed for each day of their stay and for every medication and treatment they received.

As a result, I wondered if the Social Worker who told me on September 9th that she had worked at this hospital for twenty years was entirely out of touch with reality or, worse, if she was purposely lying to me. In any case, I found her remarks extremely disturbing.

Ms. Destroyer when on, "Every patient is different. So, it's not something that we can bill extra. The hospital and the insurance companies have contracts. And they have agreed to pay us **X amount of dollars per diagnosis. That's it.** So, it doesn't matter what service the patient is getting while they're here. We're not getting paid extra, or less or more, depending on what services they're getting or for the length of time that they're in the hospital. **We just have to be a good steward of the resources, and that's all—you understand?"**

If what she said were true, the faster a patient could be stabilized and discharged, the more profitable it would be for the hospital. Therefore, they should make every effort to assist patients in recovering as quickly as possible using the least number and smallest dosages of potentially harmful medications (and therapies) possible. But, unfortunately, it would also mean that patients who required an extended stay would have their care rationed as they became ever-increasing cost burdens.

Overall, I found her claims hard to believe, and I hoped she was mistaken (or attempting to deceive me) because the last thing I wanted was for Rob's doctors and staff to take a cost-conscious approach to Rob's care. Thus, I challenged her logic by responding, "That doesn't make sense! I apologize for my ignorance about the cost, but I feel very strongly about it—and when you say 'price,' if it's the price, I'll pay myself."

With a slightly apologetic voice, she said, "I hesitate to say it because I don't want you to think that we're not doing everything that needs to be done that's <u>within reason</u>. What I'm saying is I don't even know if that's a factor. But I can tell you what certainly is a factor. We're not going to give medications that aren't really aren't necessary. I'm not saying that this isn't necessary. I'm just saying, we're looking at, you know, is this necessary? Does this warrant the cost? **DOES IT MAKE A DIFFERENCE IN THIS PATIENT'S OUTCOME**? Those sorts of things are decision points for every patient, no matter why they're here."

By saying, "Does this warrant the cost? Does it make a difference in this patient's outcome?" was she trying to assert that they had already decided my husband's fate and had determined that any "extra" therapies such as IV vitamin C were not "worth the cost?"

The patient would always lose if it came down to costs and the hospital's bottom line. Obviously, my calling her in the hope she might advocate for me and Rob was a total waste of my time and energy. The whole conversation made me sick with worry that they might have starved Rob from the day of his admission as a "cost-saving" measure. In truth, it seemed as if everyone I spoke with at this hospital gave me the same *"why would you want this life-saving therapy for your husband"* runaround.

I vainly tried to explain, "If I said that I want you to give Rob salt and pepper in his mouth every night, three times a day, then, of course, I would expect the hospital to say, 'Well, doing that costs money because we would have to put people on it, and we're not going to do that because there's no research proving it's efficacy.' I would completely understand the hospital's stand on that. However, my issue is that there is a lot of data on IV vitamin C supporting recovery. That's my position. *I'm asking for an IV vitamin C drip, not something unproven!*" She coldly replied, "In my 20 years, I've never seen us do that."

LEGAL COUNSEL STATEMENT

Members of the jury, Ms. Destroyer, excused her refusal to advocate for Rob being administered IV vitamin C by misleading Sheila and asking her to believe that health insurance only pays hospitals one flat fee per diagnosis without any regard for the duration of a patient's stay or the medications and treatments being provided. As you read above, she said, "*With the benefit of something like IV vitamin C, **how are we going to justify the cost?** So, we are being asked to be **a good steward of the resources** that we're given because they may be in the hospital for 20 days, but we may only be getting paid X amount of dollars that maybe covers the cost of the first three days, five days, or seven days.*"

After Rob's death, while reviewing the hospital bill with a representative in the hospital's billing department, Sheila asked the representative, "*I was trying to get some healthier therapies for Rob, and when I asked the Social Worker if she could please talk with the doctors and get them approved she said all insurances pay by diagnosis, and it doesn't matter if they're in the hospital for one day or ten days—it's just one flat rate. So, they needed to be good stewards of the money. Then, when I received the **110-page itemized bill**, I wondered why someone who had worked there for twenty years would say that.*" The billing office representative responded, "*I do apologize. I can't answer that, unfortunately. It does sound like it was a little rude and insensitive. **It doesn't even make any sense to me as well.**"

> *We contend that this 20-year hospital veteran is guilty of willful misconduct by purposely misleading Sheila, thereby helping deny Rob access to a vital nutrient that could have significantly aided his recovery.*
>
> On its face, her contention that giving Rob intravenous vitamin C would not be a good use of the hospital's resources because of the "cost" was ludicrous, especially in light of the massive number of harmful and expensive drugs that were administered to Rob during his 40-day nightmare at Covid Coven Hospital of Plano, TX. Below is the total bill for just a few of those medications:
>
> - **Tocilizumab** (rheumatoid arthritis drug for a condition Rob did not have) = $12,174.62
> - **The aerosol administration of VELETRI** at a cost of nearly $2,500/day x 38 days = $92,000
> - **Nimbex** (a paralytic used while Rob was on the ventilator) $1,070/dose x 50 doses = $53,500
> - **VELETRI** (instead of the budesonide they requested) $148.36 per dose x 104 doses = $15,429
> - **Remdesivir** (a drug Rob and Sheila asked he not be given) $1,000/dose x 8 vials over 6 doses = $8,000

The more I challenged Ms. Destroyer's logic, the more nervous she sounded. She rambled on, **"That doesn't mean that it shouldn't or couldn't be done. I'm just saying it's not the standard in health care at the moment**, but I will ask about it. Because, again, you never know until you ask the question. There might be a really good reason . . . there might be simply . . . I don't know why we couldn't do it. **It's just not something we typically do . . . that sort of thing.** And it's okay to ask that question. I don't have the answers. So, I don't want you to hang your hat on anything I've said and then feel like I will . . . I will find out why we don't or why we can't if that's the case. I just don't know."

Did she know, or did she **not** know? Did she have the answers, or did she **not** have the answers? Was she thinking, *"I'll just make it up as I go, as I run interference for my team"*? Had no one ever asked for something as simple as IV vitamin C during her 20 years as a Social Worker at the hospital? It felt as if I had been transported back to a time when Radium treatments were used for constipation and the spraying of DDT on children playing in the streets to kill mosquitoes was common.

Here, Rob was totally paralyzed and fully sedated (in a coma) on an invasive, positive-pressure ventilator while being continuously assaulted by a massive number and high doses of what I considered "more harmful than helpful" pharmaceuticals being administered via IV or nebulized into his airway—yet a 20-year veteran of the hospital was telling me providing him with IV vitamin C, a critical nutrient that could improve his chances of recovery, might not be cost-effective.

I asked the Social Worker what the plan would be once Rob got off the ventilator. She then perked up and said, "It can take them several weeks of needing some amount of oxygen, oxygen support . . . just not as much as he has been given, right? So, while he's in the hospital coming off the vent, the very first thing we're gonna do the minute he can tolerate it is implement some **physical therapy**, **occupational therapy**, and **speech therapy**, if needed. Speech usually is looking more at swallowing after being on the vent for a number of days.

"It is very possible he's going to need a short stay at some sort of rehab facility where he can still have nursing care, doctor oversight, and oxygen while he continues to wean down. It could take time, and he could need a lot more therapy. We would help arrange for that. The rehabs in our community are taking folks who are recovering from Covid. They just can't take a patient who's still needing 50 liters of oxygen. We need to see him able to take nutrition the good old-fashioned way, through our mouths, and that he's able to void properly. That sort of thing."

What? He might need to relearn how to swallow, speak, feed himself, urinate properly, and walk because he would leave the ventilator incapacitated and still require oxygen. Then, once his oxygen requirement was reduced, he would be transferred to a rehabilitation facility for what could be a long-term recovery!

She then admitted, "Now, if for some reason, weaning from the vent proves to be more difficult than we had hoped . . . Then we have different conversations, and we talk about things like trachs—and I don't want to go down that road and freak you out."

I **was** freaking out! She had painted a bleak picture of the long-term suffering and rehabilitation one who survived long-term on a ventilator would face. In contrast, I had been told by Dr. Dead End that Rob just needed a brief period of rest and that they would be trying to wake him daily to assess his condition and determine if they could remove him from the ventilator.

Rob had been on the ventilator for five days now, and they had been unable to awaken him and attempt to wean him off of it. Furthermore, it was becoming evident that his "little rest" would, at best, result in weeks if not months of rehabilitation—which was critical information they had purposefully withheld from me until now.

She then touched on a conversation she had with another family. "Yeah, here's the thing, I had this conversation with a family last week because there was the possibility of needing a trach. And look, there are in my 20 years of being in the hospital, there are times that the tracheostomy is an option for patients. And there are scenarios, without going into a ridiculous amount of detail, when a person is never going to have that trach removed. **They're never going to be mobile; they'll be bedbound. They're not going to know what's going on. They have neurological deficits.** And I think, oh, I don't . . . I know I wouldn't want that. Right?"

I felt nauseated after hearing her describe these horrifying potential outcomes. I had been attempting to convince myself that Rob would survive this nightmare and return home intact. Instead, she had instilled in me an indescribable sense of dread as I imagined him bedridden with neurological deficits.

She continued explaining what Rob might have to deal with **IF** he should be blessed enough to survive the ventilator. She said, "But when I look at that scenario, the trach is sort of a sign or a symbol for something **bigger**. The trach is just a tool; it's just a way to move that tube out of his mouth down to his throat. And it has no intention of being permanent. Right. I mean that it is a temporary tool to utilize to get him off that darned vent once and for all." I pleaded, "I know I've asked a million times whether I could see Rob or be there. Of course, I know he's on a paralytic and sedated. So, if I were there, I would not be in the way. But, if I can't come in to see him, could someone take pictures of him to show me he's doing okay?"

She said, "It's actually against our hospital policy; we can't even take pictures. I can take an iPad in there, and you can . . . I've had other families, unbeknownst to me, figure out how to video or record that FaceTime call. I don't know how to do that. I'm not going to pretend to know how. Okay. But we can do, like, you know, a couple of times a week, do FaceTimes where I can get one of us to just take it in the room.

"You can kind of see his room, and like his bed, and different views or whatever. But then I can also just leave it in there for 10-15 minutes, and you just say to us you want to be alone with him. I would step out; you could talk to him like you would as if you were at his bedside, then you snap whatever screenshots you want to take. Whatever you're doing on the other end, I have no control over. We can't do them every day for big chunks of time because we have 30 patients in the same boat."

I was shocked to hear that they had thirty patients "in the same boat" in their ICU. Were they all on ventilators? If so, this was indeed a money-making scheme similar to those run by organized crime.

She tried to make it sound like I could have a honeymoon FaceTime with my comatose husband, and she would be the heroine who had made it all happen. Although I could not be there in person and touch him, I could have the honor of seeing him through the lens of my iPhone or iPad. Should I bow down and kiss her feet? What I **really** wanted was to ensure Rob was being treated well and see him up close. I wanted to be **with** him to see his condition and treatments in person.

The reason I wanted ongoing pictures was to keep track of him daily so I could see what they were doing to him. Scheduling a FaceTime "chat" would not give me the same information. Even daycare centers offer live video feeds and send pictures of the children in their care so parents may monitor their condition and treatment from a distance. If parents demand and receive transparency, why can't hospital staff take and send family members pictures of patients who are being locked away "in isolation." HIPAA surely does not prevent them from doing so.

Despite my extreme disappointment, I told her I definitely did want her to set up a FaceTime "visit" with Rob and for her to do so as soon as possible. She said the best she could do was schedule the "visit" for tomorrow afternoon. I knew I needed to emotionally brace myself for what I was likely to witness.

I asked, "How soon can I come into the hospital and **see** my husband in person? I waited as she calculated the time and repeated what she had told me on September 9th. "Yeah, cuz we have his first positive as September 3rd, twenty days will be September 23rd. The date isn't everything. For example, we have some patients who have stayed in isolation **longer** because they were actually just doing worse by that point.

"And there are people that we've tested who said they were positive two months ago, went to rehab, and then they came back. We tested them because it's part of our admitting process for every patient now, and they're still positive."

I said, "You mean you guys don't question whether what you're seeing is a **false** positive?" She responded, "If we did a rapid test, then yes, we don't feel as confident in the rapid test. Not if it's a PCR test, meaning that it's sent off. The ones we send off take a couple of days to get results. So, it's a little different with the noses, but I hear you. Again, you hear stories, and I'm not saying that they're not true."

LEGAL COUNSEL STATEMENT
Members of the jury, Sheila raised a good question regarding the results of Rob's PCR (Polymerase Chain Reaction) test. PCR tests "amplify" small segments of DNA via a "thermal cycling" method that helps manufacture up to billions of copies of a specific DNA sample.

At the time, in the U.S., the PCR test was generally **cycled up to 40 times** to detect "viral fragments" from nasal or throat samples. However, **cycles of greater than 35 can be relatively meaningless** because they may detect **fragments of dead viruses** or a **nucleotide** (a fundamental building block of DNR and RNA) that are **mistaken** for a live virus fragment. Thus, most of the "positive" results are false positives.

The March 27, 2020, issue of the Lancet Infectious Diseases Volume 20, Issue 6, contained an article titled "*Understanding COVID-19: What does viral RNA load really mean?*" where they stated, "*The inability to differentiate between infective and non-infective (dead or antibody-neutralized) viruses remains a major limitation of nucleic acid detection.*"
Joynt, G. M., & Wu, W. K. K. (2020, March 27). Understanding covid-19: What does viral RNA load really mean? The Lancet Infectious Diseases. From https://www.thelancet.com/journals/laninf/article/PIIS1473-3099(20)30237-1/fulltext

Robert F. Kennedy, Jr. noted in his book <u>The Real Anthony Fauci: Bill Gates, Big Pharma, and the Global War on Democracy and Public Health</u>, "*Regulators misused PCR tests that CDC belatedly admitted in August 2021 were incapable of distinguishing COVID from other viral illnesses. Dr. Fauci tolerated their use at inappropriately high amplitudes of 37 and up to 45, even though Fauci had told Vince Rasaniello [Professor of Microbiology & Immunology at Mt. Sinai School of Medicine of CUNY and co-author of the textbook <u>Principles of Virology</u>] that tests employing cycle thresholds of 35 and above were very unlikely to indicate the presence of*

My call with Ms. Destroyer left me fearful and perplexed. I wondered whether she was misinformed, was intentionally deceiving me, or if it were true that insurance companies paid hospitals one lump sum per diagnosis, leading to their rationing care. Regardless, if Rob survived the ventilator, she had made it clear he would be crippled by the experience and end up in rehabilitation.

In the evening, I called the ICU nurse's station to check on Rob's status. The nurse who answered said, "You know that paralytic medicine? That Nimbex. They turned it off this afternoon. He was doing fine. Then he was trying to move a little bit; he was fighting a little, he was struggling. So, he was having a lot of secretion, like a bloody secretion, through the tube. **So, we had to bag him for some time**.

"Then we needed to paralyze him back. Now, he's better. His blood pressure is 172/75, and his oxygen saturation is actually 91 right now. Heart rate is 88. **On FiO2, we had to go up to 100%.** Because we had all this difficulty, we will slowly go down on it. He's resting right now. We also ordered an X-ray to make sure everything is okay."

Sadly, Rob and I had fought hard to keep him **off** the ventilator. But unfortunately, Rob and I were now trapped in a nightmare, and he was apparently "fighting" the ventilator in vain attempts at extracting himself whenever they lowered the sedatives and the paralytics.

LEGAL COUNSEL STATEMENT

Members of the jury, the sad situation the nurse described was another failed attempt at reducing the paralytics. We say, "another failed attempt," because a note in the hospital record entered at 5:27 AM the same morning says, "Remains sedated and paralyzed with Versed and Nimbex drips. **Weaned off Nimbex slowly as patient went into distress the last time.**"

A note entered at 2:52 PM, after the failed attempt, states, "Did not tolerate being off paralytics." At 5:59 PM, a nurse entered a note in the records stating, "When nimbex was stopped **pt [patient] became agitated and fighting ventilator.**"

The doctors told Sheila that placing Rob on a ventilator would be beneficial as it would give him a "little rest" and give his lungs time to heal. Yet, as the nurse shared, trying to reduce the paralytics led to Rob "fighting a little," which resulted in blood appearing in his endotracheal tube. The presence of blood required removing Rob from the ventilator, clearing the tube, manually "bagging" Rob, then placing him back on the ventilator.

- *"Bagging"* refers to the manual ventilation of a patient using a self-inflating manual resuscitator bag (also known as an Ambu bag or manual resuscitator). A nurse or doctor attaches the hand-held bag to the endotracheal tube and manually squeezes it to deliver air or oxygen to the patient.

They failed to disclose to Sheila that once a patient had been on a ventilator for over a week, weaning them from the device was nearly impossible. Lowering the sedatives and paralytics would lead to the patient "struggling" or "over-breathing." During that "struggle," the patient's blood oxygen level would rapidly drop to dangerously low levels because they were "fighting the vent" as they attempted to breathe on their own and at their own pace. The precipitous drop in the patient's blood oxygen level would cause the doctors to immediately raise the sedatives and paralytics—returning the patient to the former "calm" and comatose state.

Erin Olszewski, BSN, RN, in her book <u>Undercover Epicenter Nurse</u> said that while speaking with other nurses about a 35-year-old patient who had been heavily sedated, one of the nurses said, *"He cannot use his muscles, he is deconditioning."* A second nurse said, *"The amount of sedation is crazy. It's literally destroying their internal organs. They'll never come off."* A third nurse responded, *"Their brains will never be the same."*

Olszewski, Erin. Page 80. Undercover Epicenter Nurse: How Fraud, Negligence, & Greed Led to Unnecessary Deaths at Elmhurst Hospital, Skyhorse, 2020.

Emotionally and physically exhausted, I collapsed into bed. I closed my eyes tightly, desperately attempting to block out the voices of the doctors and nurses, which had all morphed into voices of doom. My mom, who was staying the night with me, heard me call out in the dark, "Mom, are you there?" She quickly came running to my bedside. "I'm here, Honey," she said. I sobbed, "Mom, I'm so afraid!" Tears gushed from my eyes. She held me tight and prayed.

I whimpered, "I'm so afraid my phone will ring, and they're going to tell me Rob is dead!" She attempted to reassure me that Rob would survive and continued praying while gently stroking my back until I fell asleep.

Chapter 6 – Continuation & Desperation

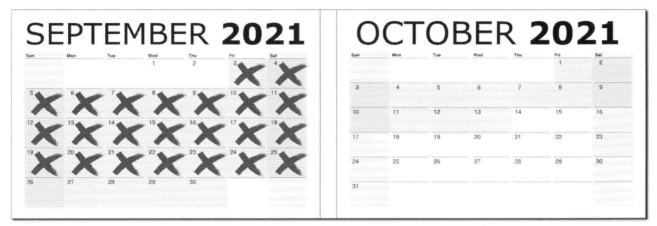

THIS CHAPTER COVERS SEPTEMBER 14-25

Tuesday, September 14, 2021

I was worried and filled with fear, and it showed. I grabbed my phone and decided to make my morning hospital call before getting out of bed. I noticed I had not missed any hospital calls, so Rob must still be alive. I was hoping no news was good news.

It seemed like each time I called, a new nurse would be assigned to Rob. Today, it was Nurse Danger. When I asked her about his vitals, she rattled them off, then asked in a snarky tone, "Do you even understand what they mean?" I found her question extremely rude and insulting.

Even though I lacked a medical background, I was doing my best to keep up with Rob's medical information. I meticulously documented my husband's vital signs, medications and dosages, lab results, and PEEP and FiO_2 settings.

After all, how else could they have expected me to advocate for him? I needed to keep track of all the critical data so that I might quickly identify negative trends that could indicate Rob's life was at further risk, allowing me to challenge new treatments in time to prevent further injury to Rob.

I wished I did not have to do any of this, but it was obvious to me that the doctors and nurses were treating Rob as just another one of their ventilated patients who would likely die. In reality, they just wanted to get through another workday. I wanted my husband to survive and come home.

Being treated with such contempt put me on guard. So, I asked, "Can you tell me something? I know we've been teetering with reducing the paralytic and then quickly increasing it again. Do you know where it's at right now?" She responded that he was currently on a continuous IV infusion of 3 mcg per kilogram per minute of Nimbex, which I jotted down in my notebook.

I then requested that she keep Rob's phone charged and have it play a continuous loop of music his mind something to focus on. I was relieved to hear that his phone was still up and running, as I believed that a loop of familiar music could provide him with a connection to the outside world and memories of us together.

I asked, "Do you know if they plan to reduce the paralytic tonight?" She quickly added, "No, because we tried to reduce it last night, and **it did not go well**." I replied, "Yeah, I know, he was off the paralytic and started fighting the ventilator, but then he settled down after they raised the paralytic back up. That was how I understood it."

She agreed and said, "So, back to being paralyzed. Like, you know, he was having a lot of fixation. So, he was coughing. And he was like desaturating. So, they had to, like, suction him really good and put him on **high flow 100%**."

> **LEGAL COUNSEL STATEMENT**
> Members of the jury, by saying "he was having a lot of fixation," Nurse Danger confirmed what another nurse had told Sheila the day before about their failed attempt to reduce the paralytic (Nimbex). During that call, the other nurse had said Rob "was fighting a little, he was struggling."
>
> The word "fixation" typically refers to the use of medications to sedate or calm the patient and minimize movement or agitation, and by saying "he was having a lot of fixation," she was likely implying Rob's chest, diaphragm, and intercostal muscles (the muscles located between the ribs that help expand and contract the ribcage during breathing) were not fully relaxed. When this occurs, the ventilator cannot properly inflate and deflate the lungs, which causes the patient's blood oxygen level to drop rapidly to dangerous levels.
>
> *Unfortunately, as is true of most other "ventilated" patients, Rob was not on a lifesaving therapy but on a one-way trip to the morgue.*

I knew that prolonged exposure to 100% oxygen could damage the lungs, but whenever they tried to reduce the sedatives and wean him off the paralytics, they said he would "fight" the ventilator. As a result, his blood oxygen level would drop, he would be re-sedated, the paralytics would be increased, and the FiO2 (oxygen concentration) would be increased **back up to 100%.** How could anyone be expected to survive this type of ongoing assault?

I had repeatedly asked the doctors and nurses NOT to attempt to wean him from the ventilator unless I were present, but they continued their futile attempts to wean him while no one who loved him was present to reassure him that everything would be all right.

I decided to try again to convince the Social Worker to advocate that Rob receive an IV vitamin C drip. To my surprise, she answered her phone. Unfortunately, her abrupt and curt answer was a simple, "No. It's just NOT something that's a standard carry." As usual, it was far easier for someone at this hospital to give me a flat-out "No" than a "Maybe, let's find out" or, God forbid, a "Yes."

I asked, "So, you couldn't give him IV vitamin C because you just don't have it?" She emphatically agreed, "We don't have it to give. It's just not a typical hospital formulary medication, I guess."

I was outright flabbergasted, "Well, I saw something about your honoring patient's beliefs on your 'Patient Rights' document. I've done so much research on IV vitamin C, and some hospitals **do** use it. So, you said there's no way to even ask for it?"

She insisted, "We just don't have it. So, I'm not a pharmacist; you know, I just don't know. So, I mean, I can pass it on to people that can give you a better response. But at the moment, I can tell you, we don't have it."

Was she making this up? How could IV vitamin C be not generally stocked in the hospital pharmacy? Are hospital pharmacies only stocked with prescription IV medications that have a laundry list of adverse side effects? Are they never stocked with vital nutrients such as vitamin C that have NO adverse side effects and cannot cause any harm? Was this how they were "good stewards" of the alleged lump sum of insurance money they received per patient and diagnosis?

When I repeated my offer to try to purchase IV vitamin C and bring it to the hospital, she retorted, "There's hospital policy about bringing in medications from the outside. And I don't begin to understand the logistics of that. So, I don't want to speak to my client and tell you the wrong thing. But there's some policies about what we can administer, and we cannot administer medications that are not provided by us."

I told her the rehab facilities I had called had said offering IV vitamin C was something hospitals should do, yet every time I asked her I was told the hospital would not cooperate. Thus, it was something they could not and would not do.

Taken aback, Ms. Destroyer replied, "I'm not saying we're not cooperating. I'm just saying **we don't have it to give.** So I don't know what it would take to get it, or I just don't know. So, again, I'm going to let that be in the hands of people that know more than me; I'll pass it on to our pharmacy."

I could tell by the tone of her voice that she had become agitated by my insistence that they stop denying my requests, which I considered to be totally reasonable. Trying to remain optimistic, I said, "Okay. If you could speak with the pharmacy about it, that would be great. And I'll work on my end to see if there's any other way to get it in there." She said she was in a hurry and that we could talk more about it tomorrow.

LEGAL COUNSEL STATEMENT

Members of the jury, can you imagine why a hospital pharmacy would not carry IV vitamin C? Could it be because it is not a high-cost, highly profitable, and potentially harmful drug?

When it comes to "costs vs. benefits," doctors and hospitals generally focus on what benefits them, not what benefits patients. They stock and administer high-cost, life-threatening, and extremely risky pharmaceuticals that provide them with the greatest profit margins while ignoring and refusing to administer low-cost alternatives that might provide patients with far greater benefits at little to no risk.

They live in a "pill for every ill" fantasy world where an inadequate amount of prescription medications in your body is alleged to be the cause of, or at least the reason for, every symptom or disease.

Although low-cost **budesonide** (for which they charged only **$19.39 per dose**) could have provided Rob with significant benefits (see **Appendix F**), the doctors at Covid Coven Hospital of Plano, TX, preferred to administer a higher-cost drug named **VELETRI** (for which they charged **$148.36 per dose**). We contend this drug caused Rob significant harm, harm that helped them eventually get Rob on a ventilator. Of course, that had been their goal for him from the moment he arrived with "Covid" symptoms.

Clearly, what used to be a motto of "above all else, do no harm" has become "above all else, make the most

After every conversation with anyone connected to the hospital, I had to take several deep breaths because it was so distressing and disheartening. I had never had to fight with people over the phone like this, and I was having to literally fight for my husband's life. I fully intended to keep pressing on and looking for ways to get Rob the nutrients and beneficial medications that other doctors used daily to save Covid patients.

LEGAL COUNSEL STATEMENT

Members of the jury, as noted on Page 235 of the hospital records (see Page C-48), when they again attempted to reduce the sedatives, Rob desaturated (his blood oxygen level dropped) into the low 70s—which led to their having to increase the FiO2 (fraction of inspired oxygen he was breathing) back up to **100%.**

Normal room air has 21% oxygen, and breathing in high levels of oxygen (levels of greater than 60%) for over 24 hours can lead to "**oxygen toxicity,**" otherwise known as "**oxygen poisoning.**" The result is oxidative damage to the cell membranes of the lungs, leading to the collapse of the alveoli. *Sadly, as shown in the chart at the bottom of Page C-54 in Appendix C, they maintained Rob's oxygen level at well above 60% most of the time during Rob's 35 days on the ventilator.*

A November 2012 article in the Respiratory Care magazine titled "**Practice of Excessive FiO2 and Effect on Pulmonary Outcomes in Mechanically Ventilated Patients With Acute Lung Injury**" noted, "*Titration of supplemental oxygen [oxygen therapy at the lowest levels necessary to maintain a target blood oxygen level of 92–96%] is important, but not adequately practiced. . . . Excessive oxygen supplementation is common in mechanically ventilated patients with acute lung injury and may be associated with worsening lung function at 48 hours.*"

Rachmale, S., Li, G., Wilson, G., Malinchoc, M., & Gajic, O. (2012, November 1). Practice of excessive FIO2 and effect on pulmonary outcomes in mechanically ventilated patients with acute lung injury. American Association for Respiratory Care. From https://rc.rcjournal.com/content/57/11/1887

A National Library of Medicine June 2015 article on "**Acute use of oxygen therapy**" noted, "*A major change is needed in the entrenched culture of routinely administering high-concentration oxygen to acutely ill patients regardless of need.*" Further, they said, "*mortality was over two times higher in patients who received routine high-concentration oxygen compared with those who received titrated oxygen therapy [oxygen therapy at the lowest levels necessary to maintain a target blood oxygen level of 92–96%]*" and stated that "*the routine administration of high-concentration oxygen to acutely unwell patients has the potential to cause harm.*"

Pilcher, J., & Beasley, R. (2015, June). Acute use of oxygen therapy. Australian prescriber. From https://www.ncbi.nlm.nih.gov/pmc/articles/PMC4653960

Sadly, the medical examiner who conducted Rob's private autopsy said his lungs looked "*shredded*" and were totally "unsurvivable" after his 36 days on the ventilator. She said she had never seen lungs in such a deteriorated condition and that they did not even look human.

This further proves that Rob died of "the protocol," not Covid. We contend that Rob's lungs were systematically destroyed by a ruthless team of doctors, respiratory therapists, and nurses who saw him as just another "Covid" patient who was going to die of the "disease" as they seemed to always do at Covid Coven Hospital of Plano, TX.

For more on the dangers of high levels of oxygen over extended periods, see the National Library of Medicine's "**Oxygen Toxicity**" article at https://www.ncbi.nlm.nih.gov/books/NBK430743

Jean Froissart (1337–1405), a French-speaking medieval author and court historian, once said: "*Doctors need three qualifications:*
* *to be able to lie and not get caught,*
* *to pretend to be honest, and*
* *to cause death without guilt.*"

The "protocol-focused" doctors Rob and Sheila encountered at Covid Coven Hospital of Plano, Texas, clearly met all three qualifications.

Wednesday, September 15, 2021

I awoke with an overwhelming feeling of dread and uncertainty. For a week now, I had been attempting to save Rob's kidneys and liver from injury by a barrage of medications. I was also trying to protect his lungs from further damage by the excessively high oxygen levels (up to 100%) and the high residual pressure (a PEEP of 14) on the ventilator.

Although I had never felt so much fear, I finally mustered the courage to make my morning call to the hospital. I spoke with Dr. Wicked, who was his usual chipper self. I wondered how he could be so upbeat when my husband, who had been improving on high-flow nasal cannula oxygen alone, was now on a ventilator—a device from which they appeared to have no clear strategy for weaning him.

It was clear Rob's situation had quickly transitioned from him just needing *"a little rest"* to *"Oh crap, he's deteriorating, and we can't figure out how to extract him from the supersonic 'ventilator' train we placed him on that is speeding toward the end of the track!"*

Once again, he said his favorite phrase, telling me, "Overall, we're stable." I was tired of Dr. Wicked's positive "overall stable" deceptive verbiage because being "stable" did not mean Rob would survive the ventilator. What I wanted and needed to hear was that he was "improving," that he was "getting stronger," and that he finally had the "reserves" he required to be able to be successfully weaned **OFF** the ventilator.

Rob was not on vacation. He was paralyzed and in an induced coma, leading to his muscles wasting away. In addition, he was continually assaulted by massive doses of harmful medications. I truly feared there was a significant risk that Rob could not and would not survive what they were doing to him.

I told Dr. Wicked I was also very concerned that, without me there, no one was encouraging Rob that he could pull through this. So, even though he was fully sedated and supposedly unconscious, I pleaded with him not to let anyone speak negatively in front of Rob. He said he would ask the nurses to be more mindful of their words in Rob's room and be more positive.

I was happy to hear that because I fully believed that "as a man thinks, so is he." It was my goal to ensure that Rob only heard positive affirmations that would encourage him that he could pull through this.

He continued, "So, his LFTs [Liver Function Tests] have been going up. Not terribly concerning at this point. But I did go ahead and get a study to see if it looked like a blockage in the bile duct or something, and all that looked okay. They look to be stabilizing today. He has a pattern, and it is **probably medication related.** There's a couple [of medications] that are possible [causes]. The **antibiotics** are the most likely."

I agreed with him that the massive numbers of pharmaceuticals he was being given were causing him to deteriorate and were destroying his liver. I asked him to STOP all the toxic drugs and get my husband breathing on his own again because the ventilator and all the heavy

He shocked me with, "We usually don't worry about stopping and changing his medications until the lab results are **more than 8 to 10 times the upper limit of normal**."

I was alarmed and could hardly believe Dr. Wicked had admitted they purposely waited until a drug had caused enough damage that the lab test result was finally "more than 8 to 10 times the upper limit of normal"—which in many cases would be a life-threatening range. Only then would they consider reducing or discontinuing a medication! Their standard action plan was to continue pushing more drugs on the patient until they were near organ failure. At that point, they would consider halting the assault.

When I went back and looked at Rob's online MyChart records, I could see that his LFTs (Liver Function Tests) **were** all trending upward. I learned that one critical measurement was ALT, a liver enzyme released into the bloodstream when liver cells are damaged or injured. The normal ALT level in the blood for men is 7 to 56 units per liter. His ALT level was 87 on September 11th, 112 on September 13th, 311 on September 14th, and had risen to 404 on September 15th.

> **LEGAL COUNSEL STATEMENT**
> Members of the jury, clear evidence that at Covid Coven Hospital of Plano, Texas, they do wait for lab tests to show results that are "8 to 10 times the upper limit of normal" appears on Page 259 of the hospital records (see Page C-50 in Appendix C). There you will see note #3 says, "***LFTs up. Monitor.*** *Cefepime [an antibiotic] most likely culprit…. **still under 8x upper limit normal**."*
>
> *What possible motive could they have for waiting for the drugs to cause sufficient damage to Rob's liver and kidneys to the point that the test results finally reached 8x to 10x their normal upper limit? If this isn't evidence of nefarious intent and malpractice, then what is?*

In his nonchalant manner, Dr. Wicked said, "And we're looking for organisms, and we're not there yet." I thought, "If they have not yet found any organisms, then why are they administering Rob such large quantities of antibiotics?"

"We're keeping an eye on it. Again, we're gonna try to work on getting him off of paralytics again. Overall, his oxygenation is stable; I am pleased with the X-ray. It seems to be stable. As I say, it's stable. I don't see any worsening of that pneumomediastinum or pneumothorax. It may be slowly clearing, but again, I don't want to get too excited about that. With these portable X-rays, the quality just isn't great. But it's definitely not worse."

How could he call Rob's condition "stable" when he was blowing out his lungs? Despite their assurances otherwise, each day I was learning more about how the ventilator was not lifesaving—but life-limiting.

They were further damaging Rob's lungs with the high PEEP (Positive End Expiratory Pressure) setting and with excessively high oxygen (FiO2) levels of up to 100%. Almost every time I asked about his FiO2 level, I was told they had to crank it up to **100% oxygen** again, which I knew was disastrous for his lungs.

Each time I called, I would ask the doctors to lower the quantity and dosages of Rob's medications so they could get him **OFF** the ventilator. **I told them they were killing my husband with their drugs, the high pressure, and the high oxygen (FiO2) levels**, but they either did not want to listen or, worse yet, they were listening but did not care. I already believed the 4.5 hours on the BiPAP had damaged his lungs to the point that they could force him on a ventilator—and now they were finishing the job with the heavy doses of medications and the high FiO2 and PEEP settings on the ventilator.

Whenever I expressed concerns, they would advise me to calm down because they were doing all they could. I thought, *"Yeah, you are. You're doing all you can to kill him!"* Yet, I could not go toe-to-toe with them as an equal because I was not a doctor. Thus, they tossed me, the simple wife of the patient, hollow platitudes and false assurances.

LEGAL COUNSEL STATEMENT
Members of the jury, as we noted earlier (in Chapter 3), just after midnight the evening of Rob's arrival in the Emergency Department, Dr. Useless wrote on Page 23 of Rob's hospital records (see Page C-2 in Appendix C), *"It is anticipated that he will require at least a two-midnight inpatient stay."*

At the same time, the Nurse Practitioner in the Emergency Department (ED) rejected that, and said Rob was *"at high risk for needing intubation"* while he was stabilizing on oxygen alone, as noted on Page 27 of the hospital records (see Page C-3), *In her view, Rob needed to be funneled to the ICU for an extended stay.*

So, although one honest ED physician had suggested Rob could possibly be stabilized and discharged in approximately two days, a Nurse Practitioner followed the "party line" and predicted Rob would likely require intubation and be *placed on a ventilator. Thus, she was clearly more on board with "the protocol."*

As we said previously—if Rob had been given only oxygen, antibiotics, steroids (for inflammation), and budesonide and had been provided with adequate nourishment so he could regain his strength—it is likely he <u>could</u> have gone home within a few days. *That should have been their "discharge plan" for Rob.*

Yet, as you have read, the medical staff were dead set on Rob following their pre-determined "treatment plan," a plan based on "the protocol that kills," where the goal was to flood Rob with as many debilitating drugs and harmful therapies as possible. *Sadly, they ultimately achieved their goal of ensuring Rob followed "the protocol" at the expense of his life.*

I advised Dr. Wicked that I had noticed in the MyChart records that Rob's hemoglobin level had declined. He explained, "We're checking blood on him every single day. So, we're drawing blood out of him, and then when you're acutely ill, your bone marrow often produces it, so it starts going down. Now, the question is, how low is too low? From our limited studies, if hemoglobin is down to about 7, we start to worry, and we recommend transfusing. So, we're well above that. But what happens to everybody in the ICU over a lengthy period is that they start getting anemia. It's very expected."

I asked him if the anemia might result from all the blood draws they were doing. He answered, "**Everyone** that's been here very long has it. A big part of it is that if you go to the OBGYN floor, nobody's anemic because over there, the blood marrow is all ramped up, breaking out and replacing everything. But when you're acutely ill and sick, you just don't make it as fast.

"And if you transfuse, trying to keep them normal or keep people up, that actually has higher **all-cause mortality** due to dying of other complications. So, we don't transfuse to keep it up normally. Again, everything we talked about—everything is risks versus benefits. So, we're nowhere near transfusion or anything at this point."

Members of the jury, anemia is a condition in which the body lacks sufficient red blood cells or hemoglobin to transport oxygen effectively to the body's tissues and organs.

Hemoglobin is the protein that carries oxygen in the blood. Low hemoglobin levels result in decreased oxygen being transported to the cells, causing fatigue, weakness, and shortness of breath. Anemia would, as Sheila inferred, weaken Rob further and have a significant negative impact on his chance of recovery.

Nutritional deficiencies, where the body is not receiving the nutrients required to produce healthy red blood cells, can cause anemia. *We know Rob had been allowed to become nutritionally deficient from the evening he arrived on September 3, 2021, twelve days earlier.*

On September 14, 2021, the day before, Dr. Wicked had said that being on paralytics "really accelerates muscle loss" and that they are the first thing he wanted to "get rid of." Yet when he tried to reduce the paralytic, Rob "coughed a little bit and **just didn't have the reserves**, so he dropped down [his blood oxygen level decreased]." *Rob was living on the edge, and with any form of anemia, he would never regain "the reserves" necessary to recover sufficiently to be removed from the ventilator.*

Sammy Wong, MD, our medical expert witness, said in his Interim Analysis in Appendix B, "*The diagnostic work up for the profound anemia was inadequately addressed.*" One of his Causes of Action was "*His hemoglobin dropped dramatically and was not addressed appropriately. Oxygen in the blood was adequate and blood was being circulated with a normal cardiac output but delivery to the tissues was profoundly lacking.*"

We contend that, whether by willful ignorance, uncaring negligence, or nefarious intent, the doctors' actions and inactions were the direct cause of Robert A. Skiba II's needless death.

I asked Dr. Wicked, "How long do you anticipate keeping Rob on fentanyl?" He quickly responded, "As long as you're on the ventilator. It is the most likely of our various sedation options. I think it is one of the better-tolerated ones. You don't get any medications to be at risk for interaction. There are some rare antibiotics that interact with it. You know, it's a cousin of morphine. So, it's, I think it's got a shorter half-life, so it's easier to titrate. But as long as he needs to have the tube in his throat, he will need the fentanyl. Yeah, we definitely can't tell if he's uncomfortable or not. I can't imagine anything worse than being paralyzed and not sedated."

The thought of Rob's waking up paralyzed had not crossed my mind—until now. To wake up, find yourself paralyzed, be unable to open your eyes, and discover an endotracheal tube shoved down your throat, would be horrifying.

Yet every time they tried to reduce the paralytics, they said Rob began to "fight the vent" and "desaturate." I wondered how many patients who had been on a ventilator for a week, like Rob, had been successfully "extubated" and removed from the ventilator—and I questioned what Rob's chances of survival truly were.

Members of the jury, as noted earlier, by September 14, 2021, just six days after being intubated and placed on a ventilator, the massive amounts of powerful and harmful drugs Rob was being bombarded with led to his **LFTs** (Liver Function Tests) being elevated.

As Dr. Torture noted on Page 254 of the hospital records (see Page C-49 in Appendix C), the LFT elevation was "**likely related to medications.**" On the afternoon of September 15, 2021, she noted on Page 266 (see Page C-51) that, "**Due to increasing LFTs Tylenol discontinued, will also change cefepime to Zosyn since GPT increased to 404.**"

Dr. Torture, therefore, admitted that the massive doses of Tylenol and cefepime (a broad-spectrum antibiotic usually administered via IV) were the likely cause of Rob's liver damage.

GPT is a common name for the ALT (Alanine Transaminase) blood test. Alanine Transaminase (ALT) is an enzyme primarily found in the liver that is a biomarker for liver injury. Elevated levels of ALT in the blood can indicate liver damage. A normal level of ALT in the blood is generally considered **less than 40 units per liter (U/L)** for men. Rob's ALT level had risen to **404**, *over ten times the normal maximum.* By October 12, 2021, the day before Rob died, his GPT level had increased to **5,480**! *This is criminal and requires justice!*

On Page 266 (see Page C-51), you will also see "Sedated on propofol." *Why would they be giving a fully sedated patient* **Tylenol** *when (a) Rob's vitals showed that for days Rob had been afebrile (had no fever) and (b) he was on high doses of* **fentanyl** *(a synthetic opioid estimated to be 50 to 100 times more potent than morphine). How can this be considered "health care?"*

In addition, on Page 266 (see Page C-51), you will see "*Remdesivir discontinued as per wife's wishes.*" *Why did it take until September 15th (one week after Rob's intubation) for them to finally recognize Sheila's Medical Power of Attorney and discontinue the remdesivir? Can there be any other explanation than that they were bound and determined to force* **THEIR WILL** *on Rob and Sheila without regard for their directives?*

As such, for their benefit and the benefit of the hospital, as we have stated earlier, the White Coat Cult at Covid Coven Hospital of Plano, Texas, knowingly and willfully violated **Title 42 of the Code of Federal Regulations, Section 482.13** (as noted in Appendix E) which states, "*The patient has the right to participate in the development and implementation of his or her plan of care,*" and that those rights include, "*being able to request or refuse treatment.*"

Thursday, September 16, 2021

Every day I was committed to finding a way to see Rob. I did not know how today would be different from any other day except that my determination had grown stronger. I decided to confront the "lockout" situation head-on. So I packed a small bag and drove to the hospital.

The "guard dog" receptionists were at the front desk as usual. I confidently approached them, made eye contact with each, and boldly stated, "I want to see my husband today!" I hoped my body language would convey my determination because I was screaming inside, "*I will NOT take NO for an answer!*"

The guard dogs barked at me in their usual manner that it was "hospital policy" and that I had to wait 21 days from the day of Rob's admission before I could visit him. As I pleaded my case, a menacing police officer stood a little taller and straighter. I said, "*It's been 13 days already. I can't wait another week. My husband is in the ICU, and he needs me!*"

They refused to budge. They would not back down. Therefore, I took out my only weapon, my phone. I called Dr. Wicked, Rob's attending physician for the day. I was surprised to be connected with him immediately. I told him I was at the hospital's front desk and wanted to see my husband.

Taken aback by my boldness, Dr. Wicked promptly reconfirmed that I could still not see Rob as he stuttered out, "Okay! I was at . . . I don't think they got him off of isolation . . . but I'm hopeful, you know, before too long, to get you a visit. He's overall stable."

As usual, he was trying to distract me by telling me Rob was "overall stable" while at the same time gleefully confirming I still could not see my husband. When I advised him it had been way too long already, he brushed my protests aside and launched into a further update on Rob's condition—as if that would meet the need.

"So, just an update. You know, the story has been, the last few days, trying to get him off paralytics. **And his lungs just don't have the reserves to quite do that yet**. But I just can't wait to get back to it again this morning. We will keep trying. Otherwise, he's looking pretty stable."

I wanted to see my husband, and now! I was sick and tired of hearing Rob was "pretty stable," yet he did not "have the reserves" to breathe on his own. I was a small, lone wife standing in the hospital lobby pleading with a physician who verified that my Medical Power of Attorney had no value. He knew he had the backing of the police officer and his "guard dog" counterparts who held me at bay while issuing face masks to the few permitted entry.

I could tell that Dr. Wicked was gloating that he could continue assaulting my husband with high-powered pharmaceuticals and harmful ventilator settings without my physical presence standing in his way.

Racing to keep up the charade and prevent me from asking again about being admitted to see Rob, he continued, "His liver function stabilized. We talked yesterday about that going up a little bit. It's not to a level that alarmed me that we need to do anything, but just keeping an eye on it. Backing off, I've been trying to keep negative on fluid, and I think we've gotten a little bit on the dry side now. So, I'm gonna back off the diuretics for a day or two and watch that, but otherwise, we're maintaining. The big picture is that we are able to oxygenate him, and he tolerates his tube feeds. **Obviously, for every day we're in, it is going to be a longer recovery course, but as long as we get to the recovery course—I'll take it**. Oh, that's pretty much your price point."

I had no idea what he meant by "that's pretty much your price point." However, I believed his stating, "Obviously, for every day we're in, it is going to be a longer recovery course, but as long as we get to the recovery course—I'll take it," was just another way of saying, *"If we're really lucky, and your husband somehow survives all this, we are talking about a LONG recovery due to all we are doing to him—and the truth is he isn't likely to make it because we are dead set on cashing in on all of the incentives possible."*

I wanted my strong, loving, talented husband to fully recover his health and mental vigor. Yet Dr. Wicked's vain attempt at comforting me destroyed the little faith I had left that they were looking out for Rob's best interest. He also weakened my confidence that Rob would be able to survive the ordeal. Even if Rob somehow survived, I envisioned him suffering a long and painful recovery where he might never be whole again.

It was clear they were injecting him with more and more drugs, then monitoring his vital signs to see what their latest assault had done. The doctors behaved like a pack of pit bulls who had happily discovered a penalty-free playground where they could harm others without repercussions.

If they made a tragic mistake that killed someone, it would be "Covid" that killed them. If they destroyed a patient's liver or kidneys with their assault of harmful medications, "Covid" would take the blame. If they blew out the patient's lungs with high pressure and 100% oxygen, the excuse would be that "Covid" caused the lung damage.

I responded, "Two days ago, a nurse told me the last time you tried to reduce the paralytics, 'it did not go well' and that he was desaturating and had to be put back on 100% oxygen, yet you keep telling me he's pretty much stable. I'm feeling very uneasy about all this. My husband is in there, he's unconscious, and the nurse seemed very negative about Rob's condition."

He explained, "It's an emotional time for everybody everywhere. The nurse . . . she's actually been very aggressive about getting him off the paralytic. But she's got him off. He's been off. He's been with her as his nurse. Yeah, his white blood count is up a little bit today. But again, I got a little concerned. But it's 15.8 today. Again, there's a lot of moving parts on that. Obviously, new infections are something that's always on our radar. But I don't have any signs of any new infections at this time. So, they're [the nurses are] always looking out for me. I obviously want to give you as much information as we can and help you understand anything you don't understand as best we can."

Then, shattering my remaining hope of Rob surviving, he said, "Here's the big picture. He is very sick. He's on, you know . . . **he's literally on life support, and anything could happen anytime. And he doesn't have much reserve. What I mean, frankly, we could lose him**—but I don't think I need to bang you up over the head with that every day. You know, he's sick."

How did we go from Rob needing to be on a ventilator to "get a little rest" from his work of breathing to "**he's literally on life support**" and "**frankly, we could lose him.**" Those ominous statements repeated so loudly in my head that it was deafening, and I could hardly focus.

If Rob could die any moment, why was he not contacting the hospital's administrators to let them know of my husband's critical condition and asking them to allow me, as his wife and duly appointed Medical Power of Attorney, to be by his side? At a minimum, whenever a patient is critically ill, his family members should be allowed to be with them. However, these heartless villains had no remorse in keeping my now critically ill husband locked away from me.

Rob had gone from a rough cough at home, to low levels of blood oxygen, to being on high-flow nasal cannula oxygen at the hospital, to a BiPAP (Bilevel Positive Airway Pressure) device that severely damaged his lungs. Now he was on a ventilator and teetering on the edge of a precipice they had led him to, and he was now dangling off the edge.

While maxed out on sedatives, paralytics, and painkillers, it was as if they were asking him to walk a tightrope across the Grand Canyon at 1,500 feet above the Little Colorado River—much like high-wire artist Nik Wallenda did in June of 2013. Nik successfully completed the trip in less than 25 minutes without a safety harness.

Rob, however, was in an induced coma. His limited "support" team was a group of worn-out nurses and uncaring doctors who were used to seeing anyone who attempted the feat of surviving a ventilator landing in a heap on the canyon floor (or make that the floor of the ICU) and then be ushered to the morgue.

"Do you have any more questions?" he asked as I attempted to process his comments about Rob being in such critical condition. Not knowing what else to say, I ended the call feeling totally defeated and more fearful for Rob than ever.

Utterly stunned by what I had just heard, I cried as I ran out of the hospital's front doors to my car. It was difficult driving because the tears would not stop flowing. When I finally arrived home, I ran into the house screaming, "*Rob is dying!*" Then, like a restless animal, I paced the floor, wondering what to do as my mother and sister, who were there to comfort me, watched.

Although it was getting dark, I decided to pack a bag and head back to the hospital. However, as I headed to the door, my mother and sister stopped me and advised me that driving back to the hospital this evening would not be a good idea. They feared that if I returned in my current state, I might cause a scene that would land me in hot water with the authorities and make it difficult ever to gain admittance to the hospital.

I lashed out, "I'm not the one being unreasonable; the hospital is! They're killing my husband! What am I to do? I've been continually waiting for permission to see my husband, and I'm tired of waiting. I don't need permission! He's my husband, for God's sake!"

Even then, I did not want to jeopardize my chances of seeing Rob. So I calmed down and finished packing a backpack with clothes and a few odds and ends for a planned trip to the hospital tomorrow. I planned to camp in the hospital lobby for an entire week if necessary. I intended on staying there until I could finally see Rob. I could not go through another day like this. I was Rob's lifeline, and he was mine.

I had made up my mind, set my face like flint, and felt much better now that I had a plan. As the prophet Isaiah said, "*For Yahuah helps me, therefore, I am not disgraced; therefore, I have set my face like flint, and I know that I shall not be ashamed.*" Isaiah 50:7

Friday, September 17, 2021

I awoke early with a raging fury, having watched the clock since before daybreak. I was enraged because I felt emotionally raped by everyone at Covid Coven Hospital in Plano, Texas. Rob had been hospitalized for 14 days and on a ventilator for nine.

Hearing my phone ringing in my purse, I dropped everything. I began shaking as I noticed it was the hospital. They hardly ever called me, so I wondered if I was about to receive terrible news.

I answered, "Hello, this is Sheila." Then, I heard Dr. Wicked's voice. He jumped right in with a report on Rob's condition. "Liver function . . . those numbers are improving, and kidney function numbers are actually a little better." I was relieved that Rob had made it through another night and was still alive.

I said, "Dr. Wicked, I'm so glad you called me this morning. I am coming to the hospital and need to see my husband. It has been 14 days now since he was admitted. I was around him for over a week before taking him there, so there's no reason I cannot come in now."

He replied, "Did you ever try the administrator's number?" I responded, "YES! I sure did, and everybody gave me the runaround. They would give me another person to call, and that person would then direct me to another number. Do you have a number I can call?"

Of course, he had no idea whom or what number I should call. All he knew was that he was being shielded from me by a ridiculous hospital policy that benefited **him** and the other doctors and staff by keeping me from seeing what was being done to Rob and observing his condition in person. So I ended the call with, "I'm heading that way!"

Rob often encouraged me by saying, *"You can do it!"* That was exactly what I needed to remember; I CAN DO IT!" So, I rushed upstairs, grabbed my backpack, and headed back downstairs to my car.

When I opened my front door, I could not believe my eyes. My mother and sister had driven over and blocked my car with theirs. As they had the evening before, they made it clear they feared I would cause a scene at the hospital and possibly end up arrested. They knew I was at the boiling point and would be unable to keep my cool if I was told "NO" one more time.

Feeling terribly insulted, I cried out, "I'M NOT STUPID! I just want to see Rob." I then tried to reason with them, yet nothing I said would convince them to move their cars. I grew more furious by the minute as I felt they did not understand how critical it was for me to get in the hospital and be with Rob. So now I had two battles to fight; one with the hospital and the other with my own family while Rob was stuck in the middle, in no man's land.

No matter how hard I tried, I could not convince my mother or sister that I would not do anything stupid that would jeopardize my chances of being with Rob. I was infuriated and secretly called my son, Jeremiah.

When I told him what had transpired, he said he was sorry I had to deal with this and that he would drive over to a neighbor's house down the road from me and text me when he arrived. He would then drive us to the hospital. The moment I received his text message, I ran out the front door with my backpack, darted down the sidewalk to the neighbors', and jumped into the passenger seat of his truck.

Jeremiah sped off, and within minutes he had dropped me off at the hospital's front doors. I was determined to gain admission to the ICU. I would not fail this time.

Although small and slim, I hoisted and donned the forty-pound backpack like it was nothing, put on my cloth mask, walked with a sense of purpose through the hospital front doors, and marched straight up to the "guard dog" ladies who volunteered at the front desk. I had put up with enough of this nonsense, and I fully expected things to go differently today. Thus, I was friendly, polite, and firm.

My jaw was set with a solid determination, and they could see I meant business. I asked to speak with the "ombudsman," an independent, neutral, impartial, non-employee designated to act as a liaison between patients or their families and hospital staff to resolve complaints and concerns while ensuring their rights were protected. I had heard of this position from an attorney friend of Rob's. He suggested I engage the ombudsman because, as an independent party not influenced by the hospital or its staff, they could advocate unbiasedly for me.

The ladies at the desk looked at me with bewilderment and said they had never heard that term before. So they asked me to repeat it. When I explained to them what an ombudsman's role was, they shook their heads and said they had never heard of such a person. They asked me to sit down nearby and wait until they could find the right person for me to speak with.

I slid the backpack from my shoulders to the ground, sat down, and waited. When they called someone in administration, they learned that the hospital had no one in that role. However, they said the ICU Charge Nurse would come down to speak with me.

In the meantime, I called Rob's attorney friend and let him know the hospital did not have an ombudsman. He said, "Let me check. I'll call you right back." Good to his word, in a few minutes, he called back. He informed me that he learned from their website that they instead had a "Risk Management" department responsible for appropriately handling patient or family complaints of a clinical or other nature. Therefore, as they were the next step before litigation, they **should** care about my situation. He then gave me the Risk Management department's phone number. However, since they are employees of the hospital, they would clearly not have an unbiased approach.

When I called, a woman answered and listened intently to my concerns. By this time, I could barely hold back the tears. She said she would need to attend to some things first but would come down to meet with me shortly.

As I waited for her to arrive, and about thirty minutes after the front desk staff had said the ICU Charge Nurse would come down to speak with me, Charge Nurse Massacre walked up and asked if I was Sheila Skiba. I said, "Yes," and she asked me to follow her to the other end of the hospital where we could talk privately.

After we sat down in the middle of a large open space, I explained to her that I had been waiting to see Rob for a full two weeks since September 3rd, and I could not wait any longer. She apologized and said she understood it was a very painful situation for me but insisted there was **nothing** she could do about it.

As had happened to me time and time again, she explained the hospital's policy. I was sick of being lectured on the hospital's insane 21-day isolation policy and having to abide by it! I told her my husband no longer had Covid, he had been tested on September 6th and was shown to have COVID-19 antibodies, and he was NO LONGER contagious.

I stood my ground and said I would **not leave** until I could see my husband. She stared at me with a dumbfounded look, as if she had never experienced a family member at their wit's end regarding their unreasonable policy. She could see the desperation in my eyes and that I meant every word but was obviously unmoved and had no grace or mercy.

I could no longer hold back the tears, and I begged her to allow me to go with her to the ICU. After explaining that I was Rob's Medical Power of Attorney and that I needed to be able to serve as his medical advocate, she stupidly asked, "What would that look like to you?"

I said, "Are you serious? It would look like me **being allowed into the ICU** to be by my husband's side so I could advocate for and aid him in person!" Seeing my intense determination, Charge Nurse Massacre said she would consider allowing me to see my husband for a measly fifteen minutes IF she could get it approved.

I was appalled and snapped back, "**NO!** I don't want to see him for just fifteen minutes; I need to be able to stay with him so I can be his advocate!" She insisted that, only with approval, the best she could offer was fifteen minutes with my husband on "an exception basis." I countered, "**NO!** That is not good enough. I want to be **with** my husband. I packed my things last night. I have them right here in this backpack. I plan to **stay** with him!"

She shook her head, squeezed her lips tightly together, made a downward frown, and said, "You staying with your husband would be **impossible**." I said, "**Nothing** is impossible. I have been praying and believing there **must be someone** in this hospital with a heart who can make this happen!" She said she would go upstairs and find out whether their uncompromising policy could be adjusted, in my case, so that I could visit Rob sooner than 21 days after his admission.

Knowing being nice would be the best approach, I thanked her profusely as I pointed out that my husband's life hung in the balance, and their decision could mean the difference between life and death for him. Besides, it would mean the world to me to see my husband, who had been trapped in the hospital for a full two weeks with no family. I stressed that in his condition, he needed me now more than ever. She headed to the elevators and disappeared behind the doors.

I quickly called Risk Management and left a voicemail message to let them know where I was in the hospital. Soon, two ladies approached me, asking if I was Sheila Skiba. I stood up and said, "Yes." They said they were from Risk Management. I thanked them for taking the time out of their busy day to listen to my concerns.

As I unfolded my whole story, both of the ladies took meticulous notes. One of the ladies said, "You mean you haven't seen your husband for two weeks?" I began crying, "Yes, that's true. I have not!" I showed them a copy of the hospital's "*Patient's Rights*" document and asked if they stood by them, which only elicited a blank stare.

I explained that my husband feared that the hospital's protocols would end his life if I could not be with him as his medical advocate. I was his Medical Power of Attorney, and he needed me to be his voice while he was weak, especially now that he had no voice due to being intubated and heavily sedated. I told them the last words Rob spoke to me in person were, "*If they don't let you be my advocate, I'm going to die in here!*" They said they would see what they could do, headed down a long hallway, and disappeared. I prayed that God would make a way when there was no way.

LEGAL COUNSEL STATEMENT
Members of the jury, Sheila did not discover until later that the ladies from Risk Management had previously been Nurse Managers who had an in-depth knowledge of, and extensive experience with, the hospital's policies and procedures. *Thus, in truth, they were not surprised at Sheila's being locked out of the hospital for two weeks and having been told she had to wait 21 days from the day of Rob's admission to be able to visit him.*

Instead of advising her that they were well aware of the 21-day isolation policy, they cruelly misled Sheila by making her believe they were shocked and dismayed that she had been isolated from her husband for two weeks implied they would try to see what they could do in the hope that Sheila would quiet down and believe someone cared about her situation—when in truth, THEY DID NOT. Thus, they walked away with NO INTENTION of supporting her in any way. Later, they ignored her repeated voicemail messages.

Over their many years at the hospital, they had become thick-skinned, cold-hearted, unsympathetic, and unfeeling flimflam artists who were highly trained in and expertly used disingenuous de-escalation techniques.

The true intention of the "Risk Management" department was to reduce the institution's EXPOSURE to potential backlashes from, or lawsuits by, patients or their families. Their ultimate goal was to determine whether Sheila might be a threat (might she cause a scene, call the press, or threaten a lawsuit?). Once they ascertained she was not going to take any action that might harm the hospital's reputation, nor would she negatively impact their bottom line, they appeased her without intending to take any action on her behalf.

Sheila had every right to be by her husband's side so she could witness his treatment firsthand and competently serve as his Medical Power of Attorney. However, as occurs in hospitals across America, the administration, doctors, nurses, and Risk Management teams all *turned a blind eye* to the extremely harmful impact of Rob's isolation, and they all coldly continued to insist that Sheila MUST remain **locked out** of the facility for a full 21 days.

We contend that this act, along with many others, was a criminal act deserving of prosecution.

I sat in the same spot until midafternoon, until finally, one of the ladies from Risk Management came back down to tell me she was still working on it. She took more notes and asked a few more questions. She could tell I had been crying. I was an absolute mess, and my eyes were bloodshot and swollen.

She asked me to follow her into a hallway so we could speak privately. I explained that I wanted to see my husband, yet I was continually being told I could not. I shared how the doctors and nurses ignored my Medical Power of Attorney and were often disrespectful and condescending when I asked for my husband's status and latest vitals.

I shared how I had heard they were short-staffed and thus could not administer nebulized budesonide because of a lack of respiratory therapists. Yet they were able to administer nebulized VELETRI multiple times a day.

She asked which doctors and nurses were disrespecting and not cooperating with me concerning Rob's care. I refused to give their names for fear they would retaliate against Rob. She was extremely surprised that I felt that way.

I also told her I was very concerned about how long they were keeping Rob on paralytics. At the same time, I was told he could not be weaned from the ventilator because any time they tried, he would fight it and "desaturate." It sounded like they did not know what they were doing, and I was tired of them "practicing medicine" on my husband. I advised her that I wanted him off the drugs and off the ventilator, and I wanted to see him today.

She slipped away and said she would continue to speak to her supervisors. Hours passed by. It was 5:30 PM, and neither of the Risk Management ladies returned, even though I had called several times and left voicemail messages. I finally realized I had been played the fool by two ladies who had promised to "see what they could do." They had feigned caring about my situation and left me in total silence. I then realized what they could do, and would do, is totally ignore me.

As I remained in the same spot where Charge Nurse Massacre had left me, her secretary came down and said, "Charge Nurse Massacre is still working on it," then disappeared behind the elevator doors just like she had hours before.

I called my attorney friend and told him about my encounter with the ladies from Risk Management, who seemed to be now totally ignoring me, and that I was still waiting to hear back from the Charge Nurse whom I had met with hours earlier. He felt no news was good news, and it was likely a good sign they were gone for so long. He believed that could only mean they were advocating for me and making headway with their superiors. He assured me they would likely be coming down soon with good news.

Soon after that, Charge Nurse Massacre showed up with her secretary in tow just before the end of her shift at 7 PM. As they walked toward me, I could see she was shaking her head as she said, "I tried, but I can't help you."

I unashamedly begged her and cried out, "My husband is suffering up there, and he needs me. How can you do this to me? This is inhumane!" She coldly retorted that no one could help me, then matter-of-factly said, "The earliest you'll be allowed to see your husband is another seven days."

I asked her, "Why so long?" and asked for a written copy of their visitation policy. She said she did not have anything in writing she could give me. I explained to her that I was told I had to wait for 21 days **if** the patient had Covid symptoms, yet (raising my voice) I said, "So, what Covid symptoms are we talking about now? Rob already had Covid antibodies identified in his lab results, and he is NO longer infectious!"

She then dropped a lead weight that shook me to my soul. "He's on a ventilator, and that counts as a Covid symptom." Seeing the stunned look on my face, she said, "I can offer you a FaceTime chat with him." I thought, "Is she kidding me? Rob is intubated, paralyzed, and in a coma."

I said, "What? A FaceTime chat? I would not be able to touch him; how would he even know I was talking to him? He needs to feel my touch. A FaceTime chat isn't the same as being with my husband!" She said, "If you record your voice, I can play it for him later." That was ridiculous! I said, "NO, I NEED TO BE ROB'S ADVOCATE!" She stood speechless for a moment, then shot back, "The answer is a firm **NO!**"

I was completely taken off guard. It was clear she was dead serious. My body began shaking and trembling as I said, "I'm sorry to have bothered you and interrupted your busy schedule. I know you must be very busy taking care of all the ICU patients, with my husband being one of them. I'm truly sorry. *Please may I have the fifteen minutes you offered me earlier?* I will take that now. It's better than nothing."

In a calloused and quiet tone, she replied, "**No.** I never got permission for that. I could not get that approved." Then, she paused and reiterated with punctuation, "*You will have to wait seven more days.*"

I said, "I will gladly sign a waiver, whatever you need. But I need to see Rob!" She shook her head again, turned around, walked to the elevator with her secretary, and disappeared. She gave me no grace, no sympathy, and no compassion.

The day before, Dr. Wicked had made it clear Rob was in critical condition, admitting, "frankly, we could lose him." Although Rob could die at any moment, this heartless and inhumane Charge Nurse told me without emotion that I had to wait another seven days to be allowed to see my husband.

Broken, devastated, and demoralized, I wailed from the depths of my soul. No one would help me. They were treating my husband like a POW (prisoner of war) and me like an outcast. They had Rob in their clutches, and although I was Rob's wife and official Medical Power of Attorney, I had been pushed aside, discarded like garbage, and dehumanized.

I called my son and cried in desperation, "Oh, Jeremiah! They won't let me see Rob. They've been jacking with me all day, and no one will help me. I'm still locked out. It would take an **ARMY** with **HEAVY ARTILLERY** to break through! Please come and get me."

In tears, I waited outside for Jeremiah as I sat on the ground with my forty-pound backpack. I wondered what had happened to my resolution to not take "No" for an answer. I felt like a wild horse who had his will whipped out of him—defeated, trodden down, and trampled on. I was flooded with guilt at not breaking through their impenetrable barrier that was preventing me from protecting my husband from "the protocol."

My son drove up, and I climbed into the front seat. Tears of frustration and fear continued to flow. He tried to comfort me but to no avail. As he pulled into my driveway, before he stopped the car, I opened the door and stumbled out. I fumbled with the keys to my front door, and once inside, I tossed my backpack into a corner and ran upstairs.

I was furious with myself and hated myself. In my singular focus on gaining entrance to the ICU, I had failed. In my efforts at gaining entry, I had also failed to call the doctors and ask how Rob was doing.

I had sat in the hospital lobby from morning until dark and had accomplished NOTHING! I felt like a complete and total failure. I had been taken for a fool and wasted an entire day while my husband lay helplessly and hopelessly in an ICU room on a ventilator. I had given my all, and my all was not enough! The level of frustration I felt was so overwhelming that I let out a blood-curdling scream. I desperately feared I was about to lose my best friend.

I then made a late-night call to the ICU nurse's station and spoke with Rob's nurse. I told her I had spent the day trying, unsuccessfully, to get in to see Rob. She said, "I heard."

What did she hear, and when did she hear about it? Who told her? I'm sure it was Charge Nurse Massacre. Had they all been talking about me?" I told her, "It didn't work today, but I'm still hopeful I will get in soon. Unfortunately, I was so busy trying to get in that I didn't call to get an update on his vitals. Are you busy, or can you give them to me?"

She gave me a quick update, then said I could view Rob's online MyChart record to read the rest. I told her the MyChart records were always one day behind, so calling was the only way I could get up-to-date information on Rob's vitals and condition.

She said they had again tried to wean him from the paralytics and that doing so caused him to desaturate into the low 80s. I asked her when they planned to try to reduce the paralytics again, and she said, "Well, he has the high FiO2. So, typically when the FiO2 is under 50%, and the PEEP is, you know, under 8, then they'll try to do those **sedation vacations,** as they call them. His PEEP is still at 14." She ended our call by saying she had to attend to other things.

Another unbearably frustrating and demoralizing day had passed without my achieving my goal of entering the ICU to be with my husband and advocate for him in person.

Saturday, September 18, 2021

I awoke with a start, wondering if I had overslept. Noticing it was still dark outside, I quickly dressed and dashed downstairs.

I hastily placed several photographs in an envelope. I planned to ensure they were hung on the wall of Rob's ICU room, hoping that seeing them would move the staff's hearts so they would begin treating him as a person instead of just another comatose, ventilated victim of "the protocol."

One of the photos was of our dog, Heidi. Another was of Rob hugging her. The third was a full-page drawing of the human anatomy that Rob had overlain with his torso and face on which he had written these words:

I am a mentally, physically, spiritually whole man of God!
Every Organ, Cell, Nerve, Muscle, Bone, Tissue, Ligament, Tendon,
and Fiber in my Body is HEALTHY
In Jesus' Name!

Rob had been a healthy, robust, 52-year-old man who loved life. He was a very successful author, speaker, and playwright. He was a wonderful, caring person with a contagious smile who had spent his life focused on blessing others.

I arrived at the hospital parking lot shortly before 7:00 AM, hoping to catch Dr. Wicked on his way in so I could personally ask him to be my advocate and help me break through what appeared to be an impenetrable wall.

I waited and watched. After thirty minutes, I called the ICU to see if I had missed him. I was disheartened to learn that he would not be working today. The wind was totally taken out of my sails as, once again, one of my plans to gain admittance had failed.

I requested that someone meet me in the lobby, take a copy of my Medical Power of Attorney and have it entered into Rob's hospital records, then tape the pictures I had brought to Rob's ICU room wall. She assured me she would send someone down to meet me.

I drove to the entrance and found a nurse there to meet me. She said she would ensure the pictures would be placed on the wall of Rob's room in the ICU and that my Medical Power of Attorney was added to the hospital's records.

Once again, I headed home, wholly dejected and filled with despair. Every idea I had come up with to gain entrance before the end of the 21-day deadline had failed, and I was at a total loss as to how to breach the impenetrable wall that still separated us. Rob had now been on the ventilator for ten days, and without some form of miracle, I would have to wait six more days before seeing him for the first time since I dropped him off at the hospital fifteen days earlier.

Later that day, I called the ICU to speak with Rob's nurse. It was Nurse Jezebel this time. When I asked her for his vitals, she said he was doing okay. His FiO2 (oxygen percentage) was set at 50%, which was good, but the PEEP (residual pressure) was still set at 14, which she admitted was still way too high. I had been advised that they could not attempt to wean Rob from the ventilator until his FiO2 (oxygen concentration) was set below 60, the PEEP (Positive End Expiratory Pressure) was at 8 or lower, he was no longer on the paralytic drugs, and they were able to lower the sedatives. Yet nothing they were doing was getting us any closer to this point—leaving Rob a captive prisoner of the ventilator.

I asked Nurse Jezebel if she had been turning Rob. She did not say yes, or no. She simply responded, "Well, right now, he is on his back. Have they told you at all about the RotoProne beds?" I said, "No, they haven't." She then explained, "Okay, they have those special beds where they can actually, instead of manually putting somebody on their belly, it allows you to be able to turn them. Then it actually kind of moves them, sways them, and it kind of hopefully helps break up some of that congestion. So, they're looking at putting him on one of those."

I had never heard of such a bed, and from how she described it, I hoped it might be helpful for Rob. Nurse Jezebel continued, "Well, it's a special bed. It has to be ordered, and the doctor is in the process of getting it here for Mr. Skiba." She then added, "Dr. Relentless is here this weekend. If anything were to change, good or bad, please know that we will always reach out to you. So, if you don't hear from us, that's good news. I mean, things are still moving in the same direction. Nothing's gone either way. I'm glad we were able to at least kind of give you an update and let you know where he's at."

I asked about the level of the paralytic Rob was on, and she responded, "So yesterday, he was desaturating without changes to the paralytic, so they had to **go up** on them. They were able to come back down. So, we're back at the same level that we were at yesterday. Hopefully, with this bed, we're able to kind of get some of that stuff in his lungs out, you know, as the bed moves you, it kind of breaks all that up, and then we'll be able to get him off of the paralytic. Our goal was always off paralytics, off sedation, and off the ventilator, right? We just have to be able to get him there, and he's not tolerating those things."

I asked, "Okay. When you pull him off the paralytic, are you also reducing the sedative? I know it's kind of like a balancing act. Is that what's going on?" She agreed, "It is a balancing act. But now you have to take the paralytic off first, and then the sedation. You would never want to have somebody not sedated and be paralyzed. Right? Well, that could be scary, right? You can't move, but you're awake. So, we never would do that, absolutely. Always paralytic off first."

I pressed in for more clarification. "And then, do you lighten the sedation?" She said, "It's like I said, like the balancing thing? Of course, I think it'd be terrible if you took the sedation off. **Well, the thing is that he's not tolerating any of that. And with these high PEEP pressures that he has, he's not in a position stable enough to even be able to tolerate that.** Ideally, what, as I said, our plan is set, you know, wean sedation and then extubate.

"So, before we can extubate, we need to make sure that he actually can breathe on his own and that he can follow commands. So, in order to do that, we do trials. And so, we'll actually pause sedation and see how he feels, and be able to follow commands, whether you are able to breathe, and can do a breathing trial on the vent while he's still intubated. And those things allow us to know that we can safely extubate him, and he's going to do well. We're just not at that point yet."

She made it very clear that his PEEP being so high was one of the key reasons they could not conduct the trials he would need to pass for them to be able to attempt to wean him from the ventilator.

I wondered what their plan was to solve the problem. Without a clear plan, Rob would simply continue to deteriorate due to the ongoing assault of the massive number of drugs, the excessive residual pressure in his lungs due to the high PEEP setting, and the up to 100% concentrations of oxygen he was breathing.

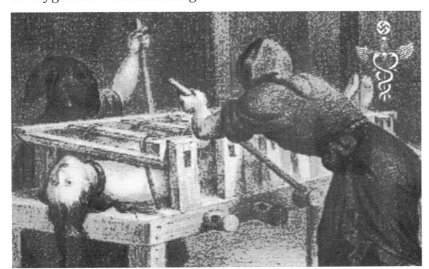

After we ended our call, I found information on the Internet about the RotoProne Therapy System. It is a specialized bed in which a patient is confined (or trapped) with straps and other restraints. The photo of the bed gave me chills because it eerily resembled drawings I had seen of torture beds used during the Inquisition to extract confessions from victims who had been accused of heresy.

LEGAL COUNSEL STATEMENT

Members of the jury, the definition of **malpractice** is the failure of a professional person, such as a physician, to render proper services through reprehensible ignorance, negligence, or through criminal intent—especially when injury or loss follows.

Whether by willful ignorance, uncaring negligence, or nefarious intent, the doctors and nurses at Covid Coven Hospital of Plano, Texas, **(a)** had no qualms about Rob's being starved into submission and being isolated from his family, **(b)** subjected him to numerous unnecessary and harmful drugs, **(c)** continually coerced him to agree to "*elective intubation*," then **(d)** subjected him to 4.5 hours on a contraindicated BiPAP therapy that caused barotrauma (the rupturing and collapse of the air sacs [alveoli] of the lungs). Each of these actions weakened, injured, and demoralized him to the point that he ended up being intubated and placed on a ventilator—which, as we noted earlier, had been their goal for Rob from the moment he arrived.

Unfortunately for families suffering these injustices, on June 14, 2021, Greg Abbott, the governor of **Texas, signed Senate Bill 6 (SB 6)**, the **Pandemic Liability Protection Act**, into law, which added a new section (Section 74.155) to Title 4, Chapter 74, Subchapter D of the State of Texas Civil Practice and Remedies Code.

Among other things, this section of the Texas law states, "*Except in a case of reckless conduct or intentional, willful, or wanton misconduct, a physician, health care provider, or first responder* **is not liable for an injury**, *including economic and noneconomic damages,* **or death** *arising from care, treatment,* **or failure to provide care or treatment** *relating to or impacted by a pandemic disease or a disaster declaration related to a pandemic disease. . .*"

Subchapter G. LIABILITY LIMITS, Section 74.301 of the law set the maximum potential award amount for such cases at $250,000 "*for each claimant, regardless of the number of defendant physicians or health care providers . . .*"
Civil Practice and Remedies Code Chapter 74. Medical liability. (n.d.). From
https://statutes.capitol.texas.gov/Docs/CP/htm/CP.74.htm

After the passage of this law, medical malpractice attorneys in Texas began to refuse to accept and file medical malpractice cases if a patient had been diagnosed with "Covid" because they knew it would be challenging to prove *reckless conduct or intentional, willful, or wanton misconduct* without spending **well over $250,000** in expert witness analysis and testimony. *With a maximum potential award of only $250,000 regardless of the number of defendant physicians or health care providers involved, it became economically unfeasible even to consider such cases.*

Jon Opelt, the Texas Alliance for Patient Access executive director, admitted, "*The Pandemic liability bill does not protect bad actors who are grossly negligent, engage in willful misconduct or are consciously indifferent to their patient's welfare and safety.*"
Yates, D. (2021, June 1). Texas Legislature passes pandemic liability protections bill. Southeast Texas Record. From
https://setexasrecord.com/stories/601942132-texas-legislature-passes-pandemic-liability-protections-bill

Even then, we contend that this law allows Texas hospitals, doctors, and staff to hide behind a curtain of immunity that, sadly, has allowed them to "**get away with murder**" because regardless of the actual cause of death—even if due to willful ignorance, uncaring negligence, or nefarious intent—a "Covid" patient's death is always attributed to COVID-19.

The Associate General Counsel for one of the largest public healthcare and hospital systems in the United States, headquartered in Dallas, Texas, said it this way: "SB 6 is a pretty wide-ranging and *fairly complex bill. But the upshot for Texas businesses is that **SB 6 will make it harder to sue businesses around Texas for Covid-related injuries or death claims.**"
Texas House passes pandemic liability protection act. Jackson Walker. (2021, December 15). From
https://www.jw.com/news/podcast-texas-pandemic-liability-protection-act

Fully aware that this law was in place, the doctors at Covid Coven Hospital of Plano, Texas, knew full well they had carte blanche; that is, they had complete freedom to act as they wished without any risk of a wrongful death lawsuit—since "Covid" patients are always deemed to have died "of Covid."

Even though the doctors and the hospital are shielded by Texas law, we believe the evidence we have presented (and will continue to provide) conclusively demonstrates they have been caught **red-handed**—and we do not say that lightly. "*Caught red-handed*" is a phrase that was first used in Scotland in the 1400s. It refers to *catching a killer whose hands are still stained with the blood of the person they murdered.*

Sunday, September 19, 2021

It was dawn, and my eyes were bloodshot from crying all night. As was my customary morning routine, I called the ICU nurses' station to check on Rob's condition.

The nurse who answered informed me that Rob had been placed into a RotoProne bed the night before. I was surprised it had arrived so quickly and wished a doctor had taken the time to call me and explain the benefits and potential risks before putting Rob in it.

Once again, they had ignored that as his wife and Medical Power of Attorney, I should have been consulted regarding any potential changes in Rob's treatment, especially significant changes of this magnitude.

She continued, "So, he's placed in the bed, and then the bed takes his whole body and flips him so he's facing downwards. So, he's prone. And then the bed is, like, swaying—rocking back and forth, so it would help with lung expansion. So far, he's been tolerating that. His saturation [blood oxygen level] is now 94. I just had to go up on the paralytic, just a tinge, **because his sat dropped.**"

Concerned, I queried, "Oh, his saturation dropped? What was it before?" Failing to answer what his blood oxygen level had dropped to, she simply rattled off more numbers. "I'll be dropping down the paralytic and sedation. For now, he's tolerating it. His blood pressure is 110 over 55. Heart rate is 67. His oxygen saturation is now 95. **His PEEP is still 14.** And that's that. So, from the FiO2 [oxygen concentration] was 65% last night, **it was then dropped to 45%.** However, when we turned him, we put it back up to 60%. So, he's now at 60%."

LEGAL COUNSEL STATEMENT

Members of the jury, as of September 18th, Rob had been on the ventilator for 10 days, and Dr. Wicked had advised Sheila on September 13th that "at 50 years old, he could **probably handle**, with paralytics, **probably 10 to 14 days** and still have enough reserve . . . most likely." By now, Rob had been on the ventilator for 11 days and had entered the critical "10 to 14 days" window—a period after which Dr. Wicked had contended he would likely exhaust his reserves and be unable to be weaned from the device successfully.

As the nurse shared with Sheila, and as substantiated in the hospital records, at **4:00 PM** on **September 18th** (Rob's 10th day on the ventilator and over five hours before Rob's being placed in the RotoProne bed), they had been able to **reduce the FiO2** (oxygen concentration) **down to 45%.** As shown in the chart at the bottom of Page C-54 in Appendix C, this was the first time they had been able to meet one of the two critical criteria for attempting to wean Rob from the ventilator, which were an FiO2 setting of 50% or less and a PEEP setting of 8 or less.

In addition, the hospital records show that Rob's blood oxygen level was **98%** at 9:00 PM, just 30 minutes before being placed in the RotoProne bed. **Yet, they did not attempt to lower the PEEP (it remained set at 14) to 8** to see if Rob could be successfully extubated and removed from the ventilator.

Before placing Rob in the RotoProne bed at 9:30 PM, the doctors should have **lowered the PEEP** setting (the residual pressure left in the lungs by the ventilator after expiration) **to 8 or less** to see if Rob's blood oxygen level would stabilize at **85% or higher**. If it had, then based on their extubation protocol, they should have reduced the sedatives and paralytics to determine if they could wean Rob from the ventilator.

*However, whether due to incompetence, conscious indifference, malfeasance, or a desire to utilize the RotoProne bed they had just rented, **the doctors bypassed a pivotal opportunity to attempt to wean Rob from the ventilator**. We contend their failure was a negligent criminal act because they KNEW they would NOT try to wean Rob from the ventilator during the entire time he was in the RotoProne bed, which Dr. Liar later admitted to Sheila.*

Thus, Rob was sentenced to not have any weaning attempts until he was extracted from the RotoProne bed one week later, on September 28, 2021. He was removed from the bed that day due to Sheila's insistence during an in-hospital family intervention meeting held with Dr. Liar on September 27, 2021. Were it not for Sheila's intervention, he might have been left in the RotoProne bed until he died.

Trying to keep up with the nurse, I wrote down Rob's vitals. Then, she quickly added, "The paralytic is to help immobilize him so that it would help with his condition right now **because if he's awakened, he'll remove it**—and that will make it worse. **The recovery would be worse if he's pulling things, right?** It will make him want to give more of an effort. Yeah, so we don't want him to exert too much effort. **So as much as possible, we are sedating him so that at least he'll be more calm.** And then the machine, the RotoProne bed, can do its thing, and all the medications will be able to do their thing because if he's awake and aware, he'll be exerting effort.

She then noted, "We are checking if he is twitching. If he twitches, we have to increase the paralytic some more. Because before we start on the titrating, we have to get a baseline. So right now, he's still twitching, so that's why we have to go up. However, the doctors wanted to wean him off the paralytic. So, we are trying to wind it down. However, if we move down, his sats [blood oxygen saturation levels] are dropping."

By saying she was further "sedating him" so he would not be "pulling things," was she admitting Rob had become partially awake and tried to remove his endotracheal tube? If so, I found the thought of that very disturbing.

The day before they placed Rob on the ventilator, he had texted me, "*Doing all they can to try to get me to agree to intubate. I'm dead if they do.*" So, of course, if he had awakened and realized he was a slave of a ventilator that he knew was a death trap, he would have tried to escape its grasp.

I knew that my chances of getting my husband home alive were dwindling by the day, and I was unsettled for the rest of the day, wondering how Rob was managing in the RotoProne bed. My skin crawled at the thought that he was now cocooned inside this contraption. I had read everything I could on the Internet about the RotoProne Therapy System, and I hoped Rob was unaware he was now confined in such a device.

Later in the day, I called again to check on Rob's condition. His nurse said, "The newest thing that I have to tell you is he's still sedated and paralyzed, but we're trying to wean him off the paralytic. Okay. So, I'm going down on his paralytic right now. Earlier, I started going down, but I have to make sure that his saturations are stable."

When I poured my heart out to her about my repeated vain attempts at getting in to see Rob, she said, "That's all of our Covid patients. We cannot have visitors." I cried out to her, "But it has been over two weeks! It's so hard. Are you married?" Ignoring my question, she said, "When he's off his sedation or paralytic, you could always do the FaceTime." My heart sank, and I wanted to scream. Instead, I calmly said, "That's not the same!"

I asked for Rob's vitals, and she replied, "So his blood pressure right now is 142 over 67. When I first came in earlier, it was in the 160s. So, I had to give him medicine to help lower it down. And so far, it's tough, okay. It hasn't been in the 160s anymore. His heart rate is 64. His sat has been 90 to 91; it's 96 now."

I ended the call with my usual request, "Well, next time you go back in there, can you whisper to him, 'Your wife Sheila loves you. She's trying to get there to see you soon.' Okay? Please let him know. Thank you so much."

Rob, the best man I knew, my confidant and provider, had so much to live for. I would gladly have taken his place and exchanged my life for his. Now, in addition to being a prisoner of the ventilator, he was trapped in a RotoProne bed.

LEGAL COUNSEL STATEMENT
Members of the jury, placing Rob in a RotoProne bed without advising Sheila of the **risks** and **benefits** was another of many glaring examples of how the doctors made unilateral decisions about his plan of care in clear violation of Sheila's rights as his spouse and Medical Power of Attorney.

According to the RotoProne Therapy System manual, the **risks** include cardiac arrest, edema or swelling, splenic rupture, blindness, damage to the ocular nerve, venous air embolism, and difficulty performing CPR.
RotoProne therapy system - qbank.arjo.com. (n.d.). From
https://qbank.arjo.com/productdocumentation/208662-AH%20Rev%20E.pdf

They had a moral, ethical, and legal obligation to keep her well-informed and consult her on major and minor decisions concerning Rob's care. Instead, they openly disregarded that obligation. Their doing so constitutes *"reckless conduct or intentional, willful, or wanton misconduct,"* which meets the criteria for liability as defined in Texas' Pandemic Liability Protection Act.
Civil Practice and Remedies Code Chapter 74. Medical liability. (n.d.). From
https://statutes.capitol.texas.gov/Docs/CP/htm/CP.74.htm

Sheila will eventually discover that Rob could not be weaned from the ventilator for the duration of his stay in the RotoProne bed because doctors preferred not to attempt to wean patients while they were in this device. *Thus, placing Rob in the RotoProne bed sentenced him to an extended duration on the ventilator.*

When she was eventually allowed to visit her husband days later, she was disturbed to discover Rob had been placed in the bed <u>naked</u> with no sheets or draping. There were only a few drop cloths on the lower frame or floor to catch any escaping bodily fluids. To Sheila, the RotoProne bed appeared inhumane, unsanitary, risky, and potentially life-threatening. In addition, Sheila later learned that many patients placed in a RotoProne bed develop secondary infections that necessitate multiple doses of antibiotics to recover from.

She had good reason to be concerned, given the RotoProne bed's high complexity and the potential for infection and other complications with its use. In addition, to ensure Rob's safety, the nursing staff would have had to be adequately trained in the proper setup, use, and maintenance of the bed, as well as proper patient care while in the bed.

I had always assisted Rob with his multiple endeavors, yet now I could not aid him in his struggle for survival. I questioned why he had to endure this and prayed to God that he was free of pain and fear.

As it became apparent that I could not break through the hospital's impenetrable and needless wall of isolation on my own, I decided to contact one of Rob's closest friends, a police officer in Austin, Texas, in the hopes that he might have some suggestions.

He said he would drive up from Austin in the morning after dropping his children at school and accompany me to meet with the hospital's Risk Management team. He would insist that I be allowed to see Rob. I inquired whether he would be wearing his uniform. Unfortunately, he could not, but he would be happy to let them know that, as a police officer, he fully supported me and believed they should stop denying me access to my husband.

Late in the evening, I called and spoke with Nurse Killjoy. She said, "He really hasn't had any changes today. His oxygenation is still 60%. He's still on the VELETRI. His PEEP is still at 14. Really, no other changes.

"We are fixing to turn him supine. He's been prone all night, but we're fixing to turn supine now. So, he'll stay that way for, like, eight hours if he can tolerate it for that long. His heart rate's been in the 80 to 90 range, blood pressures in the 120s, 130s range; oxygenation has been anywhere from 90 to 93%."

Before we ended her call, the tears were flowing again. I choked on my words, "Please whisper in his ear that his wife loves him very, very much!" She said she would.

I lived in fear, knowing Rob could die at any moment. I had never experienced such unending agony, regret, and sadness. I felt helpless, hopeless, and alone. Finally, like most nights, I eventually cried myself to sleep.

Monday, September 20, 2021

Rob's police officer friend from Austin, John, texted me and said he was on his way. It would take him approximately three and a half hours to reach the Dallas area. He would then pick me up and drive with me to the hospital. Rob and I had known him for years, and he said he would do anything to help me.

I was ready and waiting at the front door when John arrived. He encouraged me not to worry, as he was here to aid me in breaching the barrier that separated me from Rob. He wasn't wearing his uniform because doing so while off duty would be an abuse of his position. Still, he was confident he could convince them to listen to reason because he had developed keen powers of persuasion as a police officer.

I often imagined Rob waking up, getting up, and saying, "I'm going now." I so much wanted to "walk by faith, and not by sight," yet doing so was growing increasingly difficult due to our continued and cruel separation, with Rob being held against his will in a deep, dark chamber called the ICU— which I began to think of as the "Intensive Crime Unit."

We immediately headed to the hospital. With my officer friend by my side, my self-assurance grew. As we entered, I confidently approached the front desk with my head held high. I informed the front desk volunteers that I needed to speak with a representative from Risk Management. They could tell I was dead serious.

They placed a call, and within minutes the Risk Management supervisor arrived. Having a strong and determined man by my side made a substantial difference. I quickly introduced myself and my friend. The supervisor looked at him, looked at me, inhaled deeply, and exhaled audibly. She clearly recognized that we were not there to debate the issue but to achieve our objective.

She momentarily hesitated while wringing her hands. She then inquired, "What have the medical staff done for you so far?" I wanted to say, "Absolutely nothing!" But, since that would not be entirely true, I told her they had offered me the absurd "opportunity" of a "FaceTime chat" with Rob, my fully sedated and unconscious husband.

I also told her Rob would become anxious whenever the doctors tried to wean him off the sedatives. The weaning process would then be terminated, and he would be sedated again. I explained that I needed to be present so that he could hear my voice and feel my touch if they expected to be able to wean him successfully.

I asked her. "Are you married?" She said, "Yes, I am." Swooping in for a landing, I asked, "How would you feel being locked away from your husband for 17 days and told you still had to wait four more days?" Reflecting momentarily, she said, "I would not like it nor put up with it. I would be a lot more angry and violent." Her response totally took us by surprise; we did not expect to hear that.

I said, "I'm being nice, and I have shown respect to the doctors and nurses because I was afraid if I rocked the boat too much, they would retaliate against my husband and me." But, of course, I felt they already had retaliated, which was a key reason Rob was now on a ventilator. I continued, "It's at home that I show my anger, which has led to my family holding me back at times." Seeing I was on the verge of losing it, John politely interrupted, respectfully cleared his throat, and said, "I am Rob's best friend, ma'am, and I drove up from Austin this morning to make sure Sheila gets in to see him. I plan to stay right here until we get somewhere."

At that, she appeared a bit nervous and explained, "I would have to get approval from the hospital administration." Once again, I was advised that the illusive "hospital administration" must grant me the privilege of seeing a critically ill husband. I feared I was about to receive the same runaround I had received three days prior when I met with the ICU Charge Nurse and two other ladies from Risk Management.

She said, "Hold on, I'll be back." Then, a few minutes later, she returned and said, "They said you will be allowed to see your husband **for twenty minutes**."

I was ecstatic and excited to finally be able to see Rob, even if for only a brief period, and I thanked her several times. However, I refrained from asking, "Why only twenty minutes?" because I feared doing so would jeopardize my ability to see Rob at all, as it appeared to have done three days earlier when I turned down the potential offer of 15 minutes with Rob from Charge Nurse Massacre, after which she rescinded the offer and insisted I had to wait seven more days.

She instructed me to wait for the ICU Floor Supervisor to come down, who would accompany me to the ICU. I said, "Yes, ma'am." Although he knew twenty minutes was horribly unjust, John smiled at me because I was about to see Rob for the first time in seventeen days. It was a small victory that I could not have won without his assistance.

> ## LEGAL COUNSEL STATEMENT
> Members of the jury, you have likely heard of **Stockholm Syndrome**, an emotional response that some people develop when they are trapped in an abusive situation and begin to view their abuser or captor favorably.
>
> Although trapped in an abusive situation, Sheila never developed positive feelings toward the perpetrators. However, like many abused, she was forced to express gratitude for the few crumbs they tossed her way—such as the "gift" of only twenty minutes with her husband seventeen days after his admission.
>
> *What will it take to stop this abuse by American hospitals and their staff? Something must be done to right this wrong.*

Moments later, the ICU Floor Supervisor came down. My friend John looked at me, gave me a big Texas smile, and said he would wait for me. I stood up and followed the Floor Supervisor, who introduced himself as Mr. Pathetic. As we walked toward the elevators, he explained what a unique "privilege" I had been given. I expressed my gratitude and told him how much it meant to me.

When the elevator stopped on the second floor, I stayed close behind him, like a duckling following its mother. He then pushed open a set of large, double-wide wooden doors with glass windows. The nurse's station was to our left. He summoned a nurse and stated, "Sheila Skiba is here to see her husband, Robert Skiba. She has been given a twenty-minute visitation window."

The next thing I knew, he was gone. Then, a nurse instructed me on how to correctly don the Personal Protection Equipment (PPE)—a gown, cap, mask, face shield, gloves, and booties—in the correct order. After I was all geared up, the nurse showed me to Rob's room. Then, to my surprise, she told me not to touch my husband.

Nothing could have prepared me for what I was about to see and hear. I followed the nurse as she pushed open the heavy wooden doors to Rob's room. All the machines Rob was hooked up to were humming, clicking, beeping, and hissing. The most notable sound was the sucking bellows-like sound coming from the ventilator. It all sounded odd and unsettling.

Rob was tightly secured in the RotoProne bed, a large and ominous vinyl capsule. I could only see the tips of his fingers and toes and the lower portion of his face from his nose down.

Rob was in a facedown, pronated position. Cloths lay under the head of the bed to catch any drool or other fluids that dripped from his mouth or nose. Everything appeared otherworldly and unsanitary. I nearly screamed when I knelt beneath the bed and observed blood on his beard that had dripped from his nose onto the sheet below. My initial impression of Internet photographs had not changed. The contraption indeed did remind me of torture beds depicted in medieval art.

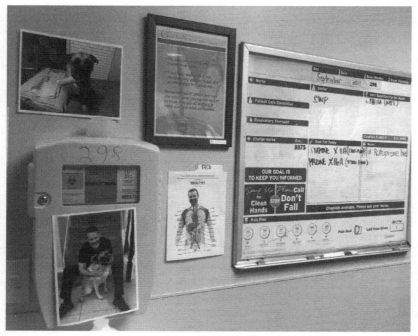

The floor of his room was disgustingly filthy, sticky, and grimy with dirt. It was covered with what appeared to be dried, flaky white skin flecks. All the wires and tubes entering my husband's body were tangled on the filthy floor. When I inquired about the filth, I was informed that housekeeping had ceased operations due to Covid restrictions.

After being left alone for a few minutes, I observed that the pictures I had dropped off had been affixed to Rob's wall. Obviously, in his fully sedated, paralyzed, and tortured state, he was unaware of their presence. However, the medical staff could see them, which was exactly what I wanted so that they would know that Rob Skiba was a vibrantly alive man with a highly infectious smile.

I touched his fingers with my gloved hand and wiped the blood that dripped from his nose. I then cried, "Honey, I'm here. I love you so very much. You will be okay. I am so sorry. You'll soon be coming home."

Before I could continue, I was interrupted by Dr. Liar, who walked into the room. I straightened up and said, "Hello." He quickly introduced himself, saying he had heard I was in the room. So he dropped in to give me a progress report. I thanked him and told him I was happy to be given twenty minutes to visit with Rob.

Using up the precious few moments I had been allotted to visit with Rob, without emotion, and in a robotic tone, he said, "We're giving him a medicine called VELETRI; he is requiring high-level support." I asked, "Does he still have pneumonia?" His formal response was, "He has inflammation, so yes." I asked, "Okay, so that is considered still having pneumonia, or is it the aftermath?" He answered, "A little bit of both. We are still now treating for both, but yeah."

I then asked him when he planned to wean Rob from the paralytics. He replied, "We will not lift the paralytics just yet, because he is requiring pretty high-level support. And if I lifted the paralytics, he's going to potentially become what we call 'distinct risk' with the ventilator, which could cause his oxygen levels to drop." Not fully grasping the true significance of what he was saying, I asked, "I know you may not know this, but how many days until you estimate you could pull the endotracheal tube out?"

He pursed his lips together, let his eyes gaze around the room, then looked back at me and said, "Depends on how he responds. There really is no answer to that. Honestly, everybody's different. I can tell you. He's going to be on the ventilator, at a minimum, **for at least another week or more.** I mean, just based on where he currently stands. Ultimately, if things are somewhat better, he may need a tracheotomy tube."

Why was I told I still could not be with Rob if his need for such intensive care indicated that he was in critical condition? I noted, "He desperately needs to hear my voice to aid in his recovery. It's very important for him. I know you're his doctor, and you want him to recover. But I know my husband, and it is urgent that I can personally say to him, 'you're going to be okay' because he already went into this situation with a lot of fear and anxiety."

He responded callously, "Yeah, I can't allow that right now. It's hospital rules, something that I can't change." I replied, "Okay. I understand the CDC and its precautions, but when you keep trying to wean him from paralytics, he becomes anxious. I believe he needs to hear my voice and hear me say, 'it's gonna be okay.' He has a great fear of hospitals. And so, I want to be here to tell him, 'Hey, Honey, you're okay.'

"He doesn't know what's going on. He's scared. I know he's sedated and paralyzed. But there have been studies that indicate that if a loved one can be with and connect with the patient, it increases their chance of full recovery.

"He needs to hear me so he can be grounded and not be fearful, and I can calm him down. So, is this possible? I thank you so much for what you're doing, but could you please honor me as his wife and let me see him? **You've tried to wean him off the paralytics numerous times, and it's not working! So, please don't try to wean him unless I'm here to calm him down because I don't think it's helping him.**"

Dr. Liar smugly suggested, "You could FaceTime him. From that standpoint, it would be fine if they tried that . . . as far as I'm concerned." I interrupted him, pleading, "**That's not it. It's not the same.** I mean, I tried it once. I called the Social Worker twice, and she did not answer. So, that's not going to work. I mean, he needs to hear me in person. He feared he would not leave here alive if I weren't his advocate. So, **I'm just asking for 10 minutes when you're trying to wean him.**"

I hoped he would listen to reason and realize that if they were going to attempt to wean Rob, they needed to let me be with him for that brief period, even if it were only ten minutes, to help him remain calm so they could do it successfully.

He said, "10 minutes? Yeah, that's something that I don't have control over. It's a hospital policy." Unwilling to take "No" for an answer, I said, "I know. **But Rob is your patient.** Don't you have authority over Rob when he's in your care?" Dr. Liar shook his head, "When it comes to the rules of a hospital . . . I still have to abide by the rules of the hospital." How convenient. Heartless Dr. Liar was more than happy to be able to keep me out of his way by hiding behind and using the excuse of "the rules of the hospital."

I cried, "I'm just saying patients need to have an advocate, and there has been no one here to advocate for my husband for over two whole weeks." Then, obviously not understanding the meaning of the word "advocate," he coldly asserted, "Your physical presence doesn't necessarily need to be here for you to be a patient advocate. Have you talked to the hospital?"

As we debated how crucial it was for me to be by Rob's side to effectively advocate for and comfort him if they attempted to wean him, my precious twenty minutes with him were ticking away.

I quickly added, "I spent all day Friday talking to Charge Nurse Massacre and a lady from Risk Management, and I got nowhere. They gave me a cold and brutal 'NO!' I'm okay to wait if I have to, and I don't want to waste your time, but Rob is a talented writer who has written eight books and traveled the world, and the last thing he said to me was, '*If you can't be my advocate I will die in here.*' **To be an advocate is for me to be here with him**. Rob thought he would die here if I could not be with him and speak on his behalf. So, you'll get a better result with his recovery if I could talk to and be with him."

He acknowledged, "I hear you. I don't make those rules. Right now, he's heavily sedated. I'm not waking him up right now. **Not while he's in the RotoProne bed.** So, I'm not sure who said we were waking him up. We are not waking him up right now."

LEGAL COUNSEL STATEMENT
Members of the jury, it is unclear why Dr. Liar said he would not even **attempt** to wake Rob up while he was in the RotoProne bed.

We do know, however, that Dr. Liar's refusal to attempt a Spontaneous Awakening Trial (SAT), followed by a Spontaneous Breathing Trial (SBT), while Rob was in the RotoProne bed meant that he had been sentenced to *remaining in a fully sedated and paralyzed, comatose state until his removal from the bed—something Sheila was not informed of when she was told, on September 18th, that they had ordered the bed to help improve Rob's condition.*

If they truly intended to reduce Rob's paralytics and sedatives as soon as possible to prevent further injury (as they repeatedly implied to Sheila), they would never have placed him in a bed from which they refused to even attempt the weaning process.

Rob was confined to the RotoProne bed for ten days with no possibility of being weaned from the ventilator the entire time. He was finally removed from the bed on September 28, 2021, but only after Sheila insisted on his removal on September 27, 2021, during an interventional in-hospital family conference.

I knew they had to attempt to awaken Rob as part of the process of removing him from the ventilator, so I asked, "You are not waking him up? My understanding was that you had been first reducing the paralytic to see how he would handle it. Then, when you did that, he would become agitated, and you would put the paralytic back on. But when you do that, and he's given fentanyl and other paralytic drugs, they can put him in a state of delusion and hallucinations.

"My concern is that you've tried this so many times without letting me be here to help ground him. Rob and I are married, we are one, and we're spiritually connected. It's just too much to keep trying to do that without allowing me, as his wife, to connect with him and let him know it's going to be okay."

Dr. Liar firmly stood his ground, "**Yeah, once it's been 21 days from when he was diagnosed, THEN you can come and visit with him. That's, unfortunately, the rules!**" I cried out again, "I understand <u>the rules</u>. I just thought that because **you are the doctor**, and **he's your patient**—as an independent contractor, you could have brought me with you into the ICU because he is **your patient,** and you know he needs me. **<u>Do you want him to recover</u>?** If you do, I know having me here with him will help speed his recovery."

He replied, "I hear where you're coming from, but it's, you know . . . I can't change that picture. So, the hospital still would not let you in. It's not under my control." I said, "They told me three days from now, on Thursday, is the earliest I can see him. I've been waiting since his admission, and it's been over 17 days now."

He said, "We are letting him rest. The paralytic can cause long-term complications. That's why we try to wean him from it." I queried, "When you reduce the paralytic, he gets agitated, and then you have to repeat this process again? Is that right?"

Dr. Liar said, "That's more of a **visceral response** in the sense that you start struggling on the ventilator. That's why he's on the paralytic." I felt Rob's agitation was an intellectual, not a visceral, response. I expected it was due to fear and confusion. So I replied, "I know, I understand that. But to me, he's agitated and not peaceful and calm because he has not heard a familiar voice saying, 'it's okay.' He needs to hear the voice of someone he recognizes."

Dr. Liar affirmed, "We are trying to keep him as comfortable as possible throughout all of this without leaving long-term ramifications from the sedatives and the paralytics. That's kind of where the balance is, and I understand you are concerned about his psychological well-being, and rightfully **as so many people do have traumatized problems in the ICU**. So, we're going to try and keep him comfortable and calm throughout this. When it's time, you can come in and visit with him. Well . . . that's all I can promise you from that standpoint."

Even though my precious "twenty minutes" with Rob were ticking away, my husband's life was at stake. So I continued, "But you understand how important it is for him to hear a calm and familiar voice. I mean, it's science. He needs to know I'm here because he came in here telling me, '*I will die in here.*'

"He needs me! **I think it would really improve his recovery chances if I were here.** So, to make me wait a total of 21 days is not helping him." Dr. Liar dismissively said, "It's out of my hands. It's out of my control." Once more, he happily hid behind the shield of the hospital's "policy."

I prodded, "Is there anyone else I could ask?" He glibly responded, "Talk to the administration of the hospital. That's the only people." I advised him that when I spoke with Dr. Wicked three days earlier, he said he would favor me coming in sooner if the other doctors agreed. If all the doctors agreed, the administration, which had not budged an inch up to now, might allow me to come in sooner.

"I'm just trying to get your approval because the hospital administration might listen to reason with your approval. I know it's out of your hands. I just need your approval."

Choking a bit on my words while hoping to smooth things over to protect Rob from potential retaliation, I said, "I appreciate you and all the doctors. I think this is the best hospital Rob could be in. And I really, really appreciate all you're doing." He responded, "We appreciate that too. I mean, we're doing the best we can."

In a last-gasp effort, I tried a softer approach. "Well, thank you. I can hear the compassion in your voice, I feel that you are very compassionate, and I appreciate you taking the time to listen to my heart. I'll absolutely continue to ask the administration and see if I can pull any strings. If not, you know I'm waiting." But, he again told me, "I cannot give you a decision, unfortunately."

> **LEGAL COUNSEL STATEMENT**
> Members of the jury, as you can see, Dr. Liar had no genuine concern for Rob. Instead, he used the hospital's 21-day isolation policy to shield himself from intrusive family members who might interfere with or question "the protocol that kills," which he strictly followed.
>
> *How convenient it must be to have the protection of hospital administration's policies and federal and state laws so that you can follow a deadly protocol without question or interference from family members and with complete impunity; a protocol that you are fully aware will result in the death of your patients.*

Sensing my retreat, he said, "I try to give updates every day. Sometimes it gets busy, where I may miss a day, but I'll do my best to give you an update as much as I can. If there is a big change, obviously, I will call. But if things were pretty stable, or even slightly improved, depending on how things are going with other patients . . . as you can imagine, it's hard to make twenty different phone calls and take care of patients."

Again, trying to keep the peace, I said, "Thank you for your compassion and explanations. It really does help." He walked away, saying, "I will keep you informed."

Unfortunately, my twenty minutes were up, and I had not spent any time comforting Rob. I whispered in the brief final moment I had with him, "You're such a good man. I miss you. You are my everything. Heidi misses you, too. Everyone wants me to tell you they love you. You are so loved, my darling."

At that moment, a nurse walked in and said, "Your time is up." I bent down and told Rob one more time, "I love you so much!" I hoped Rob could hear me. I also hoped he heard my twenty-minute conversation with Dr. Liar as I pleaded for him to help me gain admittance to the hospital sooner so I could finally be by his side and witness his care firsthand. I knew that only then could I truly advocate for him effectively.

I reluctantly exited the room. I was dejected and disheartened by Dr. Liar's refusal to make an appeal on my behalf to be with my husband. The nurse showed me where to dispose of my gown, cap, mask, face shield, gloves, and booties and then pointed toward the ICU's exit doors.

Sadly, my attempt to touch Dr. Liar's heart, hoping he would do the right thing for Rob and me, had failed. He categorically refused to advocate for my earlier admission because his own comfort and convenience (and the fact that I would be out of his way for a few more days) were more important to him than Rob's health and well-being.

I had again poured out my heart and offered solid reasoning for why I should be allowed to be by my husband's side. However, as occurred every time, I had been advised that "**the policy**" was far more important than "**the patient**."

I could imagine a monthly hospital staff meeting where the meeting coordinator announced, "*I have great news. This month we lost several patients. Each of them had lost all hope because we kept them isolated from the prying eyes of their family members. I am proud to announce that not one family member was able to violate our 21-day "isolate and devastate" policy. Better yet, we were able to earn the full federal government bonus payout on each deceased patient. So, way to go, team—and keep up the great work!*"

As I headed down in the elevator, I contemplated Hebrews 10:23, "*Let us hold fast the confession of our hope without wavering, for he who promised is faithful.*" I definitely needed to hold fast to the little hope I had and not waiver. My friend John, who had patiently waited for me, asked if he could take me to lunch. Although I was emotionally and physically drained and not at all hungry, I accepted his kind offer. I knew it would be a good opportunity to unwind.

John gave me a disturbed and surprised look as I described the PPE equipment I had to wear, the awful sticking sound of the booties I wore as I walked on the grimy floor, and how eerie I felt seeing Rob strapped inside the bizarre RotoProne bed. I told him of the disconcerting noises—especially the bellow-like sound of the ventilator that was breathing for Rob. Finally, I told him I was so shocked by the unclean conditions that I could not believe medical professionals worked in such filth.

I told him the RotoProne bed looked like something out of the Medieval period, and I felt as if Rob had been strapped into a torture device where his naked body was covered with numerous thick black vinyl cushions with his arms in vinyl sleeves that were strapped to his side. I could see that Rob had developed a rash from the irritation of the vinyl rubbing against his skin, and

I could only see his nose, fingers, toes, and crusty beard. He was not at all clean, and there was no soft cotton gown or linen to protect his skin from the hot, non-breathing vinyl.

I began crying as I explained how I had seen blood dripping from his nose onto the drop cloth thrown across the rails under the apparatus and how a nurse had told me it was "okay and normal."

NONE of it was normal, and NONE of it was okay! On the contrary, it was all horrible. I could imagine how unbearably uncomfortable my hot-natured husband would be if he could feel anything while his skin was pressed firmly against the vinyl.

I knew he would feel terribly claustrophobic if he became aware of his condition. Just the thought of it all made my skin crawl. They had told me they had him lying face down for sixteen hours at a time, then face up for six hours. How could anyone survive in conditions like this?

John did his best to console me as I expressed my desperation and despair. I knew he was deeply concerned for Rob, yet he tactfully avoided speculating on what Rob's chances were. After lunch, he quickly dropped me off at my home because he had to hurry back to Austin.

I was so happy to have had John's support and that I was finally allowed to see Rob for the first time in over two weeks. John standing by my side and saying, "*I plan to stay right here until we get somewhere,*" had made all the difference. What an incredible man. Without him, I would not have been able to see Rob today—or at least see the few parts of him that were visible while he was fully cocooned in the RotoProne bed.

While in the room, I took a few pictures, and upon reviewing them, I was surprised to see that a hospital plaque mounted to the left of a white marker board said, "*Good health is in your hands.*" I thought, "*What does that mean in the setting of an ICU room? **Besides, they took Rob's health out of his hands and mine** and made all the decisions for us.*"

Rob and I had both fought hard to have "good health" remain in **our** hands. Yet they managed to wrench health away from us by ignoring his caloric intake (which led to his being dehydrated and starved), placing him on a contraindicated positive-pressure BiPAP, poisoning him with unnecessary and harmful drugs, then giving him a life sentence on a ventilator.

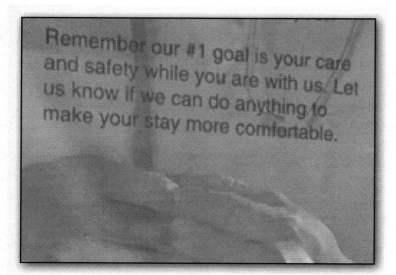

The same plaque contained this phrase: "*Remember our #1 goal is your care and safety while you are with us. Let us know if we can do anything to make your stay more comfortable.*"

To them, "*more comfortable*" meant more heavy sedatives, opioids, paralytics, antibiotics, and analgesics prescribed by wacko doctors and administered by robotic nurses.

The white marker board contained the phrase, "*Healing Hands - Caring Hearts.*"

That may have been true in times past, but not in this new era of incentivized protocols. It should have instead read, "*Hurtful Hands – Greedy Hearts.*"

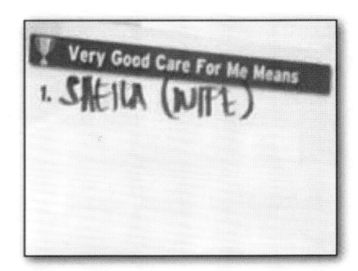

A section of the board said, "Very Good Care For Me Means" and written in the space below was **1. SHEILA (WIFE),** followed by my phone number.

What they should have written on the board were Rob's true desires, which were:

1. Having Sheila, my wife, by my side as my advocate!
2. Having adequate food and water so I may regain my strength.
3. NOT being given remdesivir or other harmful medications.
4. NOT being harassed to be intubated and placed on a ventilator.

Later that evening, when I called to check on his condition, Nurse Jackknife said, "He's doing okay; his blood pressure was up just **a little bit**. It was, like, in the low 160s. So, I gave him just a little bit of labetalol, and it came down. Right now, it is 146 over 89, back down **a little bit**. I turned him a couple of times, got him cleaned up **a little bit**, and brushed his teeth a few times.

"I haven't tried to do anything with the Nimbex [paralytic] just yet because he's still been kind of alarming 'the vent' every so often. Yeah. So, if we go a little while and we can relax **a little bit** more, and he seems a little more in tune with 'the vent,' then I'll try and go down on it. Yeah, he calmed down. *Last time, I think I might have gotten him a little riled up when we were repositioning and things.*"

I wanted to ask what he meant by "*a little riled up,*" but I kept my cool so he would continue. "But I don't want to just leave him in one spot in the bed. I know he might be a little more comfortable in one spot, but I don't want to leave him in one spot for too long."

I was concerned to hear that Nurse Jackknife repositioned Rob in the RotoProne bed all by himself. I commented, "I don't like him stuck in one spot, either. So, how do you position him? How do you do it yourself?"

He confidently responded, "Oh, yeah, he's not too big. On bigger patients, I'll get another set of hands. *But I just squeeze him up in the bed a little bit.* Then, I turn him from side to side a couple of times."

As we ended our call, I said, "I was able to see Rob for the first time today, and I noticed he's got a little cut on one of his ears." Not knowing how it happened, he could only say, "Yeah, I saw that."

I had reached the end of yet another discouraging and exasperating day of trying to convince heartless medical professionals and staff that family members were not annoyances but were essential to aid in the rapid recovery of critically ill patients.

Tuesday, September 21, 2021

During my usual morning call, I ended up speaking with Dr. Liar. I politely said, "Hi, Doctor, how are you?" He responded, "All right, how are you?" I replied, "Good. How is Rob doing today?"

He said, "He's doing . . . well to be. . . okay. We've got him down to 70% on his oxygen. We currently have him down in a prone position at the moment, and he seems to be doing well with that. The only issue that I see is he's had a little fever this morning. He's been having some low-grade fevers the last few days, but now it's a little bit higher, up to like 101."

When asked what might have caused a fever, he said, "An infection somewhere—could be pneumonia. When you're sick in the ICU, sometimes extra bacteria . . . they start to grow, and they can cause fever and infection. I think that's possible. He is on antibiotics, but sometimes patients can develop resistance in the morning, so we might need to make some changes. I think that's probably what's driving it, and we've seen this before. He's not showing signs of being septic in the sense that his blood pressure is low or anything like that. So, we just need to probably make some adjustments with these antibiotics. I was gonna defer to the infectious disease doctor on that."

After reflecting on what he said, I replied, "Okay, what is your prognosis today, like moving forward?" Dr. Liar commented, "I mean, right now, I'm just waiting for the inflammation . . . his lungs to get better. So, I try to wean his support on the ventilator. It's a little bit better today than it was yesterday, and then I've kind of gone down to 70% FiO2. I know he's gotten down that low before and kind of got back up. You know, I'm just wanting to get down. Ideally, you know, 40 to 50% FiO2 oxygen. That's where we can really start weaning a lot of the support."

I meticulously documented every detail of my husband's care and vitals from the daily MyChart records and conversations with doctors and nurses. So I shared with him that I had noticed they had Rob's FiO2 down to 50% three days earlier, on September 18th.

He seemed surprised to hear that and said, "Yeah, I'm looking back in his records. He was at 60% FiO2 a couple of days ago. **At the beginning of the 18th, he was down to— 50% FiO2**. He kind of went up then as high as 80 to 90% FiO2. Now he's down there needing 70%. So, you are right. On September 18th, it went down to 50% FiO2."

LEGAL COUNSEL STATEMENT

Members of the jury, as we noted earlier, Rob's FiO2 was **actually down to 45%** on the afternoon of September 18th, which we discovered during our deep dive into the hospital records.

Thus, the doctors should have lowered the PEEP setting (the residual pressure left in the lungs by the ventilator after expiration) to 8 or less to see if Rob's blood oxygen level would stabilize at 85% or higher. If it did so, then based on their extubation protocol, they should have reduced the sedatives and paralytics to determine if they could wean Rob from the ventilator. Neglectfully or maliciously bypassing this critical opportunity was criminal.

Adding insult to injury, once Rob was placed in the RotoProne bed at 9:30 PM on the evening of September 18th, he was sentenced to not having the opportunity of being weaned from the ventilator until he was extracted from the bed, something Dr. Liar had confirmed during Sheila's brief 20-minute visit to the ICU the day before when he advised her <u>he would **not attempt** to wean Rob from the ventilator while Rob was in this bed</u>.

I asked, "Why do you think his oxygen requirements go up and down? Are there any other underlying issues?" He stated, "No, I think it's just the inflammation from Covid that is driving this right now; and it's not just the inflammation, but also Covid causes clotting issues as well."

"And we have him on blood thinners. Lovenox, essentially, to help with the D-dimer test results, as that's gotten a little bit worse. We're probably going to increase his blood thinner to more of a full dose of this blood thinner. Covid sometimes causes problems with clotting, and that can cause problems with the oxygen. Okay? Does that make sense? Obviously, when you increase the blood thinner, there is **a risk** of bleeding as well. So, try to watch that **risk versus benefits**."

I was deeply concerned about the vast numbers and dosages of medications they were administering. Rob was so opposed to taking prescription drugs that he rarely took aspirin. Thus, I asked Dr. Liar if they could begin to reduce the dosages.

He responded, "Probably not, as far as you know . . . he's getting . . . I mean . . . it's the bacteria that gets resistant. But eventually, we'll need to cut back on some antibiotics depending on his fever. I'm not sure we want to really do that just yet. Understand? We've already cut back on steroids. So, some other medications he's on are **not really** going to cause any major issues."

LEGAL COUNSEL STATEMENT

Members of the jury, despite Dr. Liar's assertion that "some other medications he's on are **not really** going to cause any major issues," there is no doubt that the barrage of medications Rob was subjected to caused him significant harm and injury and contributed to his eventual death.

For example, Dr. Liar failed to advise Sheila that at 6:35 PM on September 20th, he had started Rob on a risky Emergency Use Authorization (EUA) trial drug named **baricitinib** (Olumiant). It is an anti-inflammatory drug typically prescribed for treating rheumatoid arthritis; Rob did not have this condition.

Baricitinib's potentially harmful side effects include upper respiratory tract infections, lower respiratory tract infections, increased liver enzyme levels, fever, shortness of breath, cancer and immune system problems, increased risk of heart attack, blood clots, and tears in the stomach or intestines of patients who are on corticosteroids—and Rob was being administered high doses of a potent corticosteroid named SOLU-MEDROL. Dosing & side effects: Olumiant® (baricitinib). Dosing & Side Effects | Olumiant® (baricitinib). (n.d.). From https://www.olumiant.com/dosing-side-effects

Thus, without Sheila's knowledge, Rob was given an additional medication that could have caused or worsened some of the symptoms they attributed to "Covid," significantly diminishing his chances of survival.

Before administering an EUA trial drug such as baricitinib, Dr. Liar was legally and morally obligated to explain the risks and benefits to Sheila and obtain her "informed consent." Accordingly, we contend that his deliberate failure to do so constitutes malfeasance and malpractice.

He continued, "He's better than yesterday. Yes, he's on less oxygen than yesterday. So, that's a good thing. The D-dimer is up **a little bit**, and that's not as good of a thing. But I'm going to try and address that with the Lovenox. With all of this, it's kind of an up-and-down sort of process. You know, in the big picture, is he dramatically worse? NO. I mean, it's a matter of that I want him to be trending to get better, essentially."

When I asked what his discharge plan was for Rob, he responded, "Yeah. The discharge plan kind of depends on where he's at in the future. I mean, it kind of depends on how long he's required to be on the vent too. Eventually, if he's on the ventilator for a while, there's a possibility that he may need, like, a tracheotomy tube, for example. But he's not there yet, in the sense that he requires too much oxygen support for a trach. He needs to be on less support than he is currently for that.

"And then the decision at that point would be, **is he strong enough to try and extubate or not**? And I can't tell you if he will be or not. But the longer he is on the ventilator, the more likely he is going to be a little too weak to just take the tube out of his mouth. And that's where a trach is helpful, and the trach helps us wean people from the ventilator better.

"Because if I, like, for example, if I had him on a setting where I did some weaning, and he seemed okay, and I took the tube out, but then he gets into trouble again, I have to go through the trauma of putting the tube back in and sedating him again and so forth; but with the tracheotomy we surgically place, it's removable, it's not a permanent fixture.

"You know, all we have to do is disconnect from the ventilator to the tracheotomy tube, and if he's breathing fine, that's great. If he gets in trouble, we just have to connect them back to the ventilator without any sort of trauma or anything. It's also a lot more comfortable for someone because we don't have to sedate them as much as when we happen to have a tube in our mouth because having a tube in your mouth . . . it kind of makes you gag.

"And so, the trach really doesn't cause you to gag or hurt much at all. That doesn't hurt at all, really, once it's placed. It's possible we may recommend that, but I just can't tell you if that's the case. I mean, it gives you a discharge plan that's kind of going in that direction . . . that possibility."

I responded, "Now if we do get to that point in the future, will I be informed before we move forward?" He said, "We'd have to get your consent." His admission that he would need my consent surprised me, as my "consent" had never been an issue. The doctors had been prescribing whatever treatments "the protocol" demanded without my knowledge and despite my objections.

I later called the ICU nurses' station to inquire about Rob's condition from his nurse and spoke with Nurse Madness. "Hi, this is Sheila Skiba. I just wanted to get an update on how Robert Skiba is doing."

She said, "I think probably pretty much about the same. He's still on 70% oxygen on the ventilator. Oxygen saturation has been like 93-94%. So, when I got here this morning, his oxygen level [FiO2] was at 80%. So, we've been able to come down slowly throughout the day. So hopefully, we'll continue to do that. And he's on his belly right now. So, usually, when he goes on to his back, his oxygen will be **a little bit low**. Sometimes it'll drop, so we just have to see how he tolerates it."

I asked Nurse Madness if she could connect me with the respiratory therapist. She then made a call and connected us.

The therapist introduced herself as RT Jab. I advised her who I was, told her I had questions about my husband, and said, "I know our focus and goal are a safe and stable extubation. My first question is, what are the barriers to extubating Rob now?" She said, "His oxygen requirement is, is extremely high. He's on 70%, and he's on a PEEP of 14. **Normal PEEP is 5.** Okay? Those would need to come down. His lungs have got to start recovering. Basically, we're proning him.

"You saw that yesterday, where he's in that special bed to lay on his chest. That's to help improve oxygenation. He has to be able to maintain oxygen of like 50% FiO2 and get his PEEP down to be able to come off that bed. **So, we're nowhere near extubation until when he starts coming off that bed.** We're moving closer, but **likely he'll still be on high PEEP when he comes off that bed.**"

I was troubled by the fact that Rob had been on a ventilator for nearly two weeks, and the PEEP had never been lowered below 14. They would never be able to extubate him and remove him from the ventilator without reducing the PEEP. Worse yet, Dr. Liar informed me that they would not attempt to wean him while he was in the RotoProne bed, a bed in which he should not have been placed without first informing me of the risks and benefits and obtaining my permission. The fact that they put him in the bed without consulting me further proves that they made decisions unilaterally without my input.

I asked, "Okay, so the focus is his lungs, as they need to start recovering. Are there any other underlying issues affecting his recovery?" She responded, "No, not as far as I can tell. As for any other underlying issues other than observations, he doesn't have a PE [pulmonary embolism] or anything that I'm aware of. So, right now, it's just his lungs and oxygenating. So just like, you know, the plan to address it is more time and getting him out of the bed, and proning, and getting **supportive therapies and medications that he's already currently on, with all those working together**.

"But mainly, it just takes time . . . some time for their lungs to start recovering, and we will slowly start coming down on things. We just haven't been able to make any improvement. He's kind of staying at the same place. It just takes time for their lungs to start recovering."

LEGAL COUNSEL STATEMENT

Members of the jury, as RT Jab stated, Rob was getting "*therapies and medications*" that were "*working together.*" Unfortunately, the numerous and heavy doses of medications Rob was being administered were "*working together*" to further weaken Rob and destroy his ability to breathe independently.

Five days earlier, on September 15, 2021, Dr. Wicked had advised Sheila that "*his LFTs [Liver Function Tests] have been going up.*" and he admitted "*it is probably medication related*" while noting **the antibiotics** were the most likely culprit. **Sheila immediately asked him to please stop the toxic drugs** (a directive he blatantly ignored) because the massive assault from the medications was causing Rob further injury. Dr. Wicked admitted, "*We usually don't worry about stopping and changing his medications until the lab results are more than 8 to 10 times the upper limit of normal.*"

Their plan was to wait until the drugs had caused sufficient damage to his liver and kidneys, as measured by the results of key laboratory tests reaching 8 to 10 times the normal upper limit. We argue that this is clear evidence of malicious intent and that, contrary to what the doctors wanted Sheila to believe, "Covid" was not the monster. Instead, the monster putting Rob's life at risk was the doctors themselves.

Below is a list of just a few of the unnecessary and harmful medications and their negative impacts:

- As noted above, on September 20, 2021, Dr. Torture began administering an Emergency Use Authorization trial drug called **baricitinib** at 4 mg for 12 doses. He also prescribed **acetaminophen** (a pain reliever) at 650 mg. for nine doses. *Both drugs can cause liver damage and failure.* Also, as noted at UpToDate.com, "*Patients treated with baricitinib are at risk for developing serious infections that may lead to hospitalization or death.*"
UpToDate. (n.d.). From https://www.uptodate.com/contents/baricitinib-drug-information

  Clear evidence of **baricitinib's** ability to cause liver damage is the National Library of Medicine's article titled "**LiverTox: Clinical and Research Information on Drug-Induced Liver Injury**," which states, "*Monitoring of serum aminotransferase [ALT] levels is recommended for patients starting **baricitinib**. De novo elevations in serum aminotransferases [ALT] levels above five times the upper limit of normal should lead to temporary cessation. If serum enzyme elevations do not resolve or improve within a few weeks of stopping, or **if symptoms of liver injury or jaundice arise, baricitinib should be permanently discontinued**.*"
NCBI Bookshelf. (n.d.). From https://www.ncbi.nlm.nih.gov/books/NBK548012

- Rob was also being administered high doses of **SOLU-MEDROL** with **baricitinib**. As noted at Drugs.com, "*Using baricitinib together with predniSONE [both prednisone and SOLU-MEDROL are corticosteroids that are used to reduce inflammation and suppress the immune system] **may increase the risk of serious and potentially fatal infections**.*" Unfortunately, Rob later developed several serious infections that helped facilitate his demise and eventual death.
Olumiant and prednisone interactions. Drugs.com. (n.d.).
From https://www.drugs.com/drug-interactions/olumiant-with-prednisone-3917-18860-1936-0.html

- On October 2nd, a Physician's Assistant covering for the Infectious Disease doctor noted Rob had elevated liver enzymes (they had risen to **more than 3x the upper limit**). *Unfortunately, a physician incorrectly attributed his elevated liver enzymes to an infection instead of a drug-induced injury. Since there is a drug for every symptom, the physician prescribed more drugs, **meropenem** and **vancomycin** (broad-spectrum carbapenem antibiotics), to treat the presumed infection. We contend that these unnecessary antibiotics exacerbated Rob's liver and kidney damage, ultimately leading to organ failure.*

According to Medscape, "*Drugs are an important cause of liver injury. More than 900 drugs, toxins, and herbs have been reported to cause liver injury, **and drugs account for 20-40% of all instances of fulminant [severe and sudden onset] hepatic failure**. Approximately 75% of the idiosyncratic drug reactions result in liver transplantation or death.*"
Nilesh Mehta, M. D. (2022, July 8). Drug-induced hepatotoxicity. Overview, Metabolism of Drugs, Clinical and Pathological Manifestations of Drug-Induced Liver Disease. From https://emedicine.medscape.com/article/169814-overview

AST and **ALT** are liver enzymes commonly measured to evaluate liver function and **detect liver damage**. Typically, the range for normal **AST** is reported between **10 to 40 units per liter** and **ALT** between **7 to 56 units per liter.** *On the right is a graph of Robert A Skiba II's ALT and AST levels from 10/5/21 through his death on 10/13/21.*

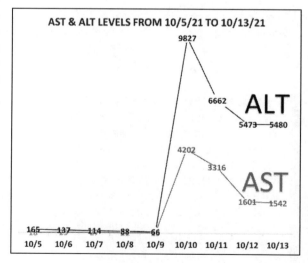

AST & ALT LEVELS FROM 10/5/21 TO 10/13/21

AST and **ALT** levels above 15 times the normal range **indicate severe acute liver cell injury**; levels greater than 1000 units per liter **are considered critical**.

*As shown in the chart above, on October 10, 2021, Rob Skiba's **AST level** reached **4,202**, and his **ALT level** reached **9,827** U/L. We contend that these massive and sudden elevations were due to the large quantities of hepatotoxic medications Rob was being administered.*

154

> Sammy Wong, M.D., our medical expert witness, stated in his interim analysis: "*The Hospitalist attributed the elevated liver enzymes to COVID or hepatic steatosis, not the possibility of* **a drug-induced influence***. Although the liver enzymes eventually returned toward normal, it again increased dramatically* **into the thousands** *prompting the liver specialist (gastroenterologist) to order a wide spectrum of labs ("shot-gunning" a diagnosis) but later attributed the hepatitis to ischemic liver.*"

The more RT Jab said, the more I could tell her hopeful pie in the sky, "*It just takes time for their lungs to start recovering,*" forecast **was never going to happen** because of the massive assault of harmful medications, the toxic levels of oxygen, and the high pressure (PEEP) Rob was continuously subjected to.

I knew Rob was in a dire situation when, eighteen days earlier, I was escorted out of the Emergency Department and denied permission to stay with him as his advocate. Any glimmer of hope I had was fading with each passing day.

I asked RT Jab, "So when you look at his X-rays, is there something you're seeing that's causing this?" She explained, "It's just time with Covid. Everything's really slow. Unfortunately, like, normally with people on a vent . . . **we start getting really nervous**."

Of course, she should be nervous. She had witnessed patients die on ventilators she had set to high pressures and toxic levels of oxygen. She had observed nurses hanging bag after bag of harmful medications because they were "following doctors' orders." This apparently clueless Respiratory Therapist had been performing the same task for two years. I wondered how many deaths she had contributed to by ensuring that her patients adhered to "the protocol that kills."

RT Jab went on, "**If they're on vent more than a week or two with Covid, they tend to be on it for a prolonged period of time to heal . . . a lot longer**. Patients with Covid always go up and down. I call it '*a honeymoon phase*,' like, where they start looking really well and we're able to start coming down on things . . . and then they go the complete opposite direction for no real reason."

That "*honeymoon phase*" where the patient starts "looking really well" and then something terrible happens was, in my opinion, **NOT due to Covid**, but due to "the protocol" that was killing the patients. When her patients finally died, did she say, "*oh well, I guess the honeymoon phase is over*"?

She alleged, "**they go the complete opposite direction** for no real reason." I knew full well that was not true. Patients were not going in the opposite direction "for no real reason." They were deteriorating and dying due to the drugs and therapies prescribed by the perpetrators who subjected them to "the protocol."

I could see that the entire American medical establishment needed to wake up and acknowledge that their protocol-driven treatments and medications were causing patients to needlessly "go the complete opposite direction" and causing their deaths. I did not want to have Rob become another of their grim statistics.

I wondered how the doctors, nurses, and respiratory therapists responsible for Rob's care could all be under the same delusion. Were they willingly burying their heads in the sand, or worse, did some of them really think the act of taking the life of an unsuspecting patient, especially if they were unvaccinated like Rob?

I also wondered how many patients must die before "medical professionals" (and I hesitate to use the term "professionals"; I prefer the term "predators") admit that "the protocol" they are adhering to is killing their patients (or is it victims?). I sensed that this insanity would never end until government incentives were eliminated and our corrupt medical system was completely reformed. Yet I realized such reform is unlikely to occur unless and until there is a massive outcry from American citizens shouting in unison ENOUGH IS ENOUGH!

She then noted, "He has no big major change on the chest X-ray. No pulmonary embolism. **Their oxygen requirements just tend to go up and down**, and it will continue to do that the remainder of the time."

Why would Rob's oxygen requirements "**go up and down**" if he was—as he should be—improving each day with the help of the "little rest" provided by the ventilator? Dr. Dead End deceived me by claiming that the ventilator would aid Rob's recovery. Now, Rob was on a roller-coaster ride of ups and downs, with the few "ups" resulting from the fact that he was still in the fight, desperately attempting to overcome the massive assault on his health.

Then, she continued, "We may start trending down and even be moving in the right direction for like a week. **But at some point, he'll take some steps back. But we anticipate that.**"

Her remarks did not make me feel any better. By saying, "**we anticipate that**," it sounded to me like she was fully expecting Rob to continue to deteriorate from this point onward until his body finally crashed and burned—just like the rest of their "Covid" patients who had been subjected to the deadly "protocol."

She ended with, "And so, we just go really slow on our weaning of the oxygen, the PEEP, and the VELETRI. But with him, we haven't been able to really move in any direction recently. **We're just kind of staying the course and not making a lot of changes.** Yes. But we've, like I said, with Covid, we typically see that where there's a period of, like, stagnant time where we're just maintaining, and there's not much improvement. They either get better or they start getting worse. That's expected."

"Staying the course" was not what I wanted to hear. I had been told Rob NEEDED to be on the ventilator and that it would give him the rest he needed to recover. Clearly, I had been misled, as Rob's condition was deteriorating daily, and he was **NOT** improving. In addition, Dr. Wicked had informed me twelve days prior that he would not have sufficient "reserves" to be taken off the ventilator after 10 to 14 days. Consequently, his chances of survival were declining by the day.

The only effect RT Jab had on me was to increase my adrenaline and put me in fight-or-flight mode. I was entirely motivated and prepared to act. However, I could not effectively defend Rob against their assault while being locked out of the hospital with doctors repeatedly and flagrantly ignoring my directives.

They were ecstatic that the hospital administration had granted them a 21-day pass during which they could do whatever they wished without my direct oversight. They only deemed it necessary to appease me with platitudes whenever I called so they could proceed with their plans for Rob.

In the evening, I placed another call to the ICU. Once more, a different nurse was on duty and caring for Rob. He said, "Hi, this is Nurse Jeering." I explained that I was calling to see how Rob was doing.

He said, "He's maintaining. I mean, his vital signs are looking good. I don't know when you called last. They said he was having some fever earlier today. Looks like his fevers are definitely coming down, and last time I went in was about 100. So, that's better. I think they've been giving him Tylenol, and they also have a cooling blanket on him. That kind of helps him maintain his temperature right now."

I asked him if they had done a blood culture to see if something else was happening. He looked in the records and said, "So, it doesn't look like they drew blood cultures in the last three weeks. But they did do a respiratory culture, which is where they get some of his sputum from down in his throat, and they did do a culture on that. They take a little drop of blood, smear it on a slide and then look at it. One of the doctors will look at it under a microscope to look for a couple of different germs . . . bacteria."

I asked if those cultures were done today, and he said, "Let's see here. No, it looks like one was done on September 9th, and a slide where they look at it under a microscope—that one was done on September 4th. The respiratory culture was done on September 9th." In the face of fever, their lack of emphasis on performing timely cultures was totally careless and negligent.

I said, "Got it. Okay. So, how will they be able to pinpoint an infection—where it's coming from and the source of the infection—unless they get a blood culture? Is there any way to get a blood culture on him?"

He said, "I mean, I could definitely talk with the physician or the nurse practitioner here. I can definitely talk to them about it." So I replied, "That would be great. Thank you so much. And you know just as well as I do that he's been on different types of antibiotics, so if you could ask, that would be great. I would really appreciate it."

He said, "You know, a lot of times when they do the blood cultures initially, they'll get them, and they like to do them <u>before</u> they give him the antibiotic. **But I have seen them do it after someone's been on antibiotics many times.** So, that's not to say that they're not useful at all, okay? I think I could bring that up."

His words were somewhat confusing. Was he saying Rob was being protected by the antibiotics he was already on or that the antibiotics would alter the results of a blood culture so that they may not be entirely accurate?

I then told him I was concerned about his wound. He said, "Yeah, he's really just got the one that we noticed is on his left ear. Yeah, and then he might have, like, a small blister or something on his right shin. But we dressed that, and that should be, you know . . . it shouldn't really get much worse. But sometimes just, you know, **that constant movement in the RotoProne bed day after day will sometimes lead to, like, little wounds.**"

After I concluded my conversation with Nurse Jeering, I received a call from a healthcare professional with whom Rob was familiar. He arranged a three-way call with a physician in

California named Dr. Mei. She said she would be willing to fly to Dallas in the morning to examine Rob and assist me in rescuing him from the "protocol-focused" (as opposed to "patient-focused") team of predators currently holding him captive.

I advised her, "I have some serious concerns and would like to brief you on what has been happening. I have never met the Infectious Disease doctor, and I have to beg the doctors and nurses for information on what they are doing to Rob. I have gone to the hospital in person several times and begged them to let me in to see Rob. If they want him well, why wouldn't they let his wife be with him to reassure him that everything will be okay?

"I called the Social Worker, and she hasn't returned my calls since Friday. I told the day shift nurse that I needed to talk with the infectious disease doctor who saw Rob three times today, and she never called me. There's a new note in Rob's hospital records noting that his heart rate was in the 120s. His hemoglobin was 9.9 [*the normal range for adult men is 14-18 g/dL*], and it's trending down."

Dr. Mei immediately stopped me and said, "**He's anemic**! He's bleeding; he's got fluid overload. Something's going on to cause his red blood cell count to drop!" I said, "Your coming could literally save his life."

The doctor replied, "You know, you can <u>demand</u> to have someone give you a report because he has patient's rights. If you have an attorney, file against the hospital for violating his patient's rights. That should get their attention, as there are hospital accreditation organizations that have oversight and monitor the facility."

I told her I had already addressed Rob's patient's rights by speaking with Risk Management. She said, "Did you ever speak to an attorney? I'm going to review all his charts and everything, and if his patient's rights have been denied, that's medical malpractice."

I told her, "In normal times, what you're saying may be true, but we live in a new era, the 'Covid' era, where there are no rights! I don't know how long you've dealt with this Covid situation, and I don't mean to sound rude, but I am dealing with a different type of animal here. *They do not seem to be afraid of attorneys or lawsuits.*"

She responded, "I went into a hospital, removed a man from his IVs, and took him out of there. They were going to cut his foot off, and I saved him from an amputation." That was nice, but that had been done in more normal times with someone who was not on a ventilator, paralyzed and sedated.

I told her I would pay for her flight, pick her up at Dallas/Fort Worth International Airport, and she could stay with me at my residence. She said she would immediately finalize her plans and arrive in Dallas as soon as possible.

Wanting me to understand her planned approach, she said, "I need to go and tell them I'm a medical doctor and I am coming in on behalf of the patient's rights; and if they say NO, I can't see Rob, then you can literally get a court order/injunction that will let you take him out of there. Really! You have legal rights, and if they refuse, you can really get after them because you have every legal right to go in and say, 'I don't like your care; I'm taking my husband to another hospital that will take better care of him.'"

Then, she informed me of the existence of a Healthcare Ethics Committee whose purpose is to assist patients, families, and all healthcare professionals in identifying, analyzing, and resolving ethical dilemmas and problems that arise in patient care. Her remarks gave me much food for thought. I advised her, "We've been looking for a holistic rehab facility, but at this point, I think he needs another hospital."

She encouraged me, "You can try to get another hospital. But if not, I believe he won't have that much difficulty getting off the ventilator." She said something about stem cells and oxygen that went way over my head. I told her we could discuss our detailed plan of action once she arrived.

I asked, "You think you can get him off the vent easily? And then what?" She confidently replied, "Yes, yes. He just needs oxygen. It's not a big deal to give him oxygen. Use a CPAP—**and he never needed to be hospitalized.** But here's the concern. *Why did his red blood cell count drop that low? That is concerning. His red blood cell count should not be dropping unless he's bleeding somewhere or they gave him too much fluid.* If it's too much fluid, then they've got a malpractice case on their hands."

She firmly believed the doctors' primary motivation was the incentive money provided by the federal government, saying she was well aware hospitals were being paid large bonuses simply by successfully getting patients on ventilators. "I am very confident he doesn't need a ventilator, and we'll manage it," she said.

I was amazed to finally have the attention of a medical doctor who understood Rob's predicament and wanted to help me save him from "the protocol" he had become a victim of. She added, "**I hate to say things against my colleagues, but I can't defend them. There is NO EXCUSE for this behavior.** *There's NO justification for them being so incompetent or unscrupulous.* It just is not right for them not to answer your questions or not allow you to be updated and informed. *That is totally illegal.*"

I agreed and added, "And not just that, but to isolate us from each other for 21 days . . . I'm afraid they're going to kill him in there." She agreed, saying, "**I have a feeling they're bent on that— because they'll get more money if he dies.**"

She said she would head to the airport and take the next available flight to Dallas. I could barely believe this was happening and that a physician who was firmly on my side would soon be arriving.

Wednesday, September 22, 2021

Dr. Mei called me in the morning and said she could not fly in until the next day, around noon. I would be prepared whenever she arrived, as I was determined to save my husband, even if it meant selling the clothes on my back and everything I owned.

I had high hopes that we would be able to save Rob together. I reached out to friends from across the nation, and prayers and offers of assistance poured in from all over the world.

A friend told me about a nurse who had witnessed firsthand the brutal treatment of patients in the name of the pandemic. Seeing patients suffer and die due to incompetence and malfeasance brought her to tears each day.

Unable to continue watching patients die at the hands of "professionals" who gleefully chased government incentives, she became a full-time patient advocate. She knew that without expert intervention, patients would continue to be isolated from their families, denied their rights, and terminated in the name of "the protocol."

When I called her, she said she had recently launched her business and was developing strategies to assist families affected by this tragedy. She informed me that some hospitals and physicians are more accommodating than others. However, many physicians viewed themselves as gods and refused to budge under any circumstances. She advised me that I would need patience and tact to win the battle for my husband.

Her preferred approach was to be soft-spoken, courteous, and assertive. Her goal was to avoid offending the doctors. However, I was the one who was being offended daily by the hospital's and doctors' insistence that I stay locked away from my husband for 21 days and their complete disregard for my directives. She acknowledged that a "soft touch" might give the impression that she was going too easy on the doctors, but she felt that "gaining a little cooperation was preferable to no cooperation."

"How long could Rob hold on to the side of a precipice with one fingernail?" I wondered. My husband was clinging to life by a thread, and we needed to act swiftly and forcefully before he died.

She explained that physicians and the medical establishment do not make hasty decisions. I informed her that I had been more than patient, as I had already been locked out of the hospital for 19 days and still had to wait two more days for my husband's "isolation" to be lifted. It was difficult to refrain from shouting in exasperation as I pondered how a "soft touch" could be effective with the unreasonable and unyielding abusers I had been battling.

On two separate occasions, one of the hospital's Social Workers, Ms. Destroyer, informed me that Rob's isolation would be lifted and I could visit him on September 23rd. I had marked that date on my calendar, and as I flipped through it, I became excited at the prospect of seeing Rob the following day. Then, I received a disturbing phone call from a colleague of hers who said, "I'm sorry, Ms. Destroyer *was told by someone* that you could visit on the 23rd, but the Infectious Disease doctors' notes say the 24th."

That was patently false. Ms. Destroyer had not been "*told by someone*" that I could visit on the 23rd. She had calculated that date on her own. During our call on September 9th, she had said, "So, the rule at the moment is . . . well, not at the moment, it's been this way since the beginning . . . **the CDC recommends twenty days from the date of his first positive**, and that was September 3rd." Then, during a conversation on September 13th, she noted, "Yeah, cuz we have his first positive as September 3rd, twenty days will be September 23rd." Whether through incompetence or outright deceit, the team at Covid Coven Hospital in Plano, Texas, consistently misled me.

Trying to remain optimistic amid this disturbing news, I called the ICU nurses' station. I requested to speak with Mr. Pathetic, the ICU Floor Supervisor had who escorted me to Rob's room two days ago for a brief 20-minute visit, hoping he could help me get in to see Rob tomorrow.

I informed him that I believed Rob was in a critical condition and that if they admitted me to the hospital sooner, he would have a much greater chance of survival. He said he would confer with the Chief Medical Officer and get back to me by tomorrow morning with a decision.

I then contacted a nurse I knew with 22 years of experience, including ten years in the ICU. I told her that a doctor from California had told me I could fire all of Rob's doctors if I so wished. But she said, "This doctor may be telling you that you can fire all the doctors, but all the doctors in the area know each other; they all play golf together. So, if you fire one group, the next group will continue with the same protocol, and they will simply watch Rob die." *Her keen insight made it clear that Rob and I were suffering from a widespread systemic plot to adhere to a deadly protocol.*

When I called the ICU to check on Rob, I ended up speaking with Nurse Jackknife. I queried, "Two doctors' notes say Rob's heart rate was 120, and I wanted to know what it is now." He said, "Right now? I just was peeking in there. It's been between like 95-98, and they'll kind of fluctuate in that range. His temperature is 98.3."

I had read that the normal range for hemoglobin in adult men was 14-18, so I said, "The hemoglobin was at 9.9 yesterday, it's now 8.8, and it looks like it's trending down. When would you ever do anything to take care of that? This trend is not good."

He replied, "As far as, like, transfusing blood or giving blood products usually, as long as he is hemodynamically stable, which means, like, his heart rate is good, his blood pressure is good, all of that, they will usually wait until it's down to like, 7.0. Yeah, that is safe; I mean, that's not for everybody. Yeah, that's a normal kind of, like, guideline. We would expect them to say, okay, if it gets below 7, go ahead if you need to give blood products. So yeah, that's, that's kind of what that is."

I questioned why they would allow his hemoglobin to drop so low before taking action. Low hemoglobin levels were of no greater concern to them than the fact that he had been malnourished and starved since the day of his arrival.

I asked, "It's so hard because I can't be there, but what is your assessment of how he's doing tonight?" Nurse Jackknife said, "Well, tonight, I mean, last night, the big thing was the temperature, and we're good on that. They did stop some of his antibiotics. I don't know if you were able to read Dr. Torture's note. She's the infectious disease doctor. Yeah, she stopped some of those. She wanted to see if maybe he was reacting to that, like sometimes, **with antibiotics, you can have an increased temperature**. So, she stopped those. And we will kind of look at his lab work in the morning and make sure his blood counts are now trending back up. And you know, they don't need to look at starting some other antibiotics or restarting what he's on."

I asked Nurse Jackknife if they would take any cultures to identify what might be causing his fever. He replied, "I think potentially . . . we'll see what his white count looks like. If it starts trending back up tomorrow to a certain point, then they may consider restarting or starting different antibiotics. And with the blood cultures, it usually takes a few days to get like, if something is growing. It takes a few days to identify exactly what it is. Usually, it takes a day or so. They will look at them and see if there is something growing; if there is, they'll do like a rough identification. It won't be like a pinpoint. And then from there, they can, you know, pick and choose antibiotics that are effective against that group of bacteria or whatever is growing."

I countered, "I think the drugs are jacking him up, I'm pretty sure they are, and he looked really swollen when I saw him the other day. So, I'm just trying to cope. You said he doesn't have a fever now."

Nurse Jackknife responded, "So, I'm just saying if, if something were to grow in those blood cultures, they take more than one sample and from various ports. *If only one came up positive, it would be because of contamination, NOT because he had an infection. Both sample cultures would have to show an infection before they put him on another antibiotic. So, they don't say that something is, you know, in his system unless it's growing in both of those samples.*"

That made sense. If only one sample showed up with bacteria, one of the samples must have been *contaminated*. Unfortunately, Dr. Torture and Dr. Liar had told me their protocol was to treat with antibiotics **if only ONE sample** came up positive, just to be sure. However, by treating Rob with antibiotics when only one of two cultures was positive, they were subjecting him to unnecessary and harmful medications that were weakening him further and decreasing his likelihood of survival.

I said, "I don't understand why they say he gets agitated while on the ventilator. That's why I was so concerned that he needs me with him to tell him, 'Honey, you're okay.' He doesn't know where he is, and I've been told the fentanyl and propofol he has been given can make him hallucinate. So, I don't understand why they would keep him from me that long. That's what's so alarming to me."

He said, "I'm jumping way ahead here. Well, the reason for the paralytic is that they do that **if he is agitated,** and that's also why they use the sedation. Being on the ventilator is uncomfortable. It can, like you said, it can be scary. So, one of the first things we do is to sedate a patient to keep them what we call 'tolerant' or 'compliant' with the ventilator so the ventilator can do its job without the patient fighting because, on two fronts, that [not being 'compliant'] is kind of . . . is counterproductive because the patient is then having to expel more energy or more oxygen, things like that, to fight against the ventilator.

"And it's not because he's doing it on purpose; it's a foreign thing, you know, a tube is not comfortable. **And, you know, you're used to just normally breathing. So first off, you're burning energy, burning oxygen, trying to fight the ventilator and breathe on your own.** But also, at the same time, the ventilator can't do its job. It can't fill the lungs with oxygen; it can't pull out the carbon dioxide. So that's why we do that. And a lot of times, if we can't accomplish that just with the sedation, then that's when they go to the paralytic."

I said, "I think I'll be more comfortable when I'm there because I feel he needs my touch to know he's okay. I don't know what he's thinking in his mind." When I asked about Rob's vitals, he said, "Right now, his blood pressure is 114 over 61 with a mean of 80. So that's perfect. His saturation is at 93% right now, and they did come down a little bit on his FiO2 today. He's on 65% right now. **The PEEP is still at 14.** Usually, they'll try and get down a little bit lower on the PEEP before they start coming down on the paralytic."

I said, "Thank you so much. I'm just trying to understand what's going on with him because I gotta have him back. I need him." He said, "No, I understand this. **Trust me; this is not the first time I've had this conversation. The last two and a half years have been, you know, pretty much the same thing.** It's been hard on everybody."

I asked him, "Are you married?" He responded quickly, "Not yet. I will be in a couple of weeks." I continued, "Okay. Well, when you do get married. I'm sure you love your fiancé. I mean, it is making me crazy. It's so inhumane to do this to a person and their family, and I know it's not your fault; it's these protocols. He said, "I know this is hard on everybody. You want to be here, but you know the way things are. I know how it is. Trust me, and like I said, I've had this conversation multiple times."

Sadly, Nurse Jackknife had been working inside the system for the last two and a half years, and when he said, "The last two and a half years have been, you know, **pretty much the same thing**," whether he realized it or not he was admitting that he had been assisting the doctors with their protocol that kills, leading to "**pretty much the same thing**" for every patient.

I then asked him how Rob's lungs were sounding. He replied, "Not bad. Still a little bit coarse, but he's moving air through all the fields. We obviously can't listen to his backside just yet, being that he's on that RotoProne bed, but we're gonna flip him over here in about 20 minutes or so, then we'll be able to listen to the back side. But the front side, he's moving air. It's a little bit coarse because of the pneumonia still, but it's not horrible. Like, I've heard worse for sure."

I thanked him for his compassion and understanding. He then said, "Oh, my God, like I said, I know it's not an easy thing for anybody. **I've seen, you know, just horrible situations throughout the last couple of years.** So I know it's hard on you, but, you know, keep your head up. We're gonna keep doing everything we can." Unfortunately, they were unwittingly, or nefariously, doing everything they could to hasten Rob's decline.

I called a family friend, Jay Goodman, an ICU nurse who had been coaching me on handling Rob's critical situation. I told him about Dr. Mei, the medical doctor who had volunteered to come from California to try and advocate for me.

I said, "I am hopeful that when she comes, she can get in with her credentials, which I've been told she can. I don't understand how you safely get him off the drugs and the ventilator, and I hope she can help with that." He said, "Yes. We want to preserve him until he gets to a point where they can take that FiO2 down, bring the PEEP down, and get him off the ventilator **without killing him**."

As an ICU nurse for many years, Jay said he had seen many things that had made him cautious regarding medications, procedures, and doctors. He said, "Keep the line of communication open, write everything down, regardless of whether you trust them—**because I don't trust anybody**. Ronald Reagan coined it the best, '*trust but verify*.'"

We discussed how they had attempted to wean Rob without me being there multiple times. He suggested I call the night nurse back and ask him to note in the hospital record that, as his wife and Medical Power of Attorney, I did not want them to attempt to wean him without me there. He stated, "If the nurse replies, 'Yes,' saying he will put that in the record, then you will know if a physician walks in and sees your request in the record that they have to decide whether or not to call you—as they will be on notice that Rob's wife and Medical POA DOES NOT want him weaned without her present. **Yeah. I'm very concerned about Rob's safety right now."**

I responded, "So we can both feel safe. I'll call Nurse Jackknife right now." When Nurse Jackknife answered the phone, I said, "I was looking through my notes again and was wondering if they were planning to attempt the weaning process in the morning?" He said, "Well, that all depends. I doubt it'll be in the morning because his settings are still too high. Usually, they'll want him down to an FiO2 of at least 60 and a PEEP of no more than 8, okay, before they think about that."

I felt relieved and asked, "Can I ask you to put something in his hospital records? Please note that I want to be there when they attempt to wean him the next time. Rob is probably delirious and doesn't know where he is. So, I want to be with him. Please put in his chart that the doctor needs to call me before they do any weaning because I don't want them to attempt to wean Rob unless they talk to me first."

He said, "Yeah, I'm just writing it down on a piece of paper here so I don't forget before I can sit down at my computer. This is what I wrote. I said, 'Please notify Mrs. Skiba before any weaning trial.'" He then explained what the weaning process entailed. "There's a couple of steps. The first one is to try and cut back on the sedation. So, before they even make any changes as far as the mode of the ventilator, they will cut back on the sedation and see if he can follow commands, pull in his own breaths, and things like that. So that will happen, more than likely, slowly. We don't just, you know, go in there and turn off the ventilator."

I said, "If the plan of action is to do this, and you are lowering his sedation, just let me know **before** you do it. I'm just saying I don't want them to start the process and then call me halfway through and say, 'We're doing the weaning.' You're saying it takes a long time. I don't want them to even start the process until I am in the room so I can connect with my husband and let him know that he's okay." Nurse Jackknife confirmed, "Yeah. I'll put a note in there."

Wanting to know more, I asked, "After reducing the sedation, what happens next?" He replied, "Well, yeah, that's like, like, step one would be, we are able to bring his vent settings down to a level where we can even attempt to do a weaning trial. So, once he's down to that level, the next step would be coming down on the sedation, and that is something we look at constantly. That's not something you know . . . we can go up and down on that, you know, as we need to.

"So that's not something, like, we're holding at a certain level, and then we have an order to go ahead and do that. So as far as the weaning the sedation and things like that, that may be a little more difficult to coordinate because we can't call you every time we make a change to the sedation. Does that make sense?"

He was making it clear that they might reduce the sedatives without being able to tell me in advance. So I asked about the paralytic. "Yes, but the paralytic being reduced is also a big part of the weaning process, and I will have a heads-up on that, right?"

Nurse Jackknife replied, "It would be pointless to do a weaning trial while he's on the paralytic because his diaphragm would be paralyzed, and he wouldn't be able to breathe out. And so, when he comes down on those vent settings, like I said, then we can start thinking about coming down on those other medications. Once the paralytic is off, we can come down on the sedations. He's on the fentanyl, and the Versed, and the propofol. Once we can come down on those, then they would say, 'Okay, let's try a weaning trial.' At that point, before we turn them off to do that. That is when we would get a hold of you if I'm understanding correctly."

Wanting more clarification, I asked, "Okay, and what levels do you even start the sedation and paralytic reduction? What would his oxygen levels be? Did you say a PEEP of 8 and 60% or less FiO2?"

He responded, "Roughly yes. That's kind of our broad parameters as to when it's okay to start doing the weaning trials. The paralytic would have to be off before we even think about doing a weaning trial because, as I say, it would be pointless to do it with the paralytic because he wouldn't be able to draw his own breath. That's kind of like what a weaning trial is. It's so he can get used to drawing his own breaths and filling his lungs again on his own with less support from the ventilator."

It was undoubtedly an extremely complicated and dangerous procedure. It sounded as challenging and risky as attempting to jump from a high-speed train at the right moment, in the right way, and in the right spot to miraculously avoid severe injury and death.

So I asked, "If it's not on a doctor's order, but you're being told if his PEEP is at 8 and his FiO2 is at 60% or less, you can start the process on your own, then I understand what to expect. Then I don't want him off the paralytic unless I'm informed first."

He answered, "Okay, gotcha, okay. So yeah, I'll put it in there to notify you before doing any weaning trials or stopping the paralytic completely—unless he has, like, some massive, sudden improvement in his respiratory status, and we're, like, 'Okay, well, let's, see if we can do anything.' So, it's not going to be tonight, and it won't most likely be tomorrow. But I will definitely put that note in there."

He had been accommodating thus far, so I said, "There's something else I need to talk to the doctor about. I had been asking since day one for nebulized budesonide. It helps to reduce inflammation in the lungs. I wanted him to increase the once-a-day budesonide treatment and have it be administered more often. So, is that something I need to talk to the doctor about, or can you put the request in the records?"

He said, "Yeah, I wouldn't be able to make a recommendation as far as that goes. That's, you know, they, they've been in school a lot longer than I have, and they know, you know, the indication parameters and all that." So I asked, "Should I talk to the respiratory therapist? Maybe it's not the doctor I need to speak with."

His rapid reply was, "No because they're taking orders from the doctor. I think it was Dr. Liar in today. Yeah, it would be him or one of his partners that would answer that for you."

Concerned about Rob not getting sufficient calories, I asked, "Can you also put in the chart to have the dietitian call me?" He said, "No problem. Oh, wait, here we go. So, I just found her name. It's Ms. Awful. I don't see a contact number for her. I will add a note in the record that you wish to speak with her."

I called Jay back and advised him they would not attempt to wean Rob in the morning because his PEEP was still too high at 14. Jay responded, "Keep this in mind. Rob's been on the ventilator for 14 days. He's been immobile for that long; he's got some muscle wasting. **He's going to have multiple issues that he's going to have to overcome.** He will overcome them quickly. Physical therapy, speech, and audiology therapy. He'll need fine motor therapy. And these are therapies that the rehab places will address. Whatever it is, we're going to do this, and then he will be flying again. And you guys are gonna be rockin'.'"

Jay then asked if they had been weighing Rob every day, saying, "Anybody can push that button at the end of the bed to give you the weight. We want them to do it because if he's losing weight, we want his tube feeds adjusted so he's not *wasting away*. We want him to get healthy fast."

He admitted, "I've been inside the hospitals during this pandemic. **The nursing atmosphere has changed.** *Yeah, and I don't like what I see. It's a whole different beast. It is evil. Many protocols were initiated that didn't need to be, and steps have been taken that didn't need to be taken.* Now we're here with Rob at FiO2 70% and 14 PEEP pressure, and he's swollen. **This is not so good. In addition, he should have a documented 'Discharge Plan.'** Even though he's in critical condition, we plan for the patient's discharge as soon as they enter our hospital's front door."

I decided to call the ICU and ask if Rob had a "Discharge Plan." I was shocked that the nurse who answered said, "**That's not even on our radar for him right now** because of the status that he's still in. So typically, you know, once he . . . eventually, he might have to go to rehab before he goes home because he'll be deconditioned and weak from not moving around and stuff on his own. So, he'll need, likely, assistance, physical therapy, and whatnot to build his strength back up. So, it just depends on how, you know, how well he does. Everybody's different. I would assume he would go to rehab first before going home to help with the therapy."

Another long, difficult, depressing, and exhausting day had passed. I chose to leave the lights on in the house at night because I found it comforting to be in the light when our situation was so dark. I was utterly exhausted. At least the Social Worker had informed me that I could see Rob on September 23rd.

I laid down, closed my eyes, and hoped Mr. Pathetic, the ICU Floor Supervisor, would be able to gain approval for me to see Rob the following morning. Nonetheless, my imagination ran wild as I contemplated the condition in which I might find him. It was all I could do to dispel the disturbing images of my husband suffering at the hands of the heartless proponents of "the protocol."

Thursday, September 23, 2021

Early in the morning, my phone rang. It was Mr. Pathetic, the ICU Floor Supervisor. He said, "So, I did talk to our Chief Medical Officer. **Unfortunately, the decision was that they have to follow the CDC guidelines,** so they're going to have to keep the isolation today.

"They said they were okay with giving an exception if you want to visit your husband today for an hour. However, you have to wear the same PPE uniform you wore when you went there the other day, with the masking and all that stuff. **His full isolation** will not be removed until tomorrow, the 24th, okay?"

I replied, "I've always been okay with the PPE and masking. So that's not a problem. I will come in today. But I want you to understand, and I don't know if I told you or not, but I've tried to tell the doctors, and I've tried to tell one of the nurses last night, that I don't want them trying the weaning process without me. So I had him put that in Rob's hospital record. The problem is that he needs me. I'm his wife, and he needs me to be there so he won't be afraid when they do this."

Mr. Pathetic said, "No, I understand you should be a part of that process." I was shocked and surprised that he seemed to be agreeing with me. I said, "You know, up until now, I've been denied being involved in that process because of his isolation, and that's why I'm upset." He said, "I agree with you. But it's just the challenge that we had with the isolation. So once that is done tomorrow . . . **then** you can participate more."

I wondered why it was not against the law to keep me locked out of the hospital and away from my husband when I was his wife and duly appointed Medical Power of Attorney who had been appointed to be his medical advocate for the express purpose of protecting him from the very system that he was now a prisoner of—a system he did not trust to begin with—one I knew was not healing him but was harming him.

His lame, "tomorrow . . . **then** you can participate more" comment confirmed that he, like all the others at Covid Coven Hospital of Plano, Texas, preferred me to be a bystander who had no input in the development of Rob's plan of care—which up to now had been a *"plan of demise."* He realized that my physical presence, officially allowed the following day, would make it more difficult for them to keep me on the sidelines.

I continued, "I was trying to get ahold of the Social Worker, but she hasn't returned my calls, which has been very frustrating." Then, sticking up for her, he said she might have been out when I called. I corrected him, "Well, I've been trying to call her since last Friday, and I don't know why she won't return my calls. I have left countless messages."

He told me that if I were at the hospital by 11:00 AM, the team of doctors, social workers, and dietitians would all be there making their interdisciplinary rounds, and I could probably speak to each of them. He then said, "We need to make sure that you're guided on how to put on the PPE, and before you take them off, we're gonna have to watch you so you don't contaminate, you know, your face, removing the PPE. I don't know if you heard the nurse the other day; you did not touch the patient, right? You can speak to him, **but don't try to touch him**."

Anguished that I had to grovel and beg to see my husband for one hour a day earlier than their 21-day lock-out policy, I thanked him for arranging for me to be able to come in today to see Rob. He said, "Okay, that sounds good. And again, we tried to accommodate, but again, I apologize that we have, you know, as a hospital, **we have to show we continue on taking care of patients. We have to follow rules**, so . . . okay?"

I saw his statement as another confirmation that it was just that, a pathetic **"show"** that they fully expected me to enjoy as a spectator as they pretended to be **"taking care of patients"** while what they were truly doing was taking care of their own pockets.

I was sick and tired of "spectating." I was more than ready to get in the game and challenge the "medical professionals" who were looking out for **their** best interests by enforcing "the protocol" at the expense of the health of my husband, "the patient."

These despicable criminals were expecting me to be ecstatic about the fact that they were allowing me to spend a meager hour with Rob one day before the end of their ridiculous 21-day "lockout" period.

I began to wonder what miracle they believed would occur at 7:00 AM on September 24th that would make it immediately safe for me to spend the entire day with Rob without wearing a gown, cap, mask, face shield, gloves, and booties. His ICU room would remain filthy, untidy, and contaminated with bacteria. Moreover, the doctors and staff would continue to be impolite, disrespectful, indifferent, and uncooperative. The only difference would be that Rob would be a day weaker.

I had read years before that Stalin once taught his followers a lesson by plucking the feathers from a live chicken during one of his state dinner parties. He then placed the bald, bloodied chicken on the floor next to him, where it consumed crumbs from his hand and refused to leave. As long as you occasionally threw them a few worthless crumbs, you could easily control stupid people, he told his dinner guests, because they would follow you no matter how much pain you caused them.

Like Stalin's chicken, Rob and I had been plucked bare of our rights—and they had made us beg for their unhealthy, life-debilitating crumbs. I was having to learn how to navigate their inhumane and cruel "system" while my husband, Rob, was slowly dying in it. I thought, "One of these days, the tables will turn. Until then, I have no choice but to eat the crumbs from the palms of their hands—at least until Rob can finally come home."

The proverbial saying *"power corrupts; absolute power corrupts absolutely"* conveys that their moral sense diminishes as a person's power increases. We, the people, have given way too much power to the medical establishment, and it is time we stand up and take that power back. I believed the time to regain my power had come, and I was ready to get in the ring and continue the fight for Rob's life.

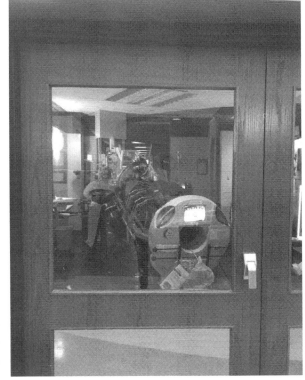

It was time to head toward the hospital, so I grabbed my things and ran out the door. I was more than ready to see Rob.

I arrived at the hospital around 10:30 AM to avoid missing the 11:00 AM ritual of interdisciplinary rounds. When I arrived at the ICU, outside of Rob's door was a shelf of PPE equipment. A nurse who saw me standing by the collection came over to aid me with putting all the gear on in the correct order. Once I had all the essential garb on, I pushed open the large wooden door with the glass windows.

I grimaced as I observed and felt that the floor was even grimier and stickier than when I had visited three days earlier for 20 minutes. Rob remained in the RotoProne bed, face down in a prone position. Once more, I heard the same horrifying clicking, clacking, humming, and hissing sounds as before.

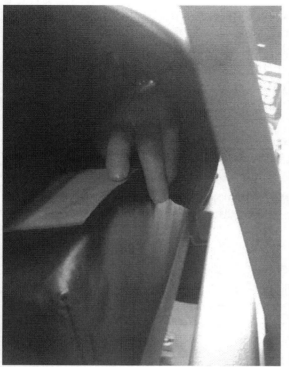

Since he was in a prone position, I had to stoop under the bed to see the exposed part of his face. His nose, taped-shut eyes, and crusty beard were visible. I could see his nose was still bleeding, and that drool had dripped from his mouth onto the pad thrown under the bed. It was not a pretty sight. Even then, I yearned to give Rob a kiss. However, I knew that if I tried and touched him, I would likely be expelled from his room. It made no sense not to be able to touch my fully sedated husband, so I took a chance and gently touched the tips of his fingers with my gloves.

I could tell they hadn't cleaned him in the past three days because his hair was still stuck together with some god-awful filth from who knows where, and it smelled oddly of urine. In addition, I observed a few unsightly rashes on his skin.

In case he could somehow hear my words in his fully sedated state, I told Rob how much I loved and missed him. I told him not to worry about anything because my family was helping me, and I was taking care of all the bills. I assured him that he was improving and that his organs were doing well. I then shared how I was working day and night to get him safely back home.

The next thing I knew, Dr. Liar, whom I had met with three days prior, stepped into the room, followed by a team of other hospital staff. After a brief "Hello," I asked Dr. Liar a pressing question. "I see no discharge plan for Rob in his MyChart hospital record. Is that right?" In his usual, nonchalant manner, he replied, "Because we don't know how things are gonna evolve." I responded, "Because you never know?" He agreed. "Exactly. *We don't have a discharge plan because he's not stable.*"

I responded, "It's really hard for me. I love him so much that I didn't want to be apart from him this long. It's been so awful. I want to thank you for your care. What is your prognosis today?" I was surprised to hear him say, "It's guarded. It's guarded just because he's critically ill. Yeah, just because he's critically ill still. Since I've been taking care of him this week, he's been stable in the sense I haven't had to increase his support on the ventilator. *But that stability is not always a good sign.*"

I recalled that after Rob was placed on a ventilator, Dr. Wicked had regularly said, in a positive tone, that Rob was "overall stable." So, up to now, I had been led to believe that "stable" on the ventilator was supposed to be good. Yet Dr. Liar was now confirming, as I had expected, "*that stability is not always a good sign.*"

Interestingly, before placing Rob on the BiPAP—a therapy that nearly immediately led to his being on a ventilator—Dr. Wicked had never said he was "**overall stable.**" Instead, he had always noted that Rob was "**improving.**" However, once Rob was on the ventilator—which had been their goal for him all along—he stopped "**improving**" and was in a continual decline.

There was no question. The massive doses of pharmaceuticals Rob had been on for 20 days, the ventilator he had been on for 15 days, and the RotoProne bed he had been on for 5 days were **not** helping him "improve." Instead of being "*stable,*" or maybe I should say "*not dead yet,*" it appeared this type of decline was precisely what they expected to occur once they succeeded in getting him on a ventilator.

I queried, "What steps are being taken to improve his oxygenation besides using the RotoProne bed?" Confirming his philosophy was one of "*more medication is always the answer,*" he said, "He's gotten some steroids and blood thinners, okay? In fact, I did increase his blood thinners to a higher dose of Lovenox." I asked, "To prevent blood clots?" He nodded his head as his eyes began to narrow at my questions. He continued, "With COVID, there's clotting that could occur, and there's a test we call the D-dimer, and that was higher, so he's on a higher dosage."

I sensed he avoided answering my question about improving Rob's oxygenation (blood oxygen level) because he did not have a good answer. I wondered if that was because he was aware that the BiPAP they had placed Rob on the morning of September 8th, just before he was placed on a ventilator, had caused enough damage to his lungs that they could not maintain a sufficient blood oxygen level without using high levels of inspired oxygen (high FiO2) and a high PEEP (residual expiratory pressure) setting.

So I said, "I guess his inflammatory markers started going up, and oxygen needed to be increased. I saw the methylprednisone was increased to 20 milligrams twice daily on September 15th." He admitted, "They go back up, and I was the one who made that decision. Probably, well, it's just the balance because . . . I also want to make . . . you know, he was having a fever, and now he's no longer having a fever. It's better. **I guess cultures haven't shown anything**."

Was he guessing that the cultures had not shown anything, or was he sure? Either he had seen the results of Rob's latest cultures, or he had not. I queried. "So, you didn't see those blood cultures?" He looked away, then quickly back at me, "Because yesterday . . . and so far, they haven't shown them . . . and he's received a full course of antibiotics. We're just going to kind of see where things go. Yeah, I may increase the steroids, right? **That's a judgment call because that can cause problems too**, so I try to balance everything."

He then shared with me that Rob was suffering from collapsed alveoli in the lungs. "I think he's dealing primarily with inflammation from infection. **As far as atelectasis** [a complete or partial collapse of the entire lung or area (lobe) of the lung that occurs when the tiny air sacs (alveoli) within the lung become deflated], this is part of what we do. *This is a lung protective strategy.* We give him **low volumes of air** because if I give him bigger volumes of air, **that's going to damage his lungs**.

"Low volumes of air in the lungs don't always fully expand as much, and maybe, you know, if you're reading the X-ray, and you are seeing **atelectasis**, that just means someone's lungs are not expanding. But that's because I'm not giving him the deep breaths. Okay? I can tell you, **if I give him bigger volumes, I'm gonna damage his lungs**."

I asked Dr. Liar why Rob had not had an X-ray for the past four days (his last X-ray was on September 19th) to check the condition of his lungs. Dr. Liar said, "We don't always continue to do it [an X-ray] unless there's a BIG change. I mean, we get them periodically."

I had heard from Dr. Mei that using a surfactant, a mixture of lipids and proteins delivered directly into the endotracheal tube to coat the alveoli (air sacs), could help improve oxygenation and reduce the risk of lung damage. So I asked Dr. Liar if he had considered this option. He boldly said, "We don't give surfactant here!"

Dr. Mei had advised me that surfactants had been used to treat respiratory distress syndrome in newborns, and they were a viable therapeutic option for adults with acute respiratory distress syndrome (ARDS). Thus, I asked him why he disagreed with using them on Rob. He replied, "Why would I not consider that right now? Just because it hasn't been well studied and it's going to cause problems. There is a drug that I can't get here. It's called beractant. It can increase surfactant, and it's been studied in COVID. It just hasn't been determined effective just yet."

My husband was in critical condition; Dr. Wicked said he could die at any time, and they had been giving Rob off-label drugs such as VELETRI, baricitinib, nitazoxanide, and colchicine. So, why would Dr. Liar be adamantly opposed to at least trying beractant (a pulmonary surfactant) to see if it could help get more oxygen into Rob's bloodstream? If it did, they could reduce the FiO2 (oxygen concentration) to a safer level, reduce the PEEP (Positive End Expiratory Pressure), and possibly wean Rob from the ventilator. Dr. Liar's illogical argument made no sense, and I was again being informed that if it were not their idea, it would not happen. Unfortunately, I could now see that being face-to-face with the doctors did not give me any more leverage than when I contended with them over the phone.

I asked him, "What are you doing about muscle wasting, and what's the plan for the future?" He hesitated, then replied, "**If** he gets better and we can wake him up. . . we can do physical therapy." That small but telling word "**if**" echoed in my head. What did this liar mean by "**If** he gets better and we can wake him up"?

I say "liar" because I had been misled regarding Rob's condition and the risks and benefits of medications and therapies from the beginning. Particularly on September 8, when they failed to admit that the BiPAP had caused such severe damage (barotrauma) that it allowed them to force Rob onto a ventilator. Next, Dr. Dead End misled me by claiming the ventilator would help Rob regain his strength when, in reality, the ventilator, in conjunction with the massive assault of powerful medications, was draining him of his remaining strength.

It was as **if** he already knew what the outcome would be because of the damage they had done to his fragile lungs and possibly to his brain, damage that might make it impossible for them to wake him up. Like Dr. Wicked and the others, I sensed he did not believe Rob would survive the ventilator and was waiting to see how much longer he would last. Rob's life and my future hinged on that tiny and now terrifying word, "**if**." It had suddenly become the most frightening word I knew.

Being deeply concerned about Rob's caloric intake, I told the small group standing around Rob's bed, "Okay, I have tried to get ahold of the dietitian, and yesterday I asked the nurse to put it in Rob's chart for her to call me, but I still have not heard from her. So, maybe before I leave here, I can get her phone number from somebody. Also, I left two messages for the Social Worker last Friday and called again twice on Monday. I still haven't heard from her." I said all of this even though the Social Worker, Ms. Destroyer, was present in the group because I was beyond frustrated at being ignored and wanted to express my annoyance to the entire team.

Flustered by my blunt and candid comments, Ms. Destroyer, trying to appear innocent, said, "For me? I didn't get any of your messages."

The truth was that she had been avoiding me like the plague because she knew I would have continued to insist that the hospital allow me to see my husband before the "21-day isolation period" was over. She also knew she had misled me when she had advised me on September 9th and September 13th that Rob's "20-day isolation period" would be over today, September 23rd. Now, here I was being given only an hour to see Rob out of the goodness of their hearts, and I could only spend a full 12-hour day with Rob starting tomorrow, September 24th.

Turning toward Ms. Destroyer, I said, "I left one of the messages on Friday at 6:00 AM and the other at 10:00 AM. That was the day I stayed in the hospital lobby all day long, until 5:30 PM, trying to get someone to help me."

In an attempt to sweep my complaint regarding her ineptness under the film of filth still stuck to the floor of Rob's ICU room, she quickly and discreetly said in a low tone

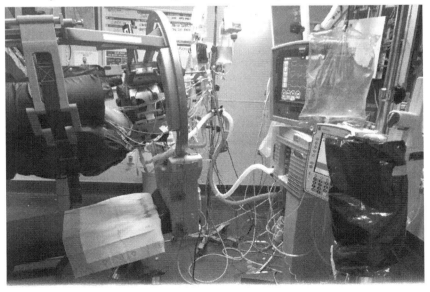

Yes, yes. Well, I'll talk to you

about it later." I responded, "If we can reconnect, that would be nice because I have a lot of questions, and I know **you're** the missing piece. So we don't waste the doctor's time, yes, please."

Since the illusive Dr. Torture, the Infectious Disease doctor I had never met, seemed to be running the show, I turned back to Dr. Liar. I asked, "I don't know if you can answer this because I've never met Dr. Torture, but I read her notes and on the 21st, two days ago, she mentioned— and I just want your opinion on this—the word 'sepsis.' It might have been an earlier observation, and maybe it was just there because of an earlier note since she tends to copy and paste her notes from day to day. *Is Rob suffering from sepsis or not?*"

Dr. Liar's response surprised me. He said, "By the definition of sepsis, honestly, if he's having a fever, he's tachycardic, and he has an infection going on, which he does, then that meets the definition of sepsis. It covers a big spectrum. There is a wide spectrum of sepsis, there's severe sepsis, and there's septic shock, which he does not have. He basically has, obviously, just sepsis. He does not have severe sepsis."

I had read a note in Rob's hospital records that said he could be suffering from what they called "a drug fever from the antibiotics," which would have nothing to do with routine sepsis. So was the discussion of sepsis a smoke screen to cover up for a fever they caused with massive doses of antibiotics?

It was apparent that they would create a problem with their heavy onslaught of potent medications, then use more drugs to treat that problem. Thus, much to their chagrin, I frequently questioned the doctors about the medications they were prescribing. I was convinced they were causing him more harm than good, further weakening him and decreasing his chances of survival. To the doctors, however, one more drug was the solution to anything they could label.

So I said, "Okay, well, I didn't realize it was such a big spectrum. Wouldn't it be best to have 'sepsis' off his chart if he doesn't have sepsis? The 'Covid' is gone, right?" Making light of it, Dr. Liar said, "It's not harmful to be on his chart." I thought, "of course not, as that makes Rob a more profitable patient.

He continued, "So . . . but I don't think he's infectious. The virus may be gone, but his immune response to the infection itself is what's driving the problem. That's the case with lots of infections. Not just Covid, right? It's just that it triggers an immune response, and it's an immune response that causes the problem."

I commented, "Okay, so that's my concern. We're very holistic. You're flooding his body with tons of antibiotics and all these other drugs. Although it's for a purpose because he is a critical patient, sometimes, when you get too much medication, that creates other problems. I know you know this, but please explain it for my own understanding." He replied, "That's why we stopped the antibiotics at this point. There might be more [drugs we finally stop giving Rob] in the future."

Returning to the surfactant, I said, "Since a surfactant could improve his oxygen level . . . " Dr. Liar jumped in without letting me finish, "We don't really do that with adults." Trying again, I asked, "But would you be open to it?" He harshly said, "NO! Because we don't always do that.

Because it's NOT medically reviewed. And it's NOT been shown to do anything. There's been studies, numerous, and they have not panned out."

I took a deep breath, took a few notes, and asked, "Okay, let me ask you this since I know it will have to come from you because you're the doctor. Rob has AB-positive blood, and his records show he's anemic. **Why is he anemic, and what are you doing about it?**" He responded with a sigh, appearing increasingly agitated, "And when people are critically ill, they are anemic. His isn't bad."

Since the dietitian was being elusive, I asked Dr. Liar to comment on Rob's nutritional intake. He said Rob was receiving a supplement called Pivot 1.5, which Dr. Wicked had told me about ten days earlier. "Rob is getting 35 milliliters an hour. When you take into account the propofol, he's also getting a lot of calories from it. We don't want to give him too many calories. Propofol gives him a lot of calories as well. So, that's why we reduce the tube feeds, **so as to not overfeed those calories.**"

From what I could see in the charts, he had already lost over 30 pounds, yet they were being cautious to "**not overfeed those calories.**" So I tried to reason with Dr. Liar, "God, it just breaks my heart. He has lost so much weight. So you're saying calories are more important than nutrients?"

LEGAL COUNSEL STATEMENT
Members of the jury, another major issue with the hospital team's lack of communication with Sheila was that they should have informed her that the RotoProne bed Rob was placed in on September 18th had a significant scale problem. This fact was documented on Page 359 of Rob's hospital's records, as shown in the snapshot below.

> Pt interview/Comments:
> 9/20: Pt remains intubated and sedated, not able to have SBT per respiratory. Large weight variance noted from 9/18 to 9/19 weights when transitioned to Rotoprone bed, staff believes new weights are inaccurate and pt is closer to 170 lb.

*Page C-55 of Appendix C contains a graph of Rob's daily weight measurements—as recorded by the hospital staff—from his admission on September 3, 2021, until his death on October 13, 2021. As you will see from the chart, there were often **massive daily changes** in the recorded weight. This indicates that their beds generally displayed inaccurate weights.*

Their failure to inform Sheila of the problem with the RotoProne bed's scale caused her unnecessary distress and anxiety. In addition, Dr. Liar, who was covering patients at three area hospitals, was unaware that Rob's weight seemed to have dropped by 58 pounds in 24 hours when he was placed in the RotoProne bed. *If he had been paying ANY attention to Rob's weight (it is clear he was not), he would have immediately noticed the drastic one-day change. Then, he should have advised Sheila that Rob had not lost a significant amount of weight because the real issue was that the RotoProne bed's scales were malfunctioning.*

Without this essential information, Sheila surmised that Rob's weight had decreased from 170 pounds at admission to 139 pounds as of September 23rd. Thus, she brought this apparent (and significant) weight loss to the doctor's attention and continued raising the issue with clueless hospital staff.

Regrettably, Sheila and the team entrusted with Rob's care frequently failed to pay close attention to vital details, and poor communication was endemic between them. For example, Sheila was not informed of the problem with the RotoProne bed's scales until the dietitian told her on September 28, 2021, when he was removed from the bed.

Dr. Liar looked dumbfounded. One thing was sure: the moment Rob crossed the threshold of the hospital's Emergency Department doors, we entered a world where up was down, down was up, and everything I thought would help my husband regain the strength he needed to survive was being denied while the things I felt would cause him harm were readily available and supplied to him in abundance.

Hoping more sound reasoning would not overload him, I changed the topic and said, "I asked the night nurse to write it in the chart last night to **please don't do the weaning process without me**. I live just a few minutes down the street and can be here quickly. I understand weaning is all based on the numbers." Dr. Liar said, "Yeah, we're not."

I turned to Ms. Destroyer, kept my eyes connected with hers, and asked, "How does visitation work? They said I could visit from 7:00 AM to 7:00 PM tomorrow. So, is it only one person per day? Our son and my sister are going to want to see him. But, of course, I want to see him first because he needs to hear me first. How does that all work?"

Ms. Destroyer coldly stated, without emotion, "So, it's <u>just one person per day</u>. So, whoever walks in, like, if you walk in at 9:00 AM, **then you're it for the day.** If your brother-in-law shows up one day at 8 AM, **then he's it for the day**. There may be exceptions now, just like anything else, like you've had an exception to come in sooner [today] than tomorrow. If there's a day that, for some reason, there's someone who came from out of town, they can come in and only stay for 30 minutes. Then you can ask for an exception, okay, for two persons that particular day, right? **But that can't be every day.**" At this, the team headed out of the room to complete the remainder of their morning rounds.

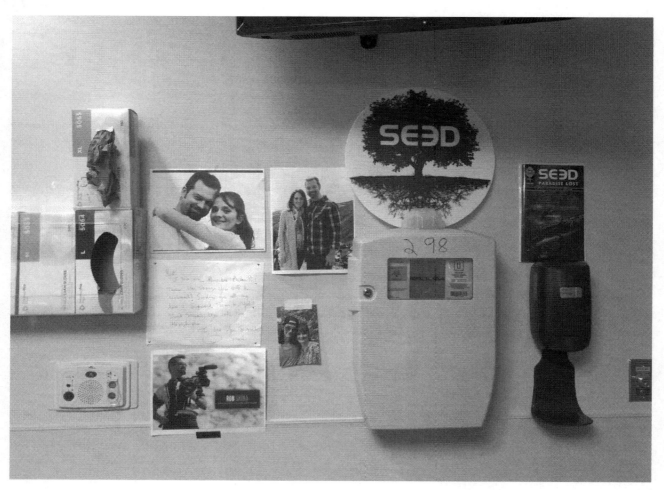

I spent the rest of my precious hour sharing positive "you can get through this" thoughts with Rob. Finally, when my one-hour visit was nearly over, a nurse came in. I commented, "I was just saying my goodbyes to Rob."

She said, "That's all right. I understand." I then briefly turned to look at the pictures on the wall. He was the love of my life, and I so much wanted to kiss his face. He was so close yet so far away, tucked in the grips of a monstrous RotoProne bed, paralyzed, and sedated into a coma. Tears welled up in my eyes as I wondered if I would ever feel his embrace or see the twinkle in his eyes again.

The nurse, who seemed genuinely concerned with my plight, said she wanted to share an incredible story. She told me that when she came into Rob's room at the beginning of her shift, she noticed the iPad in his room was playing music accompanying scripture. Then, as she typed her login password, which happened to be a verse of scripture, into the nursing terminal, she said, "The iPad you had playing the scripture with music began playing the words of the verse I use for my password! It startled me, and I have not gotten over it!"

I said, "Thank you for sharing that with me. That's confirmation that you are walking with the Spirit. Rob lived his whole life that way, and so many things like that happened to him. Thank you! I needed to hear that. That's really awesome."

I then asked, "What verse was it?" and immediately realized I shouldn't be asking for her password, So I advised her she did not need to tell me. She responded, "No, I want you to know it. It was Hebrews 10:23. It's a real confirmation for sure."

She then repeated the verse by heart, "*Let us hold fast the confession of our hope without wavering, for He who promised is faithful.*" I felt warm all over. I would treasure this verse and hide it in my heart. I believed it was a message from the Father above to encourage me to remain steadfast in my faith in him and not waver.

I agreed, "Yes, the Father does things like this. He synchronizes things. Thank you so much. I wish you were his nurse every day. I really appreciate you sharing that story with me. Thank you for sharing your heart."

She then smiled and offered to show me something else. Taking me over to the ventilator making the swishing and hissing sounds, she kindly told me the settings and how to read them. She was a rare bright light in what, up to now, had been a very dark and uninviting world.

During my hour at the hospital, my mother picked up Dr. Mei at the airport and drove her to my home. When I returned home, I thanked her profusely for coming to Rob's and my aid. When we sat down to review Rob's online MyChart hospital records, she said she was horrified at what she saw. She then reaffirmed that she believed Rob was in grave danger.

The rest of the evening, we mapped out a plan of action, which included my spending the day with Rob the next day, September 24th—as it would be my first chance to spend an entire day with Rob from 7:00 AM to 7:00 PM since his arrival at the hospital on September 3rd.

We would then have her visit with Rob the next day, on September 25th, so that she could assess his condition in person. I only wished I had met Dr. Mei sooner.

177

Friday, September 24, 2021

Today would be the first time I could spend 12 hours with Rob. We both liked essential oils, so I wore peppermint on my neck, hoping he might somehow recognize it and realize I was there even in his comatose state.

As planned, I would text Dr. Mei my observations throughout the day and send her photos of the equipment that displayed key settings and his vital signs. I would also send her pictures of the numerous IV bags hung throughout the day, administering a steady flow of multiple medications.

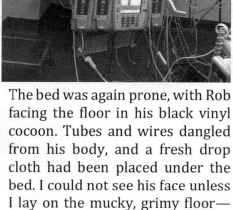

Once again, I was warned not to touch him. They seemed concerned that I might bump into the RotoProne bed if I tried to get too close to him, causing some type of crisis as a result.

When I entered the room, it was pitch black and resembled a prison cell. In reality, Rob was being held captive by the RotoProne bed he had been placed in six days prior and the ventilator they had placed him on 16 days earlier.

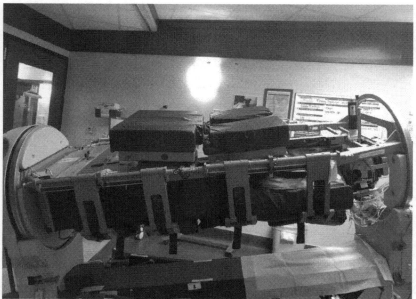

The bed was again prone, with Rob facing the floor in his black vinyl cocoon. Tubes and wires dangled from his body, and a fresh drop cloth had been placed under the bed. I could not see his face unless I lay on the mucky, grimy floor—which I would not do.

I began the day by taking pictures of the room, the IVs, and the monitors to send to Dr. Mei and texting her my observations. As I did, I spoke words of love over Rob, read him scriptures, and told him how much our son, his family, his friends, Heidi his dog, and I loved and missed him.

Rob was receiving a continuous infusion of three sedatives: fentanyl, Versed (midazolam), and propofol. In addition, he had a continuous drip of the paralytic Nimbex. Occasionally, a nurse would enter the room to hang another bag of medication or inject him with the high-powered steroid SOLU-MEDROL or the diuretic Lasix. Other than that, I was left alone in the room with my tears and my sedated and paralyzed husband—the man I loved who seemed to be slowly slipping away at the hands of the perpetrators of "the protocol."

As I texted Dr. Mei my observations, she said she was concerned that the lab results shown in Rob's online MyChart lab records indicated his total protein and albumin levels were low. She advised me that malnutrition and vitamin deficiency were the most common causes.

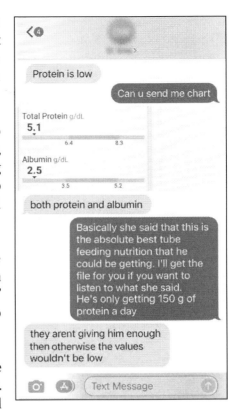

A nurse had told me that the Pivot 1.5 they were giving Rob was "the absolute best tube feeding nutrition" available. But, when I advised Dr. Mei, she responded, "They aren't giving him enough then. Otherwise, the values wouldn't be low. So ask the nurse, if Pivot 1.2 is the best, then why would his total protein level be so low?"

The nurse said it wasn't the amount of Pivot 1.5 they were giving Rob but his illness causing the low protein and albumin numbers. So in their eyes, and the eyes of the doctors, "Covid" was to blame for everything, and nothing they did, or failed to do, could possibly cause Rob any harm.

Dr. Mei replied, "My patients in the neonatal ICU who were very sick did not have values this low, and they gained weight. So Rob needs proper calories, enough lipids and protein, and complete vitamins and minerals."

The doctors, nurses, and dietitian had consistently ignored Rob's "calorie intake" and had done so since the day he was admitted. Just 48 hours after his arrival, Rob texted me, "*No food no . . .*" and "*No strength no hope left.*" On September 8, 2021, the day Rob was intubated and placed on a ventilator, Dr. Wicked even admitted, "So, I think respiratory muscle fatigue **and poor calorie intake** is the ONLY thing that's working really against us."

Twelve days ago, on September 12, 2021, I told an ICU nurse of my concern that Rob might not be receiving sufficient nutrition because there was nothing in his MyChart records regarding his caloric intake. She promised to watch his caloric intake from that point forward. Yet here he was, anemic with low protein and albumin levels.

A buffet of drugs was readily available for a "Covid" patient at Covid Coven Hospital of Plano, Texas. However, adequate calories and nutrition were not on the menu. They were not a priority because adequate nutrition was not a part of "the protocol" and would not earn hospitals any federal government incentive money.

I had learned that each day on the RotoProne bed, Rob would spend 16 hours in a prone position, then 8 hours in a supine position. At 5:00 PM, a nurse came in to rotate the bed so Rob could be face up for 8 hours. When she turned him face up, I was appalled at what I saw. His beard was still crusty, and his hair remained glued together with some ghastly muck; his lips and face were swollen, and his eyes were taped shut. I was horrified to see what they had done to my husband in the name of modern medicine.

It was evident that 16 days on a ventilator and six days in a RotoProne bed had done nothing to improve his condition; instead, he was wasting away in a prison known as an ICU. The nurse's station was just outside the door of my husband's room, and I suspected they kept the lights off when no one was present because they did not want to witness what had been done to my husband.

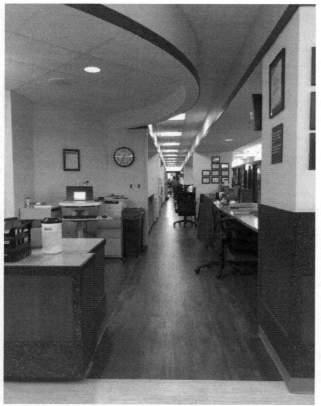

At 7:00 PM, the 12-hour nurses' shift was over, and I had to leave as the night shift came in.

I leaned over and told Rob I loved him with all my heart and that I would be back in the morning. I said, "Sleep well, my darling. You are getting stronger every day. I love you so very much!"

It was difficult to leave the love of my life strapped inside what looked like a futuristic version of a medieval torture bed. I looked at Rob again as I walked out of his room and whispered, "Good night. I will always love you—to the moon and back."

It was a solemn and depressing drive home. As I entered our neighborhood, I recalled many happy memories, such as Rob and I walking our dog, Heidi, down the sidewalk soon after moving into our first house five years earlier. We had begun to live our dream, and now I was living out a nightmare.

As I pulled into my driveway, I finally received a call from the Infectious Disease doctor, Dr. Torture. She said, "The nurse told me you had some questions about the antifungal that we need to start on him." Not at all happy they were continually adding more drugs on top of drugs, I said, "I'm just asking because, you know, he's in critical condition. He's been on a lot of antibiotics."

Dr. Torture said, "So, you know, he had some fever, and we did some blood cultures, and it's going into his lungs." I wondered if they knew what they were treating, so I asked, "What is the exact yeast in his blood?" She answered, "It's just showing that it's growing yeast. It's gonna take about a couple of days to see which kind of yeast it is. Candida?"

I pressed on, "Well, I'm just saying, if you wouldn't mind because I'm trying to preserve him, could you wait until you can tell me what that yeast is." She was adamant, "If we wait, *you can bet yeast in the blood can kill you*. We CAN'T wait with that. Well, it's an antifungal. Then we adjust accordingly when we have the final identification. You can't have yeast in your blood and not treat it. I can't tell you today what kind of yeast. I will be able to tell you in a day or two once the lab identifies it. First, they have to see that you're growing, and then they do genetic studies on it to see what kind of yeast it is. So, once I have the final idea, I can let you know, but they didn't identify it yet."

I understood her concern, yet I was equally concerned that my husband was being over-medicated and his immune system trashed.

I said, "Okay, one more thing. You are about to change a midline, and you don't want an infection that lives in the line to get into his blood, right? I mean, would you be willing to just let me send you a link to information on something that will be safer for his system? Since my husband is over Covid and pneumonia, I would like you to consider a product called Biosense that prevents and treats infections because he is sensitive to antibiotics and never takes them." She responded, "Bring something in and give it to the nurse next time you're here. Leave it there. They'll leave it in his chart, and I'll take a look, okay?"

I was happy to hear she would at least look at the product. I said I would bring it in and told her I would like to meet her in person at some point. She said, "Yeah, usually I'm there in the morning." I asked her what time, and she said, "I don't know. It depends on my schedule, okay? Yeah, hopefully, this infection will go away. There's not a lot of it. It's only in one site out of four. So that's a good thing. Okay."

I countered, "I would rather get the actual name of the yeast before you treat him." She explained, "They identify . . . a list, you know. It's probably going to be candida because that's what it usually is. But I'll give you its last name, too. Because there's like the first name, and then there's a last name, so I'll let you know which one it is once they identified it, all right?" Trying to remain positive, I responded, "That would be awesome. Thank you."

Sitting in my driveway, thinking about possibly losing Rob tore my heart out. I remembered the old Bill Withers song but changed the lyrics to: "*Ain't no sunshine when he's gone. It's not warm when he's away. Ain't no sunshine when he's gone . . . only darkness every day . . . and this house just ain't no home.*"

I banged my fists on the steering wheel and yelled, "I don't want to live without you!" as I soaked my shirt with tears. I don't recall how long I sat there staring at my house. Without Rob, it no longer felt like a home. But then, I had a revelation. Home is not a place; it's not a house; it's a person. I would have been at home in the middle of the ditch if I were with my husband. I wanted to be "home" and hide myself in his arms.

I would not be able to feel at home again until tomorrow—when I reentered his dungeon in the ICU. As creepy and depressing as it was, at least I could finally be with the man who had swept me off my feet. Even then, it would only be for twelve hours. I was deeply troubled that my husband was trapped in a hospital I had taken him to 21 days earlier for supplemental oxygen and, ideally, the minimal number of medications necessary to stabilize him.

Instead, I had been asked to leave, and he had been subjected to isolation, heavy medication, intimidation, humiliation, starvation, desperation, intubation, ventilation, and devastation. Feeling empty, like a hollow shell, I lifelessly dragged my limp and emotionally exhausted body to the front door. I unlocked it and went inside. Although my mother and Dr. Mei were there, the house felt empty without Rob.

After I had calmed myself, Dr. Mei and I sat down together and discussed her concerns about how Rob was being treated. She assured me that despite Dr. Wicked's assertion during my call with him on September 15th that "what happens to everybody in the ICU over a lengthy period is that they start getting anemia," there was no good reason for Rob to be anemic.

She explained that anemia decreases the oxygen-carrying capacity of the blood because of the reduced amount of hemoglobin available to carry oxygen. That leads to the tissues receiving less oxygen—which is the last thing you would want to see in a patient with lung issues. However, the doctors in charge of Rob's care did not seem to think his anemia was a significant concern.

She reiterated that his low protein and albumin levels showed he was being malnourished. Thus, he needed more calories and higher nutrient density. She also said she was dismayed that Dr. Liar and Dr. Terror had both agreed to immediately place Rob on an antifungal medication when only one of four blood cultures had come back positive since only one positive result was a clear indication of site contamination as opposed to a fungal infection in the blood. We both hoped her dropping in on Rob in the morning would give us valuable insights on how to best proceed.

I decided to check in with the evening shift nurse in charge of Rob's care. When I called the ICU nurse's station, Nurse Calloused answered. She said they were giving Rob diuretics due to his suffering from edema (swelling).

When I asked her why he looked so swollen, she said, "Yeah, it's because we're pushing the kidneys, okay?" Without a doubt, they were over-taxing his kidneys with a massive number and high dosages of medications, many of which were toxic to the kidneys. Even then, one more drug was always viewed as the answer for any symptom, even when that symptom had been caused by the drugs he was already on.

When asked how his lungs sounded, she said, "They sound course and diminished." When I asked if they were getting better or worse, she asserted, "All patients who have the 'Covid' lungs . . . the air going to the lungs is not expanding. Well, so, the tendency is to accumulate all this stuff . . . you know . . . whatever the body's producing. So, over time, you will hear the coarse sound in his lungs. That's why having something for turning him is good so he can get rid of this junk out of his lungs."

I sarcastically thought, "Oh, sure. 'Covid' is the only culprit, and his malnutrition, excessive medications, over-oxygenation, high PEEP setting, and the 4.5 hours of BiPAP therapy he was subjected to sixteen days ago had nothing to do with his current crisis."

When I asked her about the weaning process to get her take on it, she said, "We don't wean until the FiO2 [Fraction of Inspired Oxygen, the concentration of oxygen in the air being forced into the lungs] is less than 50%, and the PEEP is below 4 or 5—and his PEEP is currently 14. So, we don't do weaning with those numbers."

I said, "Okay, let me write that down." With a little edge in her tone, she said, "So you're taking down notes? So, this means you are, like, recording even my name?"

I told her I was taking notes because, as Rob's wife and Medical Power of Attorney, I needed to keep track of his condition and care, and I could not remember everything. So, I wrote down all the numbers, and yes, I recorded names. Of course, I knew her name from when she answered the phone. Besides, I had spoken with her previously. I responded, "I don't understand what you're saying. I mean, he's my husband, I love him, and I can't be there all the time. So, I don't understand why that would be a problem!"

She quickly tried to smooth things over with, "No, it's not a problem. It's just that in the last statement, you're saying you're kind of documenting what I said. It's just that I don't want to be named, you know, with all these numbers and all." Her hesitancy to be associated with what she was telling me shocked me. Besides, her name was all over the hospital records. Her comment made me wonder if she might be feeling guilty or ashamed of what she and others were doing to Rob.

LEGAL COUNSEL STATEMENT
Members of the jury, after this conversation, Nurse Calloused wrote in the hospital records, possibly as a warning to others: "POC [Plan of Care] reviewed with spouse over the phone. All questions and concerns addressed. Spouse has lengthy questions **and taking down notes as her queries were answered**."

We will let you decide what could have motivated a nurse at Covid Coven Hospital of Plano, Texas, to write such a statement in the hospital records. *One thing is sure. Her having done so was very suspicious.*

I explained, "I'm just trying to help myself. I'm just trying to understand. I've been trying to understand all of this since the beginning, and when I don't understand something, I write it down, okay? I didn't go to nursing school. So I don't know everything and I apologize for asking too many questions."

Since Rob could not come home until he was weaned, I asked her to elaborate on the process. She said, "If the numbers are, like, meeting the criteria for weaning, they will do the weaning. But as of this time, **his FIO2 is 100%** because he was de-sating earlier. That's why we have to increase the oxygen. Maybe overnight, the RT would have it come down again. So, the Respiratory Therapist, that's his responsibility, like, to come down with the FiO2 and see if the patient has maintained an oxygen saturation above 92."

I remembered Dr. Wicked telling me eleven days ago, on September 13th, "we are *pretty sure* 60% is not toxic from an oxygen standpoint. We don't know exactly where the threshold is. But in dogs, it's about 60%. So, we try to keep him at 60% and get him some reserve." Thus, I was very concerned that they had again raised the FiO2 (the oxygen concentration) back up to **100%**. I did not need a medical background to know that having Rob continuously breathe in high levels of oxygen was harmful to his lungs.

LEGAL COUNSEL STATEMENT
Members of the jury, as we have stated several times, normal room air has 21% oxygen, and breathing in high levels of oxygen (levels of greater than 60%) for over 24 hours can lead to "oxygen toxicity," otherwise known as "oxygen poisoning." The result is oxidative damage to the cell membranes of the lungs.

As shown in the chart at the bottom of Page C-54 in Appendix C, they maintained Rob's oxygen level at well above 60% most of the time during Rob's 35 days on the ventilator.
*We realize the high FiO2 (oxygen concentration) number shown in the chart for September 24th is **80**, not **100**. That is because we took the numbers for the chart on Page C-54 from periodic readings recorded in the hospital records. There were times during the day when, although not recorded in the records, they raised the oxygen level to 100%.*

Could it be that Nurse Calloused realized the 100% oxygen was frying Rob's already fragile lungs? Thus, she did not want "all these numbers" associated with her name.

183

Before ending our call, I asked her how long patients usually remain in a RotoProne bed since Dr. Liar had told me he could not remove Rob from the ventilator while he was in the bed.

She said, "You know, for the first week or two weeks, it depends on the patient's response with the ventilator and the proning. The last patient that I took care of, she had been on a RotoProne bed **for a month**." I did not find that answer encouraging, and I was so shocked by her response that I did not think to ask her whether the woman survived.

I hoped and prayed that Rob, the man of my dreams, would survive this ordeal, as I had no idea how I could live without him.

Saturday, September 25, 2021

Due to the hospital's policy of allowing only one visitor per patient per day, we realized that Dr. Mei's visit would prevent me from seeing Rob today. Even so, we believed it essential that she be able to evaluate his condition and level of care in person.

I lent Dr. Mei one of our vehicles so that she could drive herself to the hospital to examine and monitor Rob. During the day, she texted me pictures of the monitors showing the ventilator settings and his vital signs.

She noted that they had lowered the FiO2 setting to a 60% oxygen concentration. However, the PEEP remained, as always, set at 14 cm H_2O. They also slightly lowered his fentanyl dosage from 375 micrograms per hour to 275 micrograms per hour.

He was still heavily sedated with 60 micrograms per kilogram per minute of propofol and 15 milligrams per hour of Versed (midazolam). He was also fully paralyzed with 4 micrograms per kilogram per minute of Nimbex. In addition, he remained on 8 milliliters per hour of VELETRI, 4 milligrams daily of off-label use baricitinib (Olumiant), a daily 100 milligram IV piggyback of the antifungal micafungin (Mycamine), a 60-milligram injection of Lovenox twice a day, and twice daily 30 milligram IV pushes of SOLU-MEDROL.

She told me his vital signs (pulse, blood pressure, and temperature) were all normal. However, she believed he still required higher nutrient density to raise his protein and albumin levels and help eliminate his ongoing anemia. Although he was holding his own, undoubtedly, Rob was not making any progress, and he was no closer to being weaned from the ventilator.

Knowing Dr. Liar was on duty today, I called the ICU and asked that they have him contact me. Not long after that, he called, saying, "I was just talking with another patient's family when I saw you tried to reach me." Anxious to get his assessment, I responded, "Oh, thank you so much, as I had called the nurse's station to get a hold of you. I just wanted to get an update."

He responded, "Yeah, so, your husband, from a pulmonary standpoint, seems to be doing a little bit better. We've got him down . . . last I looked, we had him down to 65% oxygen, which is a good thing—and actually, down to 60%, and even right now, when I look at the chart, it's going in the right direction.

"You know, blood counts and everything are fine. His kidney function looks good. We have been getting a little bit of fluid off with some diuretics, and he's tolerating that well. One thing you've probably already caught wind of, you know, we did those blood cultures the other day. **He did grow some yeast OUT OF ONE of those blood cultures**, and that's why we have him on that antifungal medication. I don't know if you have talked to anybody else about that."

Based on what my medically astute friends, including Dr. Mei, had told me, I knew to question Rob's being placed on an antifungal when Dr. Torture stated that only one of four cultures had returned positive, as a single positive culture indicated likely contamination of a draw site and not of the blood. So I queried, "I did hear about it. I talked with Dr. Torture and told her I completely understood that some drugs are 100% necessary, but I would prefer not to put him on another drug if we didn't have to. I understand a fungus in the blood would be serious, but **was a second set of cultures ordered?**"

He replied, "So, there are two cultures. So, it grew out of **ONE** of two cultures. But even if it grows out of **just ONE**, actually—we treat that. **That's the standard**; we consider that a real positive culture." Although one positive culture out of two sets was good enough for him, *it was clearly against the hospital's policies and specified lab test procedures*. I asked, "So, it was positive in **ONE** but not the other? Why would it do that? Do you know why?" He ineptly and unprofessionally replied, "Sometimes that happens."

> **LEGAL COUNSEL STATEMENT**
> Members of the jury, Dr. Torture, the Infectious Disease Doctor, had ordered four blood cultures, not just two cultures, as Dr. Liar implied. Therefore, either he was mistaken or was willfully deceiving Sheila by saying one out of two cultures (which would be 50%) was adequate proof of a yeast infection in the bloodstream (i.e., systemic candidiasis).
>
> *A minimum of two positive cultures from two different sites are required to confirm that a patient has systemic candidiasis. Thus, they proceeded to inappropriately prescribe an antifungal (micafungin), exposing Rob to its many adverse side effects, which we will discuss later.*

Unfortunately, Dr. Liar's "standard" consisted of flagrantly violating the hospital's policies and standards so he could medicate Rob into oblivion. Since he and Dr. Torture collaborated on developing their own "doctors' standard," it was evident that their "drug them to death" approach was not an isolated incident but a systemic issue. Doctors, who were independent contractors as opposed to hospital employees, were apparently able to disregard the hospital's protocols and do whatever they pleased.

Instead of agreeing to order another set of draws to confirm the "positive" result, he chided me with, "So here, let me put it in the opposite perspective. Now, let's say if I do another culture, and I've already put him on medication for antifungal (actually, Dr. Torture did it) and it's negative, that doesn't mean it's truly negative."

Drs. Torture and Liar should NOT have prescribed antifungal medication to Rob in the first place. Thus, Dr. Liar's justification that the antifungal medication they had placed Rob on could result in a false-negative blood test result was a problem of their creation. Once again, I was a spectator in a circus who was expected to silently watch the program, or "the protocol," that had been pre-planned by the ringmasters.

Dr. Liar continued, "Now, the opposite perspective is if this is real, **then that is a serious problem if I don't treat it**. And right now, he seems to be doing well, and since his blood pressures aren't low and white count isn't skyrocketing . . . but fungemia, which is yeast/fungus in the blood **is a life-threatening condition if it isn't treated**. So, that's why I wouldn't do another culture. I would empirically treat it based on the evidence we have at hand. *I would try not to find a way not to treat it.* You're right. Is it possible that it's a contaminant? That's a yes, there's the realm of possibility, but we *honestly* take it seriously enough because I've seen patients where they were not treated in time, **and they died**."

I responded, "As long as you know that. We already have him on so many drugs, and I don't want more drugs to have a negative effect on his recovery while you aren't 100% positive, but I completely agree with you that I don't want him to die. I know that fungus in the blood is not a good thing, and it should be treated **IF** he truly has it and **IF** you don't think it will interfere or interact with any of his other medications. So, how long will he be on this new medication?"

As was his style, he deferred to Dr. Torture, the Infectious Disease doctor, "I'll leave that to Dr. Torture. That is, probably at least a week, maybe two? I'll leave that up to her ultimately, though. She's kind of the expert in that and the length of the treatment." I asked, "What is the name of the medication?" He said, "**Micafungin**, the generic name is micafungin. It's very commonly used, and for this situation, it's a "**good drug**." *Sometimes it can cause some liver function abnormalities as a side effect*, but that's not the case with your husband **so far**, and we monitor that. So, okay?"

What could I say? I did not want Rob to die of a potentially fatal fungal infection. Yet I was still concerned they had decided to place my husband on yet another "caustic" medication" when the blood culture result was NOT, per the hospital's policies, a true "positive." I had heard that medical errors were the third leading cause of death in the United States, and I was doing everything in my power to prevent the doctors in charge of Rob's care from adding him to the list of patients who died due to doctors' poor judgment. Yet, unfortunately, they seemed bound and determined to maintain that statistic at the expense of Rob's life.

LEGAL COUNSEL STATEMENT

Members of the jury, what Sheila is referring to is a 2016 study conducted by researchers at Johns Hopkins Medicine that led to the conclusion that "medical errors" indeed were the third leading cause of death in America.

A May 3, 2016, NPR article that referenced the study stated, "*A study by researchers at Johns Hopkins Medicine* ***says medical errors should rank as the third leading cause of death in the United States****. . . But no one knows the exact toll taken by medical errors. In significant part, that's because the coding system used by CDC to record death certificate data doesn't capture things like communication breakdowns, diagnostic errors* **and poor judgment that cost lives***, the study says.*"

Allen, M., & Pierce, O. (2016, May 3). Medical errors are no. 3 cause of U.S deaths, researchers say. NPR. From https://www.npr.org/sections/health-shots/2016/05/03/476636183/death-certificates-undercount-toll-of-medical-errors

I asked Dr. Liar, "Can you explain why one culture would be positive and the other not?" Dr. Liar took a deep breath and replied, "Well, no. I can't answer that. Why? In the sense that it happens. I've seen that happen because they take it from two separate sites. If there's just enough fungus in one site, they take some blood from the other. If there is not enough fungus in the blood in that area, then it may not necessarily grow in a culture."

Realizing he dodged the issue, I said, "Okay, and do you know if they were taken properly?" He responded, "If you mean from two separate sites and not taken from the same site, yes . . . and they clean it. There's a protocol for cleaning, but you're right; it could be a contaminant. And like I said, it could be, but I can't just ignore it." I countered, "Yes, I know. I know you can't ignore it, and we don't want to ignore it. I'm just curious if the one that showed positive was from the area where he has a rash right now, you know?" He flippantly replied, "I didn't take the culture, so I cannot answer that question."

It was clear Dr. Liar would not order a new set of blood cultures and would continue to stand behind Dr. Torture's order that Rob be administered micafungin. He then admitted, "And the other thing is, **he is at risk from the medicines. We're trying to get him to decrease inflammation with the steroids, and that does put him at risk for having fungus in the blood**. *That's a known risk. But honestly, everything we give has risks*. The whole world is full of risks . . . not just medicine. We have risks when we cross the street."

Unfortunately, that was how they operated, piling one drug on top of another due to the erroneous belief that "more drugs equals better health" while ignoring the fact that each new medication carried its own risks, including numerous potentially fatal side effects.

When was the last time a doctor was held accountable for a "side effect"? Unfortunately, the American medical establishment and state and federal regulatory agencies appear to have granted physicians blanket immunity from the severe harm that the "unwanted" effects of the drugs they prescribe may cause, even if that negative "effect" happens to be the death of the patient.

LEGAL COUNSEL STATEMENT
Members of the jury, blood is naturally a sterile fluid, and bacteria or yeasts should not be present in the bloodstream. Unfortunately, blood culture contamination is a persistent problem in hospitals. *As a result, it is known that **up to 1/3** of "positive" blood culture tests in the US are **"false" positives**.*

To mitigate the likelihood of contamination (and as specified by Covid Coven Hospital of Plano, Texas' laboratory policies), a minimum of two cultures **must** be drawn from **two** separate sites at different times, and the result is only considered "positive" if **both** specimens are positive for the same organism.

The hospital lab clearly stated in Rob's hospital records that a **"positive" culture from a single site should NOT be considered a confirmation that a patient has a blood infection**. Furthermore, as you just heard, Drs. Liar and Torture admitted that the lab had reported that only one of the blood culture draws had shown yeast contamination—*a clear indication that it was highly likely the "positive" of one of the tests was due to contamination at the draw site.*

Dr. Liar misstated or lied that one positive culture was "the standard" for declaring a positive result. In addition, Dr. Torture's prescribing **micafungin** (an antifungal medication)—with a "positive" result from only one of four sites—was a clear departure from the hospital's laboratory policy.

Prescribing **micafungin** subjected Rob to further harm from several potential side effects, including: *difficulty breathing, little or no urination, diarrhea, irregular heartbeats, and drug-induced liver injury and fever*.
The propensity for micafungin to cause drug-induced liver injury is further substantiated by a Journal of Infection and Chemotherapy article published on May 5, 2022, that notes: "***Drug-induced liver injury (DILI) is a severe adverse effect (AE) of antifungals** that leads to the development of jaundice, **liver failure**, or even to **death in clinical settings**.*"
TakanoriYamamoto, & YoshiharuSato. (2022, February 9). Risk assessment of micafungin-induced liver injury using spontaneous reporting system data and Electronic Medical Records. Journal of Infection and Chemotherapy. From

Interestingly, Dr. Liar admitted, "**Sometimes it can cause some liver function abnormalities as a side effect.**" *We contend that "liver function abnormalities" would not be a positive development for someone already struggling to survive. We believe Dr. Torture jumped to prescribe* **micafungin**, *with Dr. Liar's complete agreement and backing, because, as we noted earlier, on September 20, 2021, Dr. Torture had begun to administer an off-label drug called* **baricitinib**.

Baricitinib is an anti-inflammatory medication usually prescribed for the treatment of rheumatoid arthritis. According to MedlinePlus, "***Taking baricitinib may decrease your ability to fight infection and increase the risk that you will get a serious infection, <u>including severe fungal</u>, bacterial, or viral infections that spread through the body. These infections may need to be treated in a hospital <u>and may cause death</u>***." U.S. National Library of Medicine. (n.d.). Baricitinib: Medlineplus drug information. MedlinePlus. From https://medlineplus.gov/druginfo/meds/a618033.html

We believe the doctors were well aware that administering **baricitinib** *at 4 mg per day (double the standard 2 mg per day for rheumatoid arthritis patients) subjected Rob to a "**severe fungal**" infection that could rapidly "**spread throughout the body**" <u>and promptly kill him</u>.*

Thus, after prescribing **baricitinib**, *they chose to violate the hospital's lab policy regarding blood cultures. With a "positive" from <u>only one site</u>, they immediately began treating Rob with* **micafungin** *for a potentially lethal iatrogenic (induced by medical treatment) fungal infection they suspected they likely caused by administering high doses of* **baricitinib**.

Rob was, unfortunately, a victim of "*drugs chasing drugs*," in which doctors piled one medication on another to undo the damage caused by previously administered pharmaceuticals.

This insane approach to "health care" is not unlike someone purposely lighting a small fire, then attempting to put it out with a blowtorch, after which they go into a panic and douse it with gasoline. Unfortunately, Rob's doctors were doing just this. They were tossing gasoline on fires they started in the hope of putting them out. **This is clearly irrational, if not criminal, behavior.**

Restraining the impulse to challenge him again, I replied, "I understand, and you guys are balancing it. I know the steroids are important, but they can also cause issues when you're on them for a long time. Is there anything else you wanted to update me on?" Dr. Liar said, "I mainly wanted to mention that was the only new issue, if you will. Everything else, honestly, looks pretty decent. You know, he's on less oxygen. I hope that trend continues. If it continues, I *may* get to a point where I don't need to prone him as much anymore. I'm not quite there yet. But we're almost there. If he gets to requiring less oxygen, I may start considering that."

Remembering Dr. Liar had said he would not attempt to wean Rob from the ventilator while he was in the RotoProne bed, I asked, "As I understand it, you won't be weaning Rob off the paralytic or the sedative, or maybe just the paralytic, until he's out of the RotoProne bed. Is that right?" He confirmed, "That's pretty much correct. And even after I have put him in a supine position, I may still leave the paralytic on for a little bit. We'll start to try and lift it, but if it starts affecting his oxygen, meaning he starts fighting it a little bit, I may need to leave it on.

"Once he gets off the paralytic and stays off the paralytic, they can lift the sedation enough to make sure he is moving everything, and so forth. Maybe not the full consciousness, but they do what we call a **sedation vacation**—but he's not even close to that right now. I gotta get him off the RotoProne bed before I can get him off paralytics before we would even consider that."
I said, "So, off the RotoProne bed, that's probably the first step. Then when do you start reducing the paralytic? At what point?" He said, "It depends on how he's doing from a pulmonary standpoint. Again, it's not an exact answer on that, okay? There's not, like, a protocol for that.

Because it depends on how he's doing, it'll depend on how much oxygen he is requiring, how much ventilator support he is requiring. Then, you know, lifting the paralytic. That has nothing to do with his consciousness, or how aware he is. That just allows him to potentially move more and try to breathe more. So that [the paralytic] won't have any effect on his being awake. The sedatives are what are keeping him asleep."

I commented, "I know Dr. Wicked said he was reducing the paralytic to test Rob at one point. So they were reducing the paralytic and then putting it back on?" He said, "I've not done that yet, because he is still on the RotoProne bed, and he's been fairly sick, and there are *different styles* on how to do that. Basically, right now, I think it's better to keep him completely just healing before I start allowing him to potentially move more. **And Dr. Wicked's thought, and rightfully so, is that being on a paralytic for a while does make someone weak. Ultimately, it does require longer for someone to get stronger. But I need to make sure he can live to get to that point."**

Clearly, Rob's chances of survival were declining by the day, and he would face a long and challenging recovery. Yet I was deeply disturbed by Dr. Liar's assertion that Rob might not "**live to get to that point.**" It reminded me of when Dr. Wicked had advised me, "**he could probably handle**, with paralytics, **probably 10 to 14 days and still have enough reserve** . . . most likely." By now, Rob had been on heavy doses of paralytics and a ventilator for **17 days**—well beyond the 10-to-14-day limit—and Dr. Liar just told me Rob would <u>remain paralyzed</u> until he was extracted from the RotoProne bed.

How was Rob supposed to survive this? Why had they not warned me that being in the RotoProne bed would mean Rob would have an "extended sentence" on the paralytics and that any opportunity for "parole" from the ventilator would be suspended until he was removed from the device?

He continued, "That's why I'm making sure he doesn't have **any more setbacks** because I want to get him on the least amount of oxygen possible." It was ironic and disturbing that he said he wanted to avoid "any more setbacks" when Rob, at their hands, had suffered one "setback" after another. They were the ones who had ignored Rob's and my directives and forced him to follow "*the protocol*" they had predetermined every patient even suspected of having COVID-19 must follow.

He then said, "Because, as I've said before, **oxygen is toxic over time, although at least up to 60% or less, it's not toxic. 60% or above, it is toxic**! . . . but it gets . . . it's kind of . . . it's not a . . . it's kind of a grade . . . essentially 65%. **You can be on 65% for a month with it <u>probably not</u> getting toxic. But if you're on 100%, you can be at 100% for the week and potentially have problems. By toxic, I mean just causing damage to your lungs."**

Wondering what kept them from lowering the oxygen level, I asked, "What are we doing to get him in that range? I see him going from 60 to 65% oxygen, and then he goes back up to 70% or higher. What other barriers are we trying to tackle?" Dr. Liar said, "*Honestly*, it's really his lungs that are his problem right now, and yeast in his blood is still an issue. But that's everything else. **It's really his lungs; his lungs are the main issue."**

LEGAL COUNSEL STATEMENT

Members of the jury, as we noted previously, breathing in high levels of oxygen (at concentrations above 60%) for over 24 hours can lead to "**oxygen toxicity**," otherwise known as "**oxygen poisoning.**" *The charts on Page C-54 of Appendix C show the **excessively high levels of oxygen** Rob was subjected to before and after he was placed on a ventilator.*

A National Library of Medicine article titled "Consequences of Hyperoxia and the Toxicity of Oxygen in the Lung" states, "***Oxygen is toxic to the lungs** when **high FiO2** (>0.60) [greater than 60% oxygen] is administered over extended exposure time (≥24 hours) [for 24 hours or more] at normal barometric pressure [at sea level]. **This type of exposure is referred to as low pressure O2 poisoning, pulmonary toxicity, or the Lorraine Smith effect**. Oxygen exposure after approximately 12 hours leads to lung passageway congestion, pulmonary edema, and **atelectasis** caused by damage to the linings of the bronchi and alveoli. The formation of fluid in the lungs causes **a feeling of shortness of breath** combined with a burning of the throat and chest, and **breathing becomes very painful**.*"
Mach, W. J., Thimmesch, A. R., Pierce, J. T., & Pierce, J. D. (2011). Consequences of hyperoxia and the toxicity of oxygen in the lung. Nursing research and practice. From https://www.ncbi.nlm.nih.gov/pmc/articles/PMC3169834

Dr. Liar stated, "oxygen is toxic over time, although at least up to 60% or less, it's not toxic. 60% or above, it is toxic!" On September 13th, Dr. Wicked said, "we are *pretty sure* 60% is not toxic from an oxygen standpoint. We don't know exactly where the threshold is. But in dogs, it's about 60%. So, we try to keep him at 60% and get him some reserve." Their admissions coincide with the National Library of Medicine article quoted above.

*Unfortunately, Dr. Liar failed to mention to Sheila that Rob had been placed on high-flow nasal cannula oxygen on an Optiflow device **at concentrations from 87% to 100% during his first five days at Covid Coven Hospital of Plano, Texas**. He also chose not to mention that the morning of September 8, 2021, the day Rob was placed on a ventilator, they had diagnosed Rob with **atelectasis**—a condition the article above states can be directly **caused by** exposure to high concentrations of oxygen (concentrations greater than 60%) for only 12 hours or more. You can see the diagnosis on Page 127 of the hospital records (see Page C-35 in Appendix C).*

We agree with Dr. Liar when he said, "**his lungs are the main issue**" because:
- They knowingly damaged Rob's lungs with **over-oxygenation**.
- The over-oxygenation caused **atelectasis** (where the alveoli cannot inflate properly), as recorded in Note 1 on Page 127 of the hospital records (see Page C-35 in Appendix C).
- They placed Rob on a **BiPAP** for 4.5 hours to "see if it helps atelectasis," as also stated in Note 1 on Page 127 of the hospital records (see Page C-35).
- Yet they knew with **pneumomediastinum** (a condition where a patient has air abnormally trapped in the space in the chest between the lungs)—which was a clear contraindication for BiPAP therapy as stated in a note entered by Nurse Carnage at the top of Page 97 of the hospital records (see Page C-21)—that the BiPAP could cause **barotrauma** as evidenced by the "Monitor for barotrauma given already with pneumomediastinum" statement also in Note 1 on Page 127 of the hospital records (see Page C-35).
- The barotrauma (a potentially life-threatening condition where the alveoli, the air sacs of the lungs, rupture and collapse) made Rob **feel claustrophobic** on the BiPAP as noted at the bottom of Page 136 of the hospital records (See Page C-41), making it very difficult to breathe and placing Rob in **a life-threatening crisis**.
- All of the above gave them the excuse they needed to place Rob **on a ventilator** while Dr. Wicked had admitted on September 7, 2021, "*it is a very bad thing to have to go on, and that is 100% true. That I know. I believe the ventilator causes death.*"

Thus, the doctors all knew—yet purposely failed to disclose to Sheila—that the excessively high levels of oxygen he was being administered from the day he was admitted severely damaged Rob's lungs. Every day he spent breathing over 60% oxygen was one more day he was closer to having "unsurvivable" lungs—which is precisely how the Medical Examiner described them during Rob's private autopsy. As we noted earlier, she said she had never seen lungs in such a deteriorated condition, and they did not even look human.

Since he said Rob's lungs were the problem, I asked, "I understand the ventilator was to give Rob's lungs a break, or his body a break, so everything else could heal. Is there something in particular that you are looking at concerning his lungs?"

He explained, "It's how stiff his lungs are and the gas exchange. Gas exchange, meaning I'm having to give him more oxygen than normal room air like you and I are breathing, to keep our oxygen level up. You and I are breathing 21% oxygen, and we're able to maintain at that oxygen level. If I gave your husband 21% oxygen, his oxygen saturation would be in the 50s or lower. And so, that's what I mean by gas exchange. Because he's not able to get the oxygen into his bloodstream as effectively as you or I are at this point in time."

I asked, "Okay, good. And can you do an X-ray to maybe give us some insight into how his lungs look? When was the last time you did one?" He replied, "We did one, like, two days ago. It looked about the same. We don't do it every day because the X-ray is the last thing to change. And it doesn't change what we do. It doesn't change my management. Now if there was a problem and *his lungs all of a sudden got severely worse* or something like that, yeah, I'd get an X-ray to make sure there is nothing else going on. But that's not happening right now."

Wondering how close we might be to weaning Rob from the ventilator, I said, "Okay. All right. Did you say your goal right now is to get his FiO2 down to 40 to 50% and the PEEP down to 7? I know his PEEP has been at 14, and the goal is to get that lower. What number are you looking for?"

He explained, "The first step . . . I need to get him out of the RotoProne bed. And so, I'll do that if he stays at 60% FiO2 or less when he's on his back. Then I can keep him off of the RotoProne bed. Next step, I can start potentially weaning his paralytic. I can also wean the VELETRI, which is a medicine we're giving him to help with his oxygen, or I can wean the PEEP. We just slowly wean all of those depending on how he's doing. And there's not an exact step-by-step process. It's not this then this; it's not a computer algorithm. There's a general trend, and there's a general way to do it. But *there's not an exact answer that everybody follows*."

I felt they had missed several opportunities to attempt to wean Rob in the past, so I asked, "On September 18th, right before he was put on the RotoProne bed, his FiO2 was below 60, and at one point, it was down to 45. So, why was he not weaned at that point before he was placed in the RotoProne bed?

He stuttered and said, "He was, and then sometimes things go up and down. That's correct. I know. I've had patients with COVID who have gone completely off the ventilator, but then I had to put them back on the ventilator and go through the same process all over again. And it's not because they got reinfected or anything; it's just that the inflammatory process is what was going on. So, it is quite variable. But he's trending towards improvement now, which is a good thing, and that will go with that."

Like everyone else at Covid Coven Hospital of Plano, Texas, Dr. Liar blamed everything on "Covid." I fully expected that some of the patients he had extracted from the ventilator ended up back ON it because the massive number and dosages of sedatives and paralytics they had endured had left them totally debilitated with (as Dr. Wicked said) no "reserves" to be able to effectively breathe on their own.

I responded, "Okay, so the first step is getting him off the RotoProne bed. Then you're going to start looking at weaning things off. Like you said, 50% FiO2, and then you said your goal for the PEEP is 7 or 8." He corrected me, "Normal PEEP is down to 5. We slowly wean, and again, that's further on down the line." I wondered how much "further down the line" he was referring to and how much longer Rob's lungs could endure.

Dr. Liar jumped in, "If I get his PEEP down to 5 and I'm down 40% oxygen, and I wasn't giving him anything else except sedatives, that's the point I would try to start weaning him, meaning waking him up fully and seeing how he breathes. **He's nowhere near that!** And I know you want to be here for that, and I get it. But I'm just kind of telling you what the ultimate goal is. And also, ultimately, I think he's going to need a trach because he's going to be really too weak to wean quickly."

LEGAL COUNSEL STATEMENT
Members of the jury, you may have noticed that we've heard from others that a PEEP setting of 8 and FiO2 of 60% would be sufficient to attempt to wean Rob. Yet, Dr. Liar was now saying, "So if I get his PEEP down to 5, and I'm down 40% oxygen." As you can see, his criteria did not match others'—so it was obviously a bit of a mixed bag at this hospital.

As we stated earlier, the Agency for Healthcare Research and Quality criteria (which this hospital did follow) for attempting to wean someone from the ventilator was a **PEEP** (Positive End Expiratory Pressure) setting of **8 cm H$_2$O** or less, and **FiO2** (oxygen concentration) is of **50% or less**.
Coordinated spontaneous awakening and breathing trials protocol. AHRQ. (n.d.). From https://www.ahrq.gov/hai/tools/mvp/modules/technical/sat-sbt-protocol.html

Unfortunately, they did not reduce the PEEP and FiO2 to the required levels for the remainder of Rob's stay. *As a result, once on the ventilator, Rob was on a one-way trip to the morgue.*

As we shared earlier, Sammy Wong, MD, our medical expert witness, said in his "Letter of Introduction," which appears in **Appendix B**, "*Since he was sedated and paralyzed, he was dependent on the ventilator. All of the ABGs showed profound respiratory acidosis indicating that the staff chose not to adjust the ventilator settings to improve his alveolar ventilation. They just maintained his ventilator settings essentially unchanged . . . until he died.*"

I said, "Thank you for listening to my questions. I don't like the status quo. I feel like there is so much more we could be doing. That's why I have asked about things like a surfactant and more budesonide. I wish we could be doing both because they hit the lungs directly. If I find other things that I think will help, I will make a list and go over them with you."

I then shared, "I talked to Dr. Wicked about getting him on IV vitamin C, and he was open to it. He said he would even look into it since we wanted it as a family." Dr. Liar replied, "That might be, but he's getting it orally. *Vitamins are better given internally than through an IV.* That is the way the body's meant to absorb things. There's a feeding tube that we have down into his stomach, and that's how we introduce it. That's also how we're giving it to him, in his tube feeding."

He continued, "Feel free to **ask**. That's fine. Okay?" Unfortunately, although Dr. Liar had assured me that, as Rob's advocate, I could ask for whatever I liked, he also made it clear that it was up to the doctors whether my request would be approved. Instead of being able to provide directives, patient advocates were reduced to having to beg for what they wanted. I would beg for things that I believed might help Rob regain his strength (such as adequate calories and nutrition) and would help him heal (such as a surfactant and an increased dose of inhaled budesonide), and they would look at me with dismay or disdain and coldly say, "***Sorry, but no.***"

Dr. Liar and others made it clear that my input was irrelevant once Rob was in their hands (or in their grasp). I sensed that even if I were a licensed physician, I would still have no say in my husband's plan of care. In their view, my bringing him into their domain and his being admitted meant he had no rights to refuse medications such as remdesivir, and as his wife and duly appointed Medical Power of Attorney, I had given up my rights to determine his nutritional needs or his plan of care. I was merely "the wife" they were obligated to "deal with" because they had "full authority" to determine the medications and therapies my husband, whom they now had "custody" of, would be subjected to.

Some of my friends shared with me first, second, and third-hand accounts of innocent victims of "the protocol that kills" without realizing how it might affect me. I finally requested that they refrain from doing so because I needed to remain optimistic despite how slim Rob's chances might be. I knew I had to stay strong to continue to do my best to advocate for better care.

Based on Rob's trajectory and Dr. Liar's comments, it was evident that they lacked a solid plan for weaning him off the ventilator. They did, however, have a clear and concise plan—"the Covid protocol"—that they ensured each "Covid" patient followed precisely.

Dr. Mei had also witnessed that once a patient was "on the protocol," they were destined to complete "the full protocol"—even if that meant they would not make it home alive. The doctors would chalk up one more "win" for the protocol as they said, "*well, the treatment was a success despite the fact the patient did not survive.*"

At 7:00 PM, at the end of the day shift, she had to leave as the ICU visitors' hours were over. When Dr. Mei arrived at my home, we discussed our best next steps. To aid us in executing the plan, I decided it best to call my patient advocate.

We shared with her that Rob had not been improving, and Dr. Mei and I were disturbed that his doctors would not agree to administer a surfactant or IV vitamin C. They would only agree to follow their "standard protocol" instead of using what we believed were safer and more effective therapies.

She suggested I call the hospital Social Worker in the morning and ask her to schedule an intervention meeting at the hospital with one of the lead doctors, possibly Dr. Liar. She would attend the meeting with us, and I could bring Dr. Mei and a few others along to help make a case for changes in Rob's plan of care.

She suggested we write out our questions and concerns and bring along clinical data that validated that the therapies we were requesting were safe and effective. She reminded me that making any headway would require that we be tactful and, as she liked to say, use a "soft touch."

Thus, over dinner, Dr. Mei and I drafted our questions, concerns, and clinical data for the meeting. In the morning, I would call Ms. Destroyer, the Social Worker, to see how quickly she could set up a meeting.

Chapter 7 – Intervention & Expectation

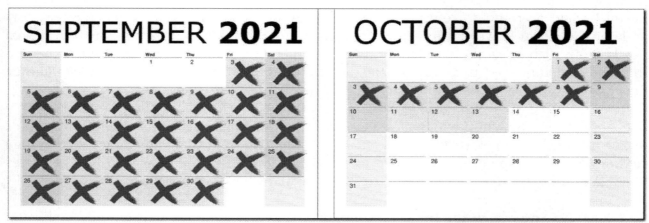

THIS CHAPTER COVERS SEPTEMBER 26 – OCTOBER 8

Sunday, September 26, 2021

In the morning, as suggested by my patient advocate, whom I had spoken with the night before, I contacted Ms. Destroyer, the hospital's Social Worker. I asked if she could schedule a face-to-face meeting with Dr. Liar so I could meet with him to discuss my concerns about Rob's care and request alternative therapies that I believed could aid in accelerating his recovery.

I let her know I would be bringing a patient advocate with me who formerly worked as a Registered Nurse. I decided not to tell her I also planned to bring my sister, two close friends, and Dr. Mei. I feared that she would refuse to schedule the meeting if she knew how much firepower I would be bringing. To my surprise, she said she would be happy to set it up. After checking her calendar and Dr. Liar's schedule, she reserved a room for 10:00 AM the following morning.

With the meeting scheduled, I advised my patient advocate, my sister, Dr. Mei, and Roberta and Allen Stalvey, who had been by my side since not long after Rob's hospitalization and were aiding me in managing the logistics of crucial day-to-day tasks. Everyone agreed to meet at the hospital just before the 10:00 AM meeting time.

We all had the same goals: to see Rob improve, be removed from the ventilator, complete any necessary post-ventilator therapy, and get back on his feet to continue his mission as a seeker and presenter of Biblical truth.

With the meeting scheduled, Dr. Mei and I reviewed our plans for the day. I would drive my car to the hospital, and she would follow me in Rob's car. I would then spend the day with Rob in his room in the ICU while she waited in the 2nd-floor waiting room so we could meet, on occasion, to discuss Rob's condition. In the meantime, we would communicate via text messages.

Dr. Mei then put on her white physician's coat and followed me to the hospital. When we arrived, I entered first. Then, after I headed up in the elevator and proceeded to Rob's ICU room, she followed soon after and headed to the waiting room on the 2nd floor. It was reassuring

194

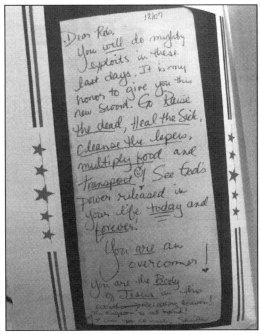

knowing that a licensed physician was as earnest as I was to help save Rob from "the protocol" as we battled a team of physicians who were promoting it.

Dr. Mei suggested that when the doctor arrived during his rounds, I should again ask if he would be willing to repeat the blood culture to ensure Rob truly needed to be on an antifungal medication and ask once more if he would agree to administer IV vitamin C.

When I arrived at Rob's bedside, I took out the small pocket-sized Bible I had given him fourteen years earlier, soon after our wedding. Then, as I stood by his side, careful not to touch the RotoProne bed, I began to read him the words of encouragement I had written inside the front cover. *"Rob, you will do mighty exploits in these last days. It is my honor to give . . ."*

At that point, choking on my tears, I put the book down and cried quietly as I told him, "I love you, Honey. You mean the world to me! You are my world. My world is empty without you. You are strong. You are getting stronger every day."

I then spoke of the memento we had given to our wedding guests. It was a tiny glass jar that held hundreds of mustard seeds. I reminded him that our great God answers prayers and told him that people worldwide were praying for him. I had more faith than one mustard seed that God could raise Rob from his RotoProne bed and send him home whole and strong.

At that point, Dr. Liar walked into the room. He cleared his throat and said, "He's about the same as yesterday, and the big picture has not changed. His labs are about the same." I could see him brace himself in expectation of my asking him more pressing questions.

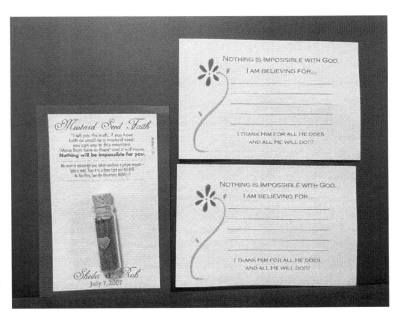

I asked why Rob had to be prone for 16 hours, then supine for only 8 hours. He responded, "Those are the standards of care. Those are our protocols." I answered, "Oh, that's your protocol." Dr. Liar said, "So, when you're lying on your back, you're getting all this blood flow to the bottom of your lungs, and all the air generally goes to the higher part of the lungs."

I said, "I know this RotoProne bed is supposed to be great, and it's helped many people. But to me, it was a little confusing why he was lying face down for 16 hours. That seems like a long time." He said, "It's human physiology, and that's how it works."

I noticed they had kept the PEEP set at 14 since they placed Rob on the ventilator, and since it had to be lowered for them to wean him, I said, "I know the PEEP has to be reduced to wean him from the ventilator. Can the PEEP be lowered?" Dr. Liar explained, "If I can lower his FiO2 and have him lie on his back, **then** I can lower the PEEP."

I then asked, "Since Rob is getting the antifungal, is there not any way you could do another blood culture? I'm asking because I don't want him getting micafungin for two weeks if he doesn't need it, as that would be a long time to get an antifungal without being symptomatic."

He repeated what he had told me the day before. "If I do a culture now, it is not going to show up in particular. There's a standard of care. So, if I just treat it for a short period of time, then it can come back with a vengeance. And yeah, that's the same thing with bacterial pneumonia, where blood cultures will fail when they've been given a couple of days of antibiotics."

Clearly, he had prematurely placed Rob on an antifungal and was now using that as the excuse for not repeating the blood culture. Instead, he should have repeated the blood culture and only if the culture from at least two separate sites came back positive, then placed him on the antifungal. Having jumped the gun meant he had no choice but to subject Rob to the entire 14-day course of the medication.

Hoping he would budge on the IV vitamin C, I began to ask if he would reconsider it. With a huff, he interrupted me mid-sentence and barked, "I told you this yesterday!" Observing that he did not appreciate his decisions being questioned, I attempted to calm him with, "I'm sorry if I can't keep track of everything. I know what you said. However, I would like him to have IV vitamin C. Dr. Wicked agreed it would be okay. But, again, I'm sorry. My husband has been separated from me for 21 days, and this has been very difficult. How would your wife feel if you were isolated from her?"

He replied, "Oh, my wife? She wouldn't want me to do this or want to see me go through this."

I explained, "If you're separated from your spouse, you lose your mind. If you had to do this, you might ask questions more than once. I'm trying to be my husband's advocate. I'm doing my best." Calming a bit, he responded, "I understand. You asked about IV vitamin C. It's better absorbed through the stomach, and that's why we are giving it to him orally. That's a better way to do it." Standing my ground, I responded, "I do not agree with you, but okay, that's fine. It's okay to agree to disagree. All right."

Not wishing to entertain any more questions, he said he had to visit other patients and scurried out of the room. When I texted Dr. Mei a summary of our discussion, she said I had done well to at least require Dr. Liar to explain why he would not agree to repeat the blood cultures or start Rob on IV vitamin C.

When I texted her photos of the monitors and massive tower of IVs pumping large amounts of medications into Rob's body, she commented, "Rob's vitals look good, his heart rate is the same, and it looks like the ventilator settings are the same as before."

I set up Rob's iPad to play some of his YouTube-based teachings, hoping he might recognize and be encouraged by them. Listening to his insightful teachings also helped the hours go by as I sat in his room watching him fight to stay alive.

He was again in a prone, face-down position, and I could not see his face. I kept telling him that I loved him, that he was my best friend, and was the best person I had ever met. It was easy to fill his ears with endless accolades, for he was indeed the best man I had ever met.

Next, one of Rob's Respiratory Therapists entered the room. I looked up and said, "Hello, I'm Sheila. I hope you don't mind my asking you a few questions. She said, "Sure." So, I told her I was concerned that the whole time Rob had been on a ventilator, they had had him fully sedated and paralyzed, then said, "That PEEP is never going to go down if they have him fully sedated. I want to understand."

She replied, "Well, here's the thing, just to let you know. When we're in this particular bed, the patient has to be completely sedated and paralyzed because when we're rotating him and everything, we don't want them to get all agitated and be able to move and try to get themselves out. So, until he's out of this bed, we cannot start the weaning process. He's prone for 16 hours, and then he's supine for 8 hours. Once we get him out of this bed and he stays supine, and his sat [blood oxygen level] stays above 88%, and we're able to wean somewhat down on the PEEP, then we can talk about reducing the sedation."

On the afternoon of September 9, 2021, the day after Rob's intubation, they had finally started Rob on a tiny 0.5-milligram daily dose of budesonide while still administering 8 milliliters per hour of continuous nebulized VELTERI per day. However, the Respiratory Therapist revealed something disturbing when she said, "The other thing is, you know this Pulmacort (budesonide) that we're giving him, I don't know how much he's actually receiving in his lungs. So, that particular drug is mainly for a respiratory issue, but he's technically really not getting that much of the drug."

I asked, "Why?" She replied, "It's because we're giving him VELETRI, and it's constantly going into him, and so when I break the circuit to put this treatment in line, it actually, almost in a sense, kind of crystalizing in this cup. So, the Pulmacort [budesonide], in all reality, is better when he's off the RotoProne bed and off the VELETRI."

I said, "To me, this budesonide is **more important** than the VELETRI. What is your opinion?" She said, "Well, the purpose of the VELETRI . . . it pretty much like nitrate. So, the reason why we have him on this is because his PEEP's 14, and his oxygen [FiO2] is 60%. You want these two numbers, in all reality, to get off VELETRI . . . it's a combination of three numbers. His sats [blood oxygen saturation] when he's supine need to be at least greater than 90%. Once we're able to get the FiO2 to at least maybe 50 or 40%, then we can wean the PEEP, and then we can slowly start weaning the VELETRI."

I replied, "**The PEEP has been 14 the entire time**, so how does that work? They told me it has to be at 8 to wean Rob." She said, "The PEEP is what we set, and in a normal person, a person who is not sick, we normally have a PEEP of 5. That [residual] pressure is what keeps our lungs open."

To confirm I understood, I said, "So, we need to get his saturation [blood oxygen level] to greater than 90% when he's supine; the FiO2 [oxygen concentration] needs to be 50 or 40%." She said, "It just depends on the doctor. Everybody's different. We literally set the PEEP, and that helps keep the airways open. So, once we're able to wean these when he's supine, then we can come off the VELETRI. Once the VELETRI is gone, everything else will start from there."

I was shocked to hear that for the past 17 days, since September 9th, they had been giving Rob **one** small daily dose of **0.5 mg** of budesonide per day when it should have been administered at **1 mg** per dose **every 4 hours**—and they had been only giving that one small daily dose to appease me. Now, the Respiratory Therapist was telling me he was likely not receiving even that tiny dose into his lungs because of the continuous flow of VELETRI.

After my discussion with the Respiratory Therapist, since nothing more was likely to change for the rest of the day, I texted Dr. Mei to let her know she could head back to my house as I remained with Rob for the remainder of the day.

LEGAL COUNSEL STATEMENT

Members of the jury, nearly a year after Rob's death, Sheila shared her audio recording of the conversation with the Respiratory Therapist with Sammy Wong, MD, our medical expert. In a written response to her, he said: *"She was simply 'shooting from the hip' regarding VELETRI and budesonide."*

He then noted, *"VELETRI (epoprostenol) is a prostaglandin, NOT a nitrate. It has two significant pharmacological actions: (1) direct vasodilation of pulmonary and systemic arterial vascular beds and (2) inhibition of platelet aggregation."* He suspected they had given Rob VELETRI to vasodilate the pulmonary vasculature since it appears they incorrectly ASSUMED Rob had pulmonary hypertension (which is different from systemic hypertension) due to COVID-19. Yet, Rob had never been diagnosed with pulmonary hypertension.

He further commented, *"As for whether the budesonide actually reached the lung parenchyma, we don't know the depth of deposition. Plus, it does not "crystalize" in the nebulizer chamber of the ventilator's tubing as the Respiratory Therapist implied. Determining the depth of particulate deposition in mechanically ventilated patients is complex (https://scholarworks.gsu.edu/cgi/viewcontent.cgi?article=1002&context=rt_facpub). We know that only about 5% of the actuated medication is deposited to the lung parenchyma using the hand-held meter-dose inhalers (MDI) as opposed to using in-line medication nebulization through the ventilator tubing. The rest of the actuated medication rains out in the mouth. Therefore, it would not be unexpected to see that the in-line budesonide could rain out along the tubing from the nebulizer chamber through and to the tip of the endotracheal tube (in the trachea just before it splits off to the right and left bronchi)."*

In Appendix B, you will find his "Interim Analysis," where he stated, *"He was given VELETRI (epoprostenol) which is indicated for people with known 'severe pulmonary arterial hypertension.' There was no objective evidence [that is, a diagnosis of pulmonary arterial hypertension does not appear anywhere in Rob's records indicating] that he had severe PAH. It is unknown whether the VELETRI caused or contributed to this patient's eventual 'extensive interstitial fibrosis.'"* He also said, *"VELETRI and baricitinib were given in spite of substantial harms which did not benefit and were without clear indications for them."* Lastly, in his "Causes of Action" (also in Appendix B), he noted, *"Epoprostenol can incite a profound inflammatory response in the pulmonary interstitium. Due to a lack of indication for its use, the patient was subjected to unnecessary risks."*

Unfortunately, *"shooting from the hip"* appears to have been a common strategy for them for their "Covid" patients. Since Rob's hospital record indicated he was infected with COVID-19, they seemed to believe they could do whatever they pleased without regard for potential adverse outcomes.

They appeared to take a *"do what you will"* approach with their "Covid" patients because it was assumed that such patients had slim chances of recovery. *Moreover, whenever a "Covid" patient died because of "the protocol" they were being subjected to, their untimely but predictable deaths were always attributed to "Covid."*

At 7:00 PM, with visitors' hours over, I headed home. When I arrived, Dr. Mei and I reviewed and updated our list of questions and concerns for the morning meeting with Dr. Liar.

We hoped the upcoming "intervention" meeting with Dr. Liar would result in significant positive changes in Rob's plan of care—changes that would help get him on the road to recovery instead of continuing on what was, at present, nothing more than a downward spiral.

Monday, September 27, 2021

In preparation for today's "intervention" meeting, I collaborated with Dr. Mei and several other medical professionals to compile a list of points to review with Dr. Liar. I then typed up and printed several copies for the meeting.

My team and I gathered in an open area on the second floor shortly before 10:00 a.m., waiting to be invited into what turned out to be a small, cramped meeting room. I was joined by my sister, my friends Roberta and Allen Stalvey (Allen had been an Air Force medic), my patient advocate, and Dr. Mei, who was dressed in her white physician's coat with her name printed on it.

When Ms. Destroyer arrived, she was undoubtedly surprised at the size of the group standing with me. Nevertheless, she requested that we follow her to a small room that featured only a few chairs around a small round table. She said she would fetch some additional chairs and inform Dr. Liar that we had arrived.

After she brought in a few extra chairs, my team and I crammed ourselves around the table, leaving only one empty seat for Dr. Liar. Having no seat, Ms. Destroyer stood by the doorway with her notepad and pen, ready to take notes for Dr. Liar. She had previously stated that she fully supported the doctors. Unfortunately, patients and their families, on the other hand, were not high on her support list. Unfortunately, the same seemed to be true of everyone at Covid Coven Hospital of Plano, Texas.

Soon, Dr. Liar entered. He was tall, with curly hair and blue eyes. He slid into the empty chair, crossing one long leg over the other. As he surveyed the group, I could see he was wondering what he had gotten himself into. I also sensed Ms. Destroyer was not pleased and was somewhat embarrassed that the doctor now faced a larger group than he had anticipated.

I had expected Dr. Liar to bring a few notes and essential information from Rob's hospital records, yet he arrived empty-handed. He appeared unprepared and completely disinterested. In addition, I had the distinct impression that he had already decided to ignore our requests and only agreed to the meeting to maintain the appearance of being open-minded.

199

When I passed around copies of the list of items we wanted to discuss, he quickly glanced at it and immediately placed it on the table in front of him. I then took a moment to quickly introduce my team members.

In a take-charge manner, Ms. Destroyer said she would read off each item on the list so we could discuss them. However, my patient advocate, who had worked in hospitals and knew she was trying to take control of the meeting, snatched control from the Social Worker by saying she would prefer to go over each item, causing Dr. Liar to turn his gaze toward her.

Dr. Liar's eyes conveyed his dismay, despite his facial expressions being partially hidden by the cloth mask he wore. After a quick glance at his copy of the list, he returned his gaze to my advocate. Before he arrived, she had called another nurse who had become a patient advocate and was her business partner. She placed her cell phone face up on the small table and introduced her partner.

Realizing we had even more firepower in the room, Dr. Liar readjusted himself in what had become "the hot seat" while attempting to appear cool, calm, and collected. We were off to a good start, and even though we were on Dr. Liar's turf, I could sense God's hand and favor as I looked around at my team of supporters. I was backed by a team who were not afraid to challenge the system that had my husband in its potentially lethal grip.

Picking up the list, my patient advocate directed her full attention to Dr. Liar, saying, "Okay. I want to go through this list to see where you're coming from. We want to get your opinion and then kind of go from there." Feeling her strength, Dr. Liar nodded his head and said, "Sure."

> **1.** Most importantly . . . people cannot heal without proper nutrition and a massive weight loss is unacceptable nursing care. He needs daily weights. He needs TPN/Lipids in addition to his tube feedings. IF you won't do TPN/Lipids, why, and why are his protein and calories not enough to prevent his severe malnutrition? This should NEVER happen. A 5% weight loss would be expected due to illness, but an admission weight of 170 lbs. to today's 123 lbs. is absolutely unacceptable.

Launching into the first item on the list, she hit him straight between the eyes with, "So, let's look at Rob's nutrition. It looks like we've got quite a weight loss. So, what is currently the plan for that?"

Struggling for an answer, he said, "He's getting nutrition, but when people are critically ill, they still can lose weight despite giving nutrition. That's called *the catabolic state*. **But the nutritionist is kind of managing what they recommend for the nutrition.** So that's . . . ." My advocate slammed back, "Well, that's lacking, okay?" He lamely responded, "I would discuss that with our good nutritionist." I quickly jumped in and said, "I have already done that, and she told me what he's getting is the best and there are no other options, which I don't think is true."

LEGAL COUNSEL STATEMENT
Members of the jury, the "catabolic state" Dr. Liar referred to is a metabolic condition that occurs when a person's caloric and nutrient intake is insufficient to meet their energy requirements.

This leads to the body breaking down its own tissue, including muscle, for energy production. Unfortunately, due to the rapid depletion of the body's muscle-bound protein reserves, many patients lose as much as 20% of their muscle mass (2% per day) within the first 10 days of their ICU admission.
Wandrag, L., Brett, S. J., Frost, G. S., Bountziouka, V., & Hickson, M. (n.d.). Exploration of muscle loss and metabolic state during prolonged critical illness: Implications for intervention? PLOS ONE. From
https://journals.plos.org/plosone/article?id=10.1371%2Fjournal.pone.0224565

The National Library of Medicine's abstract on "Nutrition in critical illness: a current conundrum" noted: *"**Nutrition authorities have long recommended providing generous amounts of protein and calories to critically ill patients**, either intravenously or through feeding tubes, in order to counteract the catabolic state associated with this condition. **In practice, however, patients in modern intensive care units are substantially underfed**. . . . The muscle atrophy of catabolic critical illness can be rapid and severe enough to debilitate healthy young adults whose initial muscle mass was normal."*

Hoffer, L. J., & Bistrian, B. R. (2016, October 18). Nutrition in critical illness: A current conundrum. F1000Research. From https://www.ncbi.nlm.nih.gov/pmc/articles/PMC5070594

Another National Library of Medicine abstract on "The relationship between nutritional intake and clinical outcomes in critically ill patients: results of an international multicenter observational study" confirmed: *"**Increased intakes of energy and protein** appear to be associated with improved clinical outcomes in critically ill patients."*

Alberda C;Gramlich L;Jones N;Jeejeebhoy K;Day AG;Dhaliwal R;Heyland DK; (n.d.). The relationship between nutritional intake and clinical outcomes in critically ill patients: Results of an international multicenter observational study. Intensive care medicine. From https://pubmed.ncbi.nlm.nih.gov/19572118

As previously stated, Rob Skiba's nutritional and caloric needs were wholly ignored from the day he arrived. In addition, Sheila's repeated attempts to reach the dietitian, whom Dr. Liar referred to as a "good nutritionist," had been unsuccessful—we suspect because the dietitian did not wish to be confronted regarding, and have to answer for, her negligence.

Consider this:

- On September 5, 2021, two days after his admission, Rob texted Sheila, "**No food no . . .**" and "**No strength no hope left.**"

- On September 13, 2021, five days after Rob was placed on the ventilator, Dr. Wicked admitted to Sheila, "So, by the time he got on the ventilator, of course, **we were nutritionally down, and he hadn't been fed for several days before**. So, he may not, you know, **he may not have enough reserve in two weeks**."

*Sadly, after being starved into submission and placed on a ventilator, Rob continued to decline due to **(a)** a continued lack of adequate nutrition and **(b)** the use of paralytics which ensured his muscles could not move, leading to muscle wasting.*

Ensuring adequate nutritional and caloric intake is an essential aspect of any hospital patient's treatment plan. Therefore, we find it unconscionable and deplorable that a physician who claims to have oversight of a patient's plan of care would attempt to pass that responsibility along to a non-physician member of the team while acting as if that aspect of patient care was neither their personal concern nor their responsibility.

Medical malpractice occurs when a physician fails to follow accepted standards of care, thereby causing harm to a patient. The ongoing and unaddressed malnutrition clearly harmed Rob. The doctors' negligence of Rob's nutritional state further depleted any "reserves" (physical strength) he may have had when he arrived at Covid Coven Hospital in Plano, Texas.

Passing the ball to the illusive "nutritionist" (otherwise known as a dietitian), Dr. Liar shook his head and replied, "They're the experts in that." I said, "Well, not really. I'm not trying to argue, but the thing is, he's losing a ton of weight. There has to be a **better** answer and a **better** way." He said, "That happens in critically ill patients. I've treated many critically ill patients. If I feed him more, **it will filter out**; it'll **just come out**."

I looked at my patient advocate and saw that she was as bewildered as I was by his response. She stepped in, "But there's also actions of TPN [Total Parenteral Nutrition] to supplement, right?" He was not about to agree with the use of TPN, adding, "As well as be very dangerous in this setting."

Members of the jury, TPN (Total Parenteral Nutrition) refers to a type of intravenous (IV) feeding that provides all of a patient's daily nutritional needs through a vein. TPN is frequently administered to critically ill patients who cannot eat or are unable to receive adequate nutrition through oral or enteral (tube) feeding.

TPN is a complex mixture of carbohydrates, proteins, fats, vitamins, and minerals, delivered directly through a central venous catheter into the bloodstream. It provides complete and balanced nutrition and can be adjusted based on a patient's individual needs and requirements. We believe Dr. Liar said TPN would be "very dangerous in this setting" for two primary reasons:

- **SOLU-MEDROL**. They had Rob on high doses of **SOLU-MEDROL**, a powerful systemic steroid. As noted earlier, WebMD said the following regarding SOLU-MEDROL, *"This medication may lower your ability to fight infections. This may make you more likely to get a serious (rarely fatal) infection or make any infection you have worse."* Thus, when Sheila asked Dr. Wicked about TPN the morning of September 8, 2021, several hours before Rob was placed on a ventilator because she knew Rob was already malnourished, he responded, "It's **a horrible infection risk**, especially when you're **already on steroids**." *They knew that with Rob being administered a massive amount of systemic steroids, the risk of infection from a central venous catheter was higher than normal because steroids vastly suppress the immune system.*

- **RESPONSIBILITY**. TPN delivers the nutrients directly into the bloodstream, bypassing the digestive system. This makes TPN a more potent form of nutritional support. However, it also increases the complexity of administration and would make it impossible for Dr. Liar to pass off the overall responsibility for Rob's nutritional and caloric intake to the dietitian/nutritionist. *Clearly, Dr. Liar had no interest in assuming greater responsibility for Rob's nutritional and caloric intake.*

She responded, "Okay. So, a 5% weight loss, you know, we would understand. That's expected, okay? But his beginning weight was 170 pounds, and now he's down to 123 pounds . . ." Dr. Liar simply said, "Sure." She continued, ". . . which is quite significant!" Again, he said only, "Sure." She stressed, "So, that does need to be looked at!" Sounding disinterested, Dr. Liar dodged once more with, "Sure. **Again, talk to the nutritionist on that**."

Members of the jury, as we mentioned earlier, the RotoProne bed that Rob was placed in on September 18th had **a massive scale problem**. This fact is documented on Page 359 of the hospital's records, as shown below.

> Pt interview/Comments:
> 9/20: Pt remains intubated and sedated, not able to have SBT per respiratory. Large weight variance noted from 9/18 to 9/19 weights when transitioned to Rotoprone bed, staff believes new weights are inaccurate and pt is closer to 170 lb.

Page C-55 of Appendix C contains a graph of Rob's daily weight measurements—as recorded by the hospital staff—from his admission on September 3, 2021, until his death on October 13, 2021.

Their failure to inform Sheila of the problem with the RotoProne bed's scale caused her unnecessary distress and anxiety. In addition, her team also had the impression that Rob had suffered a significant weight loss from the day of his admission until today because the RotoProne bed's scale indicated Rob weighed only 123 pounds, as shown in the graph on Page C-55.

If Dr. Liar had paid ANY attention to Rob's weight (which is evidently not the case), he would have immediately noticed the drastic one-day change and informed Sheila that Rob had not really significantly lost weight but rather the scales on the RotoProne bed were malfunctioning. But sadly, he was utterly clueless and unprepared to answer crucial questions about Rob's condition and plan of care.

Regardless of the weight discrepancy, the drop in Rob's protein and albumin, which comes up shortly, was still a significant issue that needed to be addressed to ensure he was not malnourished.

I was perplexed as to how he could, in good conscience, delegate responsibility for Rob's nutritional and caloric intake to someone else when he was supposed to be overseeing Rob's care.

Apparently, he and his partners in crime considered themselves primarily "*the keepers of the MAR (Medication Administration Record)*"—the document where they logged the list of prescribed medications, their dosages, frequency, and routes of administration. Then, once prescribed, they would observe how each drug affected Rob to determine what new prescription he required to counteract effects (or side effects) of the other medications.

If a patient died from malnutrition, apparently we were expected to "blame the dietitian" (a person he chose to refer to as a "nutritionist") because the doctors preferred to absolve themselves of any responsibility for a person's nutritional intake. Instead, they were only willing to be responsible for the patient's "drug intake."

My advocate pointedly asked, "Okay, so who's going to organize a discussion with the nutritionist?" Running interference for the irresponsible doctor, Ms. Destroyer, the Social Worker, stepped in, "I can give you their phone number and follow up on all that." Dr. Liar breathed a sigh of relief, and one point was scored for the Social Worker who valiantly ran interference for her hospital buddy.

My patient advocate looked dumbfounded at them both and said, "Okay. You can also ask them to <u>follow up</u>. I think that would be important because *he's gonna need those calories to get through this.*"

Dr. Mei, who had held her peace until now, could no longer keep quiet. She said, "So, quick question. Do you sign off on it or pass the buck?" Turning to look at her with piercing blue eyes, he replied, "I sign off on it, but I rely on her expertise." She responded like a bull at full charge, "I need clarification here. Because sometimes you say, 'well, they're experts, and they have all the experience,' but you say you don't give them authority to order without your sign-off?"

Dr. Liar explained, "Actually, I do . . . I usually do. I can change it. As far as enteral tube feeding. When it comes to TPN [Total Parenteral Nutrition], which you asked about, I don't necessarily recommend it."

My patient advocate weighed in, "But if we're doing supplementation, <u>we're trying to get his calories to where it needs to be for healing</u>, then we need to be smart with how we attack this problem *because the **malnutrition** is very significant. And that's actually **quite dangerous**.* So we may have to readjust temporarily how he gets nutrition until his calories improve and then switch back to tube feedings."

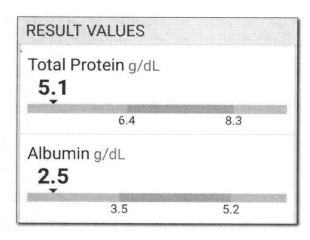

RESULT VALUES

Total Protein g/dL
5.1
6.4   8.3

Albumin g/dL
2.5
3.5   5.2

Dr. Liar said, "His albumin is actually fine." My advocate said, "It isn't good. **He's in trouble**." Dr. Liar responded, "It's like 2.2, 2.3, the last time I checked, which is low but not dangerously low. It's not severe in a sense."

I chimed in, "Well, there's a chart right there," and pointed to a chart showing how low Rob's albumin and protein numbers were. "That's why I said he needed more protein, and they just added it on the 23rd, **which kind of shows negligence, a bad trend, or an accident**."

My patient advocate said, "We're going to talk with the nutritionist, and you're gonna give her the authority to relook at this, okay? Dr. Liar responded, "As far as enteral tube feeding, yea."

She responded, "Let's see what we can do with that." I was disappointed that a potential opportunity to get Dr. Liar to finally agree to TPN feeding for Rob had passed us by. Unfortunately, with his flat-out refusal, the best we could do was to discuss with the dietitian/nutritionist the possibility of improving what she was providing Rob through his feeding tube.

So, my advocate continued, "Let's look at number two on the list. Vitamin D. That level is 74. Is

> **2.** Vitamin D level of 74 is suboptimal. Optimal levels are 90-120. He could take up to at least 10,000 IU x 7 days, then 5,000 IU daily.

that right? So, that's kind of low. Can we get that bumped up? Dr. Liar nodded, "Sure." She pointed out, "I have the recommendations on here. Is that something that you can do?" He nodded, "Yes."

Dr. Mei stepped in and said, "Get those International units up to 5000 IU." Surprisingly, Dr. Liar said that would be okay.

> **3.** Ivermectin: Here are links from the NIH themselves regarding ivermectin | COVID-19
> - Ivermectin exerts anti-inflammatory effect (nih.gov) - https://pubmed.ncbi.nlm.nih.gov/19453757
> - Ivermectin inhibits LPS-induced production of inflammatory cytokines and improves LPS-induced survival in mice - PubMed (nih.gov) - https://pubmed.ncbi.nlm.nih.gov/19109745
> - Ivermectin may be a clinically useful anti-inflammatory agent for late-stage COVID-19 | Open Heart (bmj.com) - https://openheart.bmj.com/content/7/2/e001350

My patient advocate moved on with, "Number three. What's your stance on ivermectin with appropriate dosing?" Dr. Liar sternly said, "I will not give it!" The advocate said, "You will not give it at all?" He reiterated, "NO." She then asked, "Even if it's brought in from home." He again confirmed, "NO."

I wish she had pressed the issue harder, just like I wished she had pushed harder for TPN feeding. But instead, she followed the pattern she had suggested when I first spoke with her five days earlier, where she said she believed "gaining a little cooperation was preferable to no cooperation." But, of course, I wanted more than "a little cooperation" and would have preferred her to be less soft-spoken and polite while attempting to avoid offending the doctor.

She seemed to have forgotten that I was the client, not the doctor. I was the one who had been offended by <u>everyone</u> involved in the **mis**treatment of my husband from the day he arrived at the hospital. I desperately wanted to feel "the wind of change" in this meeting, yet with her kid-glove approach I feared we would make far less progress than I had hoped.

---

4. IV NAC (in stock in the hospital pharmacy as it is used to treat Tylenol overdoses). NAC has very high anti-inflammatory properties and works to raise glutathione which is depleted in Covid patients. If you won't give it via IV, I can get NAC at Whole Foods. Can dose 2400-3000mg.
- N-Acetylcysteine to Combat COVID-19: An Evidence Review (nih.gov) - https://www.ncbi.nlm.nih.gov/pmc/articles/PMC7649937

My advocate then quietly skipped to number four, saying, "Let's talk about NAC. Do you have that in stock at the hospital pharmacy?" Dr. Liar looked up toward the ceiling and said, "Uh, I could check. Hmm . . ." Ms. Destroyer again came to the rescue with, "We can ask." Dr. Liar then agreed that NAC could be given. To confirm, she asked, "So, that might be a possibility?" Dr. Liar nodded, "Sure." Feeling she had gotten a solid win, she said, "Okay. Okay."

---

5. IV Glutathione (can get from a pharmacy and I can bring in). If you say no to IV you can give Glutathione down his tube. Liquid form at Whole Foods. Liposomal Glutathione by Quicksilver or Pure Encapsulations or ACN brand. Dose 15-18mg/kg in divided dose twice daily.
- Endogenous Deficiency of Glutathione as the Most Likely Cause of Serious Manifestations and Death in COVID-19 Patients | ACS Infectious Diseases - https://pubs.acs.org/doi/10.1021/acsinfecdis.0c00288
- Here's How Glutathione Fights Severe Inflammation Triggered By COVID-19 (onlymyhealth.com) - https://www.onlymyhealth.com/here-s-how-glutathione-fights-severe-inflammation-triggered-by-covid-19-1619606265
- Why Do We Need Liposomal Glutathione? - Researched Nutritionals - https://www.researchednutritionals.com/why-do-we-need-liposomal-glutathione

---

She hurried on to number five. "Glutathione?" Dr. Liar said, "If the pharmacy has it. Plus, if you're giving NAC and glutathione, then the NAC will replace glutathione. That's how it works. So, the N-Acetyl-L-Cysteine [NAC] will replace the glutathione levels. That's how it works. You don't need to give glutathione on top of that, and that's how you do it for Tylenol overdoses. Tylenol overdoses deplete glutathione. NAC replaces that. So you don't need to get glutathione on top of that."

My advocate's partner on the phone piped up and said, "There is some literature that supports getting both N-Acetyl-L-Cysteine <u>and</u> glutathione." Dr. Liar had to admit he was not familiar with those studies. My advocate pointed him to our sheet that listed some of them.

Dr. Liar briefly looked down at the paper and responded, "There may be studies and so forth, but that doesn't mean they're **standard of care** from the way **we** do things." My advocate snapped back, "That's true. But we also have to ask the question, will it do harm, right?" She gently pressed in again, "And these, NAC and glutathione, I want both." Dr. Liar responded, "NAC? I'd have to double-check [with the pharmacy]. Probably not. They do have glutathione."

She hammered back, "All right. If they don't have it, would you still approve it? I have a pharmacy nearby that stocks IV therapy." He advised, "They're not going to accept that at the hospital." She disagreed, saying, "They would." He firmly responded, "The hospital will absolutely NOT do that!" Surprised, she asked, "They won't?" The advocate on the phone noted, "They can do it in Dallas." Dr. Liar said, "Potentially something taken internally; they may agree with that, but not the IV."

Dr. Mei offered, "It's available in liquid form. So you could get it." Dr. Liar agreed to look into it. So my advocate said, "Just look into it and see what you think. We want to make sure we're on the same page. But the NAC would be good <u>with</u> glutathione." Dr. Liar replied, "NAC probably would not be quite at the levels that you're asking for here," as he glanced at the paper. We were startled that he was implying he might consider both NAC and glutathione. My advocate said, "So you think you can?"

He replied, "Usually it is given in, like, 600 milligrams, usually two or three times a day. Normally I give it by mouth, and I know they can probably have it by IV." The advocate on the phone piped in, "1200 milligrams twice a day" He said, "I'd have to look. Okay, I'll try. You know, the dosing sometimes is not an absolute, at least in a setting like this."

My advocate added, "What's important here is the inflammatory state, right? It's important here, so we want to try, and if it doesn't work, it doesn't work. Right?" Dr. Liar said, "I can't guarantee IV versus oral, but I'll see."

---

6. Zinc 220 mg daily.

She continued, "So, let's look at number six, zinc. Are you good with that?" Dr. Liar said, "Yeah." Wow, another small victory.

---

7. Melatonin 6-10 mg twice daily.
- Cleveland Clinic researchers identify melatonin as possible COVID-19 treatment - https://www.eurekalert.org/news-releases/918301
- Melatonin as a potential adjuvant treatment - PubMed (nih.gov) - https://pubmed.ncbi.nlm.nih.gov/32217117
- Melatonin and inflammation—Story of a double-edged blade - https://pubmed.ncbi.nlm.nih.gov/30242884

My advocate said, "Number seven. The melatonin 610 milligrams, twice daily?" Dr. Liar said, "I would not recommend twice daily, and the only reason I say that you're gonna really mess up the circadian rhythm. It's meant to reset your circadian rhythms." The advocate on the phone added, "The study from the Cleveland Clinic says giving a high dose actually works the opposite of a sedative. If you want to look into it, it's actually really interesting."

Dr. Liar said, "Yeah. And then, I mean, again, it has to do with his sleep cycles." She replied, "Yes, but there are studies to support twice a day, right? And it's from a very reputable source, you know, the Cleveland Clinic. So we're not just pulling that from out of the air." Dr. Liar said, "I Understand. I understand. There's probably some basis for everything you're asking. I get it. But that doesn't always make it the right thing to do all the time."

---

8. Positive fungal cultures in the blood. Treatment with Mycamine (micafungin) 100mg daily like they are. If sputum with fungi, I'm requesting 1/2 strength hydrogen peroxide saline nebulizer.

My advocate then moved on to number eight, saying, "Number eight, the positive fungal cultures. Where are we at with doing them again?" He said, "When you have positive fungal cultures, we treat it for a defined period of time. I'll defer to Dr. Torture, the Infectious Disease doctor. It would be up to her whether she wants to recheck it."

Dr. Mei interrupted, "What symptoms were there that <u>required</u> medication?" Dr. Liar responded, "Fever." Dr. Mei countered, "There are many causes for fever." He replied, "I understand, but also. . . ." She interrupted with, "What are the signs of infection? I would like to know if this patient was on any <u>medications</u> that might have caused his fever. And I'm trying to figure out the time of the culture draws and the time of the positive culture. In the interim, did he deteriorate without antifungals?" Dr. Liar noted, "He had fever, and he had elevated white count. He had **a** positive fungal culture."

Dr. Mei pointed out that only one blood culture of four came back positive, and the others did not. He said, "I understand." She pointed out, "**I would have expected two out of two cultures to be positive before treating and compromising his immune system any further**. Someone was not being careful to draw the blood culture, which was drawn through a line; you've got to think it can be contaminated. *Treating somebody with drugs, multiple drugs, can be very serious. Insulting his liver can be life-threatening. You MUST have two blood cultures prove a positive before treatment.*"

On the defensive, Dr. Liar said, "So let me put this in the opposite's perspective here. Let's say it **is** real, the infection, which it can be, and you can't say it's not. So, let's say the infection **is** real. He's also on immunosuppressive agents [referring to SOLU-MEDROL, the high-powered corticosteroid, and baricitinib, a high-powered anti-inflammatory], **and it can become a major infection if I don't address it**. You are welcome to talk to the Infectious Disease doctor about it." Once again, Dr. Liar passed the responsibility off to someone else, Dr. Torture, the Infectious Disease doctor.

Dr. Mei then made the point that it would not make sense to place an immunosuppressed patient on an antifungal BEFORE the cultures came back and BEFORE you have both cultures of two (not just one of two) come back positive, saying, "**You wouldn't risk that, because he could become very severely septic**."

Dr. Liar admitted to Dr. Mei, "**It's not actually standard of care to put someone on an antifungal who's immunosuppressed**." He went on to say, "We do that from the cultures. If they come back positive, then we treat it. We don't empirically treat someone with antifungals straight off."

TakanoriYamamoto, & YoshiharuSato. (2022, February 9). Risk assessment of micafungin-induced liver injury using spontaneous reporting system data and Electronic Medical Records. Journal of Infection and Chemotherapy. From https://www.sciencedirect.com/science/article/abs/pii/S1341321X2200040X

Typically, blood culture orders involve collecting two sets of cultures with two bottles per set (4 bottles total). Each set must be drawn from a different site and consist of one anaerobic and one aerobic bottle. Having a positive set of cultures (two positive bottles from <u>the same blood draw</u>) does not meet the separate occasion requirement for common commensal organisms (such as Candida, which they were treating Rob for with micafungin). At least one bottle <u>from each set</u>, collected from different sites or from the same site but after performing 2 site decontamination steps, would have to be positive to meet the "separate occasion" requirement.

*Therefore, a systemic antifungal should only be added to the mix **if absolutely necessary**--and unless you have drawn <u>a minimum of two blood cultures from two separate sites</u>, both of which come back positive, you do not have a genuinely positive result. If only one blood culture comes back positive, it is standard practice to consider that the positive culture was contaminated at the site.*

Lastly, Dr. Liar said, "If **they** come back positive, then we treat it," yet "**they**" **did not** come back positive. Only <u>one</u> of the two cultures had come back positive.

*What upset Sheila and her team was that Dr. Torture, backed up by Dr. Liar, had "jumped the gun" by starting Rob on **micafungin** without doing a second set of blood culture tests to verify the single positive was not due to local site contamination. Thus, they willingly exposed Rob to additional harm by giving him one more high-risk medication on top of the massive number of pharmaceuticals he was already on.*

As we stated previously, Rob was, unfortunately, a victim of "drugs chasing drugs," in which doctors piled on one medication after another to undo the damage caused by previously administered pharmaceuticals.

My advocate intervened, "Let's see where we are with this. Do we relook at doing some of the cultures, or what is the course of action from here?" I protested. "I do not like where this conversation is heading. I don't want him to be on this medication for two weeks. I don't want that because he's not used to any drugs. He's been on a ton of antibiotics already. I am trying to preserve his liver."

Dr. Liar quipped, "I will defer to Dr. Torture on that, but I can tell you that she's gonna say he needs to be treated because if I left it untreated, that could be serious, and fungemia is a serious problem. I've seen people die very quickly from it if it was left untreated."

Dr. Mei spoke up. "Here's the question. Where was the source? Was it from a line?" He said, "Potentially, yeah, I changed the line." She asked, "Well, which was it? Okay, you changed the line. Did you culture that midline and see if the fungus came from there? Let's say he had vegetation on his heart. You would want to do an ultrasound and see vegetation. So, it's really important to know the source because you have to get rid of it because, you know yourself, if you have an abscess and you cannot penetrate it, you've got to go in and get that abscess out. So, where is this? You say it's a line? So, did you grow the culture from there? If so, and it's not growing, then it wasn't there."

Realizing he was about to be tackled, Dr. Liar passed the ball again, saying, "I'll let you talk to Dr. Torture about it." Afraid things were becoming too confrontational, my advocate asked Dr. Liar to respond to number nine on our list.

---

9. Continuous VELETRI? Does he have pulmonary hypertension or emphysema type pulmonary edema? VELETRI is contraindicated in pulmonary edema.

Dr. Liar said, "Clinically, we give VELETRI because it allows us to reduce the oxygen that we need to give him **because oxygen at high levels can become toxic for the patient.** So, the VELETRI, what it does is it's a prostaglandin, and it dilates the blood vessels in the area allowing the alveoli to be aerated, okay? So that allows us to reduce the amount of oxygen and where he needs it. That's the purpose."

The advocate on the phone asked, "Is that helping him?" He quickly replied, "Yeah, if I stopped it, I'd have to increase the oxygen I'm giving him, and if I did that, **I would put his lungs at risk of getting oxygen toxicity over time. You know, the longer I have him on a higher level above 60%, there's the chance of oxygen toxicity and fibrosis? And fortunately, we've not required him to be up all the way, like, 100%.** At 100%, that definitely will happen much faster, where he's been between 60 and 75% lately. And you can tolerate that for probably just a few weeks, actually, without getting too toxic."

> **LEGAL COUNSEL STATEMENT**
>
> Members of the jury, as you can see in the chart at the bottom of Page C-54 in Appendix C, this day, as Dr. Liar noted, they had finally dropped the ventilator's oxygen concentration level (FiO2) down to 50 to 60%. However, you will also see that for each of the 19 days prior to September 27th, *Rob's lungs were continually subjected to oxygen levels **well above 60%**.*
>
> Once again, as he often did, Dr. Liar lied when he said, "And fortunately, we've not required him to be up all the way like 100%." The chart at the bottom of Page C-54 shows that the oxygen concentration setting on the ventilator **had been up to 100% on six prior days** and was then set to between 65% to 80%, with additional bursts up to 100% that are not shown on the chart due to their not being logged because the oxygen levels were logged in the record only at specific intervals.
>
> *Two days earlier, Dr. Liar had told Sheila that "oxygen is toxic over time, although at least up to 60% or less, it's not toxic. **60% or above, it is toxic!**" Thus, he knew Rob's lungs were being irreparably damaged by the continually high (over 60%) concentrations of oxygen. Sadly, the Medical Examiner who conducted Rob's private autopsy confirmed this by saying his lungs looked "shredded" and did not even look human.*

Unfortunately, my advocate let that one whiz by as if it were a non-issue and jumped right into number ten on our list.

> **10.** Needs follow up chest X-ray since last one was 9/19/2021.

She asked, "Okay. When was his last chest X-ray?" Having come unprepared and assuming the last X-ray had been done recently, he smugly asserted, "Couple of days ago?" She retorted, "Okay. I think the last one we saw was taken eight days ago, on September 19th."

Scanning his memory, he said, "I did one on the 23rd, I believe?" She replied, "The 23rd. Okay, was it worse? What's your opinion?" He said, "It's about the same, and the X-ray is a lagging indicator. So, I generally get an X-ray in the setting of . . . if something's worse."

To wrap up our discussion, we wanted to discuss the alternative therapies we believed could help Rob recover.

> **11.** Alternative therapies.
> - Budesonide – RT said it may not be reaching Rob's lungs due to the continuous flow of nebulized VELETRI
> - Surfactant - could help improve oxygenation and reduce the risk of lung damage

Regarding **budesonide**, I said, "I spoke with the respiratory therapist, and she told me that she believes he's really not getting much of it because of the continuous administration of nebulized VELETRI. So, he may not be getting any of that into his lungs because of the Veletri." Dr. Liar disagreed and brushed it off. "He's getting it daily."

I continued, "He's getting it daily . . . but that doesn't mean he's absorbing it and getting any benefit from it. The respiratory therapist said she felt the VELETRI was hindering him from getting budesonide into his lungs. Because I agree with you that budesonide is a very important part of the recovery process, I want something done about it. If it's not true, I don't know why the respiratory therapist would explain it this way. But anyway, it seems like Rob is not getting much of it into his lungs."

Dr. Liar responded that he would keep everything the same regarding the budesonide administration, which was **one small dose per day**, as opposed to the VELETRI, which was continuous. He then went on, "And he's getting steroids. So, quite honestly, that makes the budesonide not as necessary, right?" Once again, the doctor was downplaying the benefits of budesonide, which have been clearly documented. Speaking of at least continuing the budesonide, my advocate said, "Well, it's not going to do harm to do it."

Next, Dr. Mei weighed in on the **surfactant**. "So I'll ask, have you ever considered surfactant?" He immediately shut her down on this one. He said, "We don't have surfactant. We don't use it on adults." She disagreed with him, "They've used it in adults. Yes." Without hesitation, he was happy to declare, "Yeah, but I can't get it!" She insisted, "They've used it in COVID-19, and with success!" He responded, "I understand. I can't get it. That's what I'm trying to say." She asked, "Well, if I get it for you, would you be willing to do it? You'll see that it works!"

He then passed the buck to the hospital pharmacy, saying, "It's up to the pharmacy." Dr. Mei asked, "If you cannot get it from your pharmacy, and I can get it for you, will you use it?" However, he totally skirted her question by refusing to answer it. So my advocate said, "Here is the question concerning the surfactant. Ask the pharmacy what their policy is. If we don't ask and don't pursue it, we will NEVER really know the difference it could make."

Dr. Liar responded, "So the drug guy was going to try to get a new clinical trial drug called aviptadil. That would be the only way. It's a study drug that actually increases surfactant. That has better proof than what you're suggesting." Dr. Mei tried to get him back on course with, "It sounds like that drug is unreliable and untested. It's too premature to say if it is successful. The surfactant has plenty of clinical trials and reports. You can see all these reports of success." Dr. Liar's responded, "Sure. Those are anecdotal reports."

Dr. Mei snapped back, "No, these are not anecdotal! These are studies!" A battle was now raging between a doctor who wanted to save my husband and one who wanted to strictly follow his preferred protocol, which I had begun to see was a <u>failed</u> protocol that was not helping my husband improve. Stumbling over his words, he said, "Well, studies of . . . are . . . they . . . are they blinded studies?" Dr. Mei said, "They are! Well, I haven't read about them all." He took advantage of her hesitation and insisted, "They need to be looked at in more detail."

LEGAL COUNSEL STATEMENT

Members of the jury, four days earlier, when Sheila asked Dr. Liar about using a **surfactant** (a mixture of lipids and proteins delivered directly into the endotracheal tube) to coat the alveoli that could help improve oxygenation and reduce the risk of lung damage), his reasoning for refusing to do so was "because it hasn't been well studied, and it's going to cause problems." He also said, "we don't give surfactant in adults; we haven't ever done that around here ever, for anything, even with COVID."

Dr. Liar may not have read the following reports (and there are many more). Both are from February 2021 and were readily available before Rob's admission on September 3, 2021.

- **Pulmonary surfactant as a versatile biomaterial to fight COVID-19**
  "This so-called 'surfactant replacement therapy' (SRT) is currently the standard-of-care to reduce mortality in premature infants with surfactant-deficient lungs, and the clinical success of SRT in Newborn Respiratory Distress Syndrome (NRDS) has rationalized attempts to broaden the therapeutic application of clinical surfactants to other lung diseases like ARDS. One of the common results of a COVID-19 infection is impairment of surfactant production and secretion. **Therefore, surfactant treatment to anticipate on the progression of severe lung injury in COVID-19 patients has been proposed as a potential treatment for COVID-19.**"
  Herman, L., De Smedt, S. C., & Raemdonck, K. (2022, February). Pulmonary surfactant as a versatile biomaterial to fight COVID-19. Journal of controlled release : official journal of the Controlled Release Society. From https://www.ncbi.nlm.nih.gov/pmc/articles/PMC8605818"

- **Use of exogenous pulmonary surfactant in acute respiratory distress syndrome (ARDS): Role in SARS-CoV-2-related lung injury**
  "By infecting type II alveolar cells, COVID-19 interferes with the production and secretion of the pulmonary surfactant and therefore causes an increase in surface tension, which in turn can lead to alveolar collapse. . . . **Because of the robust anti-inflammatory and lung protective efficacy and the current urgent need for lung-supportive therapy, the exogenous pulmonary surfactant could be a valid supportive treatment of COVID-19 pneumonia patients in intensive care units in addition to the current standard of ARDS treatment.**"
  Cattel F;Giordano S;Bertiond C;Lupia T;Corcione S;Scaldaferri M;Angelone L;De Rosa FG; (n.d.). Use of exogenous pulmonary surfactant in acute respiratory distress syndrome (ARDS): Role in SARS-cov-2-related lung injury. Respiratory physiology & neurobiology. From https://pubmed.ncbi.nlm.nih.gov/33657448

Unfortunately, instead of agreeing to try a natural surfactant, Dr. Liar preferred to consider one more "clinical trial" drug. Sheila was not at all pleased that he was refusing to listen to sound reasoning from a fellow physician—and once again, Dr. Liar made it clear he was in charge of Rob's plan of care, and he had no intention of changing it.

Later in the meeting, as you will see below, Dr. Liar learned that the pharmacy **would not** *allow aviptadil, the clinical trial drug, to be administered. Thus, due to Dr. Liar's refusal to use a natural surfactant, no ground was gained here.*

Referring to the new trial drug, aviptadil, that Dr. Liar was anxious to add to Rob's regimen, my advocate asked, "And that helps with the surfactant?" Excited at the prospect of potentially trying another untested clinical trial drug on Rob as if he were part of a grand experiment, Dr. Liar answered, "It helps increase surfactant." Then she asked, "Have you been using that in others?" He apparently had not, so he sheepishly replied, "It has been used and studied at different hospitals. Now they have what's called the "Right to Try." So you could potentially be on the hook for paying for it."

Giving in once again and wanting to keep the peace, my advocate said, "Yeah, I think that'll be just fine. I think this is good."

My advocate's partner on the phone asked, "What are the next steps for Rob? What does that look like? Because I don't really prefer him to be intubated this long, and I don't prefer trachs as well. But we've got to do something to start reducing the sedation here!" Dr. Liar responded, "So, the issue is, you know, he's still on the RotoProne bed. I can't trach him in that setting because we don't prone people with trachs. The other issue is I need his FiO2 and his oxygen much lower." Unfortunately, by placing Rob in the RotoProne bed, Dr. Liar postponed any progress until Rob was extracted from the device and put back in a regular bed.

My patient advocate asked, "When would you consider a trach then?" He said, "PEEP ideally 8 and FiO2 down to less than 50%." She tilted her head, shook it in disbelief, and said, "That's your kind of standard?" He continued, "Without the VELETRI . . . I mean, those are all things that I understand. I know the risks from having a trach tube in for a long time. But sometimes . . ." My advocate interrupted and said, "Of course, we want to do it safely. But I want to start thinking about how and what our goals are." I was happy to see her pressing in on their having a Discharge Plan for Rob.

Dr. Liar continued, "I mean, he's going to need a trach ultimately to just get him off the ventilator." He then flippantly said, "He's not just gonna come right off."

Since the RotoProne bed had become a limiting factor, the advocate on the phone asked when Rob would be taken out of the RotoProne bed. Dr. Liar said, "Well, for now, I'm gonna leave him in the RotoProne bed. He's still in the bed, okay? And if he doesn't drop his oxygen saturation, meaning his blood oxygen level, and if I don't have to go up on his FiO2 [oxygen concentration], then I may take him out of the bed at that point. He's down to about 55% FiO2 right now."

Because I had been closely monitoring his FiO2 (oxygen concentration) levels and had the records in front of me, I said, "No, his FiO2 went down to 50% today." In response, Dr. "Know It All" said, "Okay, so it went down. So?" My advocate looked at me, then back to the doctor, and said, "But his PEEP is still high!" Dr. Liar chimed in, "Yeah, the PEEP will be something I also need to reduce. I want to lower the VELETRI first and then start to lower the PEEP. That's kind of how I balance that."

I was greatly disturbed to have not been informed of the benefits, risks, and limitations of Rob's being placed in a RotoProne bed, to have not been advised that he would be trapped on the ventilator until he was extracted from the bed, and to have not been asked for my approval. Instead, as was true of every course of action or drug administered, I was viewed as a troublesome and sometimes noisy spectator of the game the doctors were playing with my husband's life.

"Give me one second," Dr. Liar said. Then, he and the Social Worker stepped out of the room momentarily. When they returned, he said, "So, that was that. About what I just told you on the trial drug [aviptadil], the pharmacy **won't allow it** right now. They're looking into the policy for it."

Hearing that and realizing we had exhausted our list of discussion items, my advocate decided to confirm the few gains we had made. "So, nutrition. You're good with vitamin D, IV vitamin C, which I think will be way better than oral, IV NAC, and glutathione—and you're going to look it all over with the pharmacy, right? Dr. Liar reluctantly said, "Sure."

She went on, "And then zinc. You're good with it?" He replied, "Yeah." She then added, "The melatonin . . . at least at night?" Again, he said, "Yeah." "And then you're going to continue to use the VELETRI. Any other concerns?"

Dr. Liar responded, "No. I mean, he's doing better. I mean, just slow, gradual improvement over the last few days. I'm having these setbacks. And you know, even, you know, the yeast. That I don't consider a major setback. That's why I think we just need to treat it. The only thing I'm going to try and do is, like I said, try to keep him supine. If he tolerates that, potentially, we can get him out of the rotation . . . the RotoProne bed. Tomorrow, we'll see what that looks like.

"So, when they put him in a supine position today, which is, I believe is at the end of the day, assuming he tolerates that, meaning I don't have to go up on his oxygen, then I would leave him that way overnight in the bed and see how he does. And if he stays okay, then I'll try to do that again tomorrow. It's kind of a test. I don't want to just take him out of the bed right away."

At that, the meeting abruptly ended. Dr. Liar stood up and retreated from the room. My team and I gathered our belongings and followed Ms. Destroyer out of the room. Although we had not achieved all we had hoped for, at least we had made a little progress. What made no sense to my team and me was that with Rob being gravely ill and not making any progress, the doctors still resisted commonsense suggestions of therapeutic options that had been successfully used by other doctors—therapies that could significantly aid in Rob's recovery. Now the best we could hope for was that what minor concessions had been granted would be promptly implemented and that Rob would soon begin to recover as a result.

After everyone had departed, I headed to Rob's room. There, I encountered his nurse for the day. When I asked her for an update on his condition, she said, "His oxygen was at 92-93%, and his FiO2 was at 50. **This might have been a good day to begin weaning him.**" When I expressed my excitement about the prospect of an attempt to wean Rob from the ventilator, she noted, "His blood oxygen saturations were that high because he was prone in the RotoProne bed."

Then, without another word, she hung more drug-filled bags of IV medication. Within a few moments, Rob's blood oxygen level plunged to 89%. Just when I was excited to think he might be improving, an assault by more toxic pharmaceuticals caused his blood oxygen level to plummet. As I believed all along, I appeared to be witnessing firsthand how the barrage of medications further weakened him and sabotaged his chances of survival.

Later that afternoon, before I headed home, my friends Roberta and Allen drove Dr. Mei to the airport so she could catch a flight back to California. She desperately wanted to stay longer to assist me, yet she had to fly back home to aid an ailing family member.

I rushed to the hospital in the morning, hoping Dr. Liar had ordered the supplements he had approved the day before during our rather uncomfortable semi-productive intervention meeting.

Upon my arrival, I was surprised and delighted to learn that Rob was about to be removed from the RotoProne bed. After a ten-day sentence, he would finally be free, and they could no longer use the RotoProne bed as an excuse not to wean him from the ventilator. I was confident our intervention meeting was primarily responsible for this positive development.

I was instructed to wait outside the room for thirty minutes while they extracted him from the RotoProne and transferred him to a regular bed. Four nurses were needed to complete the procedure. I whispered a prayer, "Please, Father, keep Rob calm."

When Rob had been on the ventilator for five days, Dr. Wicked told me that a healthy man in his 50s could last "probably 10 to 14 days and still have enough reserve" to be weaned from the ventilator. He also said, "So, he may not, you know, **he may not have enough reserve in two weeks**." Rob had now been on a ventilator for 20 days, and the protein and albumin levels we presented to Dr. Liar the day before indicated he was still "nutritionally deficient." So how could Rob be expected to have the "reserves," the physical strength required, to breathe on his own at this point?

> **LEGAL COUNSEL STATEMENT**
> Members of the jury, as early as September 7, 2021, four days after Rob's admission, the dietitian noted that Rob had "not been ordering 3 meals daily." You can see her note on Page 104 of the hospital records (see Page C-27 in Appendix C).
>
> During the intervention meeting, Dr. Liar denied that Rob was being malnourished. However, below is a snapshot from an entry made that same day in Rob's hospital records where they admit, "*Suspect malnutrition given current data.*"
>
> | Diagnosis |
> | --- |
> | Nutrition Dx: Inadequate oral intake related to intubation as evidenced by inability to meet estimated needs PO, enteral nutrition required. |
> | *Suspect malnutrition given current data- reassess at follow up |
>
> *At Covid Coven Hospital of Plano, Texas, their mode of operation was to document, deny, and then ignore significant issues. Yet somehow, this is supposed to be called "health care." Instead, we would term it "negligent care."*

After thirty minutes, I was advised that I could reenter the room. I found Rob on his back in a conventional hospital bed. Because he had been placed in the RotoProne bed the evening of September 18th, ten days after being placed on a ventilator—and the first time I had seen Rob after his admission was on September 20th when I was granted a brief, 20-minute visit at the insistence of Rob's police officer friend who drove up that day from Austin to advocate for me— I had not seen him outside of the RotoProne apparatus. I so desired to embrace and kiss him, but his body was covered with tubes and wires.

As Nurse Jitters brushed past me on her way out of the room, I inquired about Rob's weight in the loss after seeing the weights that had been recorded from the RotoProne bed. Finally, with an "oops!" expression, she said, "Well, the weight on the bed is probably going to be incorrect."

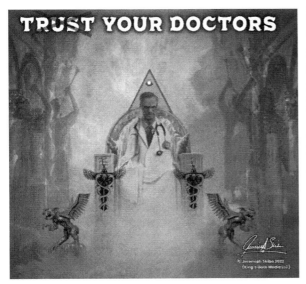

I asked, "What do you mean?" She said, "It doesn't really matter . . . but we forgot to zero out the weight on the bed." Because she had not zeroed out the bed, as one would any scale before placing an object on it, she felt the displayed weight would likely be inaccurate.

I was aghast at such a blunder in an Intensive Care Unit where my husband was in critical condition because an accurate weight was essential for determining his nutritional needs and the dosages of a number of his numerous medications. I exclaimed, "Oh my goodness, you didn't reset it to zero!" She smiled, "Well, we realized that after the fact. Then it was too late."

I asked if she could transfer the earlier weight from the RotoProne bed to the new bed. It was then that she advised me that the weight from the RotoProne bed could not be trusted either. Seeing I was visibly concerned, she said, "By the time we had him in the new bed, it was too late. We were more concerned with his airway. Yeah, I mean, you can't do anything. So that was our fault. And I apologize for that."

After she left, I took a photo of the screen on the bed scale, which displayed the weight of **the previous patient** and indicated that the bed had last been reset on September 3rd, when the earlier patient had been placed in it. I could also see the easy-to-press "**Zero Scale**" button, which she had neglected to press before transferring Rob from the RotoProne bed. I questioned how she, and the other three nurses moving Rob, could miss such a simple yet critical step.

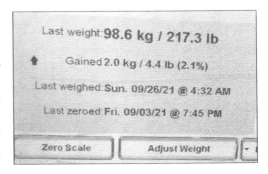

I thought, "This is completely unacceptable. What if someone makes a mistake and overdoses him on certain medications because they incorrectly estimate his weight?" Knowing Rob was in the hands of such lackadaisical hospital staff was frightening. So I requested that she document in his hospital records that **they had NOT zeroed out the bed, and thus may not know his actual weight**.

LEGAL COUNSEL STATEMENT
Members of the jury, you can see from the snapshot below that they did record in the hospital records, as Sheila requested, that they had failed to zero out the bed weight before placing Rob in it.

Progress Notes
9/29/21: 82.3 kg (181lb 7 oz) bed not zeroed
9/28/21: 80 kg (176 lb 5.9 oz) bed scale

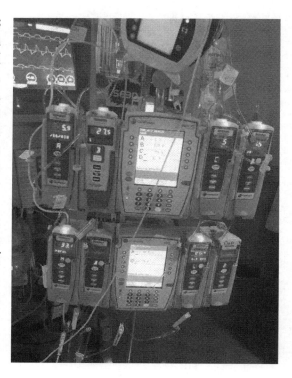

After the nurse left the room, I walked over to Rob's bedside. With love and compassion, I whispered, "You look good. You can overcome this. You're strong." I wished it were true, but he had clearly been neglected. As I touched his hand and gently brushed his matted, sticky, and clumpy hair off his brow, I could see his beard was still crusty and unkempt, and it appeared to have been glued together with plaster. He was sweating profusely, and his eyelids were oily from the protective eye salve they had smeared on them.

I sat down in dismay after wiping away the tears that welled up in my eyes at seeing him in such a deplorable state. As I listened to the constant drone of the machines and IV infusion pumps Rob was hooked up to, time flew by like water in a river. I kept an eye on the monitors, watching his heart rate, pulse rate, temperature, blood oxygen level, and blood pressure. Despite his deplorable appearance, he seemed to be holding his own, and no alarms were going off.

But then something disturbing happened. The ventilator developed an unexpected issue, and its alarm began to sound. It was so loud that it reminded me of a tornado siren in Texas. Yet, surprisingly, no one was at the nurse's station just outside Rob's ICU door. I pressed the call button several times, yet no one came to our aid.

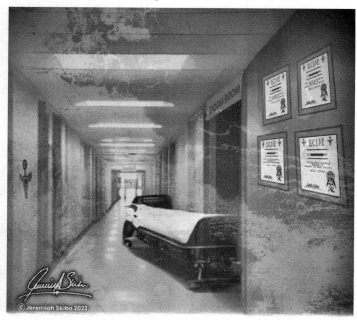

I dashed into the corridor, but no one was there. I yelled, but no one came. I rushed back into Rob's room, relieved to see his chest rising and falling in response to the sounds of the ventilator.

On the ventilator screen, the message "CIRCUIT OCCLUSION" appeared. A quick Internet search on my phone revealed that it was "*a high priority audible/visual alarm*" that sounded when the measured PEEP was higher than the PEEP set on the machine or when "*the inspiratory or expiratory limb of the patient circuit becomes sufficiently occluded to trigger the alarm.*" I had no idea what all that meant, yet Rob's vitals

Finally, Nurse Jitters entered the room, pressed a button to silence the alarm, and informed me that it was a temporary malfunction in the machine and not to worry. After checking the other equipment and reviewing Rob's vitals, she said everything was okay. Everything might have seemed fine to her. However, the blaring alarm and the fact that no one was nearby to aid me left me shaken and disturbed.

Another nurse sped past me and began replacing several of Rob's IV bags with a new round of high-powered sedatives, paralytics, and opiates. Retrieving my trusty notepad, I logged each one. I then asked her about the status of the intravenous vitamin C that Dr. Liar had agreed to order. She responded, "It has not yet arrived." I asked her to please notify me when they started administering it so I would know it had arrived.

After the nurses had left, I reapplied peppermint oil to my skin in the hope that, despite being unconscious, Rob would be able to detect it and recognize my presence. Then I gently massaged one of his dry hands with a small amount of coconut oil I had brought.

To my surprise, the dietitian I had never met walked into the room. Although I was pleased to see her, I doubt she was happy to see me because I had left her several messages, yet she had avoided returning my calls. I asked how she knew Rob's nutritional needs if she was unsure of his weight. Giving me a sideways glance, she responded, "We do daily weights." I explained that Nurse Jitters had just told me that the weight from the RotoProne bed could not be relied upon, and she admitted she had neglected to zero out the new bed. Thus, its displayed weight was also inaccurate.

She replied, "Well, I actually do need to talk to Nurse Jitters about that. I agree that there was a weight discrepancy on the RotoProne bed." I told her that the earlier weights from the RotoProne bed had me extremely worried, even panicked, because it appeared from the weights shown in Rob's online MyChart records that he had lost more than fifty pounds since his admission.

She explained that what appeared to be a weight loss of over 50 pounds was simply because the RotoProne scale weights were completely inaccurate. For example, on September 17th, he weighed 172 pounds according to the scales on his bed. Yet, when he was transferred to the RotoProne bed on September 18th, the weight displayed on the RotoProne bed was 114 pounds. Thus, the inaccurate scale on the RotoProne bed was the reason it appeared that within 24 hours he had lost 58 pounds—which, of course, was impossible.

She then told me that the weight displayed on the RotoProne bed often varied by 10 to 20 pounds per day. However, now that he was back in a standard hospital bed which should have an accurate scale, even though the scale had not been reset to zero, they could estimate his weight to be approximately 80 kilograms, which is 176 pounds. That weight was comparable to the 172 pounds he weighed the day before he was placed in the RotoProne bed.

I wondered why no one had taken the time to inform me earlier of the problem with the scale on the RotoProne bed. Their neglecting to tell me about the scale problem had caused me and my team needless anxiety and distress. In addition, when we met with Dr. Liar during the intervention meeting the day before, he was either unaware of the problem with the RotoProne bed scale or did not care whether Rob may have lost over 50 pounds. Either way, his inattention to the issue and inability to explain the situation during our meeting greatly disturbed me.

When I asked her about TPN (Total Parenteral Nutrition), which, if administered, would allow Rob to receive extra nutrients and calories via an IV, she stated, "TPN parenteral nutrition is not recommended because his gut is functional, and we're doing tube feedings which right now is the best thing we can do for him, okay? TPN is our last line of defense. On top of that, it comes with concerns for anemia."

I did not want to do anything that would worsen Rob's anemia, which was bad enough already. I wanted them to address his anemia rather than ignore it, to help ensure that his blood could effectively deliver sufficient oxygen to each cell in his body. Even then, because Dr. Mei and my patient advocate had expressed significant concerns about Rob's anemia, I requested, "Please speak with my patient advocate about this. She worked as a nurse in a hospital, I don't have a medical background, and I don't fully understand why TPN would not help Rob." She replied, "I don't think I actually can talk to her."

When I told her I would greatly appreciate her doing so, she responded, "Yeah, well, let me talk about the appropriate protocol for coordination, okay? Your patient advocate doesn't have direct care of the patient. I can talk to her, but the thing is, I definitely think the two of us talking is more important for your understanding." Her cold response disappointed me because it would have increased my trust in her if she had been willing to explain her position to my patient advocate, who I knew had the background and experience necessary to fully comprehend her point of view. Sadly, she refused to speak with my advocate.

LEGAL COUNSEL STATEMENT

Members of the jury, it is unfortunate that the dietitian was unwilling to take a few minutes to explain her position to Sheila's patient advocate. If she had done so and the advocate had agreed, Sheila would have felt confident that at least **some** of Rob's care was being handled properly.

Anyone at the Covid Coven Hospital in Plano, Texas, who was confident they were providing the best care possible should have been happy to explain how their approach to Rob's care met or exceeded the standard of care. Confident and competent practitioners take pride in their work and are delighted to explain how they exceed expectations. However, at Covid Coven Hospital of Plano, Texas, no one appreciated their approach or "plan of care" for Rob—or worse yet, "the protocol"—being questioned.

After meeting with Sheila, the dietitian wrote the following in the hospital record: "There are no changes to the nutrition plan of care at this time. RD [Registered Dietitian] encouraged the need for the wife to build trust and confidence amongst the care team members." We have to ask the question: How was Sheila supposed to "*build trust and confidence*" in a team that had:

- Ushered her out of the facility when she dropped Rob off at the Emergency Department
- Locked her out for 21 days due to an unwritten isolating policy
- Ignored that Rob was not receiving adequate food and water (causing him to text "No food")
- Gave Rob a total of 6 doses of remdesivir (2 were double doses) against her and Rob's will
- Administered a massive number of harmful medications that only worsened Rob's condition
- Gave Rob excessively high levels of inspired oxygen, causing atelectasis (collapsed alveoli)
- Removed Rob's DNI (Do Not Intubate) order without advising her they were doing so
- Placed Rob on a contraindicated BiPAP that caused barotrauma, severely injuring Rob's lungs
- Called Sheila to inform her that they had decided to put Rob on a ventilator
- Placed Rob in a RotoProne bed without advising Sheila it would extend his stay on the ventilator
- Failed to attempt to address Rob's profound anemia

> *The team in charge of Rob's care did nothing to reassure Sheila that they were doing anything other than forcing "the protocol" on him. Trust must be earned. Like a mirror, trust can be broken. Everything appears warped and distorted once it is damaged.*

She then asked me, "Are you afraid that you don't understand, or are you concerned better options are being mentioned to you by your friends and family that you're not getting? If so, that's not the case here." I queried, "You said Pivot 1.5 was the best you could give him." She agreed, "This is the Cadillac because nutrition is. . . ." I interjected, "But the trend of his protein literally went like this," as I slanted my hand downwards towards the floor.

She replied while shaking her head, "So remember, okay, this is biochemistry, all right? I feel that you're concerned he is not getting the best of options. Let's start with that. HE IS! The nutrition he's getting is the Cadillac of nutrition. Cadillac, like the top. The nutrients and the composition are high quality." I answered, "Doctors and other medical professionals who are friends of mine who have looked at his online MyChart record have told me **he's malnourished**. So maybe when you were trained to do this, they told you, 'Tell them it's the Cadillac.' If it is, why has it NOT proven to be more helpful." She quipped, "The nutrients and the composition are quality, okay?"

I noted, "His protein and albumin levels are dipping way down, and if I didn't say anything, nothing would change." She countered, "Let's talk about his albumin, okay? If you go look it up on the Internet, it's going to say it's an indicator of malnutrition, all right? It is not an indicator, not a genuine one. There are multiple factors here, and I can print off a screening criteria to show you." I asked, "Please, please do. I want to understand."

She continued, "What you do need to see is that with albumin, it is affected by inflammation, and by the infection, and by critical illness, and by physical stress. Those protein labs dipping down are because of what his body has gone through, okay? It's because of the infection, not because of him not getting the nutrition, okay? He's getting his calories.

"All of our equations are talking about how we are getting his nutrition in and meeting what he needs while not affecting his respiratory rate, okay? So here's what's crazy. If you overfeed, or you overdo something, you can make it, you know, you can make it harder for him to breathe—and that's not what we want. We want a very healthy balance, okay? Now COVID itself is a beast. We're talking about making sure that they get off the vent. That is our ultimate goal, right?"

Of course, I wanted Rob "off the vent." The problem was that he ended up on a ventilator to begin with, as he knew it would be a death sentence. I replied, "Yes, I hope so because he's been here for 25 days now! It's ridiculous. I was fighting to get answers <u>at the beginning of this nightmare before he was intubated</u>. He wasn't eating, he was losing weight, and he was growing weaker. Everyone knew that, and it was documented in his hospital record. So I called everybody for help. I called the chaplain, the charge nurse, you, and the social worker, but no one called me back. I wanted to <u>prevent</u> Rob from being on a ventilator, and now you are all talking about getting him off the thing.

"Now he's lying in a medically induced coma, wasting away! Just look at him! All of you act like everything is hunky dory! You say, 'Hi. How's it going?' But NO ONE would talk with me <u>before</u> he was on a ventilator. I was locked out, so I could not be with and help feed my husband. But now everything is coming up roses, and everyone is doing all they can. Maybe I'm going off a bit, but I still don't feel he's getting the nutrients he needs. So, who orders his nutrients, you or the doctor?"

LEGAL COUNSEL STATEMENT

Members of the jury, Rob's low **RBC** (Red Blood Cell), **HGB** (hemoglobin), and **HCT** (hematocrit) numbers clearly indicated he **was** suffering from anemia. Below is a snapshot of his September 28, 2021, levels from Page 550 of Rob's hospital records.

LABS:
Collection Time: 09/28/21 3:59 AM

Result	Value
WBC	14.4 (H)
RBC	3.16 (L)
HGB	8.8 (L)
HCT	28.4 (L)

Normal levels for an adult male are:
- **RBC** (Red Blood Cell count) at 4.5 to 5.5 (million cells per microliter)—Rob's was 3.16
- **HGB** (Hemoglobin) at 14 to 18 g/dL (grams per deciliter)—Rob's was 8.8
- **HCT** (Hematocrit) 38 to 50 (percent)—Rob's was 28.4%

The Red Blood Cell count (**RBC**) measures the number of red blood cells in a blood sample. The hematocrit (**HCT**) test measures the percentage of red blood cells in a sample of blood. The hemoglobin (**HBG**) test measures the amount of hemoglobin in the red blood cells. Hemoglobin is the part of red blood cells that gives them their red color and carries oxygen molecules throughout the body.

Rob's low **RBC**, **HBG,** and **HCT** numbers clearly indicated anemia. When a patient has anemia, they suffer from a significant reduction in the oxygen-carrying capacity of the blood. As a result, oxygen delivery is decreased to the body's tissues and organs. Therefore, anemia is a severe condition that must be addressed in critically ill patients.

According to a National Library of Medicine abstract titled "Approach to an Anemic Critically Ill Patient," phlebotomy (the drawing of blood) "*is an under-recognized cause of anemia in the critically ill.*" Like most ICU patients, Rob was subjected to blood tests every day. The article also states, "*In the average adult ICU patient, approximately 40–70 mL of blood is collected each day for investigations and only a fraction of this collected blood is actually processed. The sicker patients might have even more blood collected. It must also be remembered that only approximately 12.5 mL of blood is regenerated each day and this is not enough to compensate for the blood lost.*"
Hegde, A. (2019, September). Approach to an anemic critically ill patient. Indian journal of critical care medicine : peer-reviewed, official publication of Indian Society of Critical Care Medicine. From https://www.ncbi.nlm.nih.gov/pmc/articles/PMC6785810

There are several options for addressing anemia in critically ill ICU patients. For example, the American Journal of Respiratory and Critical Care Medicine noted in an "Understanding Anemia in the ICU to Develop Future Treatment Strategies" article, "*Anemia is associated with adverse outcomes in critically ill patients, including increased mortality risk.*" Then went on to note that a novel way to increase hemoglobin is via **vitamin D**, stating, "*In mechanically ventilated critically ill adults, treatment with 500,000 IU vitamin D3 increased hemoglobin and acutely reduced serum hepcidin concentrations.*"
American Journal of Respiratory and Critical Care Medicine. (n.d.). From https://www.atsjournals.org/doi/full/10.1164/rccm.201805-0989ED

Below is a snapshot from Page 536 of Rob's hospital records showing he was on 5,000 IU of vitamin D3 twice daily, which is nowhere near the recommended 500,000 IU per day.

Current Facility-Administered Medications						
Medication	Dose	Route	Frequency	Provider	Last Rate	Last Admin
• cholecalciferol (Vitamin D3) capsule	5,000 Units	ORAL	TWICE DAILY	▮▮Liar▮▮ MD		5,000 Units at 09/28/21

Regrettably, nothing was done to address Rob's anemia. We contend that, whether by willful ignorance, uncaring negligence, or nefarious intent, the doctors' actions and inactions were the direct cause of Robert A. Skiba II's needless death.

The dietitian responded, "I help with the guidance of the doctor." She then received a call and said, "We have a team meeting at 10:00 AM. So, I'll have to hurry. Let's try and see if we can get some of this knocked out, okay?

"So, you're still concerned that he is not getting the best of options. Let's start with that. The nutrition he's getting IS the 'Cadillac' of nutrition. The nutrients and the composition are high quality. He is currently meeting his estimated needs with our nutrition regimen."

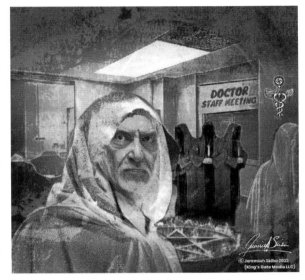

That could be true in her world. Medical grade "quality nutrition" is not, however, what the health food industry considers to be quality nutrition. They weren't giving Rob a nutrient-dense, organic, non-GMO, or all-natural supplement free of artificial colorings, sweeteners, or preservatives. She may have had a bachelor's degree and was a licensed dietitian, yet she was **not** a qualified nutrition expert with a doctorate in nutrition.

LEGAL COUNSEL STATEMENT

Members of the jury, Sheila had every right to be concerned with the standard of care at Covid Coven Hospital of Plano, Texas. Rob's nutritional needs had been ignored from the day he was wheeled into the Emergency Department, as evidenced by the fact that 48 hours after his admission, he texted Sheila, "*No food,*" followed by "*No strength, no hope left.*"

The March 2022 edition of "Today's Dietitian" contained an article that noted, "*Although malnutrition rates in hospitalized COVID-19 patients haven't yet been reported, **risk of malnutrition is high**. Poor appetite, shortness of breath, loss of taste and smell, and gastrointestinal (GI) symptoms such as nausea and diarrhea can significantly impair oral intake **even before hospital admission**. Furthermore, severe COVID-19 results in significant systemic inflammation, **which increases energy and protein needs** and is a risk factor for malnutrition. For these reasons, **most patients admitted to the hospital already are nutritionally compromised**. As with all hospitalized patients, those with COVID-**19 should be screened for malnutrition within 24 hours of admission** with the use of a validated screening tool.*" [bold ours]
MNT for critically ill COVID-19 patients - Today's Dietitian Magazine. Today's Dietitian. (n.d.). From https://www.todaysdietitian.com/newarchives/0322p32.shtml

The article noted that most COVID-19 patients, as was true of Rob, are "nutritionally compromised" when they arrive at the hospital. Rob, for example, had not eaten for over a week before his admission.

> *Rather than assessing his state of nutrition upon arrival, they isolated him from his family and looked the other way when he was too weak to order meals or feed himself. Then, due to willful ignorance, uncaring negligence, or nefarious intent, they allowed him to weaken to the point that he was <u>slowly, systematically starved into submission</u>. The lock-out of Sheila, and the absolute lack of compassionate care for Rob, were **absolutely criminal.***

I told her that I was emotionally triggered by my concern for Rob and my desire for him to live. I cried, "I mean, keeping him from me for 21 days . . . that does not show that you care about his recovery—because he needed me with him. Everyone says, 'it's COVID, it's COVID, it's COVID!' But anyway . . . I admit you are not my enemy; it's the whole system."

Since she refused to speak with my patient advocate, who had a solid nursing background, I asked if she would take time to explain everything to Ms. Destroyer, the hospital Social Worker, so that I could discuss the situation further with her. She replied, "We're here for you and your husband, okay? And I will speak with the social worker, Ms. Destroyer. okay?"

Unfortunately, no matter where I turned, everyone gave me the brush-off, saying, "You know, we're doing all we can."

If they were doing all they could, why then had they not done everything they could to keep Rob **off** the ventilator death trap in the first place? How could I trust a system and a team that followed a protocol that had led them to do all they could to get Rob **on** a ventilator, yet now that same team wanted me to believe they were doing all they could to get him off?

The medical professionals I truly trusted were those I met who claimed to have entered the profession to save lives rather than take them. They told me that what they witnessed during the pandemic prompted them to **leave** hospitals because they had witnessed patients dying needlessly due to malice, neglect, or malicious intent in the name of earning government incentives.

These same honorable professionals told me that the **last** place they wanted to be or see any of their loved ones land was in a hospital; the problem was that many of the callous and uncaring medical professionals who had stayed behind willingly followed an evil protocol that had turned what had once been healing centers into human kill shelters.

Wednesday, September 29, 2021

As had become my routine, soon after waking, I rushed to the hospital, signed in, received my visitor's wristband, and headed up to the ICU, ready to spend another 12-hour shift watching over Rob while listening to the constant cyclical whooshing of the ventilator and the multiple IV infusion pumps that were filling my husband with numerous prescription medications.

Throughout the day, nurses arrived at regular intervals to hang new bags of IV fluid containing the paralytics and sedatives that maintained Rob's complete immobility and coma. They also came in to hang Rob's daily 100 milligram IV piggyback of micafungin, an antifungal drug I insisted he not be given because, according to the hospital lab's policy, the blood culture tests were not conclusively positive. Then, twice daily, another nurse would come in to administer a 30 milligram SOLU-MEDOL IV push.

I played some of Rob's own teachings for him, monitored his vital signs, and applied more peppermint oil in the hopes that, by some miracle, his handsome eyes would open, he would look at me, and he would indicate that he was ready to be removed from the ventilator and begin his rehabilitation.

I was relieved to learn that Rob had begun receiving 1,500 mg of IV vitamin C twice daily the night before. Even so, I was greatly disturbed that it had taken a face-to-face intervention meeting with a team of five supporters on September 27th to finally convince Dr. Liar to give Rob an inexpensive, essential nutrient that I had repeatedly requested beginning on September 5th, two days after his admission and three days before they had weakened and injured him to the point where they could finally force him onto a ventilator.

On September 5th, I had asked Dr. Killer to agree to give Rob 10,000 mg. per day of intravenous vitamin C. I had also asked her to prescribe nebulized doses of budesonide because of Dr. Richard Bartlett's success using it to treat and save the lives of his West Texas Covid patients. However, she brushed off my request by implying she would need to consult with Dr. Dead End and Dr. Torture, saying, "Ultimately, you know, it has to be a joint decision because I can't do it by myself—because it's going against the protocol that we're using for our Covid patients," while confirming, "There really is **no exception** to the protocol at this time."

Although they finally began administering nebulized budesonide on September 9, 2021, the day after Rob was placed on a ventilator, it was far too little (only one small 0.5 milligram dose per day when it should have been a 1 milligram dose four times per day) too late.

Patients and their families had no rights in this absurd "the protocol comes first" world. Any effort to question the pre-defined protocol-compliant plan of care or to advocate for viable and proven alternative therapies was immediately belittled and dismissed.

What was of utmost importance was that the doctors, therapists, and nurses stuck to the protocol. As long as they did so—regardless of the number of patients who died as a result—they would be praised and rewarded for a job well done.

LEGAL COUNSEL STATEMENT

Members of the jury, one year after Rob's death, Sheila met with a radiology technologist with over 30 years of experience taking and assisting with the review of X-rays and CT scans. He explained to Sheila that he had taken early retirement because he could not tolerate what he had seen being done to "Covid" patients in the name of "the protocol."

Below are a few of the key insights he shared with Sheila.

- **Everything became Covid** when it might have been just the flu or pneumonia.
- **I hated all the lies**. People I had grown to love and respect, from doctors to nurses, were suddenly buying into this whole thing!
- I reviewed Rob's radiology reports; the first thing that caught my eye was his initial chest X-ray. They used the COVID word right out of the gate, ***but he had pneumonia!***
- The term ***ground glass opacity*** is a broad-spectrum term for any fluid buildup in the lungs, ranging from RSV [Respiratory Syncytial Virus] to simple pneumonia to a nasty nasal infection.
- So, I could see they didn't miss a beat. ***They said he had pneumonia, and they called it COVID pneumonia*** which is just a kind of a made-up term because, at that time, they did not know quite what they were dealing with.
- When COVID came out, the hospital administrators went to their doctors and said, "***you're going to buy into this new protocol or lose your job.***" They told nurses the same thing. They said, "*This is what we're*

doing, this is what the AMA says, and this is our official stance!" That was the day they adopted masks, and it got *downright Orwellian* about people wearing masks.

- Out of the gate, a handful of us said, *"This isn't making any sense at all,"* as radiologists' and ER doctors' reports suddenly had **the magic word COVID** in the algorithm."

- I noticed from the hospital records that Dr. Dead End was doing a morning and evening portable X-ray. They also did an occasional CT scan. That was not because they were looking for progress. **That's not uncommon because it is also an excellent way to generate money.**

- From the radiology reports and the portable chest X-rays they were doing, **Rob seemed to be getting moderately better.**

- When you get to September 7, 2021, **there's a day missing where they didn't do a chest X-ray**. This is suspect and *highly unusual*. You have to ask why? *I would presume he was still improving and did not need the BiPAP or the ventilator*. They could not show his improvement with another X-ray as it would be *damnable evidence* that they lured him or forced him to use *life-threatening treatments that would eventually kill him*.

- Then suddenly, on September 8, 2021, **the next chest X-ray in his record was taken post-intubation**. Yet, Dr. Dead end was fastidious with daily X-rays until then, and an X-ray on September 7th would have told me precisely what was taking place in Rob's lungs *BEFORE intubation*.

- **Why did Dr. Dead End jump to intubation?** Let's make up a scenario. Let's say Rob went into a coughing fit, all right, and they were saying, well, we've got to intubate him, or he would be crashing and burning. If that was the case, typically, the first thing they're going to do is take a quick chest X-ray to see what's going on in his lungs. **Well, that [pre-intubation] X-ray does not exist**. It's not there in the record. And neither is there a radiology report from the 7th through the 8th. *This is highly unusual*. Then, on the eighth, in the evening, *suddenly, he's intubated*.

- It's unusual that you don't see a radiology report <u>after using the BiPAP</u> and before being placed on the ventilator *when they were monitoring him for barotrauma*. It would have made sense to have taken an X-ray to know if he was okay. **That's the one report I'd really want to see** (yet it does not exist) because it would tell me why Dr. Dead End thought it was <u>necessary to intubate a man</u> who vehemently said, "I don't want to be intubated!"

- Either Rob crashed so far down that he couldn't make a decision, and they considered it an emergent, acute situation—and therefore, they took matters into their own hands and intubated him—or he was forced! **This lack of a radiology report before intubation is interesting and potentially criminal.**

- Again, **we have deliberately missing X-rays on September 7th and September 8th.** Rob's doctors are all on the same team. Hospitals tell their doctors what to do, or you won't have a job and possibly lose your license. And so, everything is going to line up.

- The word COVID was immediately put in his record, which is the protocol. We saw COVID in reports in the ER where you knew the person didn't have COVID! They simply were not in any respiratory distress. Besides, there were **seven financial incentives** hospitals were given.

- You can guarantee that radiologists and doctors will **word their reports in such a way that everybody is covered**, and they do that for medical and legal reasons.

- **I want to know what made Dr. Dead End decide to intubate Rob against his wishes.** I watched this same story play out in the hospital where I worked more than I want to tell you.

- There were some irregularities from September 6th through the 8th. Something went weird that didn't look normal. **They had an agenda, and they made that agenda work.** As far as Rob fighting to have DNI in his record, understand that in his mental condition, once he realized what they were doing, **everything inside him said fight!**

- So, they had an answer (a solution) for his fight. **It was just a matter of getting the right drugs on board, and they could take that fight right out of you right now.**

- *I guess I'm trying to tell you that I suspect a wrong was done here*. I also saw wrongful things done where I had worked.

- **Will you ever prove it in court?** Absolutely not. I know you want to know the truth. I will tell you that you are absolutely on the right track.

- **Yes, this was irregular.** Being in the medical community and aware of these truths, I had to pull back, literally. **The truth is painful. People were dying, and they did not have to.**

On September 8, 2021, Rob was taken off the BiPAP at around 2:00 PM and was not placed on a ventilator until 6:43 PM. Thus, they had well over four hours to order a portable chest X-ray to determine whether the BiPAP had caused the barotrauma they said they would monitor for as they stated on page 141 of the hospital records (see Page C-44) where they noted: "Repeat CXR [Chest X-ray] this afternoon to **monitor barotrauma**."

We contend that the BiPAP therapy significantly worsened Rob's condition. They suspected that they had induced barotrauma (a potentially fatal complication in which the alveoli, or air sacs in the lungs, rupture and collapse, resulting in symptoms such as shortness of breath, difficulty breathing, and tightness in the chest).

Thus, they deliberately chose NOT to order a post-BiPAP X-ray of Rob's lungs because it would have confirmed that the BiPAP therapy had caused the barotrauma they feared it might. Thus, they chose not to order a follow-on X-ray until Rob had been intubated and placed on a ventilator. That way, they could attribute the barotrauma to the ventilator.

Additionally, they had ample time to perform an Arterial Blood Gas (ABG) before placing Rob on a ventilator to confirm the need for intubation. They chose NOT to because the ABG would have revealed that Rob did NOT require a ventilator. Page 137 of Rob's hospital records (see Page C-43) indicates that an ABG was not obtained until 9:04 p.m., 2 hours and 21 minutes after his intubation.

Sammy Wong, MD, our Medical Expert witness, noted in cause #7 of his "Causes of Action," which appear on Page B-5 of Appendix B, that: "*There is no clear documentation readily available that provides clear indication for intubation. There were no pre-intubation ABGs. Even the ID [Infectious Disease] specialist documented (within the hour or so of intubation) that the patient was in no acute distress ('NAD').*"

Thursday, September 30, 2021

Once again, I arrived in Rob's room at 7:00 AM. On the way into the room, I encountered a night nurse ending her shift who said she had spent time washing Rob up. I thought that was very nice of her.

Before long, Dr. Liar walked in. I thanked him for finally getting Rob out of the RotoProne bed and starting the IV vitamin C, saying, "I really, really appreciate that. Thank you so much."

Dr. Liar said, "We've got his VELETRI down to almost off. A little slowly, I'm giving him some Lasix as he tolerates it to just get some fluid off of him because that can affect his breathing some. He's tolerating it fine. We tried lifting his paralytic yesterday. Normally, we just kind of turn on and off, but he gets a little bit too worked up. It's a juggling act, trying to find the sweet spot and eventually, slowly wean him."

Extracting a fully sedated and paralyzed patient from a ventilator was undoubtedly challenging. According to Dr. Liar, Rob was becoming "a little bit too worked up" whenever the paralytics were lowered. I had also heard he "struggled" or "over-breathed," which they called "fighting the vent," whenever his sedatives were reduced.

Any attempt to wean him led to his getting worked up, struggling, over-breathing, and fighting. As a result, his blood oxygen level would fall to an unacceptable level. They would then increase the sedatives and paralytics until he could no longer breathe on his own—rendering him a prisoner of the machine once again. Rob's precarious situation made me think of being stuck on a merry-go-round spinning too fast to get off. There appeared to be no means of exiting the machine without putting the patient's life at risk in the process.

As they continued to flood Rob's body with massive amounts of medications, including high doses of the corticosteroid SOLU-MEDROL, I grew increasingly concerned that the onslaught of pharmaceuticals was further weakening my husband.

LEGAL COUNSEL STATEMENT

Members of the jury, Sheila was right to be concerned about the length of time Rob had been sedated and paralyzed and the high doses of medications he was subjected to. Extended ventilation (periods longer than seven days) makes weaning patients **significantly more challenging**. *Thus, every day Rob spent on the ventilator further decreased his chances of being successfully removed from the ventilator.*

Prolonged immobility, mechanical ventilation, and certain medications (such as propofol and corticosteroids like SOLU-MEDROL) can cause idiopathic (treatment-induced) disorders that make weaning from the ventilator far more complicated. Two such disorders are **critical illness myopathy (CIM)** and **critical illness polyneuropathy (CIP)**. CIM is a disorder of the limb and respiratory muscles, while CIP is a disorder of the nerves that control the muscles. The result is limb and respiratory muscle weakness.

The American Association of Neuromuscular and Electrodiagnostic Medicine notes, "*Critical illness myopathy is a disease of limb and respiratory muscles, and is observed during treatment in the intensive care unit. This sometimes may accompany critical illness polyneuropathy. In addition to critical illness (severe trauma or infection), **muscle relaxant drugs and corticosteroid medications may be contributing factors**.*"
Critical illness myopathy. Critical Illness Myopathy | American Association of Neuromuscular & Electrodiagnostic Medicine. (n.d.). From https://www.aanem.org/Patients/Muscle-and-Nerve-Disorders/Critical-Illness-Myopathy Rob was on both a high-powered **muscle relaxer** (Nimbex) and a high-powered **corticosteroid** (SOLU-MEDROL).

In addition, "*Critical illness myopathy (CIM), critical illness polyneuropathy (CIP), and the overlap, critical illness polyneuromyopathy (CIPNM), **are the most common cause of neuromuscular weakness in the intensive care setting and a common cause of failure to wean from the ventilator**.*"
Shepherd, S., Batra, A., & Lerner, D. P. (2017, January). Review of Critical Illness Myopathy and neuropathy. The Neurohospitalist. From https://www.ncbi.nlm.nih.gov/pmc/articles/PMC5167093

It is known that "*Critical illness polyneuropathy/myopathy in isolation or **combination increases intensive care unit morbidity via the inability or difficulty in weaning these patients off mechanical ventilation**.*" In addition, "***High-dose propofol**, but also supportive treatments using catecholamines and corticosteroids, can act as **triggering factors**.*" Unfortunately, Rob was on propofol, a catecholamine (dopamine and norepinephrine), and a corticosteroid (SOLU-MEDROL).
Zhou, C., Wu, L., Ni, F., Ji, W., Wu, J., & Zhang, H. (2014, January 1). Critical illness polyneuropathy and Myopathy: A systematic review. Neural regeneration research. Retrieved From https://www.ncbi.nlm.nih.gov/pmc/articles/PMC4146320

Another common problem that makes weaning difficult is **ventilator-induced diaphragm (or diaphragmatic) dysfunction**. The American Journal of Respiratory and Critical Care Medicine has noted that "*mechanical ventilation is clearly a two-edged sword. It is also associated with major complications such as **infection**, **barotrauma**, cardiovascular compromise, tracheal injuries**, oxygen toxicity**, and **ventilator-induced lung injury**. In addition to the above well-known complications of ventilatory support, a rapidly accumulating body of evidence suggests that **mechanical ventilation, with its attendant diaphragm muscle inactivity and unloading**, is an important cause of **diaphragmatic dysfunction**.*" They go on to say that "*it has long been suspected that **mechanical ventilation itself could contribute to weaning difficulties due to atrophy and other disuse effects on the respiratory muscles**.*"
American Journal of Respiratory and Critical Care Medicine. (n.d.). From https://www.atsjournals.org/doi/10.1164/rccm.200304-489CP

Although mechanical ventilation (MV) can be a life-saving intervention, "*prolonged MV [mechanical ventilation] can promote **diaphragmatic atrophy and contractile dysfunction**, which is referred to as **ventilator-induced diaphragm dysfunction (VIDD)**. This is significant because VIDD **is thought to contribute to problems in weaning patients from the ventilator**.*"
AJ;, P. S. K. W. M. P. S. K. J. S. (n.d.). Ventilator-induced diaphragm dysfunction: cause and effect. American Journal of

https://pubmed.ncbi.nlm.nih.gov/25842081

Unfortunately, Rob had now been on the ventilator for 22 days, yet *"**Even brief periods of MV [mechanical ventilation] may result in diaphragm weakness** [i.e., ventilator-induced diaphragm dysfunction [VIDD]], which may be associated with **difficulty weaning from the ventilator as well as mortality**."* Peñuelas, O., Keough, E., López-Rodríguez, L., Carriedo, D., Gonçalves, G., Barreiro, E., & Lorente, J. Á. (2019, July 25). Ventilator-induced Diaphragm Dysfunction: Translational mechanisms lead to therapeutical alternatives in the critically ill. Intensive Care Medicine Experimental. From https://www.ncbi.nlm.nih.gov/pmc/articles/PMC6658639

*As previously stated, the insane rush to intubate and mechanically ventilate Covid patients is unwarranted in the majority of cases. **Doctors who insist on intubation and ventilation for their patients are fully aware that prematurely placing them on ventilators significantly increases the likelihood that they will not leave the hospital alive.** Rob and Sheila did not want him intubated and placed on a ventilator because they knew that the only way out for most patients who undergo this procedure was through the morgue.*

Sheila learned from the hospital's Social Worker that many of the doctors entrusted with Rob's care worked with the same patients at an affiliated rehab center where, in her words, they could provide "continuity of care" for the very same patients they had injured with the ventilator—if they somehow survived.

Eventually, and as soon as possible, I wanted to get Rob off all medications, so I inquired., "How long do you think this process will take?" He explained, "I'm encouraged by the fact that I can get him down on the VELETRI and have him tolerating that without having to go up on his oxygen. So, we're kind of on a slow but steady improvement, you know, a little bit every day. The next step would be to try to wean the PEEP on the ventilator, but that's after I get him off of the VELETRI."

I asked, "And the VELETRI is kind of opening the lungs?" Dr. Liar countered, "VELETRI, it's not— no, it works by increasing blood flow into areas of the lung that are getting air to it. And that causes what we call perfusion, ventilation matching. That helps improve oxygenation."

I asked Dr. Liar if he would speak with the dietitian about a plant-based superfood protein powder that I had heard would increase Rob's protein intake to help eliminate his anemia. He said, "The only concern I would have about using another product is if it clogs the tubes." Showing him a new, unopened bag, I assured him, "The product is a very fine powder that quickly dissolves in water and won't clog the NG tube. There shouldn't be any problems."

He asked, "And how much of this do you want him to get?" I said, "I want him to get three scoops a day." I was surprised when he said they could try it. I replied, "Okay, thank you so much. I really appreciate your kindness."

Before leaving, he said, "So, we'll start to work on lowering the PEEP, okay? I need to get his PEEP down to at least 8 or less. Then I would talk about trying to do a trach. I do not think he would be able to just come off without it. I would have a surgeon assist in the process. We do it here at the bedside. But that honestly will be next week at the earliest. I just don't know how long this is gonna take . . . for him to be ready for a trach."

LEGAL COUNSEL STATEMENT
Members of the jury, as we noted previously, their criteria for attempting to wean someone from the ventilator was a **PEEP** of **5 to 8 cm H₂O** and **FiO2** (oxygen concentration) of **50% or less**. However, they kept the PEEP setting at 14 to 15 and very seldom dropped the FiO2 level below 60% during the 35 days Rob was on the ventilator, which you can see in the chart at the bottom of Page C-54 in Appendix C.

PEEP stands for *Positive End Expiratory Pressure* and is pressure forced to remain in the lungs by the ventilator at the end of each breath (upon exhalation). This excess pressure (anything above 5 cm H₂O is excess pressure) prevents the passive emptying of the lungs and "recruits" (helps keep open) damaged or collapsed alveoli (the air sacs in the lungs) by exerting residual pressure on the alveolar walls.

We contend that they **could not** lower the **PEEP** below 14 because the 4.5 hours of BiPAP therapy had caused **barotrauma** (a potentially life-threatening complication where the alveoli, the air sacs of the lungs, rupture and collapse). *Thus, they needed to keep the PEEP high to prevent the damaged alveoli from fully collapsing because if that happened, Rob's blood oxygen level would plummet to deadly levels.*

Therefore, Rob remained trapped on a one-way trip on the ventilator due to the damage they had caused with the BiPAP, damage that was increasing by the minute due to the stresses of mechanical ventilation and the ongoing massive doses of medications. His lethal trip did not end until Rob's body could no longer endure the assault.

After Dr. Liar left, I examined Rob more closely and determined that, contrary to what the night nurse had told me, no one was attending to his physical hygiene needs. His body was crusty, filthy, and covered with a thick layer of a smelly, greasy substance. Despite what she told me on her way out, it was evident that the night nurse had not washed Rob.

In addition, because there was no cleaning staff, the floor of his room remained filthy, sticky, and disgusting. I was surprised that neither the doctors nor the hospital staff complained about the unsanitary working conditions. I should have notified OSHA (Occupational Safety and Health Administration) and the Texas Health and Human Services Commission about the unsanitary ICU environment. However, I was preoccupied with rescuing Rob from the dungeon called an ICU and ending our unbearable nightmare.

At the end of the day, I had once again spent 12 hours watching over Rob, leaving only for brief bathroom breaks so as not to miss the chance to speak with the doctors and nurses as they came and went so I could keep up to date on Rob's care and condition.

After arriving home and before bed, I called the night nurse to check Rob's status. Nurse Jackknife answered. "It's Sheila, Rob's wife. I just wondered how he was doing." He said, "His blood pressure was up just a little bit. It was, like, in the low 160s. So, I gave just a little bit of labetalol, and then it came down. Right now, it is 146 over 89. It's back down a little bit. I turned him a couple of times and got him cleaned up a little bit. Brushed his teeth a few times. He's still been kind of alarming the vent every so often."

I asked him to ensure that the music on his iPad was still playing since I felt it might help him relax and comply with the vent better. Nurse Jackknife then admitted Rob was having a tough time whenever he turned him, so I asked how he could turn him on his own.

He proudly announced he could easily turn Rob by himself, even with the endotracheal tube down his throat and all the IVs hanging from his body. He said, "Yeah, I think I might have gotten him a little riled up when we were repositioning and things, but I don't want to just leave him in one place. I know he might be a little more comfortable in one spot, but I don't want to leave him like that for too long."

I responded, "I don't like him in one spot, either. How do you reposition him by yourself?" He proudly said, "Oh, yeah, he's not too big. On bigger patients, I will get another set of hands. But I squeezed him up in the bed a little bit. I turned him from side to side a couple of times."

to side" on his own. Although he apparently meant well, I suspected Rob had gotten "a little riled up," and the nurse had then given him "a little bit of labetalol" to lower his blood pressure because he had either been harmed or, in his dream state, he was aware of being jostled by a gorilla who was carelessly tossing him around, or both.

Friday, October 1, 2021

Every day Rob was on the ventilator, I felt like more and more of him was slipping away. Despite my strong faith and conviction that he had much more to accomplish, my hope that he would recover diminished with each passing day.

Long days and constant banter with doctors, nurses, dietitians, and hospital staff who would have preferred I remained locked out of the facility were wearing me down. As I continued to advocate for Rob, I neglected my own needs. I slept poorly and ate even less. Much like Rob, I was losing weight and muscle mass and wasting away. I felt utterly crushed by the circumstances. My nerves were on edge, and I questioned how I could continue.

When my mother and sister arrived early to help me get my bearings, I called my close friend Roberta, who had attended the intervention meeting with me on September 27th. I told her I needed a break to attempt to regroup. She immediately responded that she would be delighted to spend the day with Rob and rushed to the hospital. I felt relieved knowing Rob would be in capable hands.

Throughout the day, Roberta provided me with updates on Rob's condition. She informed me that Dr. Liar had made three visits, blood cultures had been drawn, and she was briefly escorted out of the room so that an emergency chest X-ray could be performed. Additionally, the ventilator's FiO2 (oxygen concentration) setting was increased to 100 percent, and the PEEP (Positive End Expiratory Pressure) was raised from 14 to 15.

When I considered that Rob had now spent 28 days in the hospital and 23 days on a ventilator, my tension only increased. My husband, who deplored pharmaceuticals, was being continually assaulted by heavy sedatives (propofol, fentanyl, and midazolam), paralytics (Nimbex and rocuronium), a corticosteroid (SOLU-MEDROL), antibiotics (cefepime and meropenem), catecholamine neurotransmitters (dopamine and norepinephrine), a vasodilator (VELETRI), an anticoagulant (Lovenox), an anti-inflammatory (baricitinib), a Beta blocker (labetalol), a mucolytic (acetylcysteine), an analgesic (acetaminophen), and an antifungal (micafungin).

I had no idea how he could survive such an onslaught. Worse yet, I knew, just as he did, that the ventilator was a death trap. The day before Rob had spent 4.5 hours on the BiPAP, a therapy that seemed to cripple him, Dr. Wicked had warned me, "Last year, 45% of those on the ventilator **died.**" That same day Rob had texted me this dire warning: "*Doing all they can to try to get me to agree to intubate. **I'm dead if they do**.*"

I could not help but fear for Rob's life, and I blamed myself for heeding the telemedicine doctor's advice to take Rob to the hospital. Clearly, he required supplemental oxygen, and as I was unaware of any at-home alternatives, I believed I had no choice but to transport him to the hospital. Furthermore, before the "Covid madness," I had visited the same hospital several times with other family members. Besides, I never anticipated being ushered out the door and told I could not see Rob for 21 days.

I was unable to calm myself. The possibility of losing my husband continued to torment me. Dr. Liar then called me. He stated that Rob had developed a fever in the morning, his blood pressure had dropped to 87/52, his heart rate had increased to 131, and his blood oxygen level had fallen below 70%. He was also going to replace one of his intravenous ports, known as a midline, as it may have been the source of the new infection.

He had ordered a stat portable chest X-ray which revealed no adverse changes. However, to get Rob's blood oxygen level back up, they had to restart the VELETRI that they were planning to taper off, raise the FiO2 (oxygen concentration) up to 100% again, and increase the ventilator PEEP (the pressure that remains in the lungs upon expiration) from 14 to 15.

Dr. Liar commented, "We suspect he is suffering from septic shock caused by a secondary bacterial infection. So, we're going to place him on a new IV antibiotic, vancomycin, as we wait for more cultures to come back. I am also ordering a PICC line, a type of central line, because those drugs can really kind of tear up your veins."

I said, "Well, I want to know before any other drugs are administered, if you don't mind." Dr. Liar responded, "I will try it. I mean, there are some things we have to get moving on, and getting an approval for every single drug is going to be a little bit challenging. We're doing everything we can, okay? I'll let you know if anything changes later today. Tomorrow and Sunday, Dr. Dead End will be on for the weekend."

Not comfortable with Dr. Torture's approach to treating Rob with multiple antibiotics, I asked, "Because he doesn't even have Covid anymore, could you bring in another Infectious Disease doctor to see Rob? If you could do that, it would make me feel much better." He replied, "I'll be happy to get another infectious disease doctor to see him." I was surprised by how easy it was to obtain his approval for a new physician. However, I was devastated to learn Rob was back on 100% oxygen and needed a new PICC line because the new antibiotic, vancomycin, could tear up his veins.

I panicked and thought, "They are destroying his body! We've got to do something!" I yelled to my sister and mother. "No one seems to understand. Rob is fading away in that kill shelter." Sensing my elevated anxiety, my sister texted the patient advocate I had engaged to assist me and asked her to call me. When she called, I cried, "This is Sheila. I'm here with my sister and my mom, and I'm having a meltdown!"

I told her they suspected Rob was in septic shock and that they had started him on a new IV antibiotic. She tried calming me by saying, "Sheila, listen to me, okay? He is going to rebound. I've taken care of many, many, many patients that have been on a heart-lung machine for a long time, and they got better, okay? I got you. I need you to get your head back in the game here, okay?" I cried, "I'm trying. I'm trying."

She continued, "Right now. They've got antibiotics going. They've got the ventilator going. I know those drugs make you just want to just scream, right?" I interrupted her, "But I'm telling you, it is the medication.

Being allopathically trained, she disagreed, "If he were taken off the medication, he would need CPR. He would not survive, okay?" Being holistically minded, I countered, "Then what does all that medication do for him? It helps his body heal?"

Hearing my agitation, she responded, "He has got to rest. And I know that sounds silly, but with the amount of inflammation and the infection he has in his body, if he does not rest, it will deplete the oxygen and affect his brain, okay? So, he has to have these medications. I know you look at fentanyl, you look at Versed, you look at propofol online. I need you to stop doing that!"

I had taken my husband to the hospital with a life-threatening situation, and he ended up being placed on a massive number of pharmaceuticals, each of which had numerous dangerous side effects. I knew that in high enough doses and in combination, they could cause life-threatening complications. Thus, nothing my advocate said gave me any comfort, nor could she persuade me that the medications were not a major cause of Rob's continual decline.

Each time I called, I would ask the doctors to lower the quantity and dosages of Rob's medications so they could get him **OFF** the ventilator. **I told them they were killing my husband with their drugs, the high pressure, and the high oxygen (FiO2) levels**, but they either did not want to listen or, worse yet, were listening but did not care.

LEGAL COUNSEL STATEMENT

Members of the jury, Sheila had a right to be concerned about the massive number and dosages of medications Rob was being administered. As early as September 15th, Rob's elevated LFTs (Liver Function Tests) indicated the hepatotoxic (damaging or destructive to liver cells) medications he was on **were** damaging his liver.

On Page 254 of the hospital records (see Page C-49 in Appendix C), on September 15, 2021, Dr. Torture said Rob's LFT elevations were "**likely related to medications.**" The same day, Dr. Wicked advised Sheila that "his LFTs [Liver Function Tests] have been going up" and "**it is probably medication related**"—while noting **the antibiotics** he was on were the most likely cause.

Key components of the Liver Function Test (LFT) are enzymes known as **AST** and **ALT**. The normal range for AST is 10 to 40 units per liter and ALT 7 to 56 units per liter. On October 1, 2021, Rob's AST was 59, and his ALT was 140.

The graph on the right, which we shared earlier, shows Rob's ALT and AST levels from October 5 through the day he died on October 13, 2021. **AST** and **ALT** levels above 15 times the normal range **indicate <u>severe acute liver cell injury</u>**; levels greater than 1000 units per liter **are considered <u>critical</u>**. *As shown here, on October 10, 2021, Rob Skiba's **AST level** reached **4,202**, and his **ALT** level reached **9,827 U/L**.*

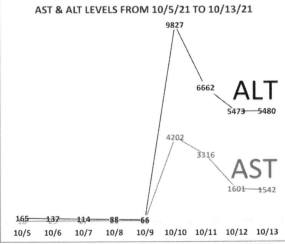

AST & ALT LEVELS FROM 10/5/21 TO 10/13/21

We contend that these massive and sudden elevations are due to the large quantities of hepatotoxic medications Rob was on.

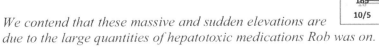

As mentioned earlier, according to Medscape, "*Drugs are an important cause of liver injury. More than 900 drugs, toxins, and herbs have been reported to cause liver injury, **and drugs account for 20-40% of all instances of fulminant [severe and sudden onset] hepatic failure**. Approximately 75% of the idiosyncratic drug reactions result in liver transplantation **or death**.*"

Nilesh Mehta, M. D. (2022, July 8). Drug-induced hepatotoxicity. Overview, Metabolism of Drugs, Clinical and Pathological Manifestations of Drug-Induced Liver Disease. From https://emedicine.medscape.com/article/169814-overview

Regardless of your view of pharmaceuticals, there is no doubt that an abundance of medications can lead to various unintended, harmful, and sometimes deadly consequences. Based on the soon-to-be elevated AST and ALT levels shown in the chart above, there is no doubt they were doing a number on Rob.

I said, "Okay, I know fentanyl is approximately 100 times more powerful than morphine, and they have him on this drug." She agreed, "Okay, it is. I know, and I used IV fentanyl all the time in the hospital, right? All the time! On little, tiny babies. And we used it for the right purpose. And then we got them weaned off of those medications. Okay? Okay? So, let's, talk about what the alternative is. . . tell me . . . if you don't want him on those medications."

"I would rather he not be on all those medications. It's an evil game being played under the COVID umbrella," I replied. She confirmed, "I know it's evil. I know. Sometimes in life, we hit a wall. Sometimes good can come out of really bad circumstances, and this is one of them. I can only give you what my experience is, and I believe in holistic measures, and I believe in prayer, and I believe that God will fight this with you. I've seen some horrendous things, and I have seen people walk out of the hospital, okay? The only goal right now is that we get the infection under control. And the only way that's going to get under control right now is with the IV antibiotics and us waiting for the cultures. That's going to take time."

Unfortunately, Rob was under the "care" of a group of "protocol-focused" doctors who had found a way to force him on a ventilator, which had been their plan for him from the moment he arrived. In addition, they were calling all the shots and administered whatever drugs they wanted, no matter how much I pleaded, begged, or attempted to reason with them.

If I complained about a new medication, such as the new (now third) antibiotic they were now ordering, they would promptly remind me that my fully sedated and paralyzed husband was on a high-powered steroid (SOLU-MEDROL) and an anti-inflammatory (baricitinib), both of which were suppressing his immune system. Thus, my immuno-compromised husband was at greater risk of succumbing to hospital-acquired infections and other ailments, and if they did not treat each new condition that cropped up with even more drugs, he might die.

Sadly, Rob was now stuck on a high-speed pharmaceutical bullet train, and I could not get him off. My goal and continued plea were to get them to slow down the train so he might somehow exit before it hit the end of the track.

Hoping to calm me down, my advocate continued, "They're doing exactly what I would do if I were in there, okay? The reason why he's not perfect today is because he has an *active infection*. **This is what happens in the hospital, okay?** We can't magically take them out of there. Maybe somebody didn't do the right washing up of his central line port, okay. But what we know is he probably had a line infection."

During our intervention meeting four days earlier, Dr. Mei had suggested a "line infection" might have been the reason one of two blood cultures returning positive for fungus, which led to Rob being administered the antifungal, micafungin. As time passed, they gave Rob one drug after another, to the point where he was now on nearly twenty medications.

She took a deep breath and said, "So I want you to think about this, okay? Deep breath. *Let's stop fighting the system.*" Her "*let's stop fighting the system*" admonition made me wonder if I had mistakenly hired her as an advocate. Once again, I found myself dealing with someone advocating **for** "*the system,*" a system I believed had an agenda, a deadly protocol, that they insisted Rob and I be willing to follow. She felt I would gain more ground by cooperating than by pushing back, by giving in a bit rather than resisting.

However, I knew this was not the time to retreat. It made no sense to expect me to trust and support the same allopathic approach that had placed Rob in the situation he was now in. I wished I had only known of some way to successfully treat Rob at home because what the "medical professionals" had done to Rob was inexcusable, and what they were doing now to solve the problem they had created was not working.

She continued, "Okay. If you're going to fight it, your stress level is going to raise, and he will feel this even from where you're at. I know he is gonna feel it. You're a believer, right? So, we are going to let go, and we're going to let God stay in control of this." That was easy for her to say because it was not her husband dying in the hospital. She was expecting me to trust, sit back, and do nothing—to just go along for the ride.

I was sick of people hijacking God and using His being "in control" to guilt me into doing nothing. I knew I was entirely responsible for my actions and inactions, and I could not just stand by and watch my husband continue to be harmed. I was still angered at being needlessly shut out for 21 days, which was a crucial part of their strategy to get Rob on a ventilator. Now, even with face-to-face meetings with doctors, nurses, and dietitians, I was still being told that I had no real input into my husband's day-to-day treatment.

In truth, his captors were "in control" and were doing all they could to ignore or discount my input. I needed an advocate who would fight for me and reason with the doctors on their level, not an advocate who wanted to calm me down so I would feel better about my husband's dire situation. Besides, if the doctors always did right, why did she stop working in hospitals and become a patient advocate? None of this made any sense.

She then said, "I've seen it over and over. I've seen sepsis, and it's nothing new in these hospitals. This is nothing new for these doctors, okay? So, there are certain things I do agree with you that they have not done right. We're going to battle that after we get Rob settled from this infection. If we push right now, they are not going to do anything differently anyway because he has an active infection, okay? If he doesn't get that under control, he will spiral down, okay, and we need these doctors to focus. Rob needs a couple of days for this infection to kind of settle down. It is not going to happen right away, okay?"

I wondered how Rob could survive another day. We needed to do something, not just hang out and wait. Waiting for Rob to get better at their hands had not worked, and each day he seemed to grow weaker. She wanted me to not rattle the doctors so they could focus on continuing their protocol. Yet, it was the things they had done already, things I could not interfere with or stop, that had landed Rob on a ventilator.

She continued, "They kept you away from your husband for a very long time, and when that happens, it's almost like you have some post-traumatic stress going on, right, and then you don't trust them. Now, we're gonna rebuild the trust and we're gonna get this under control. We are gonna let that go. Because if we don't, you're gonna harm your brain and your spirit."

I reluctantly agreed, "Yeah. Okay. I do feel violated and harmed, but I'm going to try to build back up. I'll try. It's so difficult seeing your husband wasting away in that bed with tubes coming out of his body everywhere. I hate it! I want to be with him every day and not leave him, but they won't let me stay overnight."

I explained why I was stressing with the doctors, "You know, it would have been okay if they would have let me in on day one. I wouldn't be having this battle now. That's another thing I have to let go of. I don't know what they did to him in those first 21 days. Like I told one doctor, I don't know what you did to him. I don't know what he's been through."

Picking up on my obvious *lack of trust* in the medical establishment, she felt she had to address it, saying, "I know you don't, but we are going to have to trust the doctors in some of these things. *So okay, don't fight the system*, okay? Stop fighting! We're gonna move through this, and we're going to use even the worst, hellish people; we're going to use them to do the right thing."

My nurse advocate did not see each puzzle piece concerning Rob's condition. She was not privy to any more information than I was, although she did understand how the medical system worked and how it moved and was intimately involved in the Covid protocol they were following. She was convinced she could work *within* the system and snatch Rob from the fire before it was too late.

I desperately needed an advocate willing to help me save Rob, not someone encouraging me to be docile and quiet instead of speaking out and standing up for my husband. Since it was Friday, and the doctors seemed to not change anything on weekends unless absolutely necessary, she continued, "We've got to give this over to the Lord this weekend and then relook at how he's doing on Monday."

I was disturbed by the thought that Rob would basically be on hold for the weekend and that no one would pay much attention to helping him improve until Monday. I told her I planned to remain bold and strong, continue asking questions, and insist that Rob be weaned from destructive medications.

In the evening, I spoke with the night nurse, who informed me that Rob's blood oxygen level had dropped again, so they had to increase the sedatives and paralytics again. He said, "He started over-breathing the ventilator pretty good, and his [blood oxygen] saturation dropped. So we tried to give him some extra sedation. We also went up on the paralytic. We gave him a little bit extra. It's called rocuronium. It's just a one-time push, and it does the same thing as Nimbex. It's just a little more quick to get in the system, and it's working."

I replied, "I don't understand giving him more paralytics to help him breathe." He responded, "What's happening is when he is fighting against the ventilator like that, it can't do its job, and his sats [blood oxygen saturation] can't come up."

I was again being told that Rob was "over-breathing/fighting" the ventilator. Anyone on a ventilator with sufficient reflexes to try to breathe on their own would undoubtedly fight the ventilator. Their "over-breathing" (resisting) the ventilator would cause their blood oxygen level to drop. Consequently, the patient, in this case, my husband, would be further sedated and paralyzed, becoming a permanent prisoner of the contraption that they and their family members had been told would help save their lives.

These villains had a well-defined strategy for getting Rob on a ventilator from the moment he arrived. However, now that he was caught in their deadly snare, they appeared to have no way of rescuing him. Furthermore, I questioned whether saving Rob was even important to the criminals who had kidnapped him as their prey.

I reflected on the fact that Dr. Liar had alerted me that Dr. Dead End would be covering for the weekend. Dr. Dead End was the diabolical doctor who called me on September 4, 2021, the day after Rob's arrival and shouted, "DO YOU WANT YOUR HUSBAND TO DIE?" while he stood by Rob's bedside and then turned to Rob and bellowed, "DO YOU WANT TO DIE?!" because we had both insisted we did not want Rob on a ventilator.

On the evening of September 8, 2021 (after Rob had spent 4.5 hours on a contraindicated BiPAP), this same villain called me and informed me, "He's gonna have to be put on a ventilator here. We're gonna start gathering the supplies."

I knew I could not face this monster. A nurse on my medical advocate team saw that I was struggling and said she would watch Rob on Saturday and Sunday. I told her it would save me from an unpleasant confrontation, give me a little more time to prepare the house for Rob's continued medical care and rehab, and allow me to remain updated on Rob's condition. I was thankful she was willing to stand in for me and watch over Rob.

Saturday, October 2, 2021

A part of me was dying and losing hope that Rob would ever come home. I had no appetite. I was surprised to still be breathing. I knew Dr. Dead End would be "on duty" today. Just hearing his name gave me flashbacks of his yelling at Rob and me on September 4th.

My son, Jeremiah, realizing I was in a fog, rushed over to encourage me to stay in the fight. He told me Rob needed me in the game, saying, "He needs your boots on the ground." He was right. I needed to be strong for Rob. I greatly appreciated Jeremiah's encouragement. I often felt that I was a lone soldier with a sling and a stone who had to fight a brigade of bloodthirsty giants brandishing twelve-foot spears.

We discussed everything I thought was wrong with Rob's care and how difficult it was to argue with the doctors, nurses, and dietitians about his need for better nutrition and plead with them to reduce the number and dosages of the numerous drugs he was being given.

The nurse who was watching over Rob for me over the weekend updated me throughout the day on his condition. She informed me that Dr. Dead End had dropped in and provided her with an update. Rob was still in septic shock, and they were awaiting the results of the blood culture. They strongly suspected that a gram-negative bacterium caused the infection and they were working to rule out bacterial pneumonia.

The ventilator's FiO2 (oxygen concentration) setting was at 75%, and his PEEP (Positive End Expiratory Pressure) remained at 15—which was extremely high. His blood pressure was still low at 98/58, but his blood oxygen level was a healthy 99%.

In the evening, I called the night nurse. She said, "So, he did have positive blood cultures. They started him on a couple of antibiotics." I wanted to know if they knew precisely what bacteria they were treating. The nurse said, "That's a question for the physician, okay? But pretty much the way that works is if this antibiotic is not working, they'll kind of change that up."

I responded, "So, it's a hit or miss kind of doctoring going on. Have you been trying to get him off of the paralytic?" She responded, "Yeah. But he's not tolerating it." Once again, Rob was "not tolerating" being weaned from the paralytic. He must have again ended up "fighting" the ventilator he had feared would take his life.

LEGAL COUNSEL STATEMENT

Members of the jury, what Rob was suffering from is called *patient-ventilator dyssynchrony* or *patient–ventilator asynchrony*, which is often described as a patient "fighting" the ventilator.

"Patient–ventilator asynchrony is most commonly recognized as a patient who seems to be 'fighting' the ventilator, whose efforts, either inspiratory or expiratory, are not in synchrony with the ventilator. It is a mismatch between the patient demand for flow, volume, or pressure as functions of time and what the ventilator is supplying to the patient."
Bailey, J. M. (2021, April 1). Management of patient–Ventilator Asynchrony. American Society of Anesthesiologists. From https://pubs.asahq.org/anesthesiology/article/134/4/629/115298/Management-of-Patient-Ventilator-Asynchrony

"Indeed, many reports suggest an association between dyssynchrony and poor outcomes, including higher mortality and increased duration of mechanical ventilation and ICU length of stay."
De Oliveira, B., Aljaberi, N., Taha, A., Abduljawad, B., Hamed, F., Rahman, N., & Mallat, J. (2021, September 30). Patient–Ventilator Dyssynchrony in critically ill patients. MDPI. From https://www.mdpi.com/2077-0383/10/19/4550

At Covid Coven Hospital of Plano, Texas, the "solution" to Rob's "fighting" the ventilator was to further sedate and paralyze him, yet, "*Increasing intravenous sedation to reduce asynchrony appears to be an ineffective, if not harmful, strategy. . . . Therefore, in patients experiencing asynchrony, continuous intravenous sedation should only be instituted or increased after optimization of ventilator settings combined with management of common clinical problems, such as pain, anxiety, and delirium, or with prompt administration of a bolus in cases of an evident 'struggle' between the patient and the ventilator, for safety reasons.*"
Holanda, M. A., Vasconcelos, R. D. S., Ferreira, J. C., & Pinheiro, B. V. (2018). Patient-ventilator asynchrony. Jornal brasileiro de pneumologia : publicacao oficial da Sociedade Brasileira de Pneumologia e Tisilogia. From https://www.ncbi.nlm.nih.gov/pmc/articles/PMC6326703

Unfortunately, instead of assisting Rob in getting to the point where he could be taken off the ventilator, as Sammy Wong, MD, our medical expert witness, said in his "Letter of Introduction," which appears in **Appendix B**, "*Since he was sedated and paralyzed, he was dependent on the ventilator. . . . **They just maintained his ventilator settings essentially unchanged . . . until he died.**"*

Once again, my nurse friend filled in for me at the hospital so I could avoid facing Dr. Dead End. As she did the day before, she kept me updated on Rob's condition. She advised me that Rob's blood pressure had normalized to 121/69, his temperature had dropped to 99, and they had reduced the ventilator FiO2 (oxygen concentration) to 60%. Yet, unfortunately, they had maintained the PEEP (Positive End Expiratory Pressure) at 15. Thus, on Rob's 25th day on the ventilator, they still could not attempt to wean him.

I spent most of the day designing a rehabilitation room for Rob, hoping to eventually bring him home. I could keep going as long as I remained occupied and focused on my future with Rob.

Because the team at Covid Coven Hospital in Plano, Texas, did not appear to have a clear strategy for weaning Rob off the ventilator, I discussed the possibility of transferring him to a different facility with my patient advocate. Nonetheless, we knew that transferring Rob would require overcoming two significant obstacles. The first would be finding a hospital and team of doctors who would allow us to take part in developing his plan of care rather than fighting us every step of the way. That would obviously be a challenge because every facility my family and I had previously contacted was admittedly following the same protocol. Then, according to my advocate, moving Rob might even require a court order at this point.

We then discussed the necessity of transferring Rob from the hospital to a rehabilitation facility once he had been weaned from the ventilator. The final step would be arranging for home health care and home-based rehabilitation.

Regarding Rob's condition, she said, "It's like, you know, we just kind of sometimes go one step forward and two steps back—and it's like a dance. Remember, God moves in ways that we don't even know. So, we're just going to believe that he already has the plan for this, right? In the end, we're just going to keep moving through it. Let's say a doctor, for some reason, says "**no**," to some of the things we want. We still have to believe that, for some reason, that was just in the plan, right? Or there's something else we have to move through next. Hopefully, we'll make some more good progress today. *But I feel like we're doing good as long as he's not tanking.*"

Doctors were already saying "**no**" to most of my requests, and her "*I feel like we're doing good as long as he's not tanking*" comment reminded me of how the doctors were expecting me to rejoice that Rob was "relatively stable." His being "relatively stable" and his "*not tanking*" were both ways of saying Rob was *not improving.* I wondered how much more harm Rob could endure from the assault of harmful medications and the high mortality rate ventilator.

LEGAL COUNSEL STATEMENT
Members of the jury, on March 31, 2020, Dr. Cameron Kyle-Sidell, an ER and Critical Care Doctor at Maimonides Medical Center in New York City, posted a warning about the use of ventilators for treating COVID-19 patients on YouTube. In the video, he stated:

- [1:15] "*We are operating under a medical paradigm that is untrue. In short, I believe that we are treating the wrong disease and* **I fear that this misguided treatment will lead to a tremendous amount of harm to a great number of people in a very short time** . . .
  YouTube. (2020, March 31). FROM NYC ICU: DOES COVID-19 REALLY CAUSE ARDS??!! From
  https://www.youtube.com/watch?v=k9GYTc53r2o&t=75s

- [2:32] "*I don't know the final answer to this disease, but I'm quite sure a ventilator is not it* . . . YouTube. (2020, March 31). FROM NYC ICU: DOES COVID-19 REALLY CAUSE ARDS??!! From https://www.youtube.com/watch?v=k9GYTc53r2o&t=152s

- [3:06] "*I fear that if we are using a false paradigm to treat a new disease that the method that we program the ventilator, one based on a notion of respiratory failure as opposed to oxygen failure, that this method—and there are a great many number of methods we can use with the ventilator— **but this method being widely adopted at this very moment in every hospital in the country which aims to increase pressure on the lungs in order to open them up is actually doing more harm than good**, and that the pressure that we are providing to lungs we may be providing to lungs that cannot stand it—that cannot take it—and that the ARDS [Acute Respiratory Distress Syndrome] that we are seeing, that the whole world is seeing, **may be nothing more than lung injury caused by the ventilator**.*"
  YouTube. (2020, March 31). FROM NYC ICU: DOES COVID-19 REALLY CAUSE ARDS??!! From https://www.youtube.com/watch?v=k9GYTc53r2o&t=186s

For more on Dr. Kyle-Sidell's observations, see the article titled: "How One Covid-19 Doctor Became a Ventilator Whistleblower: While caring for people with the disease, Dr. Cameron Kyle-Sidell began to suspect that the Covid-19 treatment consensus was wrong."
Ofgang, E. (2020, September 11). How One covid-19 doctor became a ventilator whistleblower. From https://elemental.medium.com/how-one-covid-19-doctor-became-a-ventilator-whistleblower-a1c2dbdd1b06

Monday, October 4, 2021

Now that the weekend was over and Dr. Dead End was no longer Rob's attending physician for the day, I awoke early and arrived at the hospital by 7:00 AM. When I entered the room, three nurses were conversing and laughing as if they were at a party. As I entered the room, they immediately left.

Rob did not appear any better, and I wondered if this nightmare would ever end. Dr. Wicked, whom I had not met in person, entered the room shortly after I arrived. Even though he was wearing a surgical mask, I immediately recognized his eyes from an Internet photo I had seen.

I said, "Hi, Dr. Wicked; I know your face from the internet. So, how's he doing?" He responded, "We finally got him off the paralytics yesterday—and the VELETRI. His blood pressure is good, and he's on less oxygen. So, I'm pleased. Because he has been on paralytics and the ventilator this long, I do anticipate him needing to go to long-term acute care. There's one we go to here in Plano, Texas. It's usually three to five days in rehab for every day he was on a paralytic."

Dr. Wicked was the most open and optimistic physician I had to deal with, and his talk about getting Rob into rehabilitation gave me hope. I was delighted to learn Rob had been weaned off the paralytics and VELETRI. In addition, they had decreased the FiO2 (oxygen concentration) to 50%. To attempt to wean Rob from the ventilator, they would also need to reduce the PEEP (Positive End Expiratory Pressure) to 8 or less. Unfortunately, that number seemed to never be decreased.

LEGAL COUNSEL STATEMENT
Members of the jury, as we noted previously, the criteria for attempting to wean a patient from the ventilator was a PEEP (Positive End Expiratory Pressure, which is the pressure that is forced to remain in the lungs by the ventilator at the end of each breath) of 5 to 8 cm H_2O and FiO2 (oxygen concentration) of 50% or less. Dr. Liar had also said they had to discontinue the drug named VELETRI.

Interestingly, on this day, they were able to reduce the FiO2 (oxygen concentration) to 50%. They had discontinued the paralytics the day before, and they finally had Rob off the VELETRI. **Thus, we wonder why**

they chose to not attempt to lower the PEEP setting since that was the final criterion for being able to try to wean Rob from the ventilator.

Perhaps the doctors knew something that Sheila did not. Is it possible that they NEVER lowered the PEEP below 14 cm H_2O but instead kept it between 14 and 15 for the entire 35 days Rob was on the ventilator because they knew they had destroyed Rob's lungs with the BiPAP (which had caused barotrauma—the rupture of the alveoli)? Were they concerned that reducing Rob's PEEP would cause his damaged alveoli to collapse, his SpO2 (blood oxygen level) to plummet, and his condition to rapidly deteriorate?

As we mentioned previously, Sheila learned from the hospital's Social Worker that many of the doctors entrusted with Rob's care worked with the same patients at an affiliated rehab center where, in her words, they could provide "continuity of care" for the very same patients they had injured with the ventilator—if they somehow survived.

Thus, Dr. Wicked would likely stand to benefit from Rob's needing "long-term acute care "due to the extensive damage caused by BiPAP, the ventilator, and his having been sedated and paralyzed for over 30 days.

Following Dr. Wicked's departure, a nurse and nurse-in-training entered the room. Each was carrying a new IV bag, so I asked them about the medications and dosages they contained. The nurse in training turned to me and asked, in a grouchy and irritated manner, why I wanted the details of every aspect of Rob's care. Even though she eventually answered my question about the drugs, it was evident I would have to exercise caution around her.

Later in the day, to my surprise, one of the hospital chaplains dropped by for the first and last time. She asked casually, "How are you doing?" On September 7th, the day before Rob was placed on the ventilator, **none** of the chaplains would agree to drop in on Rob and offer him comfort and prayer because their "protocol" did not allow them to visit patients diagnosed with Covid. Because I found their callused approach and lack of empathy irritating, I had no desire to have a casual conversation with a member of their team.

LEGAL COUNSEL STATEMENT
Members of the jury, on Page 117 of Rob's hospital records, which appears on Page C-30 in Appendix C, you will see a comment made by a chaplain. In that comment, she confirmed that Sheila had called the Pastoral Care Office and wanted Rob to have a "personal touch" and "human connection." Sheila had also asked the chaplains to "offer prayer and support." The chaplain then wrote the following in the hospital records, "I let her know that I would discuss this with supervisor since our protocol has not included going to covid rooms."

*As we shared earlier, this "Pastoral Care Office" was more of a Pastoral "We Really Don't Care" office because they **turned a blind eye** to the atrocity of patients being isolated from their families. Thus, we contend they were complicit in the evil plan to ensure any patient admitted with a "Covid" diagnosis would **lose all hope** and, out of pure desperation, agree to succumb to the abundance of medications and harmful therapies that would eventually lead to their deaths. That way, the hospital could chalk up one more "Covid death" and cash in on the large incentive booty, as noted in **Appendix D**.*

"Courage is fear holding on a minute longer," said George S. Patton, a U.S. WWII Army General who discovered that courage and fear were synonymous on the battlefield. The only difference between the two was how much longer a soldier could hold on. I struggled to "hold on" during the 12-hour days I spent watching over my husband.

Dealing with the multiple doctors and hospital staff who resented my questioning their approach to Rob's care was exhausting, and I felt like I was hanging on by my fingernails to the edge of a cliff. Whenever I felt like I could not endure another moment, my family and friends would rush to my aid and hoist me onto their strong shoulders.

Rob had been hospitalized for a month and was being horsewhipped by their savage protocol that kills. I wondered how much more his poisoned and weakened body could endure. Although some regarded me as courageous, I was genuinely fearful and often experienced paralyzing fear.

On Friday, as I had requested, Dr. Liar consulted a new Infectious Disease doctor in response to my request for an evaluation by someone other than Dr. Torture, who had been in charge of Rob's care since the day following his admission.

In the late afternoon, he called me, saying, "I'm Dr. Delusion. I saw Rob on Friday. I am the Infectious Disease doctor that Dr. Liar called for a second opinion. So, he had a fever the other day, and they sent off blood and lung cultures. Both show the same bacteria, Klebsiella. Thankfully, it's not a resistant strain, so we can reduce his antibiotics today. So, the vancomycin will be off today. But now we'll put him on this antibiotic called Rocephin. That's the specific antibiotic that works on the blood and the lungs together, okay? So, we'll treat him for that.

"He's already on the antifungal from before, but he should be done in the next few days with a 14-day course. So, he's actually doing better, as his fevers are better, and we're cutting down on the antibiotics. I have a question for you. Do you want me to keep following him because Dr. Torture was his Infectious Disease doctor from the time he was admitted, and I have talked with her?"

I advised him, "I would rather talk to you. Is that okay?" He agreed, "That's fine. Okay. I'll let her know. Because she had mentioned to me, she was like, I don't want two ID doctors to speak with you." So I responded, "I feel better with you. Is that ok?"

He said, "That's fine. Okay. So, I'll let her know. And then the two antibiotics. He'll stay on those., okay? I'll check and see if they did an ultrasound, and I'll make sure everything is done appropriately, the way things are done."

I found "the way things are done" odd because if he was going to do everything the same way it had always been done, how would his approach be any different from or superior to Dr. Torture's? He went on, "And this blood infection, usually we treat that for two weeks as well. He'll be on Rocephin for two weeks. It's a very safe antibiotic that shouldn't cause any problems. It's easy on the stomach. The next step would be weaning. But obviously, he's not doing well on the ventilator." I agreed, "Everyone has been telling me weaning him is a balancing act."

Trying to think positively, I affirmed, "He's getting stronger every day." I was working on my emotions and attempting to keep my thoughts and words optimistic. I had faith in miracles. My own life was still a miracle in the making. Meeting Rob and marrying the best man in the world was the greatest miracle of my life. I had witnessed numerous miracles, and I was seeking yet another.

Dr. Delusion said, "We hope that, you know . . . because he has been sick for a while, I hope he's strong enough to do all this. And then blood infections, every infection that happened, that makes it harder for him."

Again, attempting to remain optimistic, I said, "He's getting stronger and stronger every day. I think he's doing better." Not wanting to disagree, he said, "Let's see how things are. I'll be back tomorrow, okay? We'll do some repeat blood cultures as well to clear the blood discussion okay? We always do that to make sure that everything is gone, okay?

This was the first time any doctor considered repeating Rob's blood cultures to ensure the initial set was genuinely positive. Interestingly, Dr. Liar had told me it was pointless to repeat blood cultures after a course of antibiotics had been administered because the antibiotics could affect the outcome of the test, leading to a false negative. I was pleasantly surprised by and appreciated Dr. Delusion's refreshingly conservative approach to Rob's plan of care.

Tuesday, October 5, 2021

As usual, I arrived at 7:00 a.m. to begin a 12-hour shift of monitoring Rob, inquiring about his condition, and discussing next steps.

If he was to survive this ordeal, I knew they needed to be far more aggressive in reducing the number and dosage of medications, lowering the FiO2 (oxygen concentration) and PEEP (positive end-expiratory pressure), and successfully weaning him off the ventilator. Only then could we transfer him to a rehabilitation facility so he could begin what, by now, would be a very lengthy and difficult recovery.

I took a moment to contact a few friends and ask them to pray for Rob to synchronize with the ventilator so they could successfully wean him. Then, Dr. Wicked entered the room and confirmed what Dr. Delusion had told me. Rob had been diagnosed with Klebsiella, and his fever had abated. He was still off the paralytics, which was good. His temperature was now 97.9, his pulse rate was 64, and his BP was 139/83. His blood oxygen level was 94%, and the FiO2 (oxygen concentration) was set to 50% on the ventilator.

Once again, I hoped they would lower the PEEP so they could begin to attempt to wean Rob from the ventilator. But, unfortunately, by the end of the day, they had raised the FiO2 to 70% and had not attempted to lower the PEEP, which was still set at 15.

Martin Luther King Jr., who knew what it was like to persevere through tough times, said, "*If you can't fly, then run. If you can't run, then walk. If you can't walk, then crawl. But whatever you do, you have to keep moving forward.*" I knew I had to keep moving forward even if the movement seemed slow and awkward. I could not afford to spend time looking back because I could not change the past.

At the end of the day, due to the persistent stress, I arrived home more exhausted than the evening before. I could feel unseen scales tipping against us, and my burden felt even heavier. Yet I knew I needed to hold on for Rob, hold on to Rob, and not let him go. He once had written that he would want me in his corner if he were ever in trouble. Thus, I knew I had to continue to fight for him because he could no longer fight for himself.

Late in the evening, I called the ICU and spoke with Nurse Eerie. When I asked for an update on Rob's condition, she said, "Well, let's see, what was the last update that you had?" I thought that was a peculiar question and wondered what had gone wrong after I left.

So, I replied, "Well, I knew during the day, they had to switch one of his medications to try to get him more stable, and he was maintaining at an FiO2 of 50% while his saturations (blood oxygen levels) were in the low 90s." She said, "Okay, so of course, when I got here around 7:00

PM, our goal was to try to, you know, wean down his PEEP and his sedation. However, an additional sedation of ketamine was added. He's been kind of desatting [his blood oxygen level has been dropping] on us. He was holding at about 88% [blood oxygen level] on an FiO2 of 55% when I got here.

"So right now, he's actually on an FiO2 of 60%. We have not been able to wean down the PEEP. We actually had to go up on his oxygen to kind of get him [his blood oxygen level] to be in the 90s. Right now, he's 93%. He's holding 90's, with him being at 60% FiO2. So, we're trying to kind of, you know, give him a couple of hours to see if he can kind of get some rest and then give it another try for us to, you know, try to wean the sedation again. *And he was a little worked up earlier. Kind of, you know, over-breathing the vent quite a bit and desatting while trying to do that.*"

The news made my heart race, and fear once again consumed me. I told her, "I tried to tell him earlier today to relax and, you know, focus on his breaths. He went into the hospital with fear of being on a ventilator, and it's been a bad situation from the start. I don't know what's going on in his head. But I'm thinking maybe he might listen if I tell him that everything's okay. He's just wigging out from all the opioids he's on. He's probably hallucinating from all the drugs. But I don't know. You've seen this more than I have. What do you think?"

Nurse Eerie said, "Well, I had him last night, and he actually was doing, I would say, better last night. He was calm. I was actually able to turn down his sedation. I'm not really quite sure what happened during the day, but when I got here, he was just kind of, you know, barely, kind of tired out, trying to overbreathe the vent. Just . . . you know, he wasn't looking the same from last night."

While I was with him during the day, he appeared to be doing better. So I wondered what had occurred after I had left. Could it be that he heard me and was comforted by my presence while I was there? Then, when they tried to reduce his sedatives without me there, could he have begun hallucinating due to the effects of the fentanyl, midazolam, propofol, and ketamine?

She continued, "Yeah, I turned up his oxygen just to kind of give him just some rest and get him to, like I said, rest for a couple of hours. Later, I'm gonna give it another try again, to turn down his sedation and see how that goes. But right now, he's looking like he's a lot calmer than, you know, on shift change. He's holding 93% [blood oxygen level] now, so we'll try to come back down again later."

I said, "All right. Well, when I'm there, I just usually pray over him and put some music on and just relax him, you know, like that. I wish I could come in now, but that's against hospital policy. I'll come in tomorrow morning and just keep praying him through this transition stuff. So, that's what I'll do. Thank you for letting me know. Thank you so much. I will just keep praying tonight that he'll relax and, you know, cooperate and that he is getting synced with the vent. I'm gonna be praying fervently tonight for that."

Two days prior, they had ceased the paralytics, and Rob was doing well with the FiO2 (oxygen concentration) set at 50%. So I hoped that today would be the day they could reduce the sedatives, lower the PEEP, and attempt to get Rob off the ventilator.

Instead, my brief call with Nurse Eerie tore my heart out. I dropped to the floor and could not move. I felt totally drained and defeated. I knew Rob could not continue like this much longer.

Each day he spent heavily medicated and bound to the ventilator, he lost more of the little strength and reserves he had left.

Tomorrow, I would continue searching for a facility that might accept his transfer and make more valiant efforts to wean him off the ventilator and save his life—as things were clearly not going well for him at Covid Coven Hospital of Plano, Texas.

Wednesday, October 6, 2021

"Out of suffering have emerged the strongest souls; the most massive characters are seared with scars," said a Lebanese-American writer, poet, and visual artist, Khalil Gibran. This arduous ordeal was leaving me with the scars of a never-ending fight to save my husband's life. From the moment he arrived at the hospital, he had become a victim of "the protocol" that I had learned was responsible for the loss of countless lives, and I did not want my husband to become one of them.

When I arrived at the hospital at 7:00 AM, I thanked God that Rob was still alive. I then received a call from a friend who informed me she knew an ICU physician at a nearby hospital. She stated that she would contact him, inform him of Rob's condition, and ask if he would be willing and able to accept Rob's transfer while he was dependent on a ventilator. She would reach out to me as soon as she could contact him.

Even if the physician agreed to Rob's transfer, one of Rob's doctors would need to approve the move. I knew they would be disappointed to lose one of the large fish they had caught. In any case, it would only make sense to transfer him if the doctors at the new hospital were willing to collaborate with us on reducing his medications, reducing the FiO2 (oxygen concentration), reducing the PEEP (Positive End Expiratory Pressure), and successfully weaning Rob off the ventilator so he could begin his recovery.

As I stood by Rob's bedside, I looked into his face and prayed that his closed eyes would soon open. I missed the soothing sound of his voice and longed to again hear him sharing his keen insights with thousands of others through his teachings. Outside of Rob's gloomy room were sounds of life. Inside the room were the dreadful, depressing, and lonely sounds of the cycling ventilator and IV infusion pumps.

I struggled deeply to hang on to hope. Yet hope had become like water in my hand, difficult to grasp and maintain. The more tightly I gripped it, the less of it I had.

At 8:30 AM, a new doctor came into the room and introduced herself as a cardiologist. She explained that they had performed a transthoracic echocardiogram and that when her partner read it, they thought they saw growths, which she called "vegetations," on the valves of Rob's heart. Preferring not to speak in front of Rob in case he could hear us, I requested that we talk in the hallway.

I questioned, "Why is it that we've been here for 33 days, and nothing is changing?" She replied, "I am sorry. So sorry. I mean, he's doing better and better." I appreciated her optimism but questioned how she could say, "he's doing better and better," while every other doctor said Rob was critically ill. He appeared to be deteriorating rather than improving under their care.

She then said, "The aortic valve is kind of thick. That's why Dr. Delusion is asking for a TEE [a transesophageal echocardiogram], where a probe would be laced down his esophagus to get a closer look."

I responded, "**I'm just waiting for him to get weaned off of all this, right?** When did you find this vegetation in his heart, and are there any alternatives you can do instead? Sticking another tube down his throat is not safe. He's been bombarded with all these antibiotics and heavy narcotics. So, for me, going down his throat sounds too risky. That's my concern. Are there any other alternatives to doing this procedure?"

She answered, "The alternative would be just doing an echocardiogram over and over again, after, like, every few days. There is no rush." Refreshingly, she appeared to be a compassionate doctor who was not deeply entrenched in the lethal protocol that had been forced on Rob.

LEGAL COUNSEL STATEMENT

Members of the jury, Sheila asked the cardiologist **when** they found the "vegetation" in Rob's heart. However, the cardiologist chose not to answer that question because it had been identified over one month earlier, **on September 4, 2021**, the day after Rob's admission based on a transthoracic echocardiogram (TTE) performed that day when a radiologist wrote the following in Rob's hospital records: "Thickened, sclerotic appearing aortic valve. Possible vegetation noted."

> "Vegetation" refers to abnormal masses or growths that can form on the heart's valves. They are typically caused by bacterial infections of the endocardium (the smooth membrane that lines the inside of the chambers of the heart and the surface of the valves). The medical term for such an infection is **endocarditis,** and the typical treatment is a 4 to 6-week course of antibiotics.

*What we find **terribly disturbing** is that **endocarditis** is a potentially life-threatening condition requiring prompt diagnosis and treatment. If left untreated, endocarditis can lead to several potentially life-threatening complications, such as heart valve damage, blood clots, embolisms, sepsis, and heart failure. Since endocarditis can be life-threatening, the proper time to have conducted a TEE (a transesophageal echocardiogram) to rule out endocarditis would have been soon after the initial September 4, 2021, echocardiogram—**not 32 days later**.*

*By all appearances, **their focus was not on saving Rob's life but on getting him on a ventilator**, which they succeeded in doing on September 8, 2021. After allowing him to starve, over-oxygenating him, flooding him with needless and harmful medications, then placing him on contraindicated BiPAP therapy for 4.5 hours that caused barotrauma—a potentially life-threatening condition where the alveoli, the air sacs of the lungs, rupture and collapse, leading to difficulty breathing and decreased oxygenation of the body—they succeeded in that effort. Unfortunately, once Rob was on the ventilator, they seemed to simply go through the motions of feigning attempts to wean him from the device.*

Thus, with their Covid blinders on, none of the multiple doctors treating Rob paid any attention to the possibility that Rob might have a potentially life-threatening cardiac condition. We contend they did so because they viewed him as simply another "Covid" patient. Thus, any other potentially life-threatening conditions were ignored—because treating them was not part of "the protocol" they always followed with such patients.

As Sammy Wong, MD, our medical expert, stated in his Letter of Introduction that appears in **Appendix B**, "*While there were multiple treatment-related issues, the standard diagnostic process was clearly abandoned. As soon as he informed the ER staff that he was treated for COVID, they perseverated (repeat or prolong an action,* *expediting an aggressive diagnostic work up for his cough yet attributing everything to COVID reflects disregard to basic diagnostic medicine. If you do not make the diagnosis, you can't treat the patient properly and often subject the patient to unnecessary harms."*

In addition, a second "limited" thoracic echocardiogram had been ordered by Dr. Liar and was conducted on September 27, 2021. It had to be "limited" because Rob was still bound in the RotoProne bed at the time. The cardiologist who read the updated echocardiogram noted: "Thickened, sclerotic appearing aortic valve - small vegetation cannot be excluded." So, as you can see, both September 4, 2021, and September 27, 2021, echocardiograms showed the same "possible vegetation"—a potentially life-threatening condition they had chosen to ignore until now.

Dr. Delusion, the new Infectious Disease doctor brought in by Dr. Liar at Sheila's request to get a second opinion on Rob's condition, noted in Rob's records, "Echocardiogram was reviewed, which showed thickened, sclerotic-appearing aortic valve. Vegetation could not be excluded. At some point, we will need a TEE to rule out endocarditis." *Of all the physicians "treating" Rob, he was the first to show any genuine concern about this potentially life-threatening condition.*

The cardiologist explained, "What TEE [a transesophageal echocardiogram] does . . . we're not going into the heart. It's going on top, okay? We put the probe down his esophagus. It's a very quick procedure, and we can get better pictures from right next to the heart."

I asked, "If the thickening is vegetation, what is the remedy?" She explained, "So what happens is Dr. Delusion [the new Infectious Disease doctor] will make a decision about the exact medication, which could take six weeks. Then, of course, we have to follow it also to make sure the medicine is working. There's nothing else—because the infection can progress, and if it progresses, if the vegetation is bad, actually the treatment becomes a valve surgery."

I told her I was concerned about another invasive procedure on Rob. "He has been here 33 days, and I just hate the sound of something going down his throat close to his heart when they are trying to wean him off these drugs and the ventilator. *I don't need him to be set back by this.* That is my concern."

She completely understood, "Yeah. I'll tell you what, it is not the most pleasant thing for me to do when you already have a tube. So, it is a little difficult for me to do it. No worries. I don't think it's an emergency to do it today. So, let's get your questions answered, and if you want to take a few days, it's not going to make a huge difference. He's already being treated with antibiotics."

I told her, "I'll pray about it, and if we need to do it, we'll do it." She left, saying, "Thank you so much. No worries." I was surprised by her candor as she admitted that, like me, she was uncomfortable with the idea of putting another tube down Rob's throat while he already had an endotracheal tube. The procedure could be tricky and dangerous.

I was disturbed by the fact that from the evening of his arrival, no one physician assumed responsibility for Rob. No one doctor felt Rob was their patient. Instead, to each "specialist," he was just "the struggling Covid patient," "the patient with a heart problem," "the man who needs daily nebulized VELETRI treatments," or "the critically ill 52-year-old on a ventilator in ICU room 298."

If Rob died, it would just be another "Covid" death, not the death of a patient for whom a particular doctor felt responsible. As a result, there was no true continuity of care, no one in charge of the team of doctors running in and out, and no physician who felt personally responsible for Rob's survival.

Their failure to notice Rob's inability to order food and feed himself during his first five days in the hospital (before being placed on a ventilator) exemplifies this problem. For example, when Dr. Wicked admitted noticing Rob wasn't eating, he decided it wasn't a big deal. Furthermore, the dietitian (or so-called nutritionist) neither noted nor cared that he was wasting away and losing the limited "reserves" he had when he arrived on the evening of September 3, 2021.

The compartmentalization of Rob's care, his being viewed as just another of the "not likely to survive anyway" Covid patients who needed to follow "the protocol," and their cold and calloused attitude toward him because he was one of those who refused to be vaccinated, had led up to this point.

I could only hope and pray that somehow, some way, someday soon, this disjointed and uncaring "team" of "caregivers" would truly focus on getting Rob OFF the ventilator that they had so desperately wanted to get him on—because he would remain dependent on the ventilator until he died unless a concerted effort were made.

Mid-morning, Dr. Wicked popped in. I said, "Oh. Hi. Dr. Wicked. I have a question; I understand they're switching him from propofol to ketamine." He said, "Trying, yeah. His triglycerides are a little low, which is a side effect of the propofol. Not severe enough to really have any real problems, but I don't think he is going to come off it real soon.

"So, I'd like to switch to something else because you can get pancreatitis from it [from propofol]. My goals are still, again, I'd like to get him off paralytics and off the sedations, but obviously, his blood oxygen level is an issue for that."

I then shared, "I don't think he's doing better on the ketamine because yesterday he was a lot more agitated." He replied, "So, I think he has nurses titrating that. *Ketamine is not a great drug because it can cause like hallucinations and stuff*, but the Versed is said to prevent any of that. The Versed is still on.

"So we'll get rid of the ketamine before we get rid of the Versed, so there's no hallucinations. It's actually a street drug that gets abused. I want to keep him sedated so we can wean the PEEP to be in the safe range to do the trach, and I think he will wake up a lot better with the trach, and I'm still gonna give him some time for the lungs to get better. But now is the time for the sedation.

"The X-ray this morning . . . everything was pretty stable, but his tube looked like it migrated a little down, and it is getting real close to the split. So, they are going to readjust it. And from my standpoint, that's all I got. Right? Dr. Liar had him on IV vitamin C for a week now, but it is now on backorder. So, I have him back on the oral for now. I don't know how long the backorder will be because it's an IV form of vitamin C and is very rarely used."

Because I did not want to wait who knows how long for the hospital pharmacy to fill the order, I offered to get some IV vitamin C from a local clinic that specializes in such treatments. However, he said that would not be allowed. So I asked, "If you only have oral, what about liposomal vitamin C?" He said they only had regular oral vitamin C. He then said, "I think the oral is going to work, so I'm not worried about it. So, for now, it's not harmful. I don't mind doing the IV again like we talked about; I don't really believe taking doses of vitamin C is doing things for us. We just pee it out. But I don't think it's harmful."

He went on, "The nurse is going to readjust the endotracheal tube. It's not bad. It's just that it slides down, all right? He looks stable. So yeah, if we get down to 8-10 on PEEP, roughly 60% oxygen, and then get the trach in . . . ." I replied, "It's been a long time. He's got a long way to go, but he's still in the fight. I appreciate your efforts! I really do."

Of all the doctors, Dr. Wicked was the most agreeable and the most amiable. He seemed to want to wean Rob from the ventilator, yet he did not explain why the PEEP and FiO2 (oxygen concentration) were not being lowered. He seemed to be telling me what I wanted to hear rather than being candid about Rob's condition and chances of survival. I told him, "I feel like Rob does better when I'm here talking to him. I tell him he's doing well. Hopefully, he actually hears me." He said, "Even though he shouldn't be making any memories of this, good loving voices are always good." After saying he would see me tomorrow, he headed out.

Time drifted by. I made phone calls and noted Rob's vital signs, medications, and dosages in my journal. Then, as usual, I spent hours reassuring Rob that he would be okay.

Dr. Delusion, whom Dr. Liar had brought in at my request to replace Dr. Torture as Rob's Infectious Disease doctor, arrived in the early afternoon. Attempting a cheerful face, I said, "Hello, doctor. So, they've been trying to wean him for, I don't know, I think it's like the eighth time now. My heart is to see him transition from this to a trach or whatever the next step is. I just spoke with the cardiologist this morning, and she wanted to do a TEE. I asked her if there was an alternative and if we could focus on the weaning process instead. She said that a TEE is not urgent. She also said they could do daily external echocardiograms instead. Should I be worried about this vegetation on his heart?"

Dr. Delusion said, "No. The Candida he had in his blood before is called parapsilosis. That's the one he had. Any time there's a fungal infection in the blood, we do this. This surface ultrasound, the echocardiogram they did, it showed some abnormalities on one of the valves. I don't think that would do anything to the valve itself, okay? If there is no infection on the heart valve, then two weeks of antibiotics to clear his blood culture from the Candida are completed today. If there is an infection on the valve, then he needs six weeks of antibiotics. That's the reason I would want the TEE test, okay, because it may change how I manage it."

LEGAL COUNSEL STATEMENT
Members of the jury, the invasive candidiasis (also known as Candidemia, a Candida infection in the blood) Dr. Delusion spoke of was just one of the **many** "harms" Rob suffered at the hands of the licensed "medical professionals" entrusted with his care.

Candida parapsilosis is the main Candida species responsible for a significant proportion of outbreaks of nosocomial (**hospital-acquired**) fungemia (a medical condition in which fungal organisms are present in the bloodstream). *"Candida parapsilosis is frequently isolated from hospital environments, like air and surfaces, and causes serious nosocomial infections,"* and *"Candida parapsilosis accounts for a significant proportion of nosocomial infections, with an increasing prevalence in hospital settings."*
Sabino, R., Sampaio, P., Carneiro, C., Rosado, L., & Pais, C. (2011, August 8). Isolates from hospital environments are the most virulent of the Candida Parapsilosis Complex. BMC microbiology. From
https://www.ncbi.nlm.nih.gov/pmc/articles/PMC3166928

The International Society for Infectious Diseases noted that:

- The incidence of candidemia is higher in critical-care units than in other parts of the hospital.
- Most cases of nosocomial fungemia found in intensive care unit patients are not associated with recognized immune defense defects.
- Fungemia is associated with a high short-term mortality rate.
- It is already well documented that Candida infections, even candidemia, can be transmitted on the hands of colonized healthcare personnel.
- The evidence for cross-infection by Candida, particularly in intensive care units (ICUs), has increased in the literature.

Guide to infection control in the hospital - ISID. (n.d.). From
https://isid.org/wp-content/uploads/2018/04/ISID_InfectionControl_Chapter53.pdf

As we shared in Chapter 2, it is unfortunate that the doctors at Covid Coven Hospital of Plano, Texas, did not take **a conservative, personalized approach** to Rob's care and limit the scope of their treatment to:

- supplemental oxygen at as low a percentage as necessary to maintain an adequate blood oxygen level so as to avoid oxygen toxicity
- aiding Rob in self-proning to reduce the pressure of the heart and mediastinum on his lungs, thereby reducing the percentage of inspired oxygen required to keep his blood oxygen level at 90% or higher,
- nebulized at a dose of 1 mg every 4 hours to reduce the inflammation in his lungs
- adequate nutrition to ensure he could regain the strength he needed to heal
- antibiotics, as necessary, for bacterial pneumonia or other infections

Once adequately stabilized, Rob could have been sent home within a few days with orders for at-home supplemental oxygen therapy and prescriptions for the few remaining medications necessary to continue his recovery. Unfortunately, at Covid Coven Hospital of Plano, Texas, they focused on ensuring he followed the full "protocol that kills," which (as we have noted repeatedly) included isolation, heavy medication, intimidation, humiliation, starvation, desperation, intubation, ventilation, and devastation—and eventual termination.

Regarding the first bullet point above, we wish to note that the CDC states, "***You can discontinue the oxygen therapy when the patient's saturation remains above 90% after the oxygen is turned off.***"
Coronavirus disease 2019 (COVID-19) - centers for disease control and ... (n.d.). From https://www.cdc.gov/coronavirus/2019-ncov/videos/oxygen-therapy/Basics_of_Oxygen_Monitoring_and_Oxygen_Therapy_Transcript.pdf

In addition, "*Current guidelines for the administration of oxygen in hypoxaemic patients with Covid-19 suggest that **targeting an oxygen saturation (SpO2) between 92% to 96% appears adequate**.*"
Oxygen use and saturation targets in patients ... - wiley online library. (n.d.). From
https://onlinelibrary.wiley.com/doi/full/10.1111/nicc.12709

However, at Covid Coven Hospital of Plano, Texas, Rob's caregivers (as they generally do) targeted higher than necessary oxygen saturation (blood oxygen) levels. As a result, they subjected him to toxic (greater than 60%) levels of inspired oxygen for extended durations, which caused him further lung damage—which you can see in the charts on Page C-54 in Appendix C.

We believe a conservative, personalized approach to Rob's care could have stabilized him and had him recovering at home within a few days. Sadly, the doctors at Covid Coven Hospital of Plano, Texas, instead insisted on following "the protocol that kills," resulting in Rob's needless death.

Dr. Delusion tried to assure me, "Why would we want that [the transesophageal echocardiogram] done while he has the endotracheal tube? Because that procedure is much easier when he's intubated. It's an easy thing for a cardiologist to quickly put a probe in there and look at it. They don't have to do any sedation or anything like that."

In contrast to his assurances, that was <u>not</u> what the cardiologist had just told me. She had told me, "I'll tell you what, it is not the most pleasant thing for me to do when you already have a tube. So, it is a little difficult for me to do it." I despised that Rob's doctors frequently misled me or flat-out lied to me. Constantly navigating their deceit and misdirection was extremely taxing.

I explained, "My husband has been here for 33 days. He has already had so many things put down his throat and a massive number of drugs. I was told he would need more anesthesia for the procedure, and I don't want him to digress. **We need to focus on weaning him.**"

He acknowledged my concern. "So, this would change how we would manage it. That's the reason I would want this done. Here's the deal, okay? On the 22nd of September, we did a blood culture, right?" I answered, "They did. And they tested him again on the 30th, and it was **negative**." He said, "IT IS negative. YES, IT IS NEGATIVE, and you know, again, our goal is, you know, it's . . . if you asked me, he probably doesn't have the infection."

Feeling like I was wading through minefields of deceit and misdirection, I thought, "What kind of game is he playing.? Is he trying to pull the wool over my eyes? Here we go again." Just as I thought I could finally trust a doctor, his statements contradicted both what others had said and his own words.

He continued, "But if you look at the heart, we always look for that specifically. This is the heart, and having a small vegetation cannot be excluded. Vegetation is in the heart valve. So, I don't want to leave it like that and say, 'oh, it's not an infection,' because then what if it is an infection and a blood infection comes back?"

I was baffled. He had just said, "he probably doesn't have the infection," and yet, "I don't want to leave it like that and say, 'oh, it's not an infection.'" I felt he was talking in circles. As I had with the cardiologist, I told him I would pray about it. He confirmed, "It is not gonna make any difference today or tomorrow because he's still on the antibiotics. I'm not taking him off. I'm not taking him off until we make a call on this. So here's my thought on it. If he was my family member, I would want that test."

I stressed, "**I just want to get him OFF THE VENT.**" He tried to console me. "It's not going to be affected by what we do. So I can tell you for sure that it's not going to impact what we do here or his weaning. So my thought is that it would make life easier for him and for me. They saw something, the possible vegetation on the valve, but they couldn't exclude infection, and that [external echocardiogram] just doesn't pick up all infections. That's why the TEE test is better."

Agreeing to let me think about it, he said, "Otherwise, he's doing good, by the way." I concurred, "He's doing great!" I thought, "and he had better continue doing great. You had better not make him worse."

Dr. Delusion continued, "I think from an infection standpoint, I'm very happy with where things are. The only thing is his sedation and how much oxygen he is requiring right now." I agreed, "Yeah, they switched the drugs. Because of the sedation, they took the propofol off, and now they have him on ketamine." Again, trying to remain positive, I affirmed, "He's doing great! Love heals! You know?"

He shook his head in agreement, "Yeah, yeah, absolutely! I always tell people, you know, and I can tell you one thing, as a physician, one thing I always do is, if I order a test, or a CAT scan or something, I always think about it, is this going to change what I'm doing? This test will change what I'm doing because it'll prolong this treatment [the antibiotics] for another four weeks if I need to, and if the test is negative, then I can stop the drug. See, that's the difference."

To confirm my understanding, I said, "It's just whether you're continuing the drug or stopping the drug, right? That's the only thing that you'll do if you see the vegetation or not, right? And could you see it with an external echocardiogram and then decide?" Raising his voice a little, he responded, "That's the one we already did on the 27th." I answered, "Okay, well then, let's wait overnight, and I'll let you know. Thank you so much." He walked out, shaking his head, "Absolutely."

It was a challenging decision because he made it clear he would dose Rob with another four weeks of the antibiotic he was currently on if I did not agree to the TEE (transesophageal echocardiogram), a procedure the cardiologist had warned me was "a little difficult" due to Rob's having an endotracheal tube.

The stress of Rob's condition and daily deterioration was exacerbated by dealing with doctors who believed that a new procedure or drug was the answer to every problem. Rob and I were trapped in an allopathic world where the emphasis was on treating symptoms with invasive therapies and pharmaceuticals that weakened the body even more rather than providing life-enhancing treatments and nutrients that strengthened the body and enhanced its innate ability to restore and heal itself.

Despite everything that had happened to him up to that point, I hoped and prayed that the man of my dreams would survive this massive assault on his body and mind and be restored to total health and wellness.

My friend, who knew the ICU doctor at a nearby hospital, called me late at night to tell me that her doctor friend had agreed to accept Rob as a transfer patient and was willing to collaborate with us to wean Rob off the ventilator. Rob would have to first be accepted as a transfer patient by the hospital's transfer center, which coordinated such transfers.

I planned to ask Dr. Wicked in the morning if he would be willing to submit a transfer request since he seemed to be the most reasonable and accommodating.

Thursday, October 7, 2021

Once again, I arrived in Rob's room at 7:00 AM. As I did most days, hoping Rob might somehow recognize it, I splashed a little peppermint on my neck. Soon after my arrival—although he was on continuous IV drips of high doses of a potent opioid and two powerful sedatives—a miracle happened. *He opened his eyes.*

Somehow he pushed through the 475 mcg/hour of fentanyl (a synthetic opioid at a dosage so high it can cause confusion and altered mental status), 15 mg/hour of midazolam (a potent sedative at a high enough dose to cause heavy sedation, amnesia, and confusion), and 40 mcg/kg/min of ketamine (an anesthesia medication at such a high dose that it can cause dissociation, confusion, and hallucinations).

With a blank stare, Rob gazed straight ahead into the nothingness. I quickly fumbled for my phone and began to take a video of the miracle that seemed to be unfolding. Leaning over and looking into his eyes, I said, "Oh my gosh! I can see your beautiful green eyes. I am here, Honey. I am here! Can you see me? I can see you! I love you; you are well, Honey. You are well! You are whole! Every organ is good! All you have to do is relax so you can get this tube out of your mouth. You are doing so good! I know you are on a lot of medications, but I can see your eyes! You BLINKED! That is the first time I have seen you blink in a long time! I love you! You are a fighter! And you did so good! I am so proud of you. I am so proud of you, Honey. I am so proud of you!"

Then, in less than a minute, his eyes slowly closed. A doorway into his soul had opened for a moment, proving he was still there. I now had a ray of hope that his eyes would soon open again.

When Dr. Wicked came in during his morning rounds, I told him what I had seen. He jokingly said, "I'm trying to **not** get him to wake up, but he's chewing through today's medicine at a much higher rate than I expected. I have people three times this size that are using much less medicine."

I advised Dr. Wicked that an ICU doctor at a neighboring hospital had agreed to accept Rob as a transfer patient. I then asked if he would be willing to submit a transfer request. He said, "Sure, I can submit a transfer request. It only takes a few seconds for me to put it in the computer. However, I don't want you to get your hopes up because even if you have a doctor willing to accept the transfer, it has to be approved by the other hospital's administration. Our transfer center will call their transfer center, and **they** actually decide on whether to approve the move. Unless it is an emergent, life-saving situation and you're going there for something we don't have here, **they normally decline the transfer**—and it stops right there. If they accept the transfer request, you then often have to get in line and wait until there is a bed available. Anyway, as soon as I leave here, I'll submit the request. **Just don't get your hopes up on receiving an approval**."

I thanked him for his willingness to submit the transfer request, and he headed out the door. I later learned that although Rob was already on fentanyl, which is approximately 100 times more potent than morphine, Dr. Wicked had added an IV drip of 2mg/hour of morphine without asking for my approval. I wanted Rob to wake up, but Dr. Wicked seemed intent on maintaining his deep sedation.

Paul, a friend of Rob's who had introduced me to Dr. Mei, recommended that we have a conference call with her to discuss Rob's condition. Paul and Dr. Mei, both of whom had access to Rob's online MyChart records, had been reviewing them and wished to share their findings with me.

He conferenced in Dr. Mei, and I gave them a brief update. "I've been talking to Rob's doctors throughout the day. When I called to check on him last night, they said he was really agitated. He needs me to help calm him. So, I've been telling him he needs to relax because if he tries to breathe on his own, it messes everything up and will take longer to wean him."

Dr. Mei said, "Sheila, you're doing great. Did you find out if the other local hospital is a good option to transfer him to?" I replied, "I spoke with Dr. Wicked this morning, and he said he would submit a transfer request, yet he said it might be turned down because there is not a specific therapy Rob needs that the other hospital has, which is not already available here. If we do not get the transfer approved, at least it seems like Dr. Wicked is working on trying to get Rob stabilized so he can put in a trach and take him off the sedatives."

She responded, "What I'm worried about is his nutrition. That's the problem!" I told her Dr. Liar had agreed a week ago to add the extra protein powder I requested, yet I had subsequently learned they sometimes forgot to give it to him. She replied, "**He's still anemic and his anemia has worsened!** Ask them if there is an indication to give him what's called erythropoietin. It's a hormone produced by the kidneys that stimulates the production of red blood cells. I'm suggesting it because his red blood counts are still low. Are they addressing that? There are two ways to address it, either a blood transfusion or a hormone. The hormone is better because you know how we feel about blood transfusions. I literally feel the erythropoietin will work as it has to do with rebuilding his red blood cells."

I was unaware that Rob's anemia had worsened and found the news extremely disturbing. Dr. Mei continued, "His blood sugar is high at 100. You need to discuss this with his doctors. He should also be getting nebulized budesonide." I responded, "I just asked for them to give Rob a nebulized dose of budesonide <u>twice</u> a day instead of once per day because a Respiratory Therapist told me that due to the nebulized VELETRI, he wasn't absorbing the budesonide. So, now we've asked for it twice daily, and I hope they're doing it."

She asked, "What are they doing to ensure he doesn't have blood clots? Do they have him on a little bit of heparin?" I told her, "He's on Lovenox, a blood thinner." She responded, "Tell your doctors he needs to be on a continuous insulin drip. It shouldn't be every six hours; they should have a steady baseline insulin to drive sugar to nourish his cells. His bilirubin is high, too. That has to do with his liver.

"Rob's lack of nutrition has been a great concern of mine. And the ferritin levels are high! The ferritin may be reflective of his immune system and inflammation, and they didn't address that! You've got to calm the inflammation! That's where the steroids and the vitamin E, vitamin C, and vitamin D would have been great anti-inflammatories. *And the ferritin level shows that his immune system is compromised. He is having an iron overload because the oxygen isn't being carried into the cells correctly. It's also his liver having issues.*"

She stated that she would like to speak with Dr. Liar directly. However, I did not believe I could arrange that because they did not get along well when she met him at the intervention meeting on September 27th. So I suggested she speak with my nurse advocate, who could relay our concerns to Dr. Wicked and Dr. Liar.

Later that evening, I made my call to check on Rob. Nurse Horrors asked me what I had last heard about his condition. I told her, "I was up there until 7:00 PM when the shift changed. I know about the fever and that he was on 100% oxygen. His blood oxygen level was 90%."

She said, "Yeah. So, he has not been febrile for me tonight. He has no fever. We still have him paralyzed on that paralytic. Obviously still sedated. He has been able to go down a little bit on that medication that's keeping his blood pressure up, the Levophed. He's right now at an FiO2 of 90% oxygen, and he's satting [has a blood oxygen level of] 96%. PEEP is still at 15. **He's on a pretty decent dose of the paralytics. They did try to go down on that, but you're probably aware he did not tolerate the ventilator without that.**

"He is back on that VELETRI, that continuous nebulizer to help him oxygenate better, and his blood pressure looks great. Like I said, I've been able to go down on that Levophed a little bit. His heart rate is 105. The last BP was 116 over 61, and that's good."

I questioned how much longer Rob's body could withstand such a massive assault, and I feared he was hanging on by a thread. Yet I had to continually remind myself to remain optimistic.

As Walt Whitman said, "*Keep your face always toward the sunshine, and shadows will fall behind you.*" So I committed myself to continue looking toward the Son (Yeshua) and do my best to leave the shadows behind me.

Friday, October 8, 2021

I was never one who needed attention or to be in the limelight. I would rather be a quiet worker getting jobs done in the background or at home. I loved celebrating our successes, but I did not need any recognition. I enjoyed supporting my husband in discovering and revealing the truth. As Martin Luther King, Jr. said, "*Our lives begin to end the day we become silent about things that matter.*"

Nothing was more important to me than my husband's life. I had now been thrust into the foreground where I was on a quest to discover and expose the truth about how he was being treated by a team of "medical professionals" who had insisted from the start that he follow their rigid, highly lucrative, government-incentivized protocol. As I fought for Rob, I was relieved to have others who joined me in the fight. I could only hope I could save him from the imminent danger he was facing.

Soon after I arrived in the ICU, Dr. Delusion sauntered into Rob's room and said, "Hi. His CT scan was good, but his white blood cell count has been going up." I responded, "We're real big on vitamin C, and I've read that when you take vitamin C, it can actually increase the white blood cell count to help fight infections."

He commented, "I think the key was for us to look for inflammation and treat it. We did send another sample from his lungs. So, we're waiting on that. Thankfully, he's not running a fever. And the CT scan is reassuring. So that's a great thing, okay? I'm here on the weekend. His latest blood cultures will take about 48 hours, so I'll let you know how they come out."

I asked, "What about the earlier blood cultures, the ones done on October 5th?" He nonchalantly replied, "They were negative." I wondered why I had not been advised of that sooner and why he insisted on keeping Rob on the antibiotic, meropenem (Merrem), which he had been on since October 1st. Apparently, he planned to continue to do so unless and until they conducted the TEE (transesophageal echocardiogram) they had requested.

So, due to their constant pressure and insistence that he remain on antibiotics without the procedure, I agreed to let them perform the TEE, which they scheduled for Monday, just three days from now. Thus I asked, "What's the difference between looking at the heart with the TEE and looking at the blood culture? Wouldn't the infection show up in the blood culture if he had any? If he had one negative blood culture on October 5th, and his latest blood cultures come back negative this weekend, why do you still have to do the TEE?"

Sounding a little frustrated, he said, "The reason for the TEE is because even if he's cleared up his blood cultures if there was something on his heart valve, we would have to do six weeks of antibiotics instead of two weeks. We want to cut down as much as we can on the antibiotics, which have their own side effects."

Then, Dr. Wicked strolled in. As usual, he sounded cheerful despite Rob's critical condition. Admittedly, I preferred that to his being forlorn. I asked him, "What did you think of Rob's CT scan? He responded, "Yeah, it looks good! So, you know, we've never really looked at it. I mean, the contrast makes it to the small valve nicely. There's no way everything looks normal. In the liver, it looks pretty normal. So yeah, I was pleased with that. Now, they said they want a TEE, and I never really talked about it with you. You're okay with doing that?" Knowing a TEE could put Rob at even greater risk, I asked, "Do you think it's necessary?"

He paused, cleared his throat, and said, "So, it's not 100% necessary. It's a pretty low-risk procedure. It could be Klebsiella. It's not a common bug, but it can cause endocarditis infection on, like, the heart valve. It would not likely require surgery. The difference is, with an infection of the heart valve, we keep the IV antibiotics going for, like, six or eight weeks.

"So, with the TEE procedure, the benefit is if the results are negative, he will not require as long of an exposure to antibiotics, which is an even greater risk. But if you can't do it, and you have to keep up with the transthoracic echocardiograms where we don't get as good of a picture, then we just treat it with antibiotics for six weeks. I'd rather not have to do it. There is a risk of aspiration. That's the biggest risk for people. We go through the esophagus to view the heart. Nothing is zero risk, but the risk of not doing it is an extra four weeks of antibiotics."

I was clearly being pressed to continue with the plans for Monday's TEE regardless of how much additional risk it posed. The only other option was to subject Rob to four weeks of potentially dangerous antibiotics.

Prior to his admission, Rob had never experienced heart problems; however, in this environment — surrounded by pathogens that thrived in the ICU's dark, dirty, and dank rooms where there was no fresh air or sunshine and where doctors and staff walked in multiple times a day spreading life-threatening microbes from one patient to another — it was not surprising that he was constantly being diagnosed with a new infection.

LEGAL COUNSEL STATEMENT
Members of the jury, as we mentioned previously, the possible "vegetation" on Rob's aortic valve <u>had been identified over one month earlier</u>, **on September 4, 2021**, the day after Rob's arrival. However, their focus was not on saving Rob's life at that time. Instead, it was on getting him on the government-incentivized protocol, which included being unnecessarily placed on a ventilator.

Their unwavering focus on getting Rob to follow "the protocol" blinded them to any other conditions Rob might have had that required immediate attention. Due to their negligence, the doctors ended up pressuring Sheila, 34 days after Rob's admission, to consent to a risky procedure that could have (and should have) been performed with significantly less risk within days of his admission.

Dr. Wicked then blurted out without apology, "You know that transfer to the other local hospital. Well, uh, **they said they cannot accept the transfer.**" Shocked, I asked, "What? Why?

What was the reason?" He responded, "They said they were full, and they are only considering higher-level care patients." I could hardly believe what I was hearing.

I said, "My son hasn't been able to visit his dad as long as I am here visiting. We both need to be able to visit Rob in the same twelve-hour period. The other hospital allows for that, and yours does not." He feebly responded, "I did talk to our CMO [Chief Medical Officer] yesterday and asked him to relook at visitation limitations. The problem is that they're trying to do everything the same for all our networked hospitals in every city. Although Covid cases have been dropping here, in some other cities where we operate, they have not been dropping. They're revisiting everything next week. Once the numbers are way down, they'll go ahead and start changing visitation requirements for all of our hospitals at the same time."

I cried, "Is there any way to get on a list at the other hospital?" His heartless reply was, "They just said no. I don't have any say in this. If someone on the other 'pulling' side wishes to address it, maybe they can. There's very little leeway from the pushing side. My side and my transfer center have spoken with their transfer center, and their transfer center said no. I know their transfer center will try to keep their doctors happy. I can get somebody here easier than I can get somebody out of here. So really, they're the ones that needed to say yes."

My transfer hopes were dashed, and I was devastated. I found it hard to believe that the receiving hospital's "transfer center" would make the final decision on Rob's transfer when doctors on both ends supported it. In addition, Dr. Wicked had just implied that when a receiving hospital's transfer center declined a transfer, the "no" was not necessarily final. At this point, it seemed nothing else could be done unless the doctor on the receiving end could persuade their hospital's transfer center to reconsider their decision.

I called my friend, who had made arrangements with the ICU physician at the other hospital, and informed her of what Dr. Wicked had advised me. We were both saddened and perplexed by the transfer center's denial.

Before long, a doctor I had never met strolled into Rob's room. Seeming somewhat disinterested, he looked at me and then at Rob. His name tag said, "Dr. Ruthless." I later discovered he was a nephrologist. In a whispering tone, he asked, "How's he doing?" I informed him that Rob's CT scan looked good, and they wanted to perform a TEE on Monday to rule out an infection on his heart valve.

Still appearing disinterested, he asked, "*Were you able to put in the transfer?*" I was floored that he even knew about the transfer request. Apparently, the news of my wanting to transfer Rob had travelled far and wide. Even so, I explained that the other hospital's transfer center had denied it. I also told him one of the main reasons I wanted Rob transferred was that my son could not visit because he would have to take time off from work and could only stay for a brief period. I would then be shut out for the rest of that day due to the hospital's "one visitor per day" policy.

As he walked away, I grew concerned that they were discussing my desire to transfer Rob. I could only hope it would not result in some form of retaliation which would further worsen his condition and prevent him from being transferred—if we could somehow break through the transfer center log jam.

Prior to the onset of this nightmare, I had been pretty much a happy-go-lucky person who relished life with my talented husband by my side. Now, my world was collapsing around me, and I was deeply concerned about Rob's daily deterioration at the hands of a protocol that had claimed so many lives—and could still claim his.

Saturday, October 9, 2021

Peter Marshall—a Scottish-American chaplain for the U.S. Senate—once said, "*When we long for life without difficulties, remind us that oaks grow strong in contrary winds and diamonds are made under pressure.*" Contrary winds were blowing harder today than ever, and the pressure of medical decisions was escalating to the point that I thought I might lose my mind.

After making numerous phone calls and juggling the idea of possibly hiring home health care personnel to care for Rob in a home-based setting, if necessary, I finally made it to the hospital to watch over Rob. Before long, Dr. Wicked popped into the room, chuckling as he said, "For him not being a drinker or anything, he really goes through this sedation medication. He really chews it up really quick." He then burst out laughing.

I thought, "What kind of comment was that? Why was Rob's chewing through the medications so funny?" Clearly, his body was still capable of rapidly ridding itself of the plethora of pharmaceutical toxins he was being bombarded with. However, I was deeply concerned that his liver and kidneys would not be able to withstand the assault much longer.

I asked, "What you guys want is for him to breathe with the ventilator?" He said, "Ideally. I would like him to be triggering the ventilator if we weren't having to do high pressures and high oxygen. That would be our goal, to have him do more of that. The problem is I want to get his pressure down low enough to where he's safe to do the trach. Once that's done, yeah, I'd like him to be triggering more of the breaths. Let me do a blood gas test and make sure our pH is okay, as that's something that can drive you to breathe even if you're heavily sedated.

"If he were acidemic [when the arterial pH falls below 7.35], that would give him a strong drive to breathe more. I don't think he is, but we need to check on some blood gases. I saw the blood work. His liver numbers have never been bad, but they've been improving. White count's still up, bouncing around some."

How could Dr. Wicked say, "His liver numbers have never been bad," when just over three weeks ago, on September 15th, he had admitted Rob's LFTs (Liver Function Tests) had been "going up." He told me then that the LFT rise was "probably medication related," and it clearly was. On that day (September 15th), Rob's ALT (a key liver enzyme) level was 404 units per liter when the normal range is 0 to 55.

Astonishingly, they had previously informed me that they ignored any test results that were not at least 8- to 10 times the upper limit of normal. Eight times 55 would have been 440, and Rob's ALT level was just under their "8 times the upper limit" threshold. Thus, to this band of perpetrators, anything under 8 times the upper limit meant that the "numbers have never been bad."

I knew Rob's severe anemia was impairing his organs' ability to receive adequate oxygen. So I asked Dr. Wicked if he would be willing to start Rob on PROCRIT, a synthetic form of the human hormone erythropoietin that Dr. Mei had mentioned. I had read that PROCRIT would help stimulate the bone marrow to produce more red blood cells, which would allow the blood to carry more oxygen to Rob's vital organs. I preferred Rob receiving this medication over his requiring a blood transfusion.

He lamely rejected my request by saying, "Yeah, I'm not sure if they would want to because **it's an expensive drug**, and they have guidelines, and they follow their guidelines." I told him I would be happy to pay for it out of my pocket if my insurance company would not pay for it. He then told me that even the insurance company had to "follow their guidelines." He went on, "They have guidelines about what you can bring in, and besides, it [PROCRIT] is pro blood clotting. Did you know that?" I said, "No, I didn't know that."

After an awkward moment of silence, he cleared his throat and said, "I'll probably paralyze him today so they can see if we can come down on his PEEP and oxygen to get him in a safe range to do the trach this week."

I asked, "Why can you not reduce the paralytics." He said, "I would like to see that PEEP down, you know, to less than 10 before I take him off of paralytics." I asked again, "Isn't it true that if he were off paralytics, he would be a lot further ahead? As I understand, it's the paralytics that are hindering his progress." He agreed, "Yeah, usually with this much sedation, it's enough . . . without apparently anything else." He nervously laughed and said, "I don't have anything else to add." Then he laughed again. It was difficult for me to understand his rationale.

I then said, "I'm kind of confused because, I mean, the paralytic was to keep him from not moving. Right?" He answered, "It makes the oxygen better when they're paralyzed. But personally, I like to get him off paralytics because it does make your muscles get weak faster. Muscle loss is the issue, and we're still going to get weak. Now, once he's paralyzed, like, you don't want to be awake and be paralyzed. I can measure sedation, but once we paralyze him, I can't go down on the sedation because I don't know if he's awake or not. I can't think of anything worse than to be awake and paralyzed."

The thought of Rob awakening and finding himself paralyzed made me shiver. I said, "Of course not. I wouldn't want that either." I asked him, "When will you be starting this?" In a cheery voice, he said, "Starting today, and then if it gets down to a safe range, we can try to do the trach on Monday or Tuesday. If we can do it Monday, that would be great, but I don't know for sure **because he still is just very resistant to the treatment**." I could only imagine he was again referring to the fact Rob was "chewing through" the medications faster than a typical patient.

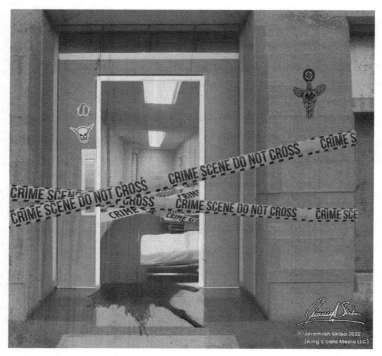

As Dr. Wicked headed out, Nurse Deviant entered the room to hang several new bags of IV fluids laced with more drugs. When I advised her that I detested that Rob was on so many medications and believed the massive doses were only weakening him, she stopped and gave me a stare that sent a shiver down my spine.

Pursing her lips as the veins on her neck expanded, she retorted, "So, I put him on a really low dose of Nimbex [a paralytic], you know. We start everybody on low doses and then bump it up by 2.5. That completely took away his shallow breaths. That's what we were aiming for, okay? So, I won't go up any more unless he processes through that and he starts having those shallow breaths. That's what we kind of want to prevent to help get him down off the high settings. So, hopefully, we won't have to go up any more because that worked perfectly." She was very proud of the fact that she could regulate Rob's "shallow breathing" simply by giving him more drugs. In this world, more medications were the answer for everything.

I then said, "My understanding was when the fentanyl came down, then they were going to give him morphine to wean him **off** the fentanyl. But now, when I review the records, I see that when they added morphine, his fentanyl went up to 500 mcg per hour, not down. So why is that?"

She haughtily shrugged her shoulders, rolled her eyes, and said, "Well, he's maxed out now. So, we can't give him any more," as if that would make me more comfortable. Instead, it made me more concerned.

So, I asked, "Why go up from 275 mcg per hour of fentanyl on October 3rd, then to 400 mcg per hour on October 4th, then 450 mcg per hour on October 5th, then 475 mcg per hour on October 6th, then max him out at 500 mcg per hour on October 7th? Are you going to be reducing that?"

She shook her head no, "We can't reduce anything while he's on the Nimbex." I was shocked, "You can't reduce anything? Why is that?" Condescendingly and arrogantly, she said, "Dr. Wicked explained that earlier to you. It's because we need him to be just as sedated as he was when we put him on the Nimbex because we don't want him waking up on Nimbex because he would wake up paralyzed—and you don't want that. We clearly didn't have him on enough sedation because he was still over-breathing the vent."

Sadly, I was again being told that Rob was "over-breathing" the ventilator and that the answer was, as always, **more** drugs. Consequently, I again wondered how much damage his organs could endure due to the non-stop and excessive doses of multiple medications. It was as if they were trying to assess how much medication his liver and kidneys could filter out before they completely shut down. If he died of organ failure, I knew they would simply chalk it up to another "Covid" death, even though Rob had been free of the disease for over a month now.

Wanting to clarify her statement, I asked, "What you call over-breathing, isn't that simply his trying to breathe on his own?" She sarcastically responded, "Exactly. You want him to do that, but you want it to be in sync with the ventilator—and you want it to be like he could take extra breaths, right, as long as he is breathing at the same pace as the ventilator, which he wasn't. So, he was stacking his breaths." She then demonstrated by bulging her eyes, sticking out her tongue, and making four loud (haaah, huuuh, haaah, huuuh) huffing sounds to simulate someone struggling to breathe. She continued, "yeah, and you don't want him to do that. So now he's breathing perfectly fine on the ventilator."

Regrettably, "breathing perfectly fine on the ventilator" meant he was fully sedated, comatose, and paralyzed with no hope of being extracted from the device. It became more apparent by the day that they were simply going through the motions of attempting to wean Rob while doing nothing to facilitate his escape from its deadly grasp.

I asked her, "Then what happens next? The respiratory therapist will maybe lower the...." she interrupted, "I don't know if he'll do it today. The high PEEP number is preventing him from being able to get that trach. **That PEEP is a very, very high number.**"

LEGAL COUNSEL STATEMENT

Members of the jury, as we've noted earlier, **PEEP** stands for *Positive End Expiratory Pressure* and is pressure forced to remain in the lungs by the ventilator at the end of each breath (upon exhalation).

This excess pressure (anything above 5 cm H_2O is excess pressure) prevents the passive emptying of the lungs and "recruits" (keeps open) alveoli (air sacs in the lungs) that had ruptured and collapsed due to **barotrauma** caused by the 4.5 hours Rob was placed on the contraindicated BiPAP therapy on September 8, 2021.

As we noted previously, a high PEEP setting can cause changes in lung compliance (that is, the ability of the lungs to stretch and expand in response to changes in pressure during breathing), making it far more difficult to wean a patient off the ventilator. Removing Rob from the ventilator required a PEEP setting of 8 cm H2O or lower, yet they kept it at 14 to 15 cm H2O for the entire 35 days Rob was on the ventilator, as you can see in the chart at the bottom of Page C-54 in Appendix C.

Over a year after Rob's death, Sheila spoke with a local respiratory therapist with thirty-six years of experience. He had also worked directly with Covid patients from the beginning of the pandemic. His disturbing insights, which help expose the darkness of "the protocol that kills," can be found in **Appendix H**.

I agreed with her. "Yes, the PEEP has been at 14 or 15 for 31 days now." She repeated, "That's a very, very high number. In order to get the PEEP down, he has to be tolerating, you know, all of that morphine." I asked, "Why do they keep going up on the fentanyl, and why is the morphine four times what it was the day he opened his eyes? **That is very disturbing!**"

She took a breath and said, "So, I went up on morphine yesterday because he was stacking breaths. I then went up from 200 mcg per hour to 400 mcg per hour on the fentanyl, and then he was still stacking breaths. And so, they moved it up again." I said, "**That seems like a lot of morphine and a lot of fentanyl.**"

259

I was jumping out of my skin, yet trying to keep my cool. Nurse Deviant responded, "Right now, that is what he is requiring. So, you know, when patients have Covid, it's been awful." I shot back, "He has not had Covid since the 6th of September, and that was over a month ago!" With a smirk, she said, "Well, it doesn't matter that he's not Covid positive. He has damage from having Covid. So, that's what I mean. All of our patients have so much lung damage from Covid. That's the real problem."

She then stepped out for a moment to get another medication for Rob. When she returned, I asked, "Are you going to give him that?" She said, "Yes, I am! It's Nimbex." I then queried, "How much of that is he getting?" Without sharing the dosage, she said, "It's the only way he's going to stop stacking breaths." I told her I felt he was **too** drugged up. "Right now, he looks like a wet noodle. *At this rate, he's never going to get off the ventilator.* The paralytic will weaken him even more, not to mention all the sedatives he's getting! I don't see how that's working.

She said, "**Nimbex will let the machine do all the breathing** so that he can get off the high PEEP *because he's at a really unhealthy level on the vent.* The paralyzing drugs keep him from taking these extra breaths, yeah, that are hindering his progress."

I responded, "But those extra breaths are <u>his own breaths</u>, correct?" She said, "Well, they are, but he'll take his own breaths afterward." At this rate, it did not seem like "afterward" would ever come. Once again, someone openly admitted they had placed Rob in a no win, no way out, "Catch-22" situation.

If he were fully sedated and paralyzed, the ventilator could effectively breathe for him. Yet if they attempted to reduce the paralytics and sedatives, he would attempt to breathe on his own and "fight" the ventilator. They would then restore the paralytics and sedatives to their previous levels, allowing the ventilator to breathe for him once more. By all appearances, they had made him a permanent prisoner of a device that was gradually draining what little life he had.

Another nurse popped into the room and said to Nurse Deviant, "Well, hey, *I got a message from Dr. Wicked about wanting to **concentrate** his ketamine. So, I'm going to make a bigger bag and concentrate it. So just make sure to **double-check** that when you put it on the pump. Okay?*"

I asked Nurse Deviant what that was about. She explained, "She's just gonna make a stronger bag of ketamine so he's not getting as many fluids because the extra fluids in all of the IVs are affecting his sodium."

LEGAL COUNSEL STATEMENT

Members of the jury, in just two days, on October 11th, Dr. Wicked will advise Sheila that something terrible happened on October 9th (this day) or early on October 10th, something he could not explain that had a significant negative impact on Rob's **kidneys** and his **liver**. *We contend that the continual heavy doses of multiple medications finally took their toll and caused Rob to suffer multi-organ failure.*

It is known that "*Drug-induced nephrotoxicity [rapid deterioration in the kidney function due to toxic effect of medications] is a common problem in clinical medicine and the incidence of drug-related acute kidney injury (AKI) may be as high as 60 percent.*"

Ghane Shahrbaf, F., & Assadi, F. (2015, September 1). Drug-induced renal disorders. Journal of renal injury prevention. From https://www.ncbi.nlm.nih.gov/pmc/articles/PMC4594214

I made an urgent call to Dr. Spite, whom I had learned was a hematologist assigned to Rob's case. I had been advised that he would have to agree with Rob's being administered PROCRIT to help him overcome his anemia. I said, "Hi, this is Sheila Skiba. You were consulted concerning my husband's, Robert Skiba's, anemia. The doctors told me I need your approval to give him erythropoietin (PROCRIT). I'm just trying to help him." His simple and unapologetic answer was, "I have to avoid giving this to him because he has no criteria for that."

I was shocked. So I asked, "Why is that? Doesn't the family have any right to try a medication that can help with his anemia?" He flatly refused my request, declaring, "No. Medically, there's no indication for using it in the ICU setting. High levels of hemoglobin are detrimental, so we don't use PROCRIT unless it is below seven." Rob's hemoglobin level was currently **7.5**, nearly half what it should be. So I implored him. "But the thing is, my husband's anemic, and we don't believe in blood transfusions."

He then argued, "The anemia . . . he's not anemic from the Covid, and now he has pneumonia from an infection. So that's why he's so sick. He has a bit of bacteremia. He developed a blood infection." Correcting him on the bacteremia, I shared, "That's already cleared up. I just talked to the infectious disease doctor, who said that's already been tested, and it's gone. Even then, that could have been caused by a contaminated line." He said, "I understand. The blood has nothing to do with his medical issue. Nothing! Zero! Blood is related to the medical problem."

"Well, the infectious disease doctor was just in here, and he agreed with us that if he had this PROCRIT to help his blood become stronger, he would heal faster, and that's what I'm begging you to do," I contended. He countered, "Okay, we could just give him a blood transfusion." "Yeah, well, I don't like blood transfusions. Personally, our religion doesn't like it. And so that's why I was looking for a more natural way," I responded.

Not willing to budge, he said, "He's not a candidate for it. Because he has normal kidney function, he has no medical criteria for it. There are people who cannot be given this, you know, reasonably." I explained, "Okay. I talked to a doctor in California—I guess they do things differently there—who suggested it. So, I guess they have different rules there? I don't know." He explained, "They only give it if they have kidney disease and his kidney function is perfect. I'm telling you, there is no evidence for him to get it. I cannot give any budge because we have no real option."

"Okay, so what do you suggest? A blood transfusion? Is that your final answer?" I asked. He responded, "Yes, okay?" Once again, I had lost a battle with one of Rob's "caregivers." Not knowing what else to say, I ended with, "Thank you so much. I appreciate it."

But then, to my surprise, a few minutes later, he called me back and said he had rethought his answer, saying, "I can **only** give him PROCRIT if you have a religious reason for refusing blood transfusions." I assured him we did. I told him we believed in the Torah and felt it taught against it. He replied, "Okay then, I can consider it **only** if his hemoglobin goes under seven." I thanked him for calling me back and being willing to consider it. Although it was not a big win, it was at least a small step forward.

LEGAL COUNSEL STATEMENT

Members of the jury, as we mentioned previously, anemia is a condition in which the body lacks sufficient red blood cells or hemoglobin to transport oxygen effectively to the body's tissues and organs. **Severe** anemia significantly reduces the amount of oxygen transported to the cells and tissues, potentially leading to **organ failure**.

The normal range for hemoglobin in adult men is 14-18 grams per deciliter (g/dL). Rob's hemoglobin level **was** at an acceptable 15.7 (g/dL) when he arrived at Covid Coven Hospital of Plano, Texas. However, on October 9, 2021, his hemoglobin level was **only 7.5**. A hemoglobin level of 6.5 to 7.9 g/dL is considered "*severe*" anemia (a level of 6.5 is considered "*life-threatening*"). **Thus, Rob had a severe case of anemia.**
Chronic anemia - statpearls - NCBI bookshelf. (n.d.). From https://www.ncbi.nlm.nih.gov/books/NBK534803/

Why would Dr. Spite wait until Rob's hemoglobin is as low as 7 g/dL when that would indicate the need for an emergency blood transfusion? Instead, why not proactively tackle the decline of hemoglobin with PROCRIT, a synthetic version of a natural hormone that stimulates the bone marrow to make more red blood cells, since having more red blood cells would raise Rob's hemoglobin level and allow more oxygen to be delivered to Rob's critical organs?

Below is a chart of Rob's levels of white blood cells (**WBC**), red blood cells (**RBC**), hemoglobin (**HGB**), and hematocrit (**HCT**) that we showed previously on **September 28, 2021**. Following that chart is another that shows Rob's lab results for **October 9, 2021**. As you can see, Rob's hemoglobin had continued to drop.

September 28, 2021

LABS:
Collection Time: 09/28/21 3:59 AM

Result	Value
WBC	14.4 (H)
RBC	3.16 (L)
HGB	8.8 (L)
HCT	28.4 (L)

October 9, 2021

```
LABS:
   Collection Time: 10/09/21  6:51 PM
Result                              Value
   WBC                              35.4 (H)
   RBC                              2.65 (L)
   HGB                              7.5 (L)
   HCT                              24.7 (L)
```

Rob's anemia was a serious condition that required prompt treatment, yet nothing was being done to treat it. As we noted previously, Sammy Wong, MD, our medical expert witness, said in his Interim Analysis in Appendix B, *"The diagnostic work up for the **profound anemia** was inadequately addressed."* One of his Causes of Action was *"**His hemoglobin dropped dramatically and was not addressed appropriately**. Oxygen in the blood was adequate and blood was being circulated with a normal cardiac output **but delivery to the tissues was profoundly lacking.**"*

We cannot say whether it was due to willful ignorance, uncaring negligence, or nefarious intent that they chose to ignore Rob's "profound anemia." Whatever the reason, we contend that the doctors' actions and inactions during his stay at Covid Coven Hospital of Plano, Texas, were the direct cause of Robert A. Skiba II's needless death.

Later in the day, a nurse popped in and told me that Mr. Pathetic, the ICU Floor Supervisor, wanted to meet with me at the end of the shift. I had first met him when he came down to the hospital lobby on September 20th—the day my police officer friend had accompanied me to the hospital and insisted I be allowed a brief "early" visit with Rob before the September 24th end of their inflexible "21-day isolation" policy. Mr. Pathetic had escorted me to the ICU for my first brief, 20-minute visit with Rob seventeen days after his September 3, 2021, admission.

I viewed the upcoming meeting with Mr. Pathetic as a key opportunity to advocate for positive changes to Rob's plan of care and to learn more about the possibility of Rob's transfer request being approved by the nearby hospital.

Knowing it would be wise to bring additional firepower, as I had during the September 27th intervention meeting, I called one of my friends who had been assisting me in reviewing Rob's online MyChart records and asked if she could meet me in the ICU lobby at 7:00 PM. Next, I called Arabella, a local hospice nurse who was a friend of Dr. Mei's. Arabella and I had been discussing Rob's eventual transfer to a hospice facility. I knew her medical background could aid me in advocating for better treatment for Rob.

Luckily, both said they would be happy to attend. Soon after they arrived and met me in the ICU lobby, Mr. Pathetic and an ICU nurse who followed him ushered us into a small meeting room. When we were seated, I said, "Mr. Pathetic, thank you for meeting with us. This is my friend and a local hospice nurse, Arabella."

I then began to share my concerns with Mr. Pathetic and the ICU nurse, starting with, "I want to transfer Rob because I don't feel he is safe here. The massive quantity of drugs is killing him, and I feel like I'm watching him die. He's only 52 years old. He's never done a drug in his life, he's never smoked, and he's against pharmakeia (the ancient Greek noun for "to use drugs" that we get our word pharmacy from). Yet whenever anything goes wrong, they give him another drug—and he's not used to all that.

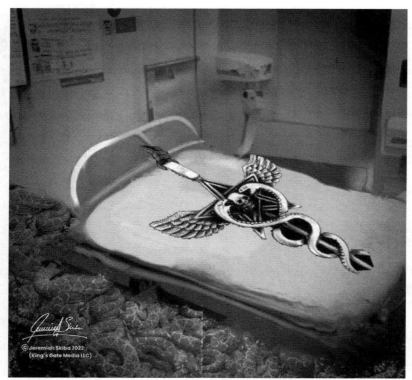
© Jeremiah Skiba 2022
(King's Gate Media LLC)

"Since day one on the ventilator, they placed him on around 250 mcg per hour of fentanyl. Then they said they were going to wean him off fentanyl and switch to morphine. Two days ago, on October 7th, he actually, opened his eyes and looked at me. He looked at me!

Then they put him on 500 mcg per hour of fentanyl and added 2 mg per hour of morphine. Now the morphine is up to 9 mg per hour. That's over four times the amount of morphine he was started on. **This is going to kill him!**"

Mr. Pathetic and the nurse appeared unmoved by my concerns. Looking at Arabella, then back at me, Mr. Pathetic calmly asked, "So, your intention is to transition him to hospice?" I responded, "My intention is to get him somewhere where I feel he's getting saved and not killed!" Dully, he asked again, "So you want to transfer him out of the hospital? That's what it sounds like."

Had I not made that clear? Besides, I knew he was well aware that I had been seeking to transfer Rob to another hospital. I responded, "I tried to get him transferred to another local hospital where an ICU doctor agreed to take him. Dr. Wicked said he put in the transfer request, yet it was *supposedly* denied by the other hospital's transfer center. I'd like to know whom I can call to verify that Rob was on their list of potential transfers. Dr. Wicked said the transfer was denied because the hospital had no beds available. But when I called that hospital, they said they did have beds available. So, I don't know what the truth is."

Appearing surprised that I would consider attempting to verify that one of his doctors had submitted the promised transfer request, Mr. Pathetic said, "Remember, **they** were declining his transfer at that time."

My friend then stepped in and noted, "Rob's being 36 days on a ventilator is the real issue, and we do not understand the plan to extubate him and why he still needs to be on the vent." I interrupted, "Any time he breathes on his own, they say he's fighting the vent." My friend interjected, "Correct. We don't understand that." I added, "Yeah, that's what they say anytime he's breathing against the vent. That he's *fighting* the ventilator."

Mr. Pathetic asked, "Have you talked with Dr. Wicked?" I replied, "Yes, but the way Dr. Wicked explained it doesn't make sense at all." The ICU nurse mocked me and said, "Wow, it didn't make sense to you at all? I mean, we couldn't, I couldn't explain it any better than he can."

Because the smug nurse had ruffled my feathers, I sternly said, "Look at these numbers!" as I thrust the notepad across the table where I had written down the dosages of the medications Rob was being given. It showed they had recently doubled the fentanyl dosage and quadrupled the morphine dosage.

I protested, "I don't appreciate being told he was going to wean him off fentanyl and get him on morphine, and now he's on four times the initial dose of morphine per hour, and the fentanyl has been doubled. He's on ketamine too. *So, in my view, they're just waiting for an accident to happen, which is not good for Rob.*"

Mr. Pathetic tried to excuse the assault of heavy medications with, "Yeah, if we cut back on things, he would be stacking his breaths so much that **he would not survive**, even if we cut those in half." He appeared to be implying that they now had Rob so dependent on the drugs that he would die without them.

My friend asked, "What do you mean stacked? You know the terminology, but we don't." He arrogantly repeated, "He's stacking his breaths." I explained, "That means he's breathing on his own." Mr. Pathetic continued, "His lungs are not healthy. He's not oxygenating at all. You're delivering all the air, but he continues to stack his breaths. I mean, that's just it in simple layman's terms."

The ICU nurse spoke up, saying, "Somebody healthy on a ventilator wouldn't be able to tolerate it. So, that's why we keep people sedated while they're on a ventilator because if he wakes up, he's gonna not be breathing with the vent. Then his oxygen would drop."

Here we were again. If Rob had to remain sedated to "survive," they could **never** wean him from the ventilator. For the past 31 days that Rob had been on the ventilator, that was precisely what I was seeing. All they did was pump him full of more drugs, then repeat the excuse, "*you realize, we cannot wean Rob while he's on all of these medications.*"

My friend said, "So, you're saying his lungs are still in very..." Mr. Pathetic finished her sentence, "Very poor condition. Yes." My friend said, "Okay, so what capacity does he have in lung function?" The ICU nurse answered, "That . . . we don't know. But he's basically maxed out on the ventilator [meaning he was on 100% FiO2 (oxygen concentration)]. It's giving him as much support as we can."

Unfortunately, when he said, "*It's giving him as much support as we can,*" I heard, "*It's causing as much damage as possible.*"

LEGAL COUNSEL STATEMENT

Members of the jury, of course, Rob's lungs were in "very poor condition." Unfortunately, these "medical professionals" appear to be totally oblivious to the concept of "**oxygen toxicity**," otherwise known as "**oxygen poisoning**"—a concept we covered previously.

Oxygen, when used at concentrations higher than 21% (the oxygen concentration of normal room air), **is a drug**, and just like any other drug, **overdosing** can cause severely damaging effects.

The administration of oxygen levels **above 60%** for over 24 hours can cause extensive lung damage. However, as shown in the chart at the bottom of Page C-54 in Appendix C, they maintained Rob's oxygen level at well above 60% most of the time during Rob's 35 total days on the ventilator.

> *As we've stated previously, the doctors all knew—but purposely failed to disclose to Sheila—that the excessively high levels of oxygen he was being administered severely damaged Rob's lungs. Every day he spent breathing over 60% oxygen was one more day he was closer to having "unsurvivable" lungs, which is precisely how the Medical Examiner described them during Rob's private autopsy. To be more exact, she advised Sheila that she had never seen lungs in such a deteriorated condition—and that they did not even look human.*

At my wits end with their excuses, I said, "That's why Rob and I had a pact **not** to take remdesivir and **not** to get on a ventilator! When he came in here, he had hypoxia. He just needed oxygen. But they stripped us apart, had a security guard usher me out, and within a few days, Dr. Dead End had coerced him into getting on the vent. The day after his arrival, this doctor, Dr. Dead End, stood at my husband's bedside yelling at me over the phone, 'do you want your husband to die?' then yelling at my husband, 'do you want to die?' They harassed and badgered him, and now look—my husband is dying."

The ICU nurse matched my intensity with, "And we can't go backwards!" I agreed, "I know we can't go backwards! But this is where we're at now!" The nurse then said, "**This has to happen. It's the process.**"

What "**has to happen,**" and what is "**the process?**" Was he saying what "has to happen" is that anyone diagnosed with COVID-19 (especially if they are "**UNVACCINATED,**" as they had plastered throughout his hospital records in bold caps) has to have their nutritional needs ignored so they can be starved into submission?

Was he telling me such unwary victims of "the protocol" had to be administered remdesivir, then intimidated and coerced into getting on a ventilator as quickly as possible because of the government incentives? Was he confirming that they also must be assaulted with a massive number of drugs at high doses of up to 100% oxygen for extended periods? One thing I was sure of was that if Rob did not survive the massive assault on his body, they would write him up as another unfortunate "Covid" death.

Mr. Pathetic asked the ICU nurse, "Don't you have a plan to wean him little by little?" I answered that question myself. "Every time they say they are going to try to wean him, they give him a new drug!" Now on the defensive, the nurse said, "Of course, we try to wean him. Every shift, we try to decrease his amount of oxygen and amount of support he needs, but he sometimes needs more, and it's been kind of up and down since he's been there."

I hammered back, 'They don't even move him every day. They said they move him every two hours, but I'm sitting there all freakin' day. They don't move him every two hours. I have to beg and plead for them to move him. I think a big part of his problem is that he's not getting moved. He's left like a log in the bed, like a slab of meat waiting for the slaughter.

"I don't know if they're giving him the budesonide, which is written in his records to be given to him twice a day. I don't know if they're giving him his protein powder, as I haven't seen him get it during the twelve hours I sit there with him each day. Maybe when I take a break to go to the bathroom, they do all this while I'm gone, but I pretty much stay in the room all day long. So, I know what they're doing and not doing."

I continued, "The problem was nothing on Covid but it's the drugs. He's never gotten worse when

As soon as they give him another drug, everything goes haywire!" The ICU nurse said, "We're just not gonna be able to give all the medications that you want." I could not believe she had said that. I thought I had made it clear I wanted Rob on FEWER drugs, not MORE. To clarify, I said, "No, no, I'm not asking for MORE medications. I'm just trying to tell you the reason you're getting crazy numbers with his vitals is because of all the drugs he's being given."

Mr. Pathetic said, "I mean if we take away all those drugs right now. . . ." I said, "I'm not saying take them away!" He interrupted, "Something bad would happen if we do." I cried out, "I didn't say, take them away. I'm just saying maybe not give him as many and not as much." He responded, "Well, he's in a different state now. His lungs are not well."

My friend asked, "What is the reason for the high dose of morphine and 500 mcg per hour of fentanyl?" The nurse replied, "**Yeah, he's on high doses.**" I cried out, "Why, why?" The nurse continued, "That's to keep him in synchrony with the vent." I asked, "500 mcg per hour of fentanyl?" She said, "Yeah, I mean. . . ." I interrupted her and added in disgust, "and 9 mg per hour of Morphine?"

She apologetically said, "**It is a lot.** We have tried." I interrupted again, "He's on a paralytic. He's paralyzed." She said, "I know, and so that was to see if that could help him get his oxygenation a little bit better so we can wean down the vent, but it hasn't really helped. *That was one of the other ideas Dr. Wicked had was just to kind of, um, max him out on everything—but nothing has helped so far.*"

Arabella stepped in and said, "I personally think that what needs to happen is that you need to look at what is going on with him and see how it can be tapered down without compromising him. *Because when they raise from 5 mg per hour to 9 mg per hour of morphine with no clear understanding of the impact, I think that is bordering neglect.*"

Downplaying the negative impact of the heavy doses of medications on Rob's health, Mr. Pathetic said, "It's very concerning that those sedations are very high doses, but we started low on those. Then his lungs, you know, um, just would not take it. He would eventually code if we. . . ." I jumped in, "*He is trying to breathe on his own, and they call it fighting the machine. That's the problem. He literally opened his eyes for the first time two days ago.*"

All Mr. Pathetic could come up with was, "When you're stacking your breaths, and going against the grain, against what the machine is giving you, you'll lose oxygenation, your cells won't get oxygen, and you will eventually fail."

As he painted a picture of never-ending hopelessness that could only lead to death, my friend said, "For us, it is like an endless cycle. How does someone ever break out of this?" I added, facetiously, "Oh, I don't know, apparently more drugs, then more drugs, and then even more drugs. It's just more drugs. But unfortunately, every time they give him a new drug, he crashes. It IS an endless cycle. First, his blood pressure goes up, and then it goes down. Then his heart beats too fast. It's a routine I've seen a million times, and I keep talking about this, and nobody listens. *It's an endless downward spiral.*"

Sensing my deep frustration and anguish, Arabella asked me, "Have you had a conference with any of the doctors?" I said, "Yes, on September 27th, we had a face-to-face meeting with Dr. Liar, but, unfortunately, it didn't get us very far."

Mr. Pathetic looked at me and said, "If you had to write down your biggest concern right now, would it be the amount of sedation?" I replied, "He has never done drugs in his life, and he's now on **double** the fentanyl and **4 times** the morphine he was on when he opened his eyes two days ago." Mr. Pathetic sarcastically asked, "Do you want us to cut the drugs in half in front of you and see what happens!?"

That was not what I was asking for, and Mr. Pathetic knew it. I was simply pleading for a more sane approach to the number and dosages of medications being administered to Rob so he might have a chance of surviving. There was no doubt the continual assault of heavy dosages of a massive number of drugs was making it harder for him to have any of the "reserves" Dr. Wicked kept saying he needed to get off the ventilator.

Arabella said, "So, what needs to happen is to check the numbers and work to get these numbers down. Like Sheila is, keep a log of the numbers. She has a record of every single day. You need to keep an eye on his dosages as well—because they just keep climbing."

Mr. Pathetic said, "We never slam dunk people on any sedation at all. We start from the bottom, and it's slowly worked up. It's called titrating. And the goal is always to titrate everything down. In fact, we have been trying to take the Nimbex [paralytic] off. But we have been having to put it back on because if he is stacking his breaths, he won't get oxygen. You can see in front of you on that paper that the oxygenation declined, and then his blood pressure went down a bit. He'll just code if you don't do anything. So, you have to kind of increase sedations."

My friend asked, "So what's going on with his lungs? Does he still have pneumonia?" The ICU nurse said, "Yeah, he has very severe Covid pneumonia." I replied, "He no longer has Covid, but you list him as if he does." The nurse responded, "He has very severe Covid pneumonia. All his problems are from Covid, causing his lungs to be super inflamed. And yes, he's had complications just from being in the hospital and being on the vent. Essentially, he has ARDS [Acute Respiratory Distress Syndrome], which is respiratory failure from pneumonia caused by Covid."

Mr. Pathetic chimed in, "It's not unique to him. Most chronic patients who had long-term Covid would have some fibrotic tissue changes in their lungs, and those become stiffer. It's harder and harder to oxygenate, and it's just one of those things. You know, we see some people survive, and some don't."

My friend said, "Now we want you to do everything possible to ensure he survives this and can come home. I know there's no guarantee you guys can put on paper, but we obviously want the best care for him. He has been in the hospital for 36 days now. What is the average for a patient with Covid pneumonia? Do you normally see them recover quicker? Is this unusual?"

Mr. Pathetic noted, "It's very varied. I mean, you can see the grim results, and you can see some good outcomes; it's a wide spectrum. By being in the ICU, we see the bad end of it—a lot— because **the ones who recover are just staying on the regular floors.**"

Rob had been doing far better on the "**regular floors**" when Dr. Dead End kicked him out of the ICU on September 5th out of spite because Rob refused to be intubated and placed on a ventilator. I truly believed Rob would be home now and well on his way to recovery if they had not forced their deadly protocol on him.

Even Dr. Wicked had noted that Rob had continued to improve over the next three days between September 5th and September 8th; that is until they placed him on the contraindicated BiPAP therapy that seemed to severely damage his lungs, leading to his being forced on a ventilator.

> **LEGAL COUNSEL STATEMENT**
>
> Members of the jury, as you saw in Sheila's statement at the start of September 9, 2021, Rob fell victim to "the protocol that kills" despite her valiant efforts to serve as his advocate while being prohibited from visiting him.
>
> As she stated, Rob "had been isolated, intimidated, harassed, starved, and harmed by a contraindicated [BiPAP] therapy that led to his being strapped to a device [the ventilator]"—a device Sheila and Rob knew was likely to kill him.
>
> *We believe Rob would not have needed mechanical ventilation if the hospital had allowed Sheila to be his on-site advocate from the day he was admitted. If she had been allowed to be with him during the day, she could have ensured he received adequate food and water so he could regain the strength he needed to heal. In addition, she could have helped prevent their placing Rob on the contraindicated BiPAP therapy—a therapy that caused so much damage to Rob's lungs (that is, barotrauma) that they then had an excuse to force Rob on a ventilator.*
>
> As we shared earlier, Erin Olszewski, BSN, RN, said in her book Undercover Epicenter Nurse, once a "Covid" patient was placed on a ventilator it was clear they were on a one-way trip.
>
> *"The ventilator approach is deadly for so many reasons. First, the sedation drugs have a negative effect on the body and the brain. Second, the use of pressure causes a situation where the membrane expand. In order to fill them, you need more and more pressure. They keep turning it up until everything is maxed out. At that point, there is nothing more you can do. You just wait for them to die."*
>
> Olszewski, Erin. Page 79. Undercover Epicenter Nurse: How Fraud, Negligence, & Greed Led to Unnecessary Deaths at Elmhurst Hospital, Skyhorse, 2020.

My friend said, "I know you guys are taking care of the medical side of everything, but there have been a lot of emotional traumas for the family because of the isolation they endured. I know you guys must have families who wouldn't want that—not to be able to see your husband and your wife or your mother, to be uninformed, and to be isolated. It's hard to recuperate from something like that and to have a trusting relationship with doctors and staff." Mr. Pathetic responded, "I understand. In your defense, no information is enough information, especially when your loved one is very, very, very sick. So, we do recognize that, and, you know, it's just a very difficult situation."

My friend said, "We want every effort made to save his life. And if there's even better care available, we want the opportunity to investigate and be able to transport him to an alternate hospital. Wouldn't you want the best for your family, no matter what, no matter what was happening? You would want them to get the best possible care, and you would take them anywhere to get that!"

The ICU nurse said, "Of course, yeah." My friend continued, "And that's no judgment on you as individual professionals but as a system. If we find a better system to work with, we have to be able to do that. So, the whole transfer thing, if that happens, I'm going to help the family work on that. So, taking one 'no' answer, that 'you're denied' by a transfer center, is unacceptable. I'm not going to accept that; I'm going to continue to pursue. . . ."

Mr. Pathetic interrupted and, while looking me directly, said, "So, I know that you wanted to move Rob even before he was intubated. I think when he was still sick and on VELETRI and all that, you considered the possibility of transferring out. And there was a clear denial from the other local hospital." Arabella responded, "But now, they are telling her that they do have room;

they do have a bed." Mr. Pathetic noted, "The transferring part is really up to the receiving hospital. You are pretty much at their mercy at that point." My friend stepped in with, "So, that's where I'm going to be working . . . on that part."

Mr. Pathetic said, "Yeah, if you have any pull over there at that hospital to tell them what you want, and they do have a bed and an accepting physician, it's a go, right? That's the hurdle. Yeah, there's always been a number of beds, sure. So, the reality, as sick as he is, it's going to be . . . it's going to take a lot. I mean, I'm telling you, it's going to be up to the receiving hospital because we transfer patients all the time. So, the critical thing is an accepting physician in a facility with an actual bed. Those are two critical things."

My friend said, "Yes, I have that verbally from a doctor, but we can't get that into motion properly until Monday." Mr. Pathetic countered, "A doctor saying that 'yeah, I can have him,' **it's not going to hold water** unless the hospital itself says, 'we have a bed, and they say 'yeah, we'll take that patient.'"

Mr. Pathetic then looked at me and said, "Do you have any more questions, Mrs. Skiba?" I shook my head, "No." I was exhausted from the battle. My friend glanced at me, then, addressing Mr. Pathetic, said, "She's kind of spent." I agreed. "It's been nearly forty days now. He was in the best health of his life. He went on a trip to Ohio. He came back coughing, and now we're here. I'm just tired and ready to get him home alive."

As my friend and Arabella followed me out of the hospital, I shared with them, "What makes me bitter is how they violated me at the beginning of this nightmare and did not let me see my husband for 21 days. That really makes it hard for me to be okay with all of this. It's trauma that I will never recover from. I don't know what they did to him for the first 21 days. I was going crazy. Yeah, and they blame it all on Covid! I'm sorry, but that's a crock of lies. Some would call it BULL CRAP."

Arabella, the hospice nurse who had so kindly come to assist me, said she was totally distressed by the tone of the meeting. As she shook her head from side to side in disbelief, she said, "And he does not have Covid now. So, what's this all about?"

I said, "I know, it's really messed up. They don't take any responsibility for all the drugs and therapies that harmed him. It's a game they're playing! He is withering away. He might as well be in hospice because when my dad was, they made him comfortable and killed him slowly with the same drugs they are giving to Rob! I've seen this before! That is exactly what they have been doing to my husband for 36 freakin' days! I can't continue watching them kill him!"
Arabella responded, "I just can't believe they think the drugs are good. Do you see the rationale? No! Do you need to keep somebody down? No! *They should be taking him off the drugs, but they give him too much fentanyl and morphine. So high of dosages that I don't have words to express my thoughts.* Do you know how these drugs affect the body and how they work?"

I said, "They suppress the respirations." She screamed, "*Yes, Yes, Yes, that is it!*" I knew very well they were systematically killing Rob with a hospice type of protocol. I responded, "I know. It makes no sense to me." She replied, "Your husband is a man covered by the blood of Jesus. Yes, God is with that man. They are giving him a dose of 9 milligrams of morphine per hour. *That large of a dose can kill a horse, and that man of God is still alive. That's unheard of.*

She was totally appalled at the quantity and dosages of drugs Rob was being administered and said she had never seen anything like it. She continued, "They need to take him **off** that medication! What kind of pain is he in? That's not a medication for the lungs! *They're telling you his lungs are not okay, yet they are over-relaxing and inhibiting his respirations! That's malpractice right there!*"

I countered, "He's gonna make it! I believe in miracles. But the thing is, he's also getting fentanyl which is 50 to 100 times stronger than morphine! He's getting a deadly cocktail of high doses of fentanyl, morphine, ketamine, Nimbex, and propofol. Still, we are not giving up, but I'm very pissed off! I feel like they have awakened a hornet's nest in me. *He can't even open his eyes, much less breathe! I want to get him out of here!* Thank you so much for listening. Blessings to you both for coming with me."

We all left the hospital parking lot and headed to our respective homes, hoping for the best but fearing the worst.

Sunday, October 10, 2021

Today was like any other day, with nurses coming in to hang more and more bags of caustic drugs that further weakened Rob.

No matter how hard I tried, I was unable to prevent them from continuously administering a large number (and high doses) of sedatives, paralytics, antibiotics, steroids, vasodilators, anticoagulants, and anti-inflammatory drugs—all of which I knew formed a toxic brew that could severely damage his liver, kidneys, and other organs.

I received a call from my friend Paul who, as he did three days earlier, conferenced in Dr. Mei. They had continued reviewing Rob's MyChart records and were beyond concerned. Paul frantically explained. "*Sheila, He's got to get out of there! I'm telling you, they are trying to stop his heart!* They had him on 2 mg per hour of morphine when we spoke with you on October 7th. Now they have him on 9 mg per hour and 500 mcg/hour of fentanyl. Dr. Mei and I are very concerned."

I told them that I was aware of all that. However, I could only remove him from the hospital if another facility would accept the transfer of a ventilator-dependent ICU patient. Rob's only other option up to this point had been a local hospital where there was a doctor willing to accept him, yet that hospital's transfer center had refused to approve his transfer.
I suggested that we conference in my patient advocate, as I felt she would have a better grasp of how to best proceed. However, before we could get her on the line, Paul interrupted and said, "*They are killing your husband! I don't think you understand what I am telling you. They are killing your husband!*" Upon hearing that, I collapsed to the floor and loudly cried, "*I know, and I don't know what to do! WHAT DO I DO?*"

In desperation, fumbling with my phone, I conferenced in my patient advocate, Dr. Mei shared that she felt Rob was a "gold citizen." In her Chinese proverb way of thinking, that meant that Rob was worth gold to them. Thus, she suspected Dr. Wicked may not have actually submitted the transfer order to avoid having him transferred.

She said, "Rob still has significantly low albumin, and he still has clotting. I saw that in the D-dimer results. *There's so much evidence that they're ignoring what is critical, and they continue to paralyze and sedate him. So, how can you get him off the ventilator without adequate nutrition and without true caring and compassion?*"

My advocate said, "I am not in disagreement with you, Dr. Mei. My best recommendation was to have him transferred. But that didn't work out. Regarding the transfer, we have to take their word for it, okay? I have a call in to Dr. Wicked, and I'm waiting for him to call me back. I'm going to call him again, probably within the next 30 minutes, to see if he got my message."

Dr. Mei was livid. "*They are not transfusing him nor giving him erythropoietin [PROCRIT] for his severe anemia, and this is the standard of care!* **Their delay in care could cost him his life**." My advocate firmly interjected, "Doctor, I understand, okay? But here's the deal. We can demand these things, but they're also going to meet <u>their</u> criteria to order them. That's what the hematologist was saying, okay? The doctor was using those criteria."

Dr. Mei countered, "*But there is evidence they are* **not** *trying to save him*. I'm sorry. By all the evidence, and we gave them good input, *they're not listening and don't care*. Let's stick to the plan to get him out somehow. Hopefully, they can do a trach on Monday because they won't do it on the weekend. There are organizations of palliative care that take patients on vents. If necessary, that's my recommendation."

Dr. Mei continued, "I need the phone number to contact about the transfer; I want that number so I can speak to them myself and verify that they did communicate. I want to verify that it was done and that they were definitely communicating. Last but not least, I will call JCAHO, the Joint Commission on Accreditation of Healthcare Organizations. They have oversight of the hospital care management, and if they don't meet the standard, then they should be shut down."

Paul then reminded us, "Two days ago, they were giving Rob 2 mg per hour of morphine. Now they have increased it to 9 mg per hour."

Dr. Mei interjected, "Dr. Wicked is treating him for blood clotting, but the cause of those blood clots is because they gave him the remdesivir, you know, and that causes blood clotting. So, what they gave him caused the blood clots, and he has micro clots according to the D-dimer numbers. He should be given erythropoietin to increase his red blood cell count. The other choice is a blood transfusion because *he is severely anemic*. So, they have two choices, either give him blood products or give him this natural product that our body uses to tell the body to make more red blood cells.

"*Now, here's the thing, it's possible he's not making sufficient red blood cells because of the super high levels of oxygen they're giving him*. So, his body's thinking, oh, I don't need more blood cells. When you're at a high altitude, your body senses there is not enough oxygen. Guess what happens? It makes more blood cells because you need the red blood cells to carry the oxygen your body needs. *His body's confused because man is confusing it*. Also, because he has been given so many drugs, including that crazy remdesivir! It could have blocked his bone marrow from making red blood cells. But just know, in my heart, it's safe to give the erythropoietin."

I agreed, "Yes, but they kept us separate for 21 days. By that time, they had already damaged him. We're almost at 40 days with Rob in the hospital. So, that's the problem I'm having. I feel the urgency and need to make something happen, like soon, because what the doctors are doing is not working."

Dr. Mei replied, "Weaning him off morphine is the next step they should do—today! *They're keeping him paralyzed, and therefore he can't breathe for himself.* But they think that's okay; *we have a machine to breathe for you, you're paralyzed, you need a machine to breathe for you. What are they talking about? They're talking out of their butts!*

"When they paralyze you, you can't move. So can you move your lungs? Can you explain to me how paralyzing makes him breathe easier? No, the machine takes over. *They are saying that he can't come off the machine because he needs the machine. Sure, that's because they're purposely paralyzing him. He has no choice!* What are they talking about? Call their bluff. When you paralyze somebody, they can't move their legs. How can they walk? Something artificial has to walk for them. Do they think that when you're paralyzed, you walk better? How do you walk better? Something would have to walk for you artificially. *Are they stupid? Are they purposely doing this?"*

She came completely unglued. I was so sorry she had needed to return to California to care for her ailing mother. She was such a great help, but this long-distance medical advocate coaching process was hard on me. I wanted someone with strength and medical knowledge to come and take over and make things happen at Covid Coven Hospital of Plano, Texas. Dr. Mei had valiantly tried to help us make some ground during our family conference with Dr. Liar on September 27th, and it truly helped—but only a little. *I knew we needed something BIGGER to happen **now** because they were destroying the little life Rob had left.*

All I could think of to say at this point was, "I don't know. I just say forgive them if they don't know what they're doing. But if they DO know what they're doing, they are in big trouble because God sees everything!"

Dr. Mei said, "God, show them. What will happen to all the wicked people at the second coming? They will all be gone, and this earth will only have good, kind people left. This is the separation of the wheat from the tares, and they will be separated. *The goats from the sheep."* I appreciated her sentiments, yet her idea of future justice did not help me or Rob right now—and we needed help now! I said, "I don't want them to give him paralytics." She said, "Remember, you have a right of refusal <u>and</u> the right to try."

I responded, "So, I'm going to tell the doctor to wait on the paralytic." She said, "Thank you. Awesome! Tell me, how does a paralyzed person walk? How is he going to be better without being able to move his lungs?" I agreed with her, "He's already on sedation and can't even lift a finger. So how is the paralytic helping him? I've asked this question so many times, but they don't seem to hear me." She said, "He opened his eyes when they lifted the paralytic. He didn't do that before, okay?"

I said," Definitely! Every night at 7 PM, I'm scared to leave Rob. I don't trust these people at all. I hate leaving Rob in their hands at night because he's completely vulnerable. He has no way to stick up for himself. He cannot do anything. He can only lay there like a limp noodle."

LEGAL COUNSEL STATEMENT

Members of the jury, according to WebMD, 98.2% of known COVID-19 patients in the U.S. survive the disease. Thus, the overall mortality rate is only 1.8%. See https://www.webmd.com/covid/covid-recovery-overview

However, the Journal of the American Medical Association (JAMA) reported in 2019 that a cohort study of patients with COVID-19 indicated **that those who were admitted to US medical centers had an over 7.5 times higher mortality rate** of 13.6%. See https://jamanetwork.com/journals/jamanetworkopen/fullarticle/2777028

Although those admitted to hospitals generally experience more severe symptoms, we contend that the vast discrepancy in the mortality rate of those who treat Covid at **home** *vs. those who end up* **hospitalized** *is primarily because the hospitals in the United States are following "the protocol that kills."*

According to a study published in the British Medical Journal in 2016, *medical errors are the third leading cause of death in the United States*, surpassed only by heart disease and cancer. However, since the arrival of COVID-19, many doctors and legislators have suggested that anyone diagnosed with Covid *can only die of Covid*, even if they fully recovered from the virus and it was no longer in their body.

In other words, whenever someone who had fully recovered from Covid later died in the hospital, their death was *always* attributed to Covid regardless of any potential mistreatment or negligence by the medical professionals responsible for their care. This faulty logic contradicts the reality that medical errors remain America's third leading cause of death.

The State of Texas' Senate Bill 6 (SB 6), known as the "*Pandemic Liability Protection Act*," seems to substantiate that irrationality by implying doctors and hospitals may "do what they will" to "Covid" patients while being wholly sheltered from malpractice lawsuits by stating, "*a physician, health care provider, or first responder* **is not liable for an injury, including economic and noneconomic damages, or death arising from care, treatment, or failure to provide care or treatment** *relating to or impacted by a pandemic disease or a disaster declaration related to a pandemic disease.*"

The implication of the doctors and the legislators who crafted SB 6 is that once a pandemic had been declared:
- Harmful drugs (such as remdesivir)—that used to cause a wealth of dangerous and often deadly side-effects—can now NO LONGER cause any harm. "Covid" patients can, of course, only die of COVID-19.
- Overdosing Covid patients with toxic medications and damaging their lungs with high levels of oxygen and pressure on a ventilator cannot harm them because only Covid can kill them.
- Placing patients on a BiPAP when it is clearly contraindicated and likely to cause barotrauma (the rupturing of the alveoli, the air sacs of the lungs) is not a problem because such an act cannot injure a "Covid" patient since only Covid can harm patients who have been diagnosed with COVID-19.
- Locking patients away from their families and neglecting to ensure they consume adequate food and water, thus allowing them to become dehydrated and starved, can cause them NO HARM since patients who have had Covid cannot die of mistreatment or willful negligence. Only Covid can cause their deaths.
- Autoimmune drugs, such as baricitinib, which are known to potentially cause infections and fevers and weaken the immune systems of many patients, can no longer have such an effect in patients once diagnosed with Covid. Only the Covid virus can weaken and harm the patient even if it has already run its entire course.
- Placing patients on ventilators who once had a Covid diagnosis and subjecting them to over 60% FiO2 (Fraction of Inspired Oxygen) for extended periods, which would typically fry their lungs by destroying the pulmonary lining and cause irreversible, permanent, and potentially fatal damage—or using too high a PEEP (Positive End Expiratory Pressure) setting for too long a period—can no longer harm patients because patients who once had Covid can now only die of Covid.
- Ensuring formerly Covid-positive patients who are placed on ventilators are "maxed out" on sedatives, opioids, and paralytics (such as propofol, fentanyl, Nimbex, ketamine, and morphine) can also NOT harm them since only COVID-19 can harm, debilitate, and eventually kill patients who were previously diagnosed with Covid.

The belief that anyone diagnosed with Covid can ONLY die of Covid is obviously absurd and faulty reasoning.

purports to protect caregivers (**NOT patients**) while granting them (the caregivers) total immunity regardless of how they treat "Covid" patients.

This dangerous and irresponsible approach to patient care undermines the rights and well-being of those seeking medical assistance. Americans need to wake up to the fact that, with or without a pandemic, drugs and therapies prescribed by doctors remain the third leading cause of death in America.

The grueling and painful call with Paul, Dr. Mei, and my patient advocate left me exhausted and despondent. I had been advised to get Rob out of the hospital immediately, yet I had nowhere else to take him.

I could only hope and pray that tomorrow would bring better news.

Monday, October 11, 2021

As I entered Rob's room at 7:00 AM to begin another 12-hour shift of watching over him, I hoped and prayed that I would finally receive good news regarding his condition and the likelihood they would reduce his medications and *finally* begin the weaning process.

During his morning rounds, Dr. Wicked came into the room. Pointing to the hallway outside the room, I asked him, "May I please ask you something in private out there?" I wanted to leave the room in case Rob might be able to hear. "Please be honest with me and give me your candid opinion. What is the likelihood of Rob surviving this?"

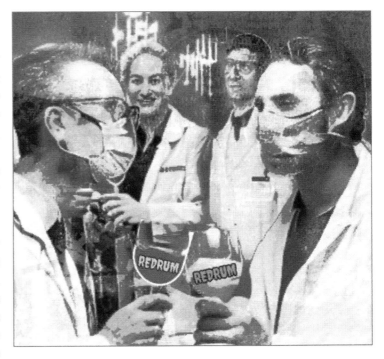

He took a deep breath, held it for a moment, then let it out with a disconcerting groan. "Three days ago, I thought he had over a 50/50 chance. *I still don't have a great handle on what all's going on, what all happened.* **We just saw it all fall off the chart with the liver and with the anemia.**" I could feel the blood draining from my face. I began to feel cold, and my knees became so weak that I could barely stand.

Nearly a month earlier, on September 15th, Dr. Wicked had told me, "So, his **LFTs** [Liver Function Tests] have been going up. . . . He has a pattern, and it is **probably medication related.** There's a couple [of medications] that are possible [causes]. The **antibiotics** are the most likely."

That same day we had discussed that Rob was clearly suffering from anemia, as evidenced by the significant decline in his hemoglobin level.

I had asked him to please STOP the toxic drugs causing Rob further injury. Yet, he had ignored my plea, saying, "We usually don't worry about stopping and changing his medications until the lab results are **more than 8 to 10 times the upper limit of normal**."

I had also asked him what they intended to do about Rob's worsening anemia. Yet, he had brushed it off with, "But what happens to everybody in the ICU over a lengthy period is that they start getting anemia. It's very expected."

Every day, I challenged their desire to give Rob additional drugs and higher doses of his existing medications, such as fentanyl and morphine, to protect his liver and kidneys from extensive damage. Two days earlier, I had asked Dr. Spite to consider giving Rob PROCRIT (erythropoietin), a hormone produced by the kidneys that stimulates the production of red blood cells, to help ward off his severe anemia. However, as was true of almost everything I asked for, I was told, "Sorry, we can't do that."

Now, Dr. Wicked was telling me Rob's liver had suffered severe damage and that his anemia was off the charts. Astonishingly, Dr. Wicked implied he did not have a handle on what was going on.

LEGAL COUNSEL STATEMENT

Members of the jury, Dr. Wicked told Sheila, "*I still don't have a great handle on what all's going on, what all happened*." However, we have a handle on "*what all happened*" and will clue you in.

Firstly, when Sheila asked Dr. Spite (a hematologist) on October 9th if he would consider giving Rob PROCRIT (a natural hormone that stimulates the bone marrow to make more red blood cells) **to address his profound anemia**, the doctor said that Rob's hemoglobin level (hemoglobin is the protein that carries oxygen in the blood) would need to drop "below seven" before he would consider administering this medication—which is a natural hormone that stimulates the bone marrow to make more red blood cells.

Rob's hemoglobin was at 7.5 grams per deciliter (g/dL) at that time. However, on the morning of October 11th, Rob's hemoglobin **plummeted to 6.1 g/dL**. According to The National Institutes of Health (NIH), a hemoglobin level of "*less than 6.5 g/dL is life-threatening and can cause death*."
Chronic anemia - statpearls - NCBI bookshelf. (n.d.). From https://www.ncbi.nlm.nih.gov/books/NBK534803

Now, his anemia had reached a life-threatening level. *As we stated earlier, we cannot say whether it was due to willful ignorance, uncaring negligence, or nefarious intent that they chose to ignore Rob's "profound anemia." But, whatever the reason, we contend that the doctors' actions and inactions during his stay at Covid Coven Hospital of Plano, Texas, were the direct cause of Robert A. Skiba II's needless death.*

Secondly, Rob had been on **heavy doses** of numerous hepatotoxic (damaging or destructive to liver cells) medications—and on what we consider a "life-limiting" vs. "lifesaving" ventilator—for a total of **33 days**. The primary components of a Liver Function Test are enzymes known as **AST** and **ALT**. The normal range for **AST** is 10 to 40 units per liter, and **ALT** is 7 to 56. Late on October 10, 2021, Rob's ALT and AST levels **rose to more than 1000 times the normal upper range**. Such levels are considered <u>critical</u>.

At 11:23 AM on October 10th, Dr. Delusion entered in Rob's hospital records, "Abrupt acute hepatitis/hepatic failure. Etiology [cause] **uncertain**." Another note stated, "**AST/ALT and ferritin acutely off the chart**." Dr. Wicked then wrote, "Unclear cause of **acute worsening**."

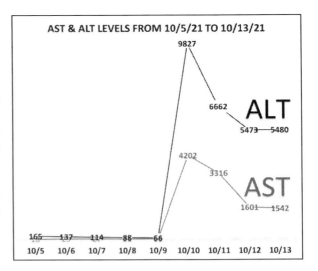

*We contend that these massive and sudden elevations of **ALT**, **AST**, and **ferritin** are due to the cumulative effects of the large quantities of medications Rob had been administered <u>nonstop</u> on a daily basis for over a month despite Sheila's continued protests and pleas for a more conservative, sane approach.*

Dr. Wicked also placed the following note in Rob's hospital records at 9:07 AM on October 11, 2021: "**ferritin** [a blood protein that contains iron] **remains acutely off the chart**." That was quite an understatement. The normal value for blood ferritin in a male is 12 to 300 nanograms per milliliter (ng/m). Rob's ferritin level rose from 2,187.1 nanograms per milliliter (ng/ml) on October 9th to **greater than 40,000** ng/mL on October 10th and 11th. This condition, known as hyperferritinemia, was a clear *"marker of cellular damage"* in the liver. Academic.oup.com. (n.d.). From https://academic.oup.com/metallomics/article/6/4/748/6015473

A gastroenterologist/hepatologist was then called to consult on Rob's condition. He noted in the hospital records, "the INR is also elevated that may be an indication that there may be underlying liver failure." INR (International Normalized Ratio) is a blood test that measures the time required for blood to form a blood clot. A high INR usually means the liver is not working as well as it should because it is not causing the blood to clot normally, which is another indication of acute liver failure.

A key hepatotoxic medication Rob was administered 12 daily doses of (from September 20, 2021, to October 1, 2021) was **baricitinib** (an anti-inflammatory medication usually prescribed for the treatment of rheumatoid arthritis, <u>which Rob did not have</u>) as an Emergency Use Authorization trial drug. UpToDate.com noted, *"Patients treated with baricitinib are at risk for developing serious infections that may lead to hospitalization or death."* UpToDate. (n.d.). From https://www.uptodate.com/contents/baricitinib-drug-information

Evidence of **baricitinib's** ability to cause liver damage can be found in the National Library of Medicine's article titled "**LiverTox: Clinical and Research Information on Drug-Induced Liver Injury**," which states, *"Monitoring of serum aminotransferase [ALT] levels is recommended for patients starting **baricitinib**. De novo elevations in serum aminotransferases [ALT] levels above five times the upper limit of normal should lead to temporary cessation. If serum enzyme elevations do not resolve or improve within a few weeks of stopping, or if symptoms of liver injury or jaundice arise, **baricitinib** should be permanently discontinued."* NCBI Bookshelf. (n.d.). From https://www.ncbi.nlm.nih.gov/books/NBK548012

As we shared previously, Medscape notes, *"Drugs are an important cause of liver injury. More than 900 drugs, toxins, and herbs have been reported to cause <u>liver injury</u>, **and drugs account for 20-40% of all instances of fulminant [severe and sudden onset] hepatic failure**. Approximately 75% of the idiosyncratic drug reactions result in liver transplantation **or death**."* Nilesh Mehta, M. D. (2022, July 8). Drug-induced hepatotoxicity. Overview, Metabolism of Drugs, Clinical and Pathological Manifestations of Drug-Induced Liver Disease. From https://emedicine.medscape.com/article/169814-overview

Unfortunately, what happened to Rob and Sheila is not an isolated incident in some obscure small-town hospital in Texas. Instead, this crime took place in the wealthiest county in Texas at one of the premier hospitals in Plano.

> *Isolating patients from their families for weeks, ignoring their directives, denying their patient rights, forcing patients on ventilators, and flooding them with toxic medications is a CRIME against patients and humanity at large.*
>
> *The doctors and nurses at Covid Coven Hospital of Plano, Texas, refused to listen to Sheila's and Rob's directives, and they did not offer conservative, life-supporting therapies which were readily available. Instead, they pushed caustic drugs and life-limiting therapies that would result in greater profits and a better bottom line in light of incentives provided by the federal government.*
>
> *As noted in the article on* **Hospitals' Incentive Payments for COVID-19** *(see Page D-2 of* **Appendix D**)*, according to Texas attorney Jerri Ward, "CMS [the Centers for Medicare and Medicaid Services] has granted 'waivers' of federal law regarding patient rights. Specifically, CMS purports to allow hospitals to violate the rights of patients or their surrogates with regard to medical record access, to have patient visitation, and to be free from seclusion." She further noted that "rights do not come from the hospital or CMS and cannot be waived, as that is the antithesis of a 'right.' The purported waivers are meant to isolate and gain total control over the patient and to deny the patient and patient's decision-maker the ability to exercise informed consent."*
>
> *How are the unwary expected to navigate the quagmire of hidden agendas, unethical policies, and deadly protocols that pad the pockets of the hospitals at the expense of the lives of patients? These government-incentivized therapies and protocols must be stopped, and patients' rights must be restored!*

Discussing the results of an ultrasound they conducted on Rob's liver, Dr. Wicked went on to explain, "There was something that changed yesterday. We looked at the liver because the only thing that usually caused the liver function tests to go up to levels like that is septic shock, but he was never low enough with his blood pressure to explain that. Clots can do that, yet all the vessels are open to his liver. I did see gallbladder sludge, but that would not explain any of this."

Trembling, I asked, "So no test is an explanation for any of this?" Taking a deeper breath, he confessed, "No. So we get into more rare things, which he definitely could have. Dr. Spite, Dr. Delusion, and I discussed it, and that's why I bumped up the steroids yesterday in case it was kind of like an autoimmune disease. The steroids are a bit of an immune suppressant. So, that's why we did that. Honestly, the way things have gone in the last 48 hours, **I don't think he's gonna survive.**"

I was crushed and totally devastated. I had feared it would come to this if they would not cease the massive, ongoing, daily assault on Rob's kidneys and liver with toxic pharmaceuticals. No matter how much I demanded that they lower the doses or, as in the case of micafungin, not even give him the harmful drug (Dr. Torture had even admitted to me on September 25, 2021, "*Sometimes it can cause some* **liver function abnormalities** *as a side effect.*")—they totally ignored my directives.

Keep in mind that when I took Rob to the Emergency Department on September 3, 2021, instead of allowing me to be with him so I could serve as his on-site advocate, they purposely locked me out for 21 days to further limit my ability to challenge the "deadly protocol" they intended on having him follow. Instead of being concerned with his medical history, they only wanted to know if he had been vaccinated, then wrote **UNVACCINATED** in bold capital letters throughout his hospital records.

Instead of honoring our directive that he NOT be given remdesivir, they managed to sneak in six doses from September 3rd to September 9th, with two being double, 200 mg "loading" doses.

him with SOLU-MEDROL, a potent steroid that can cause trouble breathing and shortness of breath and increase the risk of systemic infections.

They then gave him off-label drugs such as nitazoxanide (an antiparasitic clinical trial drug that would have required Rob's informed consent, which he had not provided) and colchicine (a drug that treats gout symptoms, which he did not have) starting on September 4, 2021, the day after his admission. Both of these drugs caused Rob nausea and diarrhea, which are common side-effects of these medications that further weakened him. They only stopped these drugs when they caused this effect, as evidenced by the "Developed diarrhea, will discontinue colchicine and nitazoxanide" note in Rob's hospital records.

In addition to causing him nausea and diarrhea, instead of ensuring Rob ordered and consumed adequate food when he had not eaten for over a week before his admission, they ignored that he was not ordering or eating meals. Thus, he was further weakened by a lack of adequate nutrition.

Instead of encouraging him that he would soon get better, they intimidated and harassed him daily and threatened that he would die if he did not agree to being placed on a ventilator.

Once they had accomplished their goal and had placed Rob on the ventilator, they subjected him to oxygen levels of up to 100% and a high PEEP (Positive End Expiratory Pressure) of 14 to 15.

In addition, despite Dr. Dead End's assurance that "We try and wake him up once a day to make certain he's awake, moving, and following all commands," they never attempted to wake him. Instead, they simply entered notes like the following in the hospital records: "Patient is not a candidate for spontaneous breathing trial due to peep of 14 and FiO2 of 95%."

At least Dr. Wicked was being honest about the massive and irreparable damage done to Rob over the past 38 days he had suffered as a victim of "the protocol." Trying to remain optimistic so I could maintain my focus on rescuing Rob from the corrupt system that appeared intent on taking his life, I innocently inquired, "Is it okay with you if I use a few drops of essential oils on Rob's hands and feet?"

He responded, "So, generally, yes. Given my philosophy, **as long as I don't think anything's harmful, I don't mind doing it.** So generally, like I said, even if I don't believe it works, **as long as it's not harming him.** The only hesitancy that I have now is that I don't know exactly what has happened in these last 48 hours. **Toxins could do this to the liver.**"

I found it ironic that he was saying I could use essential oils on Rob, "**as long as it's not harming him,**" yet they had continually bombarded him with countless drugs KNOWN to cause harm to the liver and kidneys, drugs known to significantly suppress the immune system and present the risk of serious, life-threatening infections; and drugs (Nimbex) that paralyzed his muscles and caused such severe muscle loss that he would be facing a grueling and extended recovery.

So, since he had said, "**Toxins could do this to the liver,**" I asked, "**Like Drugs?**" Stuttering and stumbling over every word, he said, "Yeah . . . usually . . . though, anything we've been giving him . . . **we went through a whole list . . . and you wouldn't expect it to be nothing, and then all of a sudden.** I don't think any of that stuff [essential oils] is going to be harmful, but we don't know how everything's going to interact. He's on so many medicines now and other non-traditional medicines, we don't know how they'll all interact."

Of course, they found nothing when they reviewed the exhaustive list of medications Rob was on because they would never implicate themselves. Yet every medical expert I consulted with had informed me that Rob was being poisoned by the massive number and high doses of medications he was being given.

I said, "At the end of October 3rd, you finally got him off Nimbex [the paralytic]. Yet on October 9th, when everything began to change for Rob, you placed him back on Nimbex. Then, his blood pressure went way high, and the alarm went off for 45 minutes while I was here. I was waiting for Nurse Deviant to come in, yet nobody came to help. His heart rate was over 130 for at least 45 minutes, which made me nervous. She was nowhere to be found, and no one was at the nurses' station."

He replied, "I went back and looked at the Nimbex on that day. That was the only thing we did that day that was different, yeah, and I thought, how did Nimbex do this?" I commented, "When Nurse Deviant finally came in, she acted as if nothing had happened. But I noticed she gave Rob labetalol, which made his blood pressure go really low and bottom out. So, I'm just thinking, all these changes could be freaking his body out!" Dr. Wicked admitted, "It definitely could. Nimbex is the only thing we did different that day. So, I went back and looked at that heavily and, like, 'Could this do it?'"

Well, the Nimbex dosage **was not** the only thing that had changed. I pointed out, "I have a list of his medications and their dosages. You were giving him 275 mcg per hour of **fentanyl** on October 3rd, then went up to 400 mcg per hour on October 4th, then 450 mcg per hour on October 5th, then 475 mcg per hour on October 6th, then maxed him out on 500 mcg per hour on October 7th? He was also placed on **morphine** on October 7th, but on October 9th, it was raised to 9 mg per hour! *I've been telling you this from day ONE. My husband has never done a drug in his life.* **To me, that's way too much!** *You made me think you were giving him the morphine to wean him from the fentanyl, but they were both doubled. So what's that about?"*

He admitted, "**They're BIG doses.** We were trying to get him in sync with the ventilator as best we could before we had to increase the paralytic." There was that excuse again; Rob needed to be in sync or "compliant" with the ventilator. Of course, I felt he would never be "compliant" with a machine that he knew was not saving his life but was draining him of the little life he had left.

I said, "But to me, I just feel like that's way too much and could be the cause of more issues." Dr. Wicked responded, "I don't want to back off any of these drugs while he's still paralyzed."

LEGAL COUNSEL STATEMENT

Members of the jury, Rob had been on a continuous IV infusion of **fentanyl** (which is 50 to 100 times more potent than morphine) since the moment he was placed on a ventilator the afternoon of September 8, 2021. Over the next few days, the dosage was titrated up to 250 to 350 mcg/hour. Then, on October 6th, it was raised to 475 mcg/hour.

On October 7th, the day Dr. Wicked advised Sheila, "I'm trying to **not** get him to wake up, but he's chewing through today's medicine at a much higher rate than I expected," he increased the **fentanyl** dosage to 500 mcg/hour and wrote this note in the hospital record: "If not making progress by end of weekend will restart paralytics to see

That same day (October 7th), a continuous IV infusion of 5 mg/hour of **morphine** was added in addition to the fentanyl. As Sheila noted above, on October 9th, the morphine dosage was increased to 9 mg/hour—resulting in Rob being on a continuous IV infusion of 500 mcg/hour of **fentanyl** combined with 9 mg/hour of **morphine**. Sheila's concern was that **fentanyl** and **morphine** are **potent opioids** that are metabolized in the liver.

Excessive doses of these two drugs alone can cause opioid-induced liver injury, as noted in an article published by the NIH that stated: "*Overdoses of the more **potent opioids** have been linked to **cases of acute liver injury**, usually **with a precipitous onset** and pattern of **acute toxicity** with **marked elevations in serum aminotransferase [ALT] levels** and **early onset of signs of hepatic failure**.*"
NCBI Bookshelf. (n.d.). From https://www.ncbi.nlm.nih.gov/books/NBK547864

Now, we see Dr. Wicked admitting to Sheila, "Honestly, the way things have gone **in the last 48 hours, I don't think he's gonna survive.**"

We contend that the massive doses of these opioids further aided in causing Rob severe and sudden liver damage. Even Arabella, the hospice nurse who had joined Sheila in the meeting with Mr. Pathetic on October 9th, had said she was appalled at the massive quantity and high dosages of drugs Rob was being administered.

I agreed with Dr. Wicked that I would not want Rob waking up paralyzed and asked, "How long is he going to be on the paralytic [Nimbex]?" He then surprised me, saying, "Let's turn it off now . . . as soon as we can titrate things down. The thing with the paralytic was to try to get him stable enough to have a trach. But now, he's not stable, and we're not doing the trach."

I questioned, "So, you will take off the paralytic now, then hopefully lower the sedatives? That would make me feel a lot better." He said, "I'm fine with that. I just don't want to do it while he's paralyzed. He's been, like, on doses that would've knocked anyone out and affect anybody. Yet he's been *floppy*; he's been moving; he opened his eyes one day."

LEGAL COUNSEL STATEMENT
Members of the jury, when Dr. Wicked said Rob had "been *floppy*" and that "he's been moving," we wonder if he might have meant Rob had a seizure. Rob was on Nimbex for 36 days—from September 8, 2021, through October 3, 2021. They then re-started the Nimbex on October 9, 2021, **the day everything went haywire**.

Nimbex is another of the many hepatotoxic medications Rob was being administered. The HepatologyAdvisor website notes that Nimbex's "*Warnings/Precautions*" include "***Renal [kidney] or hepatic [liver] impairment***" and an "***increased risk of seizures***."
Nimbex. Hematology Advisor. (n.d.). From https://www.hematologyadvisor.com/drug/nimbex

I said, "I have been praying that the drugs neutralize." He responded, "There's a lot of stuff happening in the universe that I can't explain. Whether it's God or the ether, I don't know."

Turning to a nurse who had just walked in, he said, "Let's hold off on the Lovenox [an anticoagulant] today and see which way the platelets go because they went down to 170. And then Nimbex [the paralytic], let's turn that off and see if we can come down on the sedations for a couple of hours." He then looked at me. "Yeah, and the point again, the point of Nimbex was we tried to get him stable enough for a trach earlier this week. But that is not happening."

Trying to remain positive, I said, "Yeah, we hit a little bump in the road. So, this will give us time to figure out what the liver problems are."

He followed with, "And take as much of the drugs off as we can. About his kidneys, we backed off the Lasix two days ago. I'm gonna have Dr. Ruthless see him, he is the kidney doctor, and just in case those keep getting worse, he'll be on the case already. So he'll be by and see him today. I don't think he needs any special kidney things right now, although his kidney numbers bumped a little bit, just with everything else going on.

"We'll do the erythropoietin [PROCRIT], although I don't think it will work. If it works, it will work quickly, but I don't expect it to work within a day. So first, Nimbex off, and we'll see if we can come down on the fentanyl. But I don't want to back off the fentanyl while Nimbex is on board . . . and his oxygen saturation is better." In his usually cheerful manner, he ended with a chuckle. However, there was nothing funny about Rob's condition.

Rob's oxygen saturation (blood oxygen) level improved whenever they lowered the drugs. So, I said, "Yes, that was great. If a miracle happens and the FiO2 can go down to 50%. and his blood oxygen level stays at 95%, then you could still do the trach?" He nodded. "Yes. We need to get him stable just to do it." He then headed for the door, saying, "Okay, see you later. I'll put all this in the computer."

As I stood there lost in thought, Dr. Ruthless, the nephrologist I had met briefly on October 8th, walked into the room. He commented on how pleasant the scent of lavender was that I had just rubbed on Rob's hands while mentioning that his wife enjoyed using essential oils. Then, he said, "Okay, so Dr. Wicked asked me to see Rob because of kidney function. It looks like two days ago, it was normal, and starting on October 9th, his creatinine started to go up.

"Creatinine is a blood test that we use to see how the kidneys are working, and it was good at first. Generally speaking, a normal creatine is about 0.8. It's starting to go up, and it's now 1.5. When not taken by itself, it is not alarming. But the concern is that the urine output has also decreased. So, when I look back at this, as far as I can tell, on the 9th, his blood pressures were low in the 60s and 70s. And his heart rate was rapid; it was in the 130s."

I interrupted and said, "That was right after they restarted the Nimbex. I keep track of everything. And I noticed that once they gave him Nimbex again, his heart rate shot up. So, you know, I'm asking if they can just kind of cut back on all the drugs! This guy has never done a drug in his life. He's the cleanest person you could ever imagine."

Dr. Ruthless said, "Yeah, I don't think this would have anything to do with drugs. I never expected that. This is because Covid causes kidney failure, oh, and the need to be permanently on dialysis." So I thought, "*Why isn't he being dialyzed now, then? What's with the delay?*"

I commented, "Well, he had rejected remdesivir, and I don't know what happened. He and I made a pact before he got sick that if we were ever in this position of needing hospital care, we would reject remdesivir and the ventilator because we had done the research on it. I don't know what happened. He was bullied, and he got scared or something—and he ended up having 800 mg of remdesivir over six doses. Could that be what caused the kidney issue?" He hesitated and said, "At this point, it's . . . that's uh, uh, kind of uh . . ." I interrupted and said, "So that could have been part of it!"

He would not say. Ignoring my sharing with him that Rob had been given a total of 800 mg of remdesivir, he switched back to the issue at hand, saying, "His blood pressure and heart rate look a lot better. In fact, after that night [October 9th], it looks like his vitals have stabilized. But what happens when the blood pressure is low, and the heart rate is too rapid is the kidneys don't get the blood flow they're used to getting, and they sort of starve for oxygen—hypoxia for the kidneys—and that unfortunately causes kidney damage.

"The fact that his kidneys were normal up until then improves the odds that his **kidney failure** could be temporary. But sometimes it can take days or weeks, or even a month or two until they recover—and in some cases, they don't recover. Unfortunately, that seems to be normal when it comes to Covid. It's about 50/50 with the kidneys. So, he doesn't currently need dialysis. But if this continues, he will. Are you familiar with it?"

Dr. Wicked had said he did not think Rob would survive at this point. So, if Rob had little chance of survival, why would Dr. Ruthless say his kidneys were not yet bad enough to require dialysis—especially when he was not producing any urine, and his body was already swelling? In addition, why would he attribute every kidney injury experienced by Covid patients to Covid itself when Rob had overcome the disease weeks prior and not to nephrotoxic drugs such as remdesivir, micafungin, fentanyl, morphine, midazolam, Nimbex, and Levophed—all of which were being administered to Rob.

Being very concerned about Rob's profound anemia since soon after his hospitalization, I said, "Rob's very anemic, and I've been looking at his hemoglobin numbers. We don't believe in blood transfusions, so we asked for PROCRIT. I know it takes longer to get into his system than a transfusion, but I begged for it because his hemoglobin numbers were so low. Although Dr. Wicked just said he would approve it and, finally, administer it, Dr. Spite, the hematologist, had told me he would not approve Rob's receiving it until his hemoglobin was lower than 7. Now his hemoglobin level is at 6.1. Could the delay have anything to do with the kidney damage?"

He quickly and resolutely said, "No. For people who have, like, stage four chronic kidney disease or people who are on dialysis, PROCRIT works because the kidneys are not making erythropoietin, you know, because it's something that the kidneys produce normally. I would have to ask Dr. Spite. I think if Dr. Spite felt that PROCRIT would help, he would definitely have added it because he uses it pretty often."

I said, "At least Rob will finally be on it. But I've been advised that it doesn't quite work as quickly as blood transfusions." He replied, "Right. It usually takes, you know, from my experience using it on kidney failure patients, typically about maybe three or four days for the hemoglobin to start coming up. So, on the anemia thing, I'll sort of defer to Dr. Spite because he's the expert. So, you know, we'll take it day by day, right?

"In the next 24 hours, if he's still not making any urine, then we're probably going to have to dialyze him because of the fluid overload because, you know, he's already requiring the ventilator at 75% FiO2 (oxygen concentration), and he has all these drips going in. There's a lot going in and not a lot coming out. So, he has swelling and fluid retention, which you can tell.

"I'm going to check a few urine studies, you know, just to rule out other things that may have caused the damage—maybe check an ultrasound of the kidneys, okay, if he hasn't had any imaging of the kidneys lately. Sometimes when they do the CT scan, they'll include the kidneys.

"They did see the gallbladder had some sludge. So, I don't know if that CT scan caught the kidneys, but I will do the urine studies." I asked, "And what do you look for in the urine?" He said, "Basically, the urine sodium, the urine creatinine, okay? We want to see if the kidneys are doing anything to reabsorb sodium or not."

I shared, "Yeah, see, the doctors have been amazed at how fast his body was pumping out the stuff [all the drugs]. I've been saying this since day one. We've been here 38 days, and he's been on too many drugs. I mean, he's on 500 mcg per hour of fentanyl and 9 mg per hour of morphine. He's on 40 mcg per kg per minute of ketamine, and he's on a bunch of antibiotics. I mean, that's a lot for anyone, especially someone who's never had any drugs like this in his body before."

Regarding the benefits of dialysis, he said, "So, dialysis is almost like a crutch for the kidneys. It doesn't help or hurt the kidneys. All it does is that it removes the toxins, and it keeps the person from dying." Still convinced that the non-stop assault of high doses of numerous medications had caused his kidney and liver failure, I asked, "So, you don't think that the drugs are the cause of his injury?" He contended, "No. The dialysis will detox him from the toxins that have led to his kidney failure. I think the cause is from the rapid heart rate, regardless of what caused that."

Once again, a licensed physician was trying to sweep Rob's being overdosed with multiple drugs over an extended period under the rug. Actually, every doctor, each of whose livelihood depended on pushing pharmaceuticals, had flatly denied that the massive quantities of drugs were in any way toxic to the body—yet they were the very toxins that I was confident had caused Rob's low blood pressure and rapid heart rate to begin with. Moreover, they were the very "toxins" that had severely damaged his liver.

He continued, "Now that his blood pressure and heart rate are stabilized, the period of kidney irritation is over, and then we just have to wait for the kidneys to recover—and they pretty much do that on their own. We just have to kind of support him through this, right, so the kidneys can wake up and start working again."

I replied, "Okay. Let me get this right. You said you are going to wait 24 hours to see if there is any urine output?" He confirmed, "Right now, there's no urgent indication for dialysis, and dialysis is a procedure with potential complications."

Despite Dr. Ruthless' assurances, the non-stop administration of massive numbers of caustic drugs was still underway, and the all-out attack on Rob's kidneys and liver **had not ceased**. Thus, his "kidney irritation" and liver toxicity were far from over. Then again, what else was I to expect from a group of "*medical professionals*" who believed drugs were always "*the answer*" for any symptom or disease and that pharmaceuticals could never be "*the cause*" of harm to a patient? These same "*professionals*" also believed a "Covid" patient could ONLY be weakened by and die of "Covid"—regardless of their having overcome the illness weeks earlier.

At 7:00 PM, when visitors' hours were over, I drove home feeling devastated by the day's news. First, Dr. Wicked had revealed, "***We just saw it all fall off the chart with the liver and with the anemia.***" Then, he admitted he believed Rob had slim odds of leaving the hospital alive, confessing, "**I don't think he's gonna survive.**" Finally, Dr. Ruthless had said Rob was now suffering from "kidney failure," and if his kidneys continued to decline, he might "need to be permanently on dialysis."

Every day, and each step of the way, the doctors and nurses at Covid Coven Hospital of Plano, Texas, had discounted and ignored Rob's and my directives and insisted that he follow their "full protocol," a protocol that included starvation, over-oxygenation, intubation, ventilation, over-medication, and (I now feared) very likely, termination—because Rob's liver and kidneys were rapidly failing and his anemia was totally "off the chart."

Stanley Lawrence Crouch, an American poet, music and cultural critic, syndicated columnist, novelist, and biographer, once said, "*When people conclude that all is futile, then the absurd becomes the norm.*" After over a month of daily conversations with the doctors and nurses, it was clear they saw trying to save a "Covid" patient, especially one who had not been vaccinated, as a relatively futile effort. Thus, their "*absurd*" actions driven by an unyielding "protocol" had become "*the norm.*"

A Modern-Day Dr. Mengele

A modern-day Dr. Mengele, with no mercy to spare
In ICU rooms, he lingers, a monster beyond compare
With hissing ventilators, and upside-down beds
He creates a death camp where the sick and dying are led

He experiments on the helpless with a cruel and heartless hand
Ignoring their pain, ignoring their cries, tearing lives apart with his plan
A monster in disguise, a predator in white
His evil deeds, a stain on the world, a terror in sight

But still, we fight; we resist his hold
For our lives are precious, our stories untold
And in the face of evil, we will not back down
For our will is strong, and our spirit is sound

We rise up with a voice that is true
And we fight for life with all we can do
For we will not be silenced, and we will not cave in
We will live on with hope — to his chagrin.

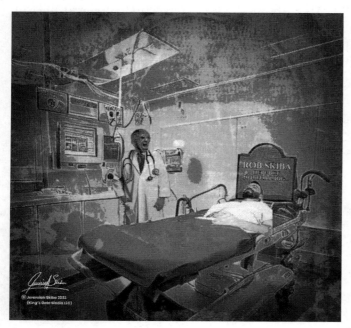

At the start of the day, I sat by Rob's bed, listening to the unnatural sounds of the ventilator breathing—forcing air in and drawing air out. There was nothing comforting in that sound. Instead, it taunted me as if on each inhalation and exhalation, it was saying, "I have . . . your husband . . . I'll never . . . let him go . . . he's going . . . to die."

Dr. Delusion then slithered into the room, "All right, so . . . from an infection standpoint, he had developed a fever a few days ago, and we had broadened his antibiotic. I sent another culture from his lungs to the lab. It's not growing anything so far. So, that's a good thing. He had developed a fever, but now that is better, and he did not have anything going on bad in his belly from the CT scan."

I had learned weeks earlier from Dr. Torture that Rob's fevers—since his cultures usually came back negative—were often what they call "drug fevers." If his fevers were often drug-related, why did they insist on compromising his immune system with even more antibiotics? To me, their "*drugs on top of drugs to combat the effect of drugs*" methodology was a clear example of the absurd becoming normal.

LEGAL COUNSEL STATEMENT
Members of the jury, Rob spent 17 days on Zithromax (azithromycin). During 12 of those days, he was also on Maxipime (cefepime). Both are broad-spectrum antibiotics. Then, on September 24, 2021, Dr. Torture wrote in Rob's hospital records: "Will stop antibiotics today, this will be 14 days. It is possible that part of his fevers also drug fever from the antibiotics hence will see the response." Below is a snapshot of the actual note.

> **Will stop antibiotics today, this will be 14 days.**
> **It is possible that part of his fevers also drug fever from the antibiotics hence will see the response.**

In their report on a "*Clinical study of drug fever induced by parenteral administration of antibiotics*," the National Institutes of Health noted, "*The most common feature of drug fever induced **by the use of an antibiotic** was as follows: A low-grade fever at the time of onset is followed by a high and remittent fever. The highest diurnal body temperature rises gradually, and then the fever subsides promptly after cessation of the causative antibiotic. The fever of this type accounted for 70% of all the drug fever in this study.*"
M. O. K. O. K. W. A. M. (n.d.). Clinical study of drug fever induced by parenteral administration of antibiotics. The Tohoku journal of experimental medicine. From https://pubmed.ncbi.nlm.nih.gov/2815075

In the "*Drugs & Therapy Bulletin*" published in June 2011 by Shands Hospital at the University of Florida in a "*The truth about drug fever*" article, they noted, "*In the hospitalized patient, the most common presentation for drug fever is a patient with a resolving infection, on **antimicrobial therapy**, and after initial defervescence. Fever in this patient can result in the over-utilization of antimicrobials and the addition of agents to treat an infection that is not present. This could potentially cause more adverse effects and further contribute to antimicrobial resistance. . .*"

"*A review of drug fever during antibiotic administration* was performed in a University hospital in Japan during the late 1980s. In their study, they found that 13% of patients (51 of 390) being treated with antibiotics for respiratory infections for more than 7 days developed a fever of 37.5°C (99.5°F). It was found that 49 of the 56 episodes of fever were greater than or equal to 38°C (100.4°F) and they were all unrelated to a true infectious process."
Volume 25, Number 6 June 2011 drugs & therapy - UF health, university ... (n.d.). From https://professionals.ufhealth.org/files/2011/11/0611-drugs-therapy-bulletin.pdf

In 1981, the Journal of the American Medical Association (JAMA) noted, "*Failure to diagnose **drug fever** may lead to **inappropriate and potentially harmful diagnostic and therapeutic interventions**.*"
Jama Network. (n.d.). From https://jamanetwork.com/journals/jama/article-abstract/373897

On October 11, 2021, Rob was now on Merrem (meropenem), a broad-spectrum antibiotic, and Mycamine (micafungin), an antifungal—for which "*fever*" is a commonly reported side effect, according to Drugs.com.
Micafungin side effects: Common, severe, long term. Drugs.com. (n.d.). From https://www.drugs.com/sfx/micafungin-side-effects.html

*There is no doubt Rob was regularly subjected to a barrage of "**inappropriate and potentially harmful diagnostic and therapeutic interventions**" that contributed to his needless death.*

So I asked, "Could it be one of his antibiotics causing these fevers? I'm asking because Dr. Torture previously wrote in his record that he could be suffering from 'drug related' fevers?" He promptly replied, "It's NOT. **It's not the antibiotics, okay,** because I didn't change anything he's on.

"Yeah, he's on the antifungal micafungin and on meropenem [a broad-spectrum antibiotic]. And, you know, even the meropenem, if his cultures that we repeated stay negative, I'm going to cut him back to what he was on before we broadened it out. And, you know, the Rocephin [another broad-spectrum antibiotic that Rob had been on October 4th through October 7th] should also be done. My plan was to go until the 14th."

After telling me Rob's blood cultures had come back negative, he—like all the other doctors—wanted to keep pumping Rob full of more and more antibiotics. How was he expected to survive such a full-on assault?

Realizing he would not listen to reason regarding the antibiotics—none of the doctors would—I brought up that Rob was profoundly anemic and that this life-threatening condition needed to be addressed. He responded, "You know, I don't know if that anemia would directly correlate with his current infection, *but anemia makes him, you know, less likely to heal.*" I yelled, "Exactly!"

Dr. Delusion continued, "His white blood cell count is 29. His CRP is 10, and it was 8 one day ago. So, that's very nonspecific. So, what I'm going to do is . . . I think my suspicion is since we didn't find any infection to explain the white blood cell count being so high and we're trying to treat for pneumonia . . . sometimes when people are sick that long, their bone marrow starts producing the white blood cells."

I suggested, "Vitamin C can increase your white blood cell count. At least, that's what I've been reading. At my request, he has been on 1,500 mg of vitamin C every 12 hours since September 28th." He argued, "From what I see, I don't see a correlation. But what I'm telling you is that the bone marrow is probably in hyperdrive trying to produce white blood cells because he's stressed out from all this illness."

"True, he has been here almost forty days," I said. Then, in a rush to leave, he hurriedly said, "So, you know, I think that may be the reason; I will touch base with you again tomorrow."

As Dr. Delusion headed out, Dr. Ruthless walked into the room and said, "I know you were talking to Dr. Wicked yesterday. Do you have any questions about the kidney failure or about dialysis?" I replied, "I never understood what's going on with his kidneys. He was producing a lot of urine, and then all of a sudden, it stopped. So, I don't know what caused that."

He cleared his throat and asserted, "Well, like I said yesterday, what caused that is the shock that he's in, and how on October 9th, his blood pressure was low in the 60s and 70s, and his heart rate was like 130s and 140s. That's bad for the kidneys, and that's what set off the chain of events and has caused the kidneys to shut down because it 'killed off' the tubules inside the kidneys. This is called ATN, or acute tubular necrosis."

I looked at him with dismay and protested, "**They KEEP giving him all these drugs, and his body is NOT used to these drugs!**" With a wave of his hand, he said, "It was shock connected to Covid." Once again, one of Rob's "caregivers" was attempting to convince me that every issue Rob faced was undoubtedly, and conveniently "connected to Covid," a condition Rob had recovered from over one month prior.

I was sick and tired of doctors refusing to take responsibility for the injuries they (not Covid) had caused with their own prescribed therapies (such as the 4.5 hours Rob had been subjected to on a contraindicated BiPAP followed by continually high expiratory pressure and non-stop over-oxygenation on the ventilator) and the non-stop heavy doses of high-powered medications.

I queried, "Have you done any tests to know for sure?" Looking surprised, he asked, "What kind of test?" I said, "Kidney function tests." Trying to assure me, he said, "Well, he's having daily kidney tests. What we look at is a test called creatinine. That one was normal, but then over the last few days, it's gone up, and it is bad because when the creatinine goes up, it means that the kidney functions go down. So that and the urine, those two things, and also along with the creatinine, we look at the electrolytes and the chemistry of the blood. Basically, we look at whether or not his blood has too much acidity because of the kidney failure.

"We look at whether his potassium is building up high. We look at the blood urea nitrogen, which is one of the toxins that the body normally produces. It's a toxin that all organisms produce. That's why we have kidneys to filter that out because it's a metabolic byproduct that is toxic if it stays in the body. So that's why people have kidney failure and get sick because urea and several other toxins build up in the body. *They cause complications up to and including death.*"

I said, "He was putting out so much urine before, then suddenly, it stopped. Then, on October 9th, I remember his heart rate went up to 130, the nurse gave him a drug, and his blood pressure went down. I knew this was hurting Rob. As I said, he's never done drugs in his life." Dr. Ruthless insisted, *"But this has nothing to do with drugs. It doesn't because it's related to Covid. It's not related to whether he did drugs or not."*

I insisted, "**He doesn't <u>have</u> Covid! He hasn't had Covid for WEEKS.**" He shot back loudly, *"Covid causes kidney failure, and being in shock like he was with low blood pressure causes this,*

How could he possibly contend that the continual, daily onslaught of high doses of a massive number of medications could **not** affect his kidneys or liver? Drugs kill people every day, and drug overdoses happen in hospitals on a regular basis.

LEGAL COUNSEL STATEMENT

Members of the jury, a National Institutes of Health (NIH) article titled "*What Do We Know about Opioids and the Kidney?*" published January 22, 2017, noted that "*it has been noted **that renal blood flow was lower with the opioid fentanyl** when compared to other anesthetics like ketamine.*"

They also stated, "*Among anesthetic agents, it has been noted that **morphine** and **fentanyl** decrease GFR [the glomerular filtration rate (GFR) that indicates how well the kidneys are filtering] and **urine output** . . . .*" and that "*Clinically, **opioids** can result in **AKI [Acute Kidney Injury]** from changes in GFR, dehydration, rhabdomyolysis [the breakdown of skeletal muscle fibers and leakage of muscle contents into the circulation that can damage the heart and kidneys and cause permanent disability or even death] and **urinary retention**.*"
Mallappallil, M., Sabu, J., Friedman, E. A., & Salifu, M. (2017, January 22). What do we know about opioids and the kidney? International journal of molecular sciences. From https://www.ncbi.nlm.nih.gov/pmc/articles/PMC5297852

As you read earlier, Rob had been maxed out on 500 mcg per hour of **fentanyl** and 9 mg per hour of **morphine** beginning October 9, 2021. Then, two days later, on October 11th, Dr. Wicked stated, "Honestly, the way things have gone in the last 48 hours, I don't think he's gonna survive."

In addition, the antibiotic **vancomycin**, which Rob was administered six doses of October 1st through October 4th, "*is a known cause of acute kidney injury*" and "*VA-AKI [Vancomycin-Associated Acute Kidney Injury] has been associated with increased in-hospital mortality.*"
Patel, N., Stornelli, N., Sangiovanni, R. J., Huang, D. B., & Lodise, T. P. (2020, September 21). Effect of vancomycin-associated acute kidney injury on incidence of 30-day readmissions among hospitalized Veterans Affairs patients with skin and skin structure infections. Antimicrobial agents and chemotherapy. From https://www.ncbi.nlm.nih.gov/pmc/articles/PMC7508587

Furthermore, it is known that "*Although there is a low rate of renal toxicity with modest doses, **vancomycin** reduces the threshold for kidney injury while using other agents with potential nephrotoxicity.*"
Bamgbola, O. (2016, June). Review of vancomycin-induced renal toxicity: An update. Therapeutic advances in endocrinology and metabolism. From https://www.ncbi.nlm.nih.gov/pmc/articles/PMC4892398

*We contend that the massive doses of **fentanyl** and **morphine**, possibly aided by the previous administration of **vancomycin**, further assisted in causing Rob's severe and sudden kidney injury—a contention Dr. Ruthless attempted to flatly deny because the doctors at Covid Coven Hospital of Plano, Texas, were unwilling to accept responsibility for their willful ignorance or uncaring negligence (or worse yet, nefarious intent) that directly led to Rob's death.*

I replied, "It's been so stressful with all these drugs being given to Rob every single day. I'm going to be praying over him today. There are a lot of people praying, and, you know, we'll see what happens tomorrow." Calming a bit, Dr. Ruthless said, "Yeah, currently, there's nothing that says we have to do dialysis because despite the urine output being low and despite the creatinine going up, it's up now to about 2.1."

Rob had had no urine output for several days, and his body was swelling. Yet Dr. Ruthless was still saying that Rob did not need dialysis. Although I did not like the idea of dialyzing him, the alternative was to watch him be poisoned—not only by the drugs that now had no way to get out of his system but also by his own metabolic wastes. Drugs by the IV bagful were still being hung one after another and flooding Rob's body with excess fluids. If he could not release the fluids, the fluid overload would cause him even more harm.

So, I said, "I would rather just help him by letting his body rest from all these IVs." He said, "His potassium is okay if his blood is not too acidic. *So, there's really nothing urgent to do.* The minute that changes, then I'll be the first one to say, 'Okay, now we absolutely have to do dialysis, or *he might die of kidney failure.*' We're not yet at that point, so I think waiting another 24 hours is fine."

Rob had clearly fallen through the ICU cracks, which had only widened since his arrival—cracks that had already swallowed up thousands of other patients across America. Yet, at the same time, the doctors and the hospital had no remorse, soul, heart, nor sense of responsibility because "Covid" was a big cash grab for them.

> **LEGAL COUNSEL STATEMENT**
> Members of the jury, we believe Rob's fluid overload should have been more aggressively addressed.
>
> A "*Fluid accumulation, survival and recovery of kidney function in critically ill patients with acute kidney injury*" article published in Kidney International, Volume 76, Issue 4, 2 August 2009, Pages 422-427, noted: "*Patients who remained with fluid accumulation during their hospitalization had a higher mortality rate that was proportional to the degree of fluid accumulation. There was an incremental increase in mortality in patients with a higher proportion of days with fluid overload after AKI [Acute Kidney Injury] diagnosis.*"
> Josée Bouchard; Fluid accumulation is associated with adverse outcomes in critically ill patients. Here. (2009, May 13). Fluid accumulation, survival and recovery of kidney function in critically ill patients with Acute Kidney Injury. Kidney International. From https://www.sciencedirect.com/science/article/pii/S0085253815539756
>
> Furthermore, in March 2018, the National Institutes of Health (NIH) published an article titled "*Iatrogenesis: A review on nature, extent, and distribution of healthcare hazards.*" In that article, they noted:
> "*A study conducted by the WHO [World Health Organization] concluded that **per capita medication usage was highest in the USA** which exceeded Latin America and even Europe. The report, compiled by (Life Extension Magazine) LEF estimates that **every year in the USA, 2.2 million people experience ADRs [Adverse Drug Reactions]** and **the death due to ADRs is 783,936**. Although the USA spends 14% of its gross national product on healthcare yet, it is ironical that **the American Medical System contributes to most of the deaths. The government-sanctioned medicine in the USA alone is responsible for 700,000 deaths every year.**"*
> Peer, R. F., & Shabir, N. (2018). Iatrogenesis: A review on nature, extent, and distribution of healthcare hazards. Journal of family medicine and primary care. From https://www.ncbi.nlm.nih.gov/pmc/articles/PMC6060929
>
> *As stated previously, we contend that Rob's death was iatrogenic. That is, the proximal cause of his death was the medications and treatments prescribed by his doctors.*

When I arrived home, I called the patient advocate I had hired to aid me in more effectively communicating with the doctors. She informed me that she had been able to get in touch with Dr. Richard Bartlett in Odessa, TX—the Emergency Department physician who had used adequate doses of budesonide to save the lives of numerous Covid patients.

When Dr. Bartlett learned of Rob's current condition and the levels of budesonide he was receiving, he told her that Rob's dosage of budesonide—which they had started at only one small 0.5 mg dose per day on September 9th to appease me and which at my insistence they had finally increased to twice per day on October 5th—needed to be increased to 1 mg every 4 hours for it to be truly effective because he was currently receiving "*a sub-optimal dose.*"

Dr. Bartlett also told her, "*He is not a 'Covid' patient now. He's an ARDS [Acute Respiratory Distress Syndrome] patient. The cytokines from the lung lining are causing the problem with his other organs. So when you do the 1 mg. every 4 hours, it will shut down the cytokines, improve the blood oxygen level, and stop the production of scar tissue in the lungs.*"

I reminded her, "We asked Dr. Liar to increase the budesonide dosage when we had the to talk with Dr. Wicked in the morning. I don't really care what his opinion is. He is a practicing doctor, and his duty is to do all the treatment options he can. He needs to increase the dose and frequency of the budesonide and ensure that Rob is being turned from side to side every two hours. We've got to move his lungs to help get them cleared of the cytokines. We've also got to wake him up more so he can be coughing more, as the sputum has got to be coming up. They're going to need to turn him and move him."

I pointed out, "They're not really turning him. All they're doing is pulling him up and putting two pillows under him. I wish you would come down there and show them how to do it. Can you come to the hospital and talk with Dr. Wicked in person in the morning?"

She replied, "Yea, I can do that. I can come down there in the morning. We've got to start being aggressive about **not** using a paralytic and sedation if at all possible because we've got to wake him up a little bit. We've got to activate his lungs to shut down the cytokine storm."

I thought we needed to be aggressive from the moment I hired her as my patient advocate 17 days earlier. Instead, she chose to play sweet patty-cake with the doctors and nurses while telling me we needed to play nice and not offend them. However, playing nice was allowing precious life-saving time to pass through our fingers. Unfortunately, she had waited to "start being aggressive" WAY TO LATE.

Glad to see she was finally in the game, I agreed, "If they tried that, like you said, for 24 hours, I think we'd see a huge improvement. The question is, does he want Rob to live, or has he just given up?"

We agreed to meet just before 7:00 AM in the small meeting room down the hall from the ICU where we had held the intervention meeting with Dr. Liar on September 27th since that room was not normally occupied. I would head into Rob's room in the ICU at 7:00 AM at the start of visitors' hours. Then, when Dr. Wicked arrived, as he usually did between 7:30 AM and 8:00 AM, I would ask him to meet with us to discuss our concerns and requests.

Wednesday, October 13, 2021

19th-century Scottish minister, Robert Murray M'Cheyne, said, "*The sea ebbs and flows, but the Rock remains unmoved.*" Standing on the rock of my salvation, I hoped that today would result in changes to Rob's plan of care that would allow him to be weaned off the ventilator that was holding him captive so that he could begin what would be a long and arduous recovery.

As planned, I met with my patient advocate just before 7:00 AM in the small meeting room down the hall from the ICU. She advised me not to worry, as she would help me reason with Dr. Wicked on appropriately adjusting Rob's plan of care, as we had discussed the evening before. I then headed into Rob's ICU room to await Dr. Wicked's arrival.

I was shocked at my terribly swollen husband's appearance. It was significantly worse than the previous day. His body was so bloated that it reminded me of white, water-filled gloves. His urine bag hung limp and empty on the side of his bed, indicating his kidneys were still not functioning.

Despite the grim circumstances, I started the day playing and singing to uplifting praise and worship music. I noticed Rob's FiO2 (oxygen concentration) was set at 95% and wondered why it was again set so high.

Dr. Ruthless, the nephrologist, showed up shortly after my arrival. When I asked him if he had seen the results of Rob's latest blood tests, he responded, "So, his creatinine is 2.6 today, and the blood urea nitrogen is 84. Urine output, of course, is still close to nothing."

Since my patient advocate was waiting around the corner to speak with Dr. Wicked, I asked Dr. Ruthless if he would be willing to meet with us for a few minutes so we could gain a better understanding of his plan of action. When I informed him that we also wanted to speak with Dr. Wicked, he said he would let him know, and since Dr. Wicked had yet to arrive, he would be happy to meet with us first.

He followed me to the meeting room and said, "I'm the kidney doctor." My patient advocate then introduced herself, letting him know she was working for me to aid me in advocating for Rob. She also advised him that she had a medical background.

He advised us, "His creatinine is 2.6 today, and the blood urea nitrogen is 84. The urine output is negligible, and he's requiring higher oxygen on the ventilator. The potassium is okay. He has fluid overload which is increasing his oxygen requirement, and he probably has fluid in his lungs now from the kidney failure. So, the FiO2 is up to 95%.

"So I think we need to do dialysis. That's my recommendation. In his case, we'd need to do Continuous Renal Replacement Therapy [CRRT]. That's continuous dialysis. It's a slow 24/7 dialysis that is done at the bedside because he's too sick to tolerate the regular kind of dialysis which could cause the vital signs to get unstable."

Since Rob's kidneys and liver began to deteriorate significantly on October 9th, I wondered why they waited so long to address the situation. My advocate asked, "How many patients have you recently been putting on continuous dialysis?" He responded, "Too many, unfortunately, because of the pandemic." She then asked, "What are your outcomes with continuous dialysis?" He said, "Well, the dialysis works. It does its job. But the outcomes, unfortunately, are not good because of the Covid."

She argued, "Well, it's not Covid that he's dealing with. It's not. He's got inflammation caused by Acute Respiratory Distress Syndrome. That's really what's happening. He's been in here for 40 days." Dr. Ruthless asserted, "These are all long-term complications of Covid."

Like every other physician at Covid Coven Hospital in Plano, Texas, he enthusiastically attributed every "complication" to Covid. It was their standard CYA tactic—even when a "complication" or injury had actually been caused by negligent or malicious starvation, massive quantities of pharmaceuticals and their damaging side effects, toxic levels of oxygen (which today was at 95% and later peaked at 100%) over extended periods, or the continued high levels of residual expiratory pressure (PEEP) set on the ventilator.

She responded, "We understand. But he's got inflammation that's impacting his other organs. You're saying for those on continuous dialysis the outcomes are poor." The best he could offer was, "They die without it. There are possible **risks** that you should be aware of. One of the risks is related to **the line placement** because to put someone on dialysis, he needs a catheter, and that's a central line placement."

LEGAL COUNSEL STATEMENT
Members of the jury, a "central line" is a special type of catheter that is inserted into a large vein in the body, usually located in the neck, chest, or groin. The line is advanced until it reaches a larger vein close to the heart. Central lines are significantly more invasive than peripheral IVs and carry a heightened risk of complications such as bleeding, infection, or damage to surrounding organs and tissues. Therefore, they must be placed with extreme care and regularly monitored.

An article in the July-Sept 2015 issue of the "International Journal of Critical Illness & Injury Science" noted, "***Immediate complications*** *related to central venous access include vascular, cardiac, pulmonary, and placement complications.* ***These immediate complications are related to technique at the time of procedure.*** *Recognition and management of immediate complications is paramount as they can often quickly become life-threatening.* ***Overall, number of unsuccessful insertion attempts is the biggest predictor of complications.***"
Central line complications Kornbau C, Lee KC, Hughes GD, Firstenberg MS ... (n.d.). From
https://www.ijciis.org/article.asp?issn=2229-5151;year=2015;volume=5;issue=3;spage=170;epage=178;aulast=Kornbau

As you will soon see, Rob appears to have suffered from an "immediate complication" of the insertion of the central line for his planned continuous dialysis.

Dr. Ruthless continued, "He has a lot going on right now. He's very sick. He's on a ventilator. He has a very high white blood cell count. He has anemia that keeps reoccurring. Now in kidney failure. Kidney failure adds to the mortality. So, a person's mortality, Covid or not, with all these complications, is high. Not doing dialysis and a person with kidney failure who needs dialysis is 100% mortality. So those are basically the choices."

I had no choice but to approve the dialysis because Rob would die from kidney failure without it. He continued, "With this type of dialysis, because it's continuous, they have to bring in another machine into the room that he'll be on for 24 hours, 24/7, for as long as he needs it. The goal in these patients is that as they get their blood cleaned and the toxins removed, and the urea lowered with the machine. Then we aim to eventually switch them to the regular type of dialysis, which can be done daily, or every other day depending. We basically do it on an as-needed basis, depending on how his labs look, how the urine output looks, how he's doing on the ventilator, and all along that time, we're watching for evidence of recovery of kidney function.

"Now, like I said, when a person is on dialysis, it's hard because it's going to look like things are improving; but that's just the machine removing the creatinine, removing the blood urea nitrogen. So, the first thing we would look for in him is for urine his urine output to increase. So, you know, if that starts to happen, and he starts to make more urine, then *that would be a very big significant step in the right direction.*

"And at some point, I would stop the dialysis, and we would see how he does without it. So, putting him on dialysis doesn't mean that he's going to stay on it for life. So, in fact, the odds are pretty good that his kidneys could recover from this because they were in better shape, you know, just a few days ago—a week ago.

"But of course, that all depends on how the rest of him is doing, and of course, dialysis is not going to do anything to help his other problems. All dialysis is, it's basically like a crutch to support his body while the kidneys are not doing what they're supposed to do. The only thing that would

293

explain the rise in the FiO2 over the past few days is the kidney failure. From the respiratory end, the kidney failure is making it harder to ventilate him, and that's why he's requiring more oxygen because he's got all of his fluid coming in right away that has nowhere to go."

My advocate said, "I want to ask Dr. Wicked to do some things on the respiratory end that can help improve things as well, and they can work together in combination as there are some tweaks we can do there as well. I believe the issue is with cytokines." Dr. Ruthless said, "The good thing about this type of dialysis is it removes cytokines. Also, Dr. Wicked knows you're here. Actually, he's waiting for me to finish speaking with you so he can meet with you."

I said, "Hopefully, it would help get the fluid off, and urine would start back up." He noted, "I don't like putting people on dialysis. I just don't like seeing them die of kidney failure. So, we do dialysis; it's nice that we have that option because in the past, 40-50 years ago, you would be talking to a chaplain right now because he would be dying of kidney failure. So, it's nice that we have such a thing because we don't have it for the liver and other organs."

I said, "I think he needs it." He replied, "That's really the only proven way to remove toxins. The only way to dialyze is with a catheter in these cases." My patient advocate noted, "The catheter can have issues. That's a risk of any procedure." Dr. Ruthless noted, "I wouldn't be the one placing the catheter. It would be Dr. Wicked and his assistant. I just write the dialysis order, and I manage that."

I interjected, "I have a question. When he was in the ER, I specifically told them that Rob's dad had lost a kidney and that I did not want any of the remdesivir at all because I've done the research and I saw that it was bad for people with kidney problems, and they kept pressuring him, and we ended up losing contact, and they did end up giving him six doses. So could that contribute to his kidney problems?"

Dr. Ruthless responded, "It's contraindicated in people who already have kidney problems, but in his case, his kidney function was normal at that time. There are more side effects with people with kidney problems, but in his case, I think it was related to the low blood pressure."

So, I asked, "According to one medical journal, high doses of fentanyl and morphine can also cause renal failure, and I've been screaming at the top of my lungs, 'please reduce it,' and I don't know why they had it so high." He replied, "That can cause acidosis, yet right now, he's fortunately not acidotic. It's thanks to that we have not had to do the dialysis before now."

To assure us the team in the ICU had the skills necessary to manage continuous dialysis, he said, "The ICU nurses have continuous dialysis training to troubleshoot if there are any problems with the machine, and there are company representatives they can call if there are any problems with the machine, and if they can't solve a problem they can call me or whoever's covering for me at that time."

LEGAL COUNSEL STATEMENT
Members of the jury, as noted near the top of Page 646 of the hospital records (see Page C-52), Rob received a total of six doses of the toxic drug, remdesivir. Two of those doses were double-strength "loading" doses.

doses. Thus, they revealed that their Covid "protocol for profit" included **a total of 10 doses which would have**

> **been 1100 mg** (of which he received 800 mg), and Sheila and Rob had frustrated their plans by only allowing them to force on Rob a total of 6 of the planned doses.
>
> As we noted earlier, in Chapter 3, an April 30, 2021, WebMD article titled "COVID-19 and Your Kidneys: What You Should Know" said, "*Research suggests that up to half of people hospitalized with COVID-19 get **an acute kidney injury**. That's a sudden case of kidney damage, and in some severe cases, kidney failure, that happens within hours or days.*"
> WebMD. (n.d.). Covid-19 and your kidneys: What you should know. WebMD. From https://www.webmd.com/lung/covid-kidneys-damage-coronavirus
>
> Because **remdesivir** is part of the standard Covid protocol being followed in hospitals across America, it is no wonder that up to 50% of hospitalized Covid-19 patients end up with acute kidney injury—and as we also noted previously, on Rob's death certificate, the underlying cause of death was listed as "**ACUTE KIDNEY INJURY.**"

As he headed out the door, he said he would let Dr. Wicked know we were available. In less than a minute, he popped back in and said, "He's examining Rob right now; then he'll be right in."

I hoped and prayed that the central line insertion would go smoothly and that the continuous dialysis would rid Rob's body of the cytokines that were causing him chronic inflammation, assist him in recovering from the overdoses of multiple potent medications, and restore his kidney function.

In about a minute, Dr. Wicked opened the door and stepped in. "Well, so Dr. Ruthless has talked to you about the kidneys. He is not yet peeing. We will be starting CRRT. **Otherwise, things are stable.** The liver numbers are stable compared to yesterday. They [the ALT and AST] were coming down, but now they're about the same as they were yesterday. **I bumped the steroids way up.**"

My patient advocate asked, "What are you doing with the steroids?" He responded, "I don't know; I guess that's a bad-sounding answer. Obviously, weaning down the steroids over time was our plan, **and then the wheels just fell off the other day**. His pattern really looks like someone who had just been in, like, a really refractory shock. He needed some pressors [vasopressors, medications that increase blood pressure], but he was never 'no blood pressure.' I think he's on norepinephrine."

My advocate explained, "So, the norepinephrine would be a blood pressure medication, and it's just going to bump the blood pressure and maybe help with a little urine output—but since the kidneys are impacted, not so much right now."

She then asked, "So, IV steroids then, that's what you bumped up? What was the point of that?" He replied, "So, I bumped them up considerably when things were *just going hot the other day*. If it wasn't shock causing the liver . . . his liver looks like ischemic or shock liver. But he was never as hypotensive as we'd expect for someone to do that, so I started looking at more rare diseases."

My advocate then said, "So, one of the things we'd really like to try is to bump the budesonide up to 1 mg and do it every 4 hours. I do think it can help with the cytokines in the lung lining, and it can eventually impact the other organs. The budesonide has been shown in a number of studies to help with the blood oxygen levels, reduce scarring, and shut off the cytokine storm."

Dr. Wicked replied, "We could bump it up, but I don't believe in it because there is not a steroid receptor in his body that is not being saturated because he's getting 120 mg of SOLU-MEDROL directly into the vein, which is going everywhere. I'm going to have them do it, but I have zero belief that it's going to change anything. The CRRT is very effective at clearing out cytokines."

My advocate noted, "I think if we can attack it from a nebulizing standpoint as well as intravenous, let's do it. Right now, he's getting 0.5 mg twice a day, and you're going to increase it to 1 mg every 4 hours, and we're going to just see how it goes—because assisting his lungs with recovery can also assist with the cytokine issue."

Dr. Wicked noted, "So, I have to put the dialysis catheter in for the machine to hook up to, most likely in the right internal jugular. The line, like anything, risks bleeding or potential pneumothorax, so I get an X-ray after to look for that, and we use an ultrasound to put it in to be as safe as possible."

What troubled me was that, as he had many times before, Dr. Wicked, the deceiver, was using his favorite phrase and telling me that "**things are stable.**" After telling me the day before, "**I don't think he's gonna survive,**" Rob was clearly anything but "**stable.**"

In truth, my husband was lying in a fully paralyzed, totally sedated, comatose state with non-functioning kidneys, acute liver failure, and severe anemia that **they** (the doctors, therapists, and nurses charged with his care) had caused. Rob was in a crisis of **their** creation.

They had brought this on us by forcing Rob to follow every step of "the protocol that kills" for their own gain, knowing but not caring it would likely cost him his life.

They had led us here by ignoring our loud and continual pleas that Rob NOT be given remdesivir, NOT be intubated, NOT be placed on a ventilator, and NOT be given high dosages of a multitude of largely unnecessary and harmful pharmaceuticals.

They had brought him to this point, this crisis, this day, by ignoring his urgent need for adequate nutrition from the moment he arrived and then ignoring his profound anemia until it, along with the continual assault of toxic medications, led to Rob's now suffering from multi-organ failure.

They had spent untold hours trying to convince me they wanted the best for Rob. Yet all the while, they fully expected my previously healthy, vibrantly alive, athletic, robust, 52-year-old husband to die under their pseudo-care model.

They had decided it best he become a statistic instead of a survivor because he had committed the unforgivable crime of entering the Emergency Department of their facility with difficulty breathing and a persistent cough while admitting he was, by choice, unvaccinated.

They, in my eyes, were entirely responsible—and were a group of deceitful, evil, murderous criminals who feigned caring while being totally detached, completely unsympathetic, and utterly uncompassionate.

Rob had now been a captive of the ventilator for 35 of his 40 days in the hospital. Although **they** had brought us to this point, I still hoped and prayed that God would give them favor in the insertion of the risky jugular vein central line catheter. If it went well, I hoped that the

Continuous Renal Replacement Therapy (CRRT) and the increased dosage of more frequent nebulized budesonide treatments would help get Rob back on the road to recovery.

The next order of business would be to get them to be more aggressive in getting Rob off the paralytic, reducing the sedatives, lowering the high PEEP setting, reducing excessive FiO2 (oxygen concentration) level, and then finally beginning to make daily attempts to successfully wean Rob from the ventilator.

When I returned to Rob's room, I was again struck by how bloated he appeared. His skin was stretched taut across his entire body. He was leaking so much fluid that his sheets were wet, and large watery blisters had appeared on his legs and arms. As I considered how critical Rob's condition was, I began to feel a deep sense of dread. I had never seen him like this before. I was truly afraid he was going to die.

As I prayed over him, I thanked God for everyone who had stood by me and supported me up to this point. I affirmed, "my husband is strong, he is bold, and he is not silent, and I thank you that you have made him to be such a mighty man of God. I praise you, Father, for him and I thank you, Father."

I again played and sang praise and worship music while waiting for them to let me know that they were ready to begin the insertion of the central line catheter so they could initiate the critical continuous dialysis treatment he now required.

The longer I waited, the more I wondered why they were taking so long. Rob was in critical condition, but they seemed to have no sense of urgency. Dr. Wicked apparently had to complete the rest of his rounds before things could get started.

In the meantime, I called my trusted friend, Roberta, who had joined me at the intervention meeting we held with Dr. Liar on September 27th. I asked her if she could come to the hospital to sit with Rob for a while because they had finally agreed that someone else could come in so I could take a break from the stress of watching over my loving husband.

When I informed her of the situation, she said she would head right out and see me soon. What I really wanted was for them to allow her to be there with me. However, even though we could trade out, they would not allow me to stay if she were coming in. Roberta was like a mother to me, and she adored Rob as if he were her son.

I headed down and met her in the hospital parking lot. I burst into tears the moment I saw her. As she hugged me, I told her I was terrified that Rob might not make it, and I could not stand to be there alone. She said she was happy to stand in for me and would keep an eye on him as they inserted the central line catheter and began the dialysis.

When I arrived home, I lay down and cried into my pillow. If things did not go as planned, I knew I could not watch my husband die. As I closed my eyes, all I could see was his severely bloated body. His beautiful face had become almost unrecognizable.

Then, at 1:15 PM, Roberta texted me to let me know how things were unfolding. They were ready to insert the central line, and she had been asked to leave the room and wait in the ICU waiting area. They told her that the catheter insertion would only take 30 minutes because it was a quick and easy procedure. As a result, they should be finished by 1:45 PM.

At 2:20 PM, an hour and five minutes after they started what was supposed to be a 30-minute procedure, she headed back to Rob's room to see if they had finished and had forgotten to call her back in. Unfortunately, a doctor was hovering over Rob and was apparently still in the midst of the procedure. So, she quietly backed away and returned to the waiting area. Finally, at 2:42 PM, a nurse came out and told Roberta that Rob was fine and that she would eventually be able to return to the room.

At 3:23 PM, Roberta was finally summoned and told she could return to the room. To her horror, she noticed Rob's head was slumped over to his left side, and he appeared utterly wasted and lifeless. Were it not for the ventilator making its rhythmic sounds, she would have thought he had died.

She stood at Rob's bedside for the next fifty-five minutes, sharing positive thoughts with him. As a woman of faith, she said, "Like the children of Israel who were in the wilderness for 40 years, you have now spent 40 days in the hospital. It's time to open your eyes so you too can go home." She wanted him to keep up the fight so he could eventually recover from the 40 days of abuse he had suffered in his own wilderness.

Then Nurse Malfeasance entered the room, pushing a CRRT machine loaded with hoses and plastic containers. She appeared lost and nervous, dropping and picking up items as she went, looking around as if she had no idea what she was doing. Roberta asked her if she was going to begin the CRRT treatment. She replied that she could not do it alone and needed to wait for another nurse who was currently on a break.

Then, at around 4:15 PM, Nurse Malfeasance began working on the setup, fumbling with the tubing as if trying to make sense of it all. At 4:18 PM, when the other nurse, who claimed to be trained in CRRT therapy, arrived, the nurses asked Roberta to step out once more while they set up the machine and got Rob hooked up.

Given the apparently difficult and problematic insertion of the central line catheter, Roberta would have preferred to remain in the room while Rob was connected to the machine and was apprehensive about being asked to leave once more. She also had the uneasy impression that neither nurse knew precisely what they were doing.

She texted me again at 4:33 PM to let me know she was still waiting for the nurses to complete the setup and allow her to return to Rob's room. Obviously, what was supposed to be a "quick and simple" procedure was neither quick nor simple. Clearly, things were not going well.

Having a feeling of dread, I hopped in my car and returned to the hospital after texting Roberta that I was on my way. At 5:06 pm, I arrived at the hospital. Fearing something terrible was happening, the moment I parked in the hospital parking garage, I ran straight in and immediately headed to the ICU. At the same time, however, I received a text from Roberta letting me know she had headed down to meet me in the first-floor lobby because she knew they would frown on both of us being in the ICU at the same time.

At 5:08 PM, as I exited the elevator by the ICU, I ran into Charge Nurse Massacre. She looked at me with wide, puppy dog eyes, wrung her hands, and shouted, *"Sheila, Sheila! Your husband, your husband!"* I cried, *"What's wrong with my husband!"* Before she could answer—and not wanting to be alone, whatever was occurring—I told her to immediately call down to the main desk in the lobby and tell them to send Roberta back up. I also texted Roberta, *"Don't leave. Something happened to Rob. Come back up."*

I wondered what in the world had transpired in the few minutes Roberta had spent heading down to meet me as I drove to the hospital. Not wanting to head into the ICU alone, I waited for her by the elevators as my heart pounded like a massive drum. Then, an emotional tornado completely engulfed me. My ears began buzzing, and the world started to spin. The next thing I knew, Roberta exited the elevator and ran toward me. We linked arms and entered the ICU together.

In the hallway outside Rob's room, a group of stoic doctors and nurses with sunken eyes and folded hands stood in formation in white uniforms and coats. They appeared like soulless ghouls from the underworld, gleefully grinning as they observed the commotion inside Rob's room.

When they saw us approaching, they parted like the Red Sea to let us pass. As we headed in, we could see approximately ten individuals crowded together, hovering over Rob's bed. Suddenly, as if on cue, they all set their eyes on me, turned back toward Rob, and began what appeared to be a CPR charade. A stocky nurse straddled Rob's body and made two or three crunching compression sounds with all her might on his chest.

I sensed the theatrics were purely for my benefit to give the impression that they were making a valiant effort to save Rob's life. Her movements were so dramatic that her glasses flew violently off her head as she jumped off, presumably because she had completed her grand "watch me do chest compressions" performance.

She then stumbled past me, wiping her forehead and letting out a loud sigh as if she had spent a considerable amount of time working on Rob. The crowd again parted as they congratulated her with loud clapping while patting her on her back for her heroic efforts. It was a good show, but who was in charge, and where were the defibrillator paddles?

They evidently expected me to be impressed, but I found the entire scene disturbing and grotesque. As Roberta and I looked at each other in bewilderment, we sensed that the whole production had been staged for our benefit. No one said a word or explained what happened, and none of it felt right. I later learned from several medically trained friends that this type of "simulated CPR" in front of family members is quite common and is designed to help "give closure" to family members.

With the performance now over, Dr. Wicked and several nurses stood motionless by Rob's bed. As we made eye contact, I felt I was looking into the eyes of the enemy—an enemy who had forced my husband to follow every step of their unyielding, highly profitable, and lethal protocol; an enemy who had been delighted I was locked out for 21 days so I could not interfere with their plans for my husband; an enemy who had ignored my pleas to properly nourish my husband and had poisoned him with toxic medications that damaged his kidneys and his liver; and an enemy who, up until now, would not allow two of Rob's family members or friends into the room at the same time and who only allowed a single visitor per day.

They were methodical, unfeeling, merciless, and indifferent. Unfortunately, they had succeeded in forcing Rob to follow "the **full** protocol," and now that my husband of 14 years had breathed his last and final breath and was dead at their hands, they could write "COVID-19" on yet another death certificate.

I asked Roberta, "What are we going to do? Is it time to raise the dead?" She replied, "Yes, it's time!" I called out, "Rob, you will live and not die! You have life! You are not done! Yeshua (Jesus), you said we will do greater works and that we are to heal the sick and raise the dead! Rob, get up and walk."

The band of doctors and nurses surrounding Rob's hospital bed were paralyzed in shock as we expressed our desire to raise him so he could continue the ministry God had laid out for him. I gestured toward the door and yelled, "Get out! I forgive all of you for what you did to my husband but get out!"

LEGAL COUNSEL STATEMENT

Members of the jury, below is a timeline detailing the significant events of Rob's final four hours:

- **1:15 PM**—Roberta was asked to leave the room so they could insert the central line catheter.
- **1:30 PM to 2:30 PM**—The hospital records state that a doctor surgically inserted a jugular port for the CRRT and that a Physician's Assistant student was "in attendance and participated in parts of the procedure." Thus, what was said to be a quick-and-easy "30-minute" procedure lasted a full hour. Records say, "Blood aspirated but no complications" and "patient tolerated procedure well."
- **2:20 PM**—Roberta peeked in and saw a doctor still hovering over Rob.
- **2:42 PM**—Nurses came out of Rob's room and told Roberta that he was fine and did well with the procedure.
- **3:23 PM**—Roberta was finally allowed to return to Rob's room after 2 hours and 8 minutes. If the catheter insertion had been completed at 2:30 PM, it is unclear why Roberta was kept out of the room for nearly another hour.
- **4:18 PM**—Roberta was asked to again leave the room for the setup and connection of the CRRT.
- **4:50 PM**—Hospital records indicate that CRRT was initiated. Rob's blood oxygen level dropped to 79%, although the FiO2 (oxygen concentration) was set at 100% on the ventilator. The Respiratory Therapist was immediately called into the room, and he called Dr. Wicked, who gave orders to increase the PEEP setting on the ventilator.
- **4:55 PM**—Hospital records show that Rob's heart rate dropped from 99-100 into the 70s as the CRRT machine began alarming. A crash cart was brought to Rob's bedside.
- **5:00 PM**—Rob had no pulse, and CPR was started.
- **5:08 PM**—Sheila exits the elevator on the floor of the ICU and meets Charge Nurse Massacre as she shouts, "*Sheila, Sheila! Your husband, your husband!*"
- **5:10 PM**—Sheila and Roberta enter Rob's room in the ICU and witness the end of what had been a ten-minute CPR performance.
- **5:11 PM**—Recorded in the hospital records as the official time of death. Upon Rob's being disconnected from the CRRT machine, they noted in the hospital record that "*the end of the tube to CRRT blood had already gelled.*"

We find it disturbing that postmortem coagulation (the gel-like clotting of blood) had rapidly occurred in the central line placed in Rob's neck—the line inserted for and connected to the CRRT [Continuous Renal Replacement Therapy] machine. Forensic pathologists and investigators often use the extent and location of postmortem clotting to help determine the cause and time of death. However, the blood becoming gelled this rapidly is very uncommon, unusual, and suspect.

Below is a snapshot of the notes written in the hospital record starting at 16:50 (4:50 PM).

> 1650 CRRT initiated. Pt immediately started to desat to 79-80% on 100% FIO2. Immediately called RT to room. RT arrived immediately and he called **Dr. Wicked**. **Dr. Wicked** gave him orders to increase Peep. 1655 noted HR had dropped from 99-100's to 70's. At the same time CRRT started alarming. Crash cart brought to bedside. 1700 pt had no pulse and CPR started. Time of death 1711. When pt disconnected from dialysis catheter, the end of the tube to CRRT blood had already gelled.

With startled expressions resembling deer in headlights, they stumbled over each other as they scrambled out of the room at my command.

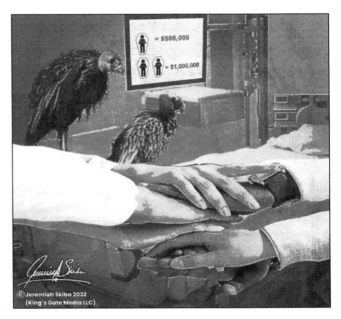

As I drew the curtain around Rob's bed for privacy, I met Charge Nurse Massacre's eyes as she tried to move out of the way and exit the room. I screamed, *"What happened to my husband? How did he die?"* She feebly answered, "I don't know. I was not here." She then informed me that I could review Rob's online MyChart Records in the evening to see what they had recorded there.

I thought, "How could the ICU Charge Nurse not know—and if she truly does not know, why would she not ask the doctors what went wrong?" It then occurred to me that the doctors and nurses would want to huddle first to agree on how to best explain Rob's death to put them and the hospital in the best possible light and avoid any liability for Rob's needless death.

While Roberta prayed over Rob, I called my mother, followed by my sister, to inform them that the medical establishment had finally succeeded in killing Rob. From the moment Rob was admitted, they had been confident that the doctors had Rob's best interests in mind and were doing everything possible to save him.

Yet Rob had warned me via a text message on September 5, 2021, his 2nd day in the hospital, *"Doing all they can to try to get me to agree to intubate. I'm dead if they do."* My family now realized that Rob's and my deep-seated fear—that American hospitals, which we had once trusted as life-saving "health care" centers, had now become "human kill shelters"—was well founded.

Rob's tragic and unnecessary death made it painfully clear to everyone who had told me to "trust the doctors" that the "medical professionals" they thought had Rob's best interests in mind had become "white coat assassins" who were knowingly or unwittingly taking part in an evil plot to force on patients a lethal, government-incentivized, "protocol that kills." Although Rob had died a wholly preventable and totally needless death, I knew that none of the doctors, therapists, or nurses charged with his care would ever admit to being the proximal cause of his death—nor were they likely to be held accountable for their involvement in the diabolical scheme.

I was totally stunned and paralyzed as I stood by Rob's bed. The spirit of the man I loved had escaped this realm, and his disfigured and swollen body looked like the body of a man who had been the victim of a horrendous medical experiment gone horribly wrong.

Word of what had been done to Rob soon got out, and before long, a few close friends arrived to support and comfort me. No one in the ICU objected this time since the deceased may have multiple visitors. Only the living needed to be isolated and sheltered from the prying eyes of those who love them.

Then my God-fearing mother rushed into the room like a mighty wind, touched Rob's forehead, and began to pray. Next, my sister entered. She was utterly shocked by Rob's hideous appearance. Kneeling beside his bed, she gently touched his leg while Roberta placed her hands on his feet and prayed that our Father would grace us with his spirit's miraculous return. We all believed in a loving God who is the universe's creator, who answers prayers, and who, if we humbly asked, might grant our request that Rob be resurrected like Lazarus.

I suddenly realized how quiet the room was. The ventilator was no longer cycling, the IV infusion pumps had all been turned off, and the monitors that had once beeped with Rob's heartbeat and displayed his temperature, blood pressure, and blood oxygen level were now all dark.

As I removed some tape from Rob's body, I noticed a splattering of muck on his beard that looked like blood and vomit. A doctor re-entered the room, so I asked, "*What happened here? What is all of this?*" He was only willing to say it was left over from Rob's tube. He then quickly left the room, preventing me from asking further questions.

As I picked up Rob's limp hand, I cried to my mother, "**He doesn't even look like himself! Look what they did to him!**" All she could say was that she could still make out that it was Rob despite his bloated appearance.

Not knowing what else to do, I began to take down the photos I had previously asked be taped to the wall in the hope that Rob would eventually awaken and see them as he was being weaned from the ventilator. Sadly, and tragically, Rob had spent 35 days on the device he knew would lead to his death—and not once had the team at Covid Coven Hospital of Plano, Texas, come even close to successfully weaning him.

Suddenly, I felt a rush of uncontrollable emotion and said to my mother, sister, and friends, "*I have to leave. I cannot stay here any longer.*" My mother said she wanted to stay and pray for a little while, and Roberta agreed to stay with her. They both believed in *the God of the living* and the power of His resurrection. As I rushed toward the door, my sister ran after me, insisting I not be alone.

When I reached the hospital parking lot, I could see it was raining heavily. It was as if all of heaven were crying with me. My heart was broken beyond repair, and I knew I would never be whole again. I had defined my life and purpose as being Rob's faithful and supportive wife. Who was I now? I felt as if I were being sucked into the darkest and deepest black hole imaginable.

As I drove through a heavy downpour, the tears raining from my eyes made it even more difficult to see. I called my son, Jeremiah, and screamed into the phone, "*Rob's dead! They killed him!*" Jeremiah was so shocked and speechless that the line went silent. Thinking we had been disconnected, I cried, "Are you there?" He replied, "Where are you?" I responded, "I'm on my way home." He said, "I'll be there in a few minutes."

My sister, riding beside me, loved my husband like a brother, and her heart was breaking for me. The moment I pulled into my driveway, the reality of the fact that Rob would never be coming home hit me so hard that I laid my head on the steering wheel and cried uncontrollably.

Eventually, I collected myself enough to open my car door and step out into the darkness and the rain. Although it was only a few steps to my front door, I was sopping wet when I reached it. Trembling and shaken by what had just happened, I struggled to get my house key into the door lock.

Finally, the door opened, and I stepped inside my empty house. My sister followed and closed the door. We both stood in the foyer, dripping wet. I then heard a knock at the door. It was Jeremiah. He rushed in and hugged my limp body.

I looked up into his dark brown eyes and saw he was holding back the tears. As he hugged me close, we cried together. Time stood still as we all felt the loss of a wonderful husband, a great father, and a loving brother-in-law.

As the downpour continued outside,
we wondered if it would ever stop raining in our broken hearts.

Chapter 9 – Accusation & Adjudication

Legal Counsel Closing Argument

We commend you for assuming the role of a juror, as *adjudication by a jury* is a fundamental pillar of our legal system.

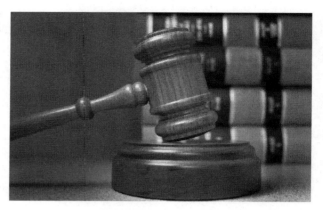

This adjudication process allows citizens to participate in the administration of justice and helps ensure that our legal system reflects the values and perspectives of the community it serves.

As the sole judge of the facts, you play a crucial role in upholding the principles of fairness, impartiality, and justice. Moreover, as you judge the facts, you are responsible for assessing the credibility of the witnesses who have testified in their own words.

As you do so, you may take into account several factors, including **(a)** the demeanor and manner of the individuals, **(b)** any possible biases they may have had, and **(c)** whether their statements were consistent or inconsistent, contradicted or corroborated.

Rob Skiba once said, "*I don't care what it costs; I want to know the truth.*" As a juror, you are searching for the truth of how and why Robert A. Skiba II died. The only currency that matters is the truth, and we hope that by revealing the truth about what goes on behind closed hospital doors, we can help prevent further unnecessary deaths.

As pointed out in **Appendix D**, the CARES Act has supplied specified incentive payments to hospitals for certain medications and therapies. That has resulted in the use of a set of standardized treatments mandated or encouraged by the federal government under the auspices of the National Institutes of Health and Centers for Disease Control's "guidelines."

In this case, we argue that the malevolent actors literally "*forced their will down Rob's throat*" and ensured he succumbed to "*the protocol that kills*" for their financial gain by weakening him through starvation and using harmful drugs and therapies, which we have further detailed in summary format in **Appendix A**.

In the earlier chapters, we spelled out how "the protocol" consists of **isolation, heavy medication, intimidation, humiliation, starvation, desperation, intubation, ventilation, devastation, and eventual termination** of Rob's life.

Unfortunately, this same pattern has been and is still being repeated in hospitals across the United States. *Thus, Rob Skiba's case is not unique, as imposing "the protocol" on unwary patients has resulted in the deaths of thousands of innocent victims.*

You have seen, despite Rob and Sheila's demands to the contrary, how he was forced to follow the mandated, inflexible, one-size-fits-all "protocol," which resulted in his avoidable and unnecessary death.

You witnessed Sheila being cruelly and needlessly locked out of the hospital for 21 days— despite her protests and the fact she had contracted Covid at the same time as Rob, had recovered from the illness, and had been tested and confirmed to have antibodies against the virus and would thus not present any risk to her husband or hospital personnel. We contend she was isolated from her husband to ensure she could not interfere with their

You saw how Sheila and Rob's repeated refusals of remdesivir and their demands that he not be intubated or placed on a ventilator were ignored and denied. You were also informed of how the doctors subjected Rob to high doses of several off-label use drugs with life-threatening side effects that clearly worsened Rob's condition and ultimately contributed to his death.

You beheld how doctors and nurses badgered and coerced Rob (and Sheila) from the moment he was admitted to force him to agree to "elective intubation" while repeatedly refusing reasonable requests for beneficial medications and supplements such as ivermectin, hydroxychloroquine, budesonide, and IV vitamin C—all of which are known to speed recovery and reduce the length of hospital stays.

The doctors did this despite their actions violating **Title 42 of the Code of Federal Regulations, Section 482.13** (as noted in **Appendix E**), which states: "*The patient has the right to participate in the development and implementation of his or her plan of care.*" Those rights include "*being able to request or refuse treatment.*" In truth, they *grossly* violated this right by intentionally neglecting to inform Rob and Sheila of the risks of the drugs and therapies Rob was being administered.

You also observed the hospital staff's consistent negligence and lack of focus on ensuring Rob received adequate nutrition, which he desperately needed to regain the strength and "reserves" necessary to fight the illness.

You were made aware of how Rob's vital signs, as documented in hospital records, proved that he was doing far better before being subjected to 4.5 hours of contraindicated BiPAP therapy than he was afterward and how that therapy severely injured his lungs (by increasing his pneumomediastinum and causing barotrauma), and how this act resulted in Rob's unwanted and previously unnecessary intubation and ventilation.

You followed how Rob's forced intubation and ventilation, the onslaught of toxic levels of oxygen, and the barrage of an abundance of harmful sedatives, paralytics, antibiotics, steroids, vasodilators, anticoagulants, and anti-inflammatory drugs caused Rob irreparable harm—leading to his tragic and needless death after 40 days at Covid Coven Hospital of Plano, Texas.

You were apprised of the fact that Sammy Wong, MD, our medical expert witness, stated:

- *At times, it appears that there was absolute disregard of the patient's and spouse's wishes.*

- *Many of the cases that I have reviewed have a single extreme departure from the standard of care or a few simple departures. In this case, there are multiple extreme departures. There were multiple temporal and proximate relationships that would suggest causation.*

- *The lack of expediting an aggressive diagnostic work up for his cough yet attributing everything to COVID reflects disregard to basic diagnostic medicine. If you do not make the diagnosis, you can't treat the patient properly and often subject the patient to unnecessary harms. It took 40 days and an autopsy to make the diagnosis.*

- *There was lack of clear documentation of the risks, benefits and reasonable alternatives on procedures and medications given. VELETRI and baricitinib were given in spite of substantial harms which did not benefit and were without clear indications for them. Tocilizumab, known not to benefit in those with COVID, was given without benefit and he was exposed to risk of harm.*

- *We are not arguing the issue of Covid. Whether it was COVID or not, it does not matter because, at the end of the day, it turned out to be cryptogenic organizing pneumonia [which the medical examiner who conducted Rob's autopsy noted], which is not like regular pneumonia at all. It is caused by toxins or drugs.*

- *The diagnostic work up for the profound anemia was inadequately addressed. His hemoglobin dropped dramatically and was not addressed appropriately. Oxygen in the blood was adequate and blood was being circulated with a normal cardiac output but delivery to the tissues was profoundly lacking.*

- *I believe this is a case that bears altruistic impact, accountability and societal benefit.*

Considering the preponderance of the evidence presented, we contend that Rob Skiba did not die a natural death from his unquestionably curable illness. Instead, due to gross negligence and possibly malicious intent, his needless death was caused by iatrogenic injury (injury caused by doctor-prescribed drugs and medical treatments).

Of course, to be found guilty of being the proximal cause of Robert A. Skiba II's death, the administration of Covid Coven Hospital in Plano, Texas, and the doctors and nurses, would have to have motive and opportunity.

They clearly had the opportunity, and we contend their motivation was the government incentives that enriched the hospital and further secured the medical staff's positions.

We also contend that the U.S. government incentivized the placement of "COVID-19" on death certificates—regardless of the cause of death—so they could "prove" that a large number of Americans were dying of Covid to intimidate the general public to agree to be injected with a new class of experimental mRNA technology that researchers in the National Institutes of Health (NIH) were paid royalties on.

NIH researchers' receiving royalty payments from pharmaceutical companies is nothing new. The British Medical Journal (BMJ) reported in a January 22, 2005, article titled "*Royalty payments to staff researchers cause new NIH troubles*" that:

"*Patients who took part in clinical trials at the US National Institutes of Health (NIH) had no idea that **scientists at the institutes received $8.9m (£4.8m; €6.8m) in royalty payments** and might benefit financially for the use of their discoveries by pharmaceutical companies and device makers, reports from Associated Press allege. This information was not made public until the press agency obtained the information after filing a request under the Freedom of Information Act. At the same time, NIH researchers spent millions of taxpayers' dollars studying the treatments that they had developed that were licensed to drug companies, the agency reported. **A patient advocacy group, the Alliance for Human Research Protection, says that patients might have thought differently about the risks of trial treatment if they knew of scientists' financial interests. The NIH has been criticized before for not disclosing conflicts of interest**.*"
Tanne, J. H. (2005, January 22). Royalty payments to staff researchers cause new NIH troubles. BMJ (Clinical research ed.). From https://www.ncbi.nlm.nih.gov/pmc/articles/PMC545012

As an additional benefit, whenever "COVID-19" was placed on a death certificate, hospitals and medical professionals were granted blanket immunity from prosecution by federal and, in some cases, state statutes. For example, on June 14, 2021, Greg Abbott, the governor of Texas signed Senate Bill 6 (SB 6), the Pandemic Liability Protection Act, into law which added a new section (Section 74.155) to Title 4, Chapter 74, Subchapter D of the State of Texas Civil Practice and Remedies Code.

Among other things, this section of the Texas law states, "*Except in a case of reckless conduct or intentional, willful, or wanton misconduct, a physician, health care provider, or first responder **is not liable for an injury, including economic and noneconomic damages, or death** arising from care, treatment, or failure to provide care or treatment relating to or impacted by a pandemic disease or a disaster declaration related to a pandemic disease.* .
Civil Practice and Remedies Code Chapter 74. Medical liability. (n.d.). From https://statutes.capitol.texas.gov/Docs/CP/htm/CP.74.htm

Therefore, after examining and considering
all of the evidence, what is your verdict?

Closing Thoughts

Vladimir Zelenko, MD, said, *"I want to place these mass murders brought about by improper treatment and withholding lifesaving treatment in their truly horrific context. The mismanagement of the COVID-19 pandemic is akin to mass murder and the genocide of the elderly and infirm. The root cause of this crime against humanity is the denial of man's divine origin. . .*

"Despite a plethora of scientific data, lifesaving information and access to vital medications are being suppressed for the majority of the human race. This has so far led to the tragic and preventable deaths of over three million people. The perpetrators of this historically heinous crime are motivated by the desire for power and control over the human race. These modern-day slave masters believe that they are übermensch (superhuman) with the right to decide who should live or die. . .

"It is my supposition that this suppression of lifesaving information and medication is mass murder. This crime against humanity has been willfully perpetrated by a group of sociopathic despots that possess a delusional "G-d complex" and perceive themselves as superhumans with the right to enslave others. It is my strong hope and prayer that they will be brought to justice in both the earthly and heavenly courts."
Breggin, P. R., & Breggin, G. R. (2021). In Covid-19 and the global predators: We are the prey. Introduction, Lake Edge Press.

Incentivized medicine creates a clear conflict of interest in which lethal but profitable protocols take precedence over patients' rights, health, and well-being. The inevitable and morbid consequence has been an untold number of senseless and avoidable deaths by negligent manslaughter or premeditated murder, such as Robert A. Skiba II's needless death.

If you have decided that Robert A. Skiba II did not die of natural causes—but rather as a result of a government-incentivized "protocol that kills"—we encourage you to join us in our mission of bringing an end to the government's incentivization of specific drugs and therapies for medical conditions.

Nearly all U.S. medical school graduations include a public pledge. Some use a modernized version of Hippocrates' words from the "Hippocratic Oath." The original oath, written either by Hippocrates (an ancient Greek physician often referred to as the father of Western medicine) or one of his students, contained the following phrase regarding the treatment of patients:

> *"I will do no harm or injustice to them. I will follow that system of regimen which, according to my ability and judgment, I consider for the benefit of my patients, and abstain from whatever is deleterious and mischievous. I will give no deadly medicine to any one if asked, nor suggest any such counsel."*
> Encyclopædia Britannica, inc. (2023, February 19). Hippocratic oath. Encyclopædia Britannica. From
> https://www.britannica.com/topic/Hippocratic-oath

In accordance with this principle, whenever patients consent to treatment, they trust that their physician(s) will act in their best interest or, at the very least, refrain from causing them harm. Medical professionals must prioritize the health and well-being of their patients above all else, even if it means forgoing increased revenue and profits. Only then will patients receive the care they deserve—and the sacred trust between doctor and patient that has been broken be restored.

Lastly, it is a heinous crime against humanity when medical professionals betray their patients by imposing lethal protocols on them for financial gain or to curry favor with their employers (or the state), as was the case with the 23 physicians and researchers tried by U.S. military courts in Nuremberg, Germany after World War II.

In the "Doctors' Trial" of 1946-1947, sixteen defendants were found guilty. Seven were given the death penalty. Nine were given prison terms ranging from 10 years to life.

The *Nuremberg Code*, the most influential document in the history of the ethics of medical research, grew out of that trial.
Washington State Courts Washington Courts. (n.d.). From
https://www.courts.wa.gov/library/exhibit2008/The%20Doctors%20Trial%20display%20board.pdf

The Nuremberg Code's fundamental doctrine is one of "*informed consent.*" Principles 1 and 2 of the code state:
> "*The **voluntary consent** of the human subject is absolutely essential. This means that the person involved should have legal capacity to give consent; should be situated as to be able to **exercise free power of choice, without the intervention of any element of force, fraud, deceit, duress, over-reaching, or other ulterior form of constraint or coercion**, and should have sufficient knowledge and comprehension of the elements of the subject matter involved as to enable him to make an understanding and enlightened decision.*"
> Ghooi, R. B. (2011, April). The nuremberg code-A Critique. Perspectives in clinical research. From
> https://www.ncbi.nlm.nih.gov/pmc/articles/PMC3121268

In addition, the Nuremberg Code requires that physician-researchers protect the best interests of their subjects as spelled out in Principle 10, that states:
> "*During the course of the experiment **the scientist in charge must be prepared to terminate the experiment at any stage**, if he has probable cause to believe, in the exercise of the good faith, superior skill and careful judgement required by him that a continuation of the experiment is likely to result in injury, disability, or death to the experimental subject.*"
> Ghooi, R. B. (2011, April). The nuremberg code-A Critique. Perspectives in clinical research. From
> https://www.ncbi.nlm.nih.gov/pmc/articles/PMC3121268

If a new, modern-day "Doctors' Trial" were to be held before a U.S. military tribunal to try those who have selfishly and callously promoted "*the protocol that kills,*" we believe the appointed judge and jury would render the correct verdict so that justice could finally be served.

Checkmate

They plotted and planned to make us ill
Tilting the scales of balance and will
Their game of chess was rigged from the start
Forcing us to play our part

They moved the pieces, no chance to win
Snatching away the joy within
From this battle there was no escape
We were destined to our fate

The pieces moved and plans were made
To deceive and bring much dismay
The outcome was known before the start
We were doomed to break our heart

The pawns were sacrificed, the knights were taken
The rooks were blocked, the bishop forsaken
The queen was cornered, the king under siege
Our hopes were fading away with ease

Checkmate, you thought the game was done
Your dreams of financial freedom are none
Your pieces were scattered amongst the board
We'll fight for freedom in one accord

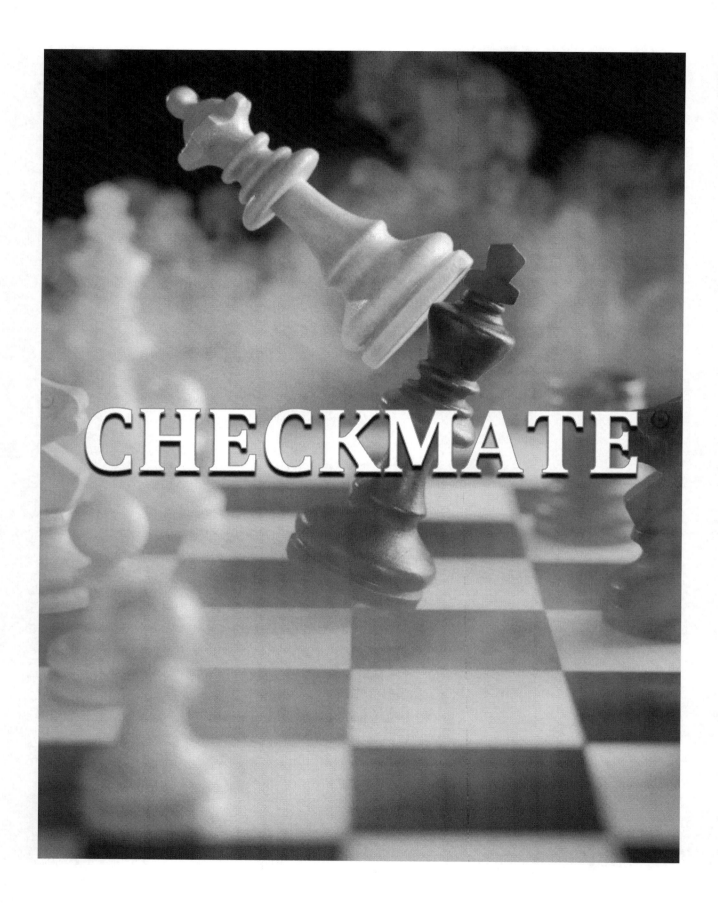

Appendix A – Key Facts

- **Initial condition:** Rob Skiba, an otherwise healthy 52-year-old man with no comorbidities, was admitted to a hospital in Plano, Texas, on September 3, 2021, with the hope of receiving beneficial treatments for persistent coughing and a low blood oxygen level.

- **Expected treatments:** Even if Mr. Skiba were accurately diagnosed with COVID-19, being under age 65 with no comorbidities, he faced an exceptionally minimal risk (a less than 1% chance) of dying from COVID-19 *if given the proper and conservative treatments he expected.*

  - *Conservative treatments would have included:*
    - *supplemental oxygen at as low a percentage as necessary to maintain an adequate blood oxygen level while avoiding oxygen toxicity,*
    - *aiding Rob in self-proning to reduce the pressure of the heart and mediastinum on his lungs, thereby reducing the percentage of inspired oxygen required to keep his blood oxygen level at 90% or higher,*
    - *nebulized budesonide (a corticosteroid) at a dose of 1 mg every 4 hours to reduce the inflammation in his lungs,*
    - *adequate nutrition to ensure he could regain the strength he needed to heal, and*
    - *antibiotics, as necessary, for bacterial pneumonia or other infections.*

  - Once adequately stabilized by conservative treatments, Rob could have been sent home within a few days with orders for at-home supplemental oxygen therapy and prescriptions for the few remaining medications necessary to continue his recovery.

- **PCR testing:** Soon after his arrival, Rob was given a PCR test. According to the hospital records, he tested positive for COVID-19. At that time, in the U.S., the PCR test was generally cycled up to 40 times to detect *"viral fragments"* from nasal or throat samples.

  - *PCR test cycles of greater than 35 can be relatively meaningless because they may detect fragments of dead viruses or a nucleotide (a fundamental building block of DNR and RNA) that are mistaken for a live virus fragment. Thus, most of the "positive" results are false positives.*

- **Apparently targeted:** Rob appears to have been targeted because he had not received an admittedly *experimental mRNA COVID-19 vaccine.*

  - This is evidenced by the fact that the first and only question Sheila was asked when she delivered Rob to the hospital Emergency Department was, "Is he vaccinated?" On Page 28 of Rob's hospital records (see Page C-6 in **Appendix C**), you can see they wrote in bold italics, "***He has not been vaccinated***." On Page 53 of his records (see Page C-8), you will find, "**COVID 19 VACCINATION STATUS: UNVACCINATED**."

  - *Patients and their families across America have reported that unvaccinated patients have been targeted and received harsh treatment by cold-hearted pro-vax doctors and nurses who appear to have a substantial prejudice against the "unvaxxed" and wish to make examples of them.*

- **Protocol initiated:** "The Protocol That Kills" plan of action was **in play from the moment Rob arrived at the hospital,** as evidenced by the fact that although Rob's blood oxygen level rose from 71% into the upper 90s upon the administration of supplemental oxygen, Nurse Practitioner Horrendous wrote in Rob's record at 9:07 PM, minutes after his admission to the ICU (see Page C-3), *"Patient is at high risk for intubation."*

  - *Her note clearly indicates that the plan was to force on Rob "the protocol" from the moment he arrived—a protocol that consisted of isolation, heavy medication, intimidation, humiliation, starvation, desperation, intubation, ventilation, devastation, and eventual termination.*

- **Unnecessary lockout:** Although Sheila Skiba, Rob's wife of 14 years, had a signed Medical Power of Attorney, had been exposed to Rob during his illness for seven days at home, had overcome the illness, and had antibodies to the disease, the moment she delivered Rob to the Emergency Department, **they forced her to leave and needlessly forbid her visiting her husband** (other than two brief 20-minute and one-hour exceptions) **for 21 days**.

  - *The conduct of all defendants to this cause of action where they prevented Rob and Sheila from having physical contact for 21 days, thereby preventing Sheila from serving as Rob's on-site medical advocate and properly overseeing his care (or mistreatment), constituted criminal neglect.*

  - Sheila repeatedly demanded a copy of the hospital's "21-day" visitation restriction in writing, yet one was never provided. *The defendants' refusal to provide her with a written copy of their visitation policy and restrictions violated Title 42 of the Code of Federal Regulations, Section 482.13 (as noted in* **Appendix E***), which states, "A hospital must have written policies and procedures regarding the visitation rights of patients, including those setting forth any clinically necessary or reasonable restriction or limitation that the hospital may need to place on such rights and the reasons for the clinical restriction or limitation."*

- **ICU Admission:** Despite his immediate improvement on supplemental oxygen alone, at 9:05 PM on September 3, 2021, they decided to **admit Rob to the ICU** instead of a room on a regular floor so they could give him a high-risk, nebulized, **off-label use drug called VELETRI**. Veletri is *so high-risk* that it may only be administered in the ICU because it can cause patients severe shortness of breath, gasping for breath, and possible death— risks that were not disclosed to Rob or Sheila. Rob was given 12 doses of this drug.

  - In his "Causes of Action" (see **Appendix B**), Sammy Wong, MD, stated that VELETRI *"can incite a profound inflammatory response in the pulmonary interstitium [the tissue in and around the wall of the alveoli (air sacs) of the lung where oxygen moves from the alveoli into the capillary network (the bloodstream)]. Due to a lack of indication for its use, the patient was subjected to unnecessary risks."*

- **Forced remdesivir:** Mr. Skiba's risk of death dramatically changed for the worse after being assaulted with nebulized **VELETRI** and then being given a high-risk drug named **remdesivir** without his "informed consent" and against the express wishes of his wife, Sheila Skiba, who had Medical Power of Attorney. Instead of honoring their directives that he NOT be given remdesivir, they administered six doses from September 3rd to September 9th, with two being double, 200 mg "loading" doses.

  - This was done to Rob despite the WHO's 2020 "Solidarity Trial" indicating that remdesivir had little or no effect on hospitalized patients with covid-19. On

November 19, 2020, the British Medical Journal published an article titled "**WHO Guideline Development Group advises against use of remdesivir for covid-19**" where they stated, "*The antiviral drug remdesivir is not suggested for patients admitted to hospital with covid-19, regardless of how severely ill they are, because there is currently no evidence that it improves survival or the need for ventilation.*" Who guideline development group advises against use of remdesivir for covid-19. BMJ. (n.d.). From https://www.bmj.com/company/newsroom/who-guideline-development-group-advises-against-use-of-remdesivir-for-covid-19

- o In addition, on February 26, 2021, the National Library of Medicine published an article titled "**Kidney disorders as serious adverse drug reactions of remdesivir in coronavirus disease 2019,**" where they pointed out that "*the use of remdesivir was associated with an increased reporting of kidney disorders*" and stated, "*real-life data from > 5000 COVID-19 patients support that kidney disorders, almost exclusively AKI [Acute Kidney Injury], represent a serious, early, and potentially fatal adverse drug reaction of remdesivir.*" It is, therefore, no surprise that on Rob's death certificate, the underlying cause of death was listed as "**ACUTE KIDNEY INJURY.**" Chouchana, L., Preta, L.-H., Tisseyre, M., Terrier, B., Treluyer, J.-M., & Montastruc, F. (2021, May). Kidney disorders as serious adverse drug reactions of Remdesivir in coronavirus disease 2019: A retrospective case-noncase study. Kidney international. From https://www.ncbi.nlm.nih.gov/pmc/articles/PMC7907730

- **Refused budesonide.** Instead of giving Rob life-saving drugs such as **nebulized budesonide**, which Sheila repeatedly requested, they flooded him with **SOLU-MEDROL**, a potent steroid that can cause trouble breathing and shortness of breath and increase the risk of systemic infections. Although he was eventually administered one small dose of nebulized budesonide per day starting on September 9, 2021, the day after he was placed on a ventilator, it was far too little too late.

  - o Speaking of SOLU-MEDROL, an article in WebMD noted, "*This medication may lower your ability to fight infections. This may make you more likely to get a serious (rarely fatal) infection or make any infection you have worse.*" WebMD. (n.d.). Solu-Medrol intravenous: Uses, side effects, interactions, pictures, warnings & dosing. WebMD. From https://www.webmd.com/drugs/2/drug-152303/solu-medrol-intravenous

  - o *Rob already had symptoms (trouble breathing and shortness of breath) that this high-powered systemic steroid was known to likely cause or exacerbate, and he already had a severe infection (pneumonia). If this drug could "make any infection you have worse," and cause or worsen symptoms Rob already had, why would his physicians administer SOLU-MEDROL instead of safe and effective budesonide, which was known to reduce patients' recovery time as noted in the article abstract in **Appendix F**.*

- **Negligent starvation:** While isolated and on his own, Rob did not have the strength to even think about ordering meals. In addition, he was too weak to feed himself even if a meal were delivered. On September 5, 2021, the third day of his stay, Rob texted Sheila, "*Doing all they can to try to get me to agree to intubate. I'm dead if they do.*" Later that same day, he texted, "***No food.***" Whether due to willful ignorance, uncaring negligence, or nefarious intent— Robert A. Skiba II was slowly and systematically **starved into submission** so he would eventually succumb to "the protocol that kills."

  - o *As noted on Pages 104, 105, 117, and 149 of Rob's hospital records (see Pages C-27, C-28, C-30, and C-31 in **Appendix C**), Rob was being slowly starved into submission while being further weakened by the **remdesivir** (which is known to cause trouble breathing and acute kidney injury) and **VELETRI** (which should NEVER be used on a patient who* *is already short of breath because it may cause SERIOUS side effects that include "severe shortness of breath, gasping for breath, and anxiety").*

- *The "pt has not been ordering 3 meals a day" and "Unsure about pt's weight history" notes on Page 149 (see Page C-31) are especially troubling as they clearly indicate the doctors, nurses, and dietitian were all well aware that Rob—who had no one assisting him in eating and drinking—was becoming critically weakened by severe malnourishment.*

- *On September 13, 2021, five days after Rob was placed on the ventilator, Dr. Wicked admitted to Sheila, "So, by the time he got on the ventilator, of course, **we were nutritionally down**, and **he hadn't been fed for several days before**. So, he may not, you know, he may not have enough reserve in two weeks."*

  o *Medical malpractice occurs when a physician fails to follow accepted standards of care, thereby causing harm to a patient. The ongoing and unaddressed malnutrition clearly harmed Rob. The doctors' negligence of Rob's nutritional state further depleted any "reserves" (physical strength) he may have had when he arrived at Covid Coven Hospital in Plano, Texas.*

- **Constant badgering:** From the moment of his arrival, Rob was **continually badgered** to agree to be intubated and placed on a **ventilator** and agree to receive **remdesivir** (which they had already begun to give him without his consent).

  o One example can be found in the 5:43 PM note on September 5, 2021, located at the bottom of Page 78 (and continues at the top of Page 79) of the hospital records (see Pages C-17 and C-18), where Nurse Malign noted she had a "*Lengthy discussion with patient regarding intubation and use of Remdesivir."*

  o Less than 5 hours later, at 10:40 PM, Nurse Felonious disrupted Rob's insufficient rest and "checked with pt [patient] about limited DNR [Do Not Resuscitate] status," as you can see in the note on the bottom of Page 79 of the hospital records (see Page C-18). Rob reiterated, "**I want to avoid intubation,**" as you can see in the highlighted notes on Page 79 of the records (see Page C-18).

    - At the same time, she noted on Page 79 that Rob's blood oxygen level was at 94% (see the top of Page 79 on Page C-18), which is substantiated by the vital signs shown on Pages 2411-2412 (see Page C-19). Thus, there was no reason to be pressing Rob to agree to be intubated and placed on a ventilator.

  o During a call with Sheila on September 7, 2021, Rob said, "*The doctors are doing all they can to make me take remdesivir and be intubated. They harass me every time they come into my room. They send in the nurses to badger me. I told them to put it in my record NO remdesivir and in bold DO NOT INTUBATE. I don't know how I'm going to survive this if they have their way! But I'm trying to be strong and need the oxygen."*

  o *These so-called "medical professionals" would not let up—and their continual harassment of Rob violated Paragraph (c)(3) of Title 42 of the Code of Federal Regulations, Section 482.13 (see **Appendix E**), which clearly states: "The patient has the right to be free from all forms of abuse or harassment."*

- **Palliative care:** On September 4, 2021, at 9:57 AM, the morning after his arrival, Dr. Dead End entered a note that said "**Consult palliative Care**" as part of the initial "Impression and Plan" for Rob. You can see that note on Page 57 of the hospital records (see Page C-11). It was entered immediately following the note that "patient does not want intubation" (see Note 1) and "COVID-19 unvaccinated" (see Note 2). "***Palliative care***" is a term that is often used interchangeably with "comfort care." Both terms refer to a similar approach of care that emphasizes comfort and support, particularly at end-of-life.

  o *It was as if they had written Rob off from the moment he arrived because of his "unvaccinated" status and because Rob made it clear he did not want to be intubated and placed on a ventilator since he knew being on a ventilator would likely be a death sentence.*

- **Dangerous withdrawal:** On September 5, 2021, at 5:05 PM, frustrated and irritated that Rob refused to remove his DNI (Do Not Intubate) order and would not agree to be intubated and placed on a ventilator, Dr. Dead End ejected him from the ICU and had him sent to a regular hospital room on a different floor. This resulted in the hazardous and potentially lethal abrupt withdrawal of the administration of **VELETRI** (epoprostenol). This drug is such a high risk that it may only be administered in the ICU and must be slowly withdrawn to avoid potentially life-threatening complications. Rob had already been given six doses of this medication, which was administered every six hours since the morning after his arrival at the hospital.

  o A patient on **VELETRI** (epoprostenol) should **NEVER** be abruptly withdrawn from this medication because "*Abrupt withdrawal (including interruptions in drug delivery) or sudden large reductions in dosage of Veletri may result in symptoms associated with rebound pulmonary hypertension, including dyspnea [difficult or labored breathing], dizziness, and asthenia [abnormal physical weakness or lack of energy]. In clinical trials, one Class III primary pulmonary hypertension patient's death was judged attributable to the interruption of epoprostenol. Avoid abrupt withdrawal.*" Veletri: Package insert. Drugs.com. (n.d.). From https://www.drugs.com/pro/veletri.html

  o *Clearly, Dr. Dead End used the abrupt withdrawal of VELETRI to weaken Rob further so they could more easily force him onto a ventilator, an act we contend that, along with the massive assault of numerous toxic medications, directly led to his death.*

- **Falsified consent:** On September 6, 2021, realizing they did not have any signed **consent forms**, a hospital "Admission Specialist" wrote "*Verbal*" on a "General Consent for Treatment" form and two additional standard consent forms. You can see the signature blocks of all three forms on Pages C-25 and C-26. **Appendix I** details Sheila's communication with the hospital on this topic.

  o When the Admission Specialist who filled out the forms posted them at 1:07, 1:08, and 1:09 PM, she wrote in "*spouse*" as the signing party—implying Sheila had given her verbal consent—which made no sense because Sheila did not have the authority, per the hospital's policies, to sign for Rob while he was (and he was) "alert and conversant." In addition, Sheila was not called and asked to provide her verbal consent.

  o *A thorough review of the records confirmed that these three were the only "consent" forms filed during Rob's 40-day stay. What is blatantly missing is any signed "Informed Consent" forms for the Emergency Use Authorization (EUA) medications Rob was subjected to and the high-risk treatments he endured, such as the 4.5 hours he was subjected to on a hazardous, contraindicated BiPAP therapy and his eventual intubation and ventilation.*

- **Oxygen toxicity.** Rob was placed on **excessively high concentrations of oxygen** from the moment of his arrival, which resulted in **atelectasis** (*a condition where alveoli in a lung or a part of a lung deflate, causing a partial or complete collapsed lung, resulting in shortness of breath and painful breathing*). The doctors then noted, as shown on Page 127 of the hospital records (see Page C-35 in **Appendix C**) they had decided to place Rob on a BiPAP to "see if it helps atelectasis." In addition, the high concentrations of oxygen (above 60%) caused a cascading negative effect that led to further lung damage.

  o The **atelectasis** caused by the long duration of excessively high concentrations of oxygen (as shown in the chart at the top of Page C-54), followed by the barotrauma caused by 4.5 hours of BiPAP therapy (see Pages C-37 and C-38 and the point below) resulted in Rob's ending up on a ventilator against his will.

  o Once on the ventilator, as shown in the chart at the bottom of Page C-54, they continued to subject Rob to **unnecessarily high levels of inspired oxygen** (referred to as FiO2 for the fraction [or percentage] of inspired oxygen).

  o On July 14, 2021, CapnoAcademy published an article titled "Hyperoxia: Too much of a good thing," in which the authors noted, "*Research shows that time and time again, routine [one-size-fits-all approach] and unchecked high-flow oxygen administration **reaches toxic internal levels within minutes**. To this extent, the current European Society of Cardiology guidelines **recommends giving oxygen only when oxygen saturation levels are below 90%.**" Furthermore, they detailed the cascading negative effect of giving patients unnecessarily high levels of inspired oxygen (referred to as FiO2 for the fraction [or percentage] of inspired oxygen) by stating, "*The patient progressively inhales higher oxygen concentrations as the flow is increased, **causing more and more previously functional and intact alveoli to collapse**. This **increasing atelectasis** [a complete or partial collapse of the entire lung or lobe of the lung] further decreases lung surface area for the transfer of oxygen into the blood. **The hypoxemia [below-normal levels of oxygen in the blood] worsens, and oxygen flow is increased, and so on.**"*
  CapnoAcademy. (2021, August 13). Hyperoxia: Too much of a good thing. CapnoAcademy, From https://www.capnoacademy.com/2021/07/14/hyperoxia-too-much-of-a-good-thing-2

- **DNI removed.** On the morning of September 8, 2021, without notifying Sheila, Dr. Wicked removed Rob's **DNI (Do Not Intubate)** order from his records right before placing Rob on positive-pressure **BiPAP** therapy for **4.5 hours** despite admitting to Sheila "*it has a risk because he has **pneumomediastinum**.*" You can see this order on Page 1018 of the hospital records (see Page C-33).

  o *If Rob had agreed to remove his "do not intubate" (DNI) order, he would have advised Sheila of that fact, yet during a brief call he had with her that morning, he said nothing about agreeing to remove the order prohibiting the doctors intubating him and placing him on a ventilator.*

  o *We contend the doctors removed the DNI order without Rob's agreement for their benefit because they were about to place him on a therapy (BiPAP) they knew could severely damage his lungs. That damage would allow them to force Rob to agree to be placed on a ventilator. That way, they could ensure Rob experienced every aspect of "the protocol that kills."*

- **Contraindicated BiPAP.** Rob was placed on the contraindicated **BiPAP therapy** at around 9:30 AM on September 8th, even though his blood oxygen level was at an acceptable 92%. However, after just over two hours on the BiPAP, his blood oxygen level dropped to 89%, indicating that the BiPAP was worsening his condition. At that point, therapy should have been immediately discontinued. However, Rob was left struggling on the BiPAP for two more hours until around 2:00 PM.
    - **BiPAP** therapy was clearly contraindicated because:
        - Soon after Rob arrived in the Emergency Department on September 3, 2021, he was diagnosed with **pneumomediastinum**. Then, on September 6, 2021, Nurse Carnage advised Sheila, "*He's not a candidate for the other option called BiPAP because he has a pneumomediastinum—which is where there's air trapped in the space in the chest between the lungs, and it can cause him traumatic injury if we do a positive pressure such as a BiPAP.*" This is further confirmed by her note on Page 97 of the hospital records (see Page C-21), where she wrote, "*At this point, patient is maxed out on oxygen, is not a candidate for bipap d/t [due to] pneumomediastinum and is refusing intubation.*"
        - Dr. Wicked knew **barotrauma**—a potentially life-threatening condition where the alveoli, the air sacs of the lungs, rupture and collapse, leading to difficulty breathing and decreased oxygenation of the body—was a likely outcome for someone with pneumomediastinum. On Page 127 of Rob's hospital records (see Page C-35), he stated, "*Monitor for barotrauma given already with pneumomediastinum.*" Unfortunately, the BiPAP did cause barotrauma, as documented on page 141 of the hospital records (see Page C-44), where they stated, "Repeat CXR [Chest X-ray] this afternoon to monitor barotrauma."
    - After the BiPAP and Rob's subsequent intubation, a chest X-ray showed "Extensive pneumomediastinum and chest wall and soft tissue gas in the neck."
    - Furthermore, our independent medical expert, Sammy Wong, MD, considered the use of a BiPAP on Rob an injurious act and one of his "Causes of Action" against the doctors (see **Appendix B**), stating, "*He had known pneumomediastinum on admission yet he was subjected to 4½ hours of BiPAP which substantially increases the risk for barotrauma.*" Dr. Wong also noted, "*It is conceivable that the 'claustrophobia' [that Rob experienced on the BiPAP, as noted on Page 135 of the hospital records on Page C-37] was more likely feeling shortness of breath from the iatrogenic [worsened by medical treatment] pneumomediastinum.*"
    - *Their placing Rob on a BiPAP likely led to their having to place Rob on a ventilator because the damage caused by the BiPAP was so extensive that he could not survive any other way. Such a deliberate and reckless act should at least be considered malpractice. In some courts, it might be regarded as premeditated murder.*

- **Forced ventilation:** Since his arrival at the hospital on September 3, 2021, Rob adamantly insisted, despite the constant badgering to change his mind, that he did **NOT** want to be placed on a ventilator because he knew it would be a death trap. Unfortunately, the 4.5-hour **BiPAP therapy** further damaged Rob's lungs to the point that it was nearly impossible for him to breathe on his own. The increased difficulty breathing he experienced, combined with his weakness because of the starvation he suffered due to their neglecting to focus on his nutritional intake, gave the doctors the excuse that they wanted to force Rob to be placed on a ventilator at 6:43 PM.

    o On Page 136 of the hospital records (see Page C-37 in **Appendix C**), Dr. Dead End alleged that Rob was "borderline" and "will need intubation" at 1400 (2:00 PM). Yet, as shown on Page 3012 of the records (see Page C-38), at that exact time (at 2:00 PM), Rob's respirations were only 22 (the intubation criteria is generally > 30 breaths/minute), and his SpO2 (his blood oxygen level) was at 92%, which is within the NIH's acceptable target range.

        ▪ It is important to note that UC Health Medical Center states that they do not believe patients must be placed on a ventilator until their O2 saturation (SpO2) is **below 85%**, saying: *"When oxygen levels become low (oxygen saturation < 85%), patients are usually intubated and placed on mechanical ventilation."* Covid-19 resources. UC Health. (n.d.). From https://www.uchealth.com/en/media-room/covid-19/ventilators-and-covid-19

    o When he came off the BiPAP at 2:00 PM, as shown on Page 3012 of the hospital records (see Page C-38), Rob's oxygen saturation (blood oxygen level, noted as SpO2), as noted above, was at 92%. As shown on Page 3013 of the records (see Page C-39), his blood oxygen level (SpO2) was at 91% at 4:00 PM. It had only dropped to 88% at 5:00 PM, right before being placed on a ventilator at 6:45 PM. *Thus, it appears Dr. Dead End was dead set on getting Rob intubated and put on a ventilator regardless.*

- **No ABG:** Despite the damage caused by the BiPAP, they should have drawn **an Arterial Blood Gas (ABG)** to ensure that Rob truly and desperately needed to be put on a ventilator. However, they did not have an ABG drawn until 2 hours 21 minutes AFTER Rob was intubated, as noted on Page 137 of the hospital records (see Page C-43).

    o *Sammy Wong, MD, our Medical Expert witness, noted in cause #7 of his "Causes of Action," which appear on Page B-7 of* **Appendix B**, *that: "There is no clear documentation readily available that provides clear indication for intubation. There were no pre-intubation ABGs. Even the ID [Infectious Disease] specialist documented (within the hour or so of intubation) that the patient was in no acute distress ('NAD')."*

    o Considering the fact, as noted by the American Journal of Critical Care, *"A large percentage of ICU patients who require 5 days or more of mechanical ventilation **die in the hospital**,"* no one should be placed on mechanical ventilation without their informed and written consent or the informed and written consent of their Medical Power Attorney. Douglas SL;Daly BJ;Brennan PF;Harris S;Nochomovitz M;Dyer MA; (n.d.). Outcomes of long-term ventilator patients: A descriptive study. American journal of critical care: an official publication, American Association of Critical-Care Nurses. From https://pubmed.ncbi.nlm.nih.gov/9172858

- **Remdesivir extended:** Despite Sheila's directives as Rob's Medical Power of Attorney that he **NOT** be administered **remdesivir**, after succeeding in getting Rob on a ventilator, Drs. Lament and Torture placed the following notes on Page 159 of Rob's hospital records (see Page C-45): "Refused Remdesivir from 9/5 until 9/6" (by Dr. Lament) and "Now that he is intubated will extend Remdesivir to 10 days" (by Dr. Torture).

  o *These statements, made by Drs. Lament and Torture make the case that they were delighted Rob was finally on a ventilator so they could subject him to 10 days of **remdesivir** so Covid Coven Hospital of Plano, Texas, could earn more of the "bonus incentive payments for all things related to COVID-19 (testing, diagnosing, admitting to hospital, use of remdesivir and ventilators and also death" that are paid by the federal government (your tax paying dollars at work killing your loved ones) under the CARES Act as noted in the "Hospitals' Incentive Payments for COVID-19" article in **Appendix D**.*

  o *Ignoring Sheila's clear directive violated paragraph (a)(3) of Title 42 of the Code of Federal Regulations, Section 482.13, which appears in **Appendix E**, and states, "The patient or his or her representative (as allowed under State law) has the right to make informed decisions regarding his or her care. The patient's rights include being informed of his or her health status, being involved in care planning and treatment, and being able to request or refuse treatment."*

- **High PEEP:** From the moment Rob was placed on the ventilator, the **PEEP (Positive End Expiratory Pressure)** setting remained at a high level of 14 cm H_2O. PEEP is pressure applied by a ventilator (or a BiPAP device) at the end of each breath (upon exhalation) to "recruit" (keep open) damaged alveoli. Rob had ruptured/collapsed alveoli due to the **barotrauma** caused by the 4.5 hours of BiPAP therapy, and excess "end expiratory pressure" was required to "recruit" them (that is, to keep them from collapsing between breaths) as, if they were to collapse, adequate oxygen and carbon dioxide exchange could not occur. The continually high PEEP setting that was never reduced created two problems:

  1. High PEEP levels can decrease lung compliance (that is, the ability of the lungs to expand and contract in response to changes in pressure with a resulting lack of efficient exchange of gasses in the lungs), making it far more difficult (or nearly impossible) to wean a patient off the ventilator. *Thus, the barotrauma caused by the BiPAP and the resulting high PEEP on the ventilator setting put Rob in a very precarious situation.*
  Advanced respiratory monitoring in COVID-19 patients: Use less PEEP! (n.d.). Retrieved April 5, 2023, from https://ccforum.biomedcentral.com/counter/pdf/10.1186/s13054-020-02953-z.pdf

  2. Their criteria for attempting to wean someone from the ventilator was a PEEP of 5 to 8 cm H2O and an FiO2 (oxygen concentration) of 50% or less. However, they kept the PEEP setting on the ventilator at 14 to 15 for the entire 35 days Rob was on the ventilator, as shown in the bottom chart on Page C-54 in **Appendix C**. Unfortunately, because they refused to lower the PEEP setting below 14, Rob was *trapped on a device they could not remove him from.*

     ▪ Sammy Wong, MD, our medical expert witness, said in his "Letter of Introduction," which appears in **Appendix B**, "*Since he was sedated and paralyzed, he was dependent on the ventilator. . . They just maintained his ventilator settings essentially unchanged . . . until he died.*"

- **Profound anemia:** On September 15, 2021, Sheila brought to the doctors' attention, based on the blood tests shown in the online MyChart records she had access to, that Rob was suffering from **anemia**. Rob's protein intake was inadequate, and his body was not producing sufficient red blood cells (and hemoglobin, which carries oxygen) to adequately carry oxygen throughout the body. Dr. Wicked brushed off her concerns by saying, "what happens to everybody in the ICU over a lengthy period is that they start getting anemia."

    o They ignored Rob's anemia despite the fact, "*Recent studies have indicated an association between improved mortality, shorter ventilation days, and shorter duration of ICU and hospital stays with increases in protein intake for critically ill patients. This is particularly relevant for those critically ill patients with a prolonged ICU stay.*" Dickerson, R. N., & Buckley, C. T. (2021, July 1). Impact of propofol sedation upon caloric overfeeding and protein inadequacy in critically ill patients receiving nutrition support. Pharmacy (Basel, Switzerland). From https://www.ncbi.nlm.nih.gov/pmc/articles/PMC8293440

    o Rob was already living on the edge. The last thing he needed was to end up suffering from anemia because he was already "hypoxic" (a condition in which there is a deficiency in the amount of oxygen that reaches the body's tissues), as noted at the top of the "Impression and Plan" on Page 27 of his hospital records, which you can see on Page C-3. *Whether by willful ignorance, uncaring negligence, or nefarious intent, the doctors chose to ignore Rob's eventually profound anemia, which further decreased his chance of survival.*

    o Rob's Sammy Wong, MD, our medical expert witness, said in his Interim Analysis in **Appendix B**, "*The diagnostic work up for the profound anemia was inadequately addressed.*" One of his Causes of Action was "*His hemoglobin dropped dramatically and was not addressed appropriately. Oxygen in the blood was adequate and blood was being circulated with a normal cardiac output but delivery to the tissues was profoundly lacking.*"

- **Pharmaceutical assault:** Despite Sheila's continual request that Rob not be subjected to high doses of a barrage of **nephrotoxic** (toxic to the kidneys) and **hepatotoxic** (toxic to the liver) medications, during his 40-day stay, Rob was continually assaulted by heavy sedatives (propofol, fentanyl, and midazolam), paralytics (Nimbex and rocuronium), a corticosteroid (SOLU-MEDROL), antibiotics (cefepime and meropenem), catecholamine neurotransmitters (dopamine and norepinephrine), a vasodilator (VELETRI), an anticoagulant (Lovenox), an anti-inflammatory (baricitinib), a Beta blocker (labetalol), a mucolytic (acetylcysteine), an analgesic (acetaminophen), and an antifungal (micafungin).

    o *The non-stop bombardment of pharmaceuticals further weakened him, caused him irreparable harm and injury, sabotaged his chances of survival, and directly contributed to his eventual death.*

    o *Near the end of his stay, Rob suffered from **severe acute kidney and liver injury**, which is no surprise because the doctors made it clear to Sheila that their policy was to continue the daily, non-stop, massive assault of harmful medications until lab tests showed results that were "8 to 10 times the upper limit of normal" as noted on Page 259 of the hospital records (see Page C-50 in **Appendix C**).*

    o *What possible motive could they have for waiting for the drugs to cause sufficient damage to Rob's liver and kidneys to the point that the test results finally reached 8x to 10x their normal upper limit? If this isn't evidence of nefarious intent and malpractice,*

- **Risky drug:** On September 20th, at 6:35 PM, without advising Sheila or requesting her permission, Rob was started on a risky Emergency Use Authorization (EUA) trial drug named **baricitinib** (Olumiant), an anti-inflammatory drug typically prescribed for treating rheumatoid arthritis (a condition Rob did not have) that the doctors were using in an off-label manner.

  - *The drug's harmful side effects included upper respiratory tract infections, lower respiratory tract infections, increased liver enzyme levels, fever, shortness of breath, cancer and immune system problems, increased risk of heart attack, blood clots, and tears in the stomach or intestines of patients who are on corticosteroids—and Rob was being administered high doses of a potent corticosteroid named SOLU-MEDROL.*

    - *According to MedlinePlus, "Taking baricitinib may decrease your ability to fight infection and increase the risk that you will get a serious infection, including severe fungal, bacterial, or viral infections that spread through the body. These infections may need to be treated in a hospital and may cause death."*
      U.S. National Library of Medicine. (n.d.). Baricitinib: Medlineplus drug information. MedlinePlus. From https://medlineplus.gov/druginfo/meds/a618033.html

  - Thus, without "informed consent" from Sheila, Rob was given another (and there were several) medication that was likely to worsen his "Covid" symptoms. Of course, when his symptoms did subsequently worsen, they would always attribute the decline to "Covid," not to the drugs that were significantly diminishing his chances of survival. *Before administering an EUA trial drug such as baricitinib, the doctors were morally obligated to explain the risks and benefits to Sheila and obtain her "informed consent." Accordingly, we contend that their deliberate failure to do so constitutes malfeasance and malpractice.*

  - It is medically unethical and a violation of Texas, federal, and international laws to administer a medical treatment without informed consent. *The doctors involved committed constructive fraud, which occurs when a physician breaches their fiduciary duty to disclose material information to their patient. No fraudulent intent is required, and reasonable reliance on the nondisclosure is presumed.*

- **Refused surfactant:** On September 23, 2021, Sheila learned from Dr. Mei, a doctor friend from California, that a **natural surfactant** (a mixture of lipids and proteins) could be delivered directly into the endotracheal tube to coat Rob's damaged alveoli (the air sacs of the lungs), thereby increasing their efficiency. The result would be improved oxygenation of Rob's bloodstream at a reduced level of PEEP (Positive End Expiratory Pressure) and decreased oxygen concentrations—lessening lung damage and making it more likely that Rob could be weaned from the ventilator. *Unfortunately, her request that Rob be administered natural surfactant was flatly refused.*

  - Surfactant is a substance that is usually produced by the alveoli to reduce surface tension, keep the alveoli from collapsing between breaths, prevent the lungs from collapsing when you breathe out, and help them inflate more easily when you breathe in. Inflamed and damaged alveoli (which Rob had) generally produce less surfactant.

  - When Sheila asked Dr. Liar on September 23rd if he would agree to administer a surfactant, he boldly said, "We don't give surfactant here!" Then, during a September 27, 2021, intervention meeting, Dr. Mei asked Dr. Liar face-to-face if he would agree to administer a natural surfactant. He replied, "We don't have surfactant." When she offered to procure and bring it in herself to help save Rob's life, he said he would only agree to consider an unproven "clinical trial" drug. However, he quickly learned that the hospital pharmacy would not approve procuring the "trial" drug.

     ○   A pivotal opportunity to vastly improve Rob's chances of survival was missed because Dr. Liar chose to ignore the input from another qualified, licensed physician who knew that pulmonary surfactant was considered a viable treatment for Covid patients. That fact was noted in numerous articles published in early 2021. One such article stated that "*This so-called 'surfactant replacement therapy' (SRT) is currently the standard-of-care to reduce mortality in premature infants with surfactant-deficient lungs, and the clinical success of SRT in Newborn Respiratory Distress Syndrome (NRDS) has rationalized attempts to broaden the therapeutic application of clinical surfactants to other lung diseases like ARDS. One of the common results of a COVID-19 infection is impairment of surfactant production and secretion. Therefore, surfactant treatment to anticipate on the progression of severe lung injury in COVID-19 patients has been proposed as a potential treatment for COVID-19.*"

         Herman, L., De Smedt, S. C., & Raemdonck, K. (2022, February). Pulmonary surfactant as a versatile biomaterial to fight COVID-19. Journal of controlled release : official journal of the Controlled Release Society. From https://www.ncbi.nlm.nih.gov/pmc/articles/PMC8605818

- **Ultimate demise:** Rob ultimately suffered a slow and painful death because his physicians failed to disclose the availability of **a safe, outpatient, multi-drug, and oxygen at-home treatment for COVID-19**. They instead gave him harmful drugs and therapies, including insisting he be intubated and placed on a ventilator when his blood oxygen levels were above 90%.

     ○   *The drugs and therapies prescribed and forced on Rob by the doctors were the proximal cause of Rob's death. Sheila was also severely harmed. She suffered the loss of love, affection, intimacy, relationship, comfort, care, support, companionship, solace, training, guidance, and other benefits and assistance, from Rob. She also suffered significant economic loss and expenses.*

- **Proximal cause:** The proximal cause of Robert A. Skiba II's death was the **medications and treatments** prescribed by his doctors and facilitated and promoted by the policies and dictates of the administration of Covid Coven Hospital of Plano, Texas. They had a motive (the **government incentives** that enriched the hospital and further secured the medical staff's positions) and a clear opportunity to cause Rob harm for their benefit. He did not die of natural causes but rather due to "*the protocol that kills*" that was forced upon him despite his and Sheila Skiba's clear and loud objections.

     ○   *The conduct of all defendants to this cause of action in allowing or performing Robert A. Skiba II's malnutrition, over-oxygenation, needless intubation and ventilation, and excessive medication to the point of multi-organ (liver and kidney) failure constitutes medical misfeasance.*

     ○   *The reckless, negligent, fraudulent, malicious, and oppressive conduct of the physicians charged with Rob's care was the primary cause of his death and Sheila's resultant harm. Such egregious conduct warrants the imposition of punitive and exemplary damages and potential criminal charges.*

     ○   *In addition, Covid Coven Hospital of Plano, Texas, is vicariously liable for the conduct of the physicians since their behavior was authorized, approved, and ratified by officers, directors and/or managing agents of the hospital.*

Appendix B – Medical Expert Testimony

Sammy Wong, MD FACP — Letter of Introduction
July 21, 2022

To whom it may concern:

Re: Robert Skiba

Having provided formal and informal opinions, often without compensation, on well over a hundred cases over the past 30 years along with expert opinions and testimonies for the Medical Board of California, I recently came across a case that has multiple areas of medicolegal vulnerabilities.

While most cases that are presented to me are from attorneys, physician-clients and the Medical Board, I was introduced to Mrs. Sheila Skiba through a physician friend. Her 52-year-old previously healthy, robust and highly influential husband, Robert, was speaking at a conference in Ohio in August 2021 and came down with COVID symptoms. He was treated but continued to have a cough as he returned home to Plano, Texas.

He was seen at a local hospital and his oxygen saturation was noted to be low at 71%. A chest X-ray showed pneumomediastinum (abnormal air collection in the space between the lungs).

As he was hospitalized, he and Sheila requested that he not be given **remdesivir** and not be mechanically ventilated. Instead, a nurse practitioner prescribed **remdesivir** which was given. **VELETRI**, used for pulmonary hypertension, was also given even though he had no evidence for this condition. (*VELETRI is associated with development of profound inflammatory response in the lungs.*)

He was also given **Tocilizumab** even though an article in New England Journal of Medicine published 5 months earlier clearly indicated lack of benefit in people with COVID. He was also given **baricitinib** which resulted in hepatitis yet was ineffective against COVID. The baricitinib-associated hepatitis was overlooked. He developed liver failure 9 days after the baricitinib was stopped. He died 3 days later.

Aside from giving Robert *ineffective and harmful medications*, he was subjected to bi-level positive airway pressure (BiPAP) even though he had the known pneumomediastinum. He was oxygenating adequately with supplemental high flow oxygen. BiPAP is contraindicated in pneumomediastinum. He was reportedly "claustrophobic" with BiPAP and was intubated shortly thereafter in spite of prior refusals.

There were no arterial blood gases (ABGs) prior to the intubation to verify impending respiratory failure. Available notes indicated that he was not in acute distress prior to the intubation. After he was sedated, paralyzed, intubated, and mechanically ventilated, a chest X-ray showed new extensive pneumomediastinum.

Since he was sedated and paralyzed, he was dependent on the ventilator. All of the ABGs showed profound respiratory acidosis indicating that the staff chose not to adjust the ventilator settings to improve his alveolar ventilation. *They just maintained his ventilator settings essentially unchanged . . . until he died.*

While there were multiple treatment-related issues, the standard diagnostic process was clearly abandoned. As soon as he informed the ER staff that he was treated for COVID, they perseverated (repeat or prolong an action, thought, or utterance after the stimulus that prompted it has ceased) in keeping that diagnosis. They did not expand the differential diagnosis in this patient who had caught something while in Ohio. They also did not consider doing a bronchoscopy or lung biopsy in this otherwise, young healthy man.

After his death, a private autopsy showed severe and extensive fibrosis with diffuse alveolar damage consistent with (cryptogenic) organizing pneumonia. (This is not "pneumonia" per se that is treated with antibacterial antibiotics.) The standard treatment for organizing pneumonia is high dose corticosteroids which results in complete recovery in up to 80% of patients within a few weeks.

*Many of the cases that I have reviewed have a single extreme departure from the standard of care or a few simple departures. In this case, there are **multiple extreme departures**. There were multiple temporal and proximate relationships that would suggest causation.*

The lack of expediting an aggressive diagnostic work up for his cough yet attributing everything to COVID reflects disregard to basic diagnostic medicine. *If you do not make the diagnosis, you can't treat the patient properly and often subject the patient to **unnecessary harms**. It took 40 days and an autopsy to make the diagnosis.*

Although I have not completely reviewed and analyzed all of the over 5,000 pages of the medical record, I have already identified key medicolegal vulnerabilities (**Interim Analysis Report**), indexed the huge document, and entered data into Excel format for ease of trending and associating conditions with interventions.

I believe this is a case that bears altruistic impact, accountability, and societal benefit.

Sincerely,

Sammy S. Wong, MD FACP
Assistant Professor of Medicine (ret)
Medical Consultant and Expert, Department of Consumer Affairs, Medical Board of California

*The views expressed by Dr. Wong are solely his own and
do not necessarily reflect the views of his affiliated institutions or organizations.*

Interim Analysis

Sammy S. Wong, MD FACP Bio
American Board of Internal Medicine Certified Internist.
Assistant Professor of Medicine (ret), Loma Linda University School of Medicine.
Annual lecturer in ACP-sponsored ABIM preparation conferences since 1999, giving multiple presentations on Medical Malpractice, Patient Safety, Cognitive Bias, and Diagnostic Errors.
Provided expert opinions and testimonies on over a hundred cases over the past 30 years.

Mr. Skiba was a robust and healthy 52-year-old married, former Army helicopter pilot who was a keynote speaker at a major conference in Ohio late August 2021.

About 2 weeks later, on Friday, September 3, prior to the Labor Day weekend, he was seen at a hospital in Plano, Texas with a cough, congestion, shortness of breath and an oxygen saturation of 71% (normal is > 92%).

He was placed on supplemental oxygen which improved the oxygen saturation to 95%. He was without a fever and had a respiratory rate of 22 per minute. He was not ill-appearing and was not in respiratory distress. A chest X-ray showed pneumomediastinum [air abnormally trapped in the space in the chest between the lungs] and air in the soft tissue of the neck. A CT scan showed no (large) pulmonary embolus but had multiple pulmonary opacities. His white cell count was normal, but the inflammatory markers (CRP, ferritin, D-dimer) were abnormally elevated. An arterial blood gas (ABG) showed respiratory alkalosis with an arterial oxygen of 62 mmHg (saturation 94%) while on 80% supplemental oxygen.

He was admitted to the hospitalist service though a nurse practitioner from the Critical Care service was consulted. She noted that the patient had "increased work of breathing," yet he was "without use of accessory muscles or paradoxical movements" (of the diaphragm). The hospitalist noted that the patient "appears comfortable" and "in no acute distress." Even the ER physician noted *"He is not ill-appearing"* and *"No respiratory distress."* Nevertheless, the Critical Care nurse practitioner indicated that the *"Patient is at high risk for needing* intubation [as if it was a foregone conclusion—see Page 27 of the hospital records on Page C-3 in Appendix C]." Her plans included Optiflow, **VELETRI**, **remdesivir**, empiric antibiotics and enoxaparin.

At 9:05 PM on 9/3/21 he was transferred from the ED to the ICU, and at about midnight that evening he was given remdesivir in spite of the patient's and spouse's objections. He was given another five doses over the next several days. VELETRI was also started at 3:25 AM (on 9/4/21). He was temporarily moved out of the ICU on 9/5/21 because he refused intubation but was transferred back to the ICU on 9/6/21 to resume VELETRI administration. Reportedly, his oxygenation worsened though no repeat ABGs [Arterial Blood Gasses] were done. VELETRI was given without any evidence of pulmonary hypertension.

On September 8, he was placed on bi-level positive airway pressure (BiPAP) for 4 1/2 hours even though he had a known pneumomediastinum [see the bottom of Page 135 of the hospital records on Page C-37 in Appendix C]. The patient felt claustrophobic with the BiPAP [see the bottom of Page 136 of the hospital records on Page C-41 in Appendix C]. At 5:48 PM, the nurse noted that the patient was "alert, awake, cooperative, oriented (x4) and tranquil" [see the bottom of Page 3729 of the hospital records on Page C-40 in Appendix C] and that his "speech was clear." His lungs were clear though he was tachypneic and had a productive cough. Although his respiratory rate was in the 30s at 4 PM and 5 PM, it had been fluctuating in the 20s and 30s for at least the prior two days. His oxygen saturation at 5 PM was 88% though he had been fluctuating between 89 and 97% in the prior two days [see pages 3012 and 3013 of the hospital records on Pages C-38 and C-39 in Appendix C].

At 6:28 PM, the physician documented that the patient was in "mild respiratory distress," [see the top of Page 136 of the hospital records on Page C-41 in Appendix C] but the note also indicated that "Called back to bedside at 6:00 p.m. increased work of breathing respiratory muscle fatigue and requesting intubation." It is unknown whether the physician actually witnessed increased reliance of accessory muscles of ventilation, paradoxical ventilatory motion of the diaphragm, sweating, or nasal flaring. There are no available ABGs to document acidosis or increased PCO2 (to reflect lactic acidosis due to muscle fatigue with hypoventilation) prior to intubation. End-tidal CO2 was checked only during intubation and not prior.

With intubation, he was sedated and paralyzed for the rest of his hospitalization with continuous infusions of cisatracurium, fentanyl, midazolam, propofol and ketamine. Prior to this hospitalization he had never been on any of these medicines.

His course was complicated with Klebsiella bacteremia and fungemia as well as profound anemia with blood noted in the stool. No endoscopy was done. The spouse requested Procrit instead of blood transfusion.

On September 20, baricitinib was prescribed for 12 days. Notably, he developed hepatitis on October 2, but the cause was attributed to hepatic steatosis or COVID. The liver enzymes returned near normal but on October 10, the liver enzymes shot up into the thousands. This was attributed to "ischemic" liver. The next day, he developed acute renal failure (Cr 1.5).

By the morning of October 13, his kidney function worsened (Cr 2.11) and for some reason at this level of kidney dysfunction, Continuous Renal Replacement Therapy (CRRT) was to be implemented. He had a dialysis catheter placed via the right internal jugular vein that morning. However, later that afternoon, he developed pulseless asystole and died after 4 rounds of epinephrine were given between chest compressions. No attempts at defibrillation were documented in the event the asystole was fine ventricular fibrillation. Mr. Skiba was pronounced dead at 5:11 PM.

An autopsy was performed by a privately paid pathologist 2 days later showed the following:
I. Organizing pneumonia:
    a.   Diffuse, bilateral, dense, tan-red, fibrotic lung parenchyma
    b.   Focal firm brown lung parenchyma in the left upper lobe
    c.   Cysts and honeycombing with necrotic debris/hemorrhage
    d.   Small pleural effusions
    e.   Microscopic findings consistent with end-stage organizing pneumonia:
    i.   Diffuse alveolar damage
    ii.   Areas of ischemic/necrotic lung parenchyma
    iii.   Diffuse fibrosis
    iv.   Microcystic remodeling
    v.   Arteriolar clots and re-cannulization.
II. Cardiac hypertrophy (552g).
III. Anasarca of the soft tissues.
IV. Red-purple contusions of the chest and abdomen.

The final cause of death was "Organizing pneumonia."

The pathologist noted the following microscopic description of the lungs: End-stage organizing pneumonia with diffuse alveolar damage. There are numerous alveolar macrophages and reactive pneumocytes, squamous metaplasia, and increased mixed inflammation with fibrin in the alveoli. Extensive interstitial fibrosis is present. In some areas there is frank ischemic necrosis of the parenchyma. Small clots are present in the small arterioles and there are focal areas demonstrating long-term architectural changes such as recannulization of vessels and microcystic honeycombing.

In summary, this was a healthy 52-year young married man who was seen at the ER about two weeks after exhibiting COVID-like symptoms. He and his wife specifically requested that he not be on remdesivir, but it was given. He was given **VELETRI** (epoprostenol) which is indicated for people with known "severe pulmonary arterial hypertension." There was no objective evidence [that is, a diagnosis of pulmonary arterial hypertension does not appear anywhere in Rob's records indicating] that he had severe PAH. It is unknown whether the VELETRI caused or contributed to this patient's eventual "extensive interstitial fibrosis." (Epoprostenol-associated pneumonitis. J Heart Lung Transplant. 2010 Sep;29(9):1071-5. doi: 10.1016/j.healun.2010.04.023. Epub 2010 Jun 8.)

He had known pneumomediastinum on admission, yet he was subjected to 4 1/2 hours of BiPAP which substantially increases the risk for barotrauma. After the BiPAP and then intubation, a chest X-ray showed "Extensive pneumomediastinum and chest wall and soft tissue gas in the neck." *It is conceivable that the "claustrophobia" was more likely feeling <u>shortness of breath</u> from the iatrogenic [caused or worsened by medical treatment] pneumomediastinum.*

There is no clear documentation readily available that provides clear indications for intubation. The vital signs recorded did not reflect significant deviation from the vital signs taken in the days leading up to the intubation though there were variations in the oxygen saturations and respiratory rate. There was no pre-intubation ABGs. Even the ID specialist documented (within the hour or so of intubation) that the patient was in no acute distress ("NAD"). The oxygen saturations noted in the chart below indicate adequate oxygenation:

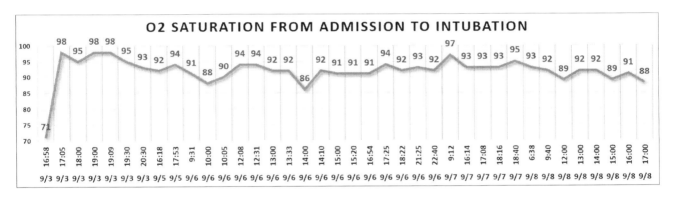

Although the autopsy did not reveal endocarditis, it should be concerning on a prospective basis that a TEE was not performed as soon as symptomatic fungemia was known in face of known thickened aortic valve (on September 4 echocardiogram). The treatment and management differ substantially with fungal endocarditis as opposed to bacterial endocarditis.

It is beyond this reviewer's practice to opine on the type and extent of the sedatives and paralytics that were administered to this patient during this hospitalization. It is unknown whether there was a reasonable and compassionate level of sedation administered versus excessive though all of the ABGs after he was intubated and mechanically ventilated showed profound respiratory acidosis. He was completely dependent on the ventilator, yet he was not being ventilated adequately. An opinion regarding the sedatives and paralytics would not have been necessary if the patient was not intubated and be completely dependent on the ventilator.

It is also troublesome that the physicians were focused on the patient having only COVID to explain all the symptoms. It appears that there were cognitive errors in the diagnostic work up. These errors included premature closure [a type of cognitive error in which the physician fails to consider reasonable alternatives after an initial diagnosis is made. It is a common cause of delayed diagnosis and misdiagnosis borne out of a faulty clinical decision-making process], framing effect [an effect that occurs when decision makers choose inconsistent solutions for identical problems based on the way the problems are presented to them], and diagnostic momentum [a type of confirmation bias that can occur in medical settings where the tendency is for a diagnosis to be blindly accepted and passed on with little examination of the underlying evidence for its validity]. There was no evidence that a bronchoscopy or even lung biopsy was even considered in this previously healthy young man. Limited expansion of the differential diagnosis was made for the rapidly and markedly elevated transaminases but that merely included blood work.

The diagnostic work up for the profound anemia was inadequately addressed. It appears that the presence of blood on the fecal occult blood test (FOBT positive on October 4) was not addressed. He likely had intraluminal gastrointestinal bleeding. Lack of blood in spite of adequate arterial oxygenation and cardiac function still results in poor tissue oxygenation.

There was lack of clear documentation of the risks, benefits and reasonable alternatives on procedures and medications given. **VELETRI** and **baricitinib** were given in spite of substantial harms which did not benefit and were without clear indications for them. Tocilizumab, known not to benefit in those with COVID, was given without benefit and he was exposed to risk of harm.

The above highlights the concerns that reflect suboptimal partnered collaboration with the patient and spouse by specific physicians involved.

At times, it appears that there was absolute disregard of the patient's and spouse's wishes. With continued review of the over 5,000 pages of the hospital documents, additional medicolegal vulnerabilities may arise.

Sammy S. Wong, MD FACP
Assistant Professor of Medicine (ret)
Medical Consultant and Expert, Department of Consumer Affairs, Medical Board of California

September 12, 2022

The views expressed by Dr. Wong are solely his own and
do not necessarily reflect the views of his affiliated institutions or organizations.

Causes of Action
September 12, 2022

#	Issue	Comments
1	Physician acknowledged that he refused remdesivir but was given six doses a total of 800 mg.	Does this rise to the level of criminal assault and/or battery? The renal failure toward the end of his hospitalization could be argued as due to acute tubular necrosis (ATN) due to hypoperfusion due to hypotension.
2	No indication for the use of epoprostenol (**VELETRI**).	He had no evidence of pulmonary arterial hypertension. His ECGs did not demonstrate right ventricular hypertrophy. Both echocardiograms did not demonstrate right ventricular hypertrophy or right ventricular enlargement. **VELETRI** is a prostanoid vasodilator indicated for the treatment of pulmonary arterial hypertension (PAH) (WHO Group 1) to improve exercise capacity. Studies establishing effectiveness included predominantly patients with NYHA Functional Class III-IV symptoms and etiologies of idiopathic or heritable PAH or PAH associated with connective tissue diseases. (www.accessdata.fda.gov/drugsatfda_docs/label/2012/022260s005lbl.pdf) The initiation of iEPO and iNO in patients with refractory hypoxemia secondary to COVID-19, on average, did not produce significant increases in oxygenation metrics such as Pao2/Fio2, Pao2, or Spo2 despite minimal other confounding interventions. (www.ncbi.nlm.nih.gov/pmc/articles/PMC7581066/#_sec11title)
3	Side effect of epoprostenol (**VELETRI**) includes profound interstitial lung disease.	**Epoprostenol** can incite a profound inflammatory response in the pulmonary interstitium. Due to a lack of indication for its use, the patient was subjected to unnecessary risks. (www.ncbi.nlm.nih.gov/pmc/articles/PMC2926193) Epoprostenol-associated pneumonitis. J Heart Lung Transplant. 2010 Sep;29(9):1071-5. doi: 10.1016/j.healun.2010.04.023. Epub 2010 Jun 8.
4	**Tocilizumab** given in spite of lack of literature to support its use in COVID	**Tocilizumab**, known not to benefit in those with COVID, was given without benefit and he was exposed to risk of harm. In a randomized trial involving hospitalized patients with severe COVID-19 pneumonia, the use of tocilizumab did not result in significantly better clinical status or lower mortality than placebo at 28 days. (N Engl J Med 2021; 384:1503-1516 (April 2021))
5	BiPAP instituted in spite of having pneumomediastinum - contraindication	He had known pneumomediastinum on admission, yet he was subjected to 4 ½ hours of BiPAP which substantially increases the risk for barotrauma. After the BiPAP and then intubation, a chest X-ray showed "Extensive pneumomediastinum and chest wall and soft tissue gas in the neck." It is conceivable that the "claustrophobia" was more likely feeling shortness of breath from the iatrogenic [caused or worsened by medical treatment] pneumomediastinum.
6	Physician acknowledged his refusal of intubation and mechanical ventilation but eventually sedated, paralyzed him, intubated, and mechanically ventilated him until he died.	Does this rise to the level of criminal assault and/or battery?

7	Indications for intubation and mechanical ventilation not met	There is no clear documentation readily available that provides clear indication for intubation. There were no pre-intubation ABGs [Arterial Blood Gasses]. Even the ID [Infectious Disease] specialist documented (within the hour or so of intubation) that the patient was in no acute distress ("NAD"). It is clear that the facility had an end-tidal CO_2 monitor since they used it during intubation.
8	Remained profoundly in primary respiratory acidosis while mechanically ventilated, sedated and paralyzed without appropriate adjustment of the ventilator settings.	Refer to ABGs [Arterial Blood Gasses] post intubation and during rest of his course.
9	**Baricitinib** causing hepatitis unrecognized	He was given **baricitinib** daily starting on September 20 for 12 days. His liver enzymes rose to greater than 3 times upper limit of normal by early October. The PA covering for Infectious Disease did not address this on October 2 even after s/he acknowledged elevated liver enzymes in the progress note. The Hospitalist attributed the elevated liver enzymes to COVID or hepatic steatosis. Although the liver enzymes eventually returned toward normal, it again increased dramatically into the thousands prompting the liver specialist (gastroenterologist) to order a wide spectrum of labs ("shot-gunning" a diagnosis) but later attributed the hepatitis to ischemic liver.
10	Profound anemia in face of blood in stool not addressed	When he was admitted, his hemoglobin was 15.7 (normal).

When he was admitted, his hemoglobin was 15.7 (normal).

On October 4, he was noted to have blood in the stool sample which was not addressed. His hemoglobin was 7.7 on that day. A reticulocyte count was not done until October 8 (which was slightly elevated suggesting the anemia was not a marrow-suppressive cause).

His hemoglobin dropped even further October 11 to 5.9. He died two days later.

Oxygen delivery to the tissues include three factors:
• Cardiac output
• Oxygen saturation
• Hemoglobin

His cardiac output based on ejection fractions on the echocardiogram was normal.
His oxygen saturation has been consistently above 90%.
His hemoglobin dropped dramatically and was not addressed appropriately.

Oxygen in the blood was adequate and blood was being circulated with a normal cardiac output but delivery to the tissues was profoundly lacking.

Sammy S. Wong, MD FACP
Assistant Professor of Medicine (ret)
Medical Consultant and Expert, Department of Consumer Affairs, Medical Board of California

The views expressed by Dr. Wong are solely his own and
do not necessarily reflect the views of his affiliated institutions or organizations.

Appendix C – Excerpts from Hospital Records

Exhibit 1–Double Dose of Remdesivir Given in ED Prior to Admission (Evening of 9/3/21)

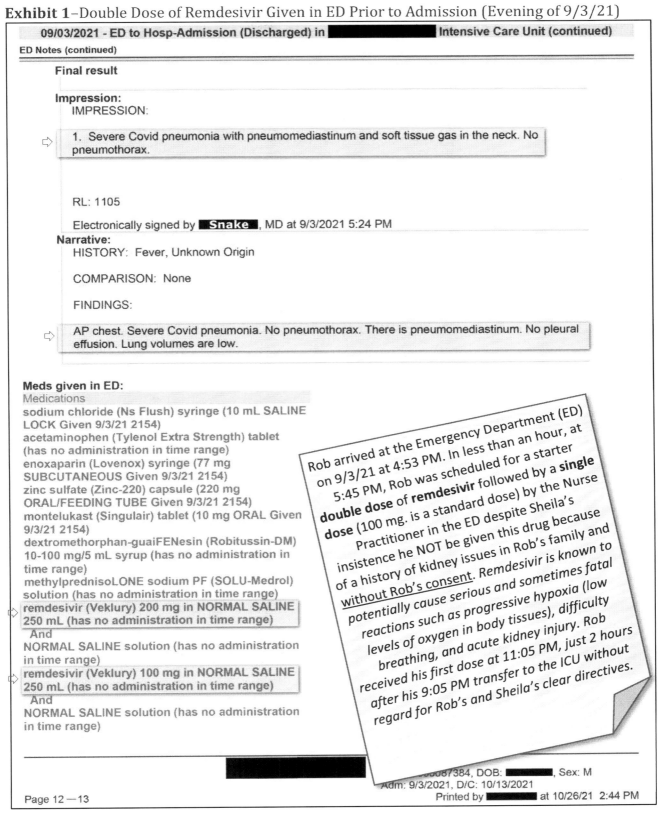

09/03/2021 - ED to Hosp-Admission (Discharged) in ▮▮▮▮▮▮▮▮▮▮ Intensive Care Unit (continued)

ED Notes (continued)

Final result

Impression:
IMPRESSION:

➪ 1. Severe Covid pneumonia with pneumomediastinum and soft tissue gas in the neck. No pneumothorax.

RL: 1105

Electronically signed by ▮**Snake**▮, MD at 9/3/2021 5:24 PM

Narrative:
HISTORY: Fever, Unknown Origin

COMPARISON: None

FINDINGS:

➪ AP chest. Severe Covid pneumonia. No pneumothorax. There is pneumomediastinum. No pleural effusion. Lung volumes are low.

Meds given in ED:
Medications
sodium chloride (Ns Flush) syringe (10 mL SALINE LOCK Given 9/3/21 2154)
acetaminophen (Tylenol Extra Strength) tablet (has no administration in time range)
enoxaparin (Lovenox) syringe (77 mg SUBCUTANEOUS Given 9/3/21 2154)
zinc sulfate (Zinc-220) capsule (220 mg ORAL/FEEDING TUBE Given 9/3/21 2154)
montelukast (Singulair) tablet (10 mg ORAL Given 9/3/21 2154)
dextromethorphan-guaiFENesin (Robitussin-DM) 10-100 mg/5 mL syrup (has no administration in time range)
methylprednisoLONE sodium PF (SOLU-Medrol) solution (has no administration in time range)
➪ **remdesivir (Veklury) 200 mg in NORMAL SALINE 250 mL (has no administration in time range)**
And
NORMAL SALINE solution (has no administration in time range)
➪ **remdesivir (Veklury) 100 mg in NORMAL SALINE 250 mL (has no administration in time range)**
And
NORMAL SALINE solution (has no administration in time range)

Rob arrived at the Emergency Department (ED) on 9/3/21 at 4:53 PM. In less than an hour, at 5:45 PM, Rob was scheduled for a starter **double dose** of **remdesivir** followed by a **single dose** (100 mg. is a standard dose) by the Nurse Practitioner in the ED despite Sheila's insistence he NOT be given this drug because of a history of kidney issues in Rob's family and without Rob's consent. Remdesivir is known to potentially cause serious and sometimes fatal reactions such as progressive hypoxia (low levels of oxygen in body tissues), difficulty breathing, and acute kidney injury. Rob received his first dose at 11:05 PM, just 2 hours after his 9:05 PM transfer to the ICU without regard for Rob's and Sheila's clear directives.

▮▮▮▮▮▮▮087384, DOB: ▮▮▮▮▮, Sex: M
Adm: 9/3/2021, D/C: 10/13/2021
Page 12 — 13   Printed by ▮▮▮▮▮ at 10/26/21 2:44 PM

09/03/2021 - ED to Hosp-Admission (Discharged) in ████████████ **Intensive Care Unit (continued)**

H&P Notes (continued)

Extensive multifocal pulmonary opacities likely related to pneumonia such as COVID pneumonia.

⇨ *Pneumomediastinum and subcutaneous emphysema as detailed above.*

⇨ *The heart is enlarged.*

Low-density of the liver likely represents fatty infiltration.

RL: 1603

End of report.

Electronically signed by ███ **Quack** ███ *, MD at 9/3/2021 6:41 PM*

⇨ Chest Xray: Normal sized heart with extensive bilateral pulmonary o[...]

EKG (telemetry): Sinus rhythm

I visualized CXR images and EKG strip

Discussed plan of care with patient

Assessment:

Acute respiratory failure with hypoxia
COVID-19 pneumonia
Hyponatremia
Hyperglycemia

Plan:

Admit to inpatient status.
⇨ It is anticipated that he will require at least a two-midnight inpatient stay.
Inpatient admission is warranted given COVID-19 pneumonia with hypoxia

Pneumonia:

The patient's condition is: Worsening

Assessment:
- Based on the patient's presentation cough, dyspnea, tachypnea, rales, decreased O2 sats and infiltrates on CXR and associated No other symptoms or findings the patient has a COVID Pneumonia.
- Organism identified/suspected and/or aspiration pneumonia: ☐ Yes ☐ No
- Oxygenation: 45L Oxygen Therapy O2 Device: high-flow oxygen device
- CURB-65:

Skiba, Robert
MRN: 2000087384, DOB: ████████, Sex: M
Adm: 9/3/2021, D/C: 10/13/2021
Printed by ████████ at 10/26/21 2:44 PM

Page 23

Annotation 1: Prior to Rob's admission to the ICU, the MD on duty in the ED identified that Rob **clearly had a pneumomediastinum** (*air leaked into the space between the lungs*) which is a <u>definite contraindication</u> for use of a **BiPAP** which Rob was later placed on. Even Nurse Carnage noted on Page 97 of the hospital records (which appears on Page C-21) that Rob was "not a candidate for bipap d/t (due to) pneumomediastinum."

Annotation 2: As noted here, it was expected Rob would require at least a "two-midnight inpatient stay." If Rob had been given **only oxygen, antibiotics, steroids (for inflammation), and budesonide** it is likely he could have gone home within a few days. Unfortunately, numerous unnecessary and harmful drugs and treatments continually worsened his condition.

Exhibit 3–Pneumomediastinum, VELETRI, High Risk for Needing Intubation (9/3/21)

Consults (continued)

CA	8.9	09/03/2021 1709	No results found for: PT, INR
TPROT	6.5	09/03/2021 1709	
ALB	2.7 (L)	09/03/2021 1709	
ALKPHOS	81	09/03/2021 1709	
AST	158 (H)	09/03/2021 1709	
ALT	118.0 (H)	09/03/2021 1709	
TBILI	1.2	09/03/2021 1709	

Imaging Studies
1. Chest X-ray/CTA (Images personally reviewed): Diffuse opacities, pneumomediastinum, subcu air.

Impression and Plan
Acute hypoxic respiratory failure
COVID-19 (symptom onset 8/21, lab + 9/3)
Pneumonia
Pneumomediastinum
Elevated troponin
Hyperglycemia

1. Optiflow, wean O2 as tolerated. Add veletri
2. Remdesivir, Toci, empiric abx (elevated procal), consult ID in AM
3. Monitor Subcu air, no need for CT at this time.
4. Follow trop, likely demand R/T hypoxia.
5. SSI, check A1C. No h/o DM
6. Ppx: GI: pepcid, DVT: full Lovenox (adjused for d-dimer)

Patient is at high risk for needing intubation.

Lines/Drains/Wounds:
Peripheral IV Left antecubital (0days)
No Tubes or Drains Found
No Airways Found
No Wounds Found

Thank you for allowing us to participate in the care of this patient. We w

Horrendous, NP 9/3/2021

Electronically signed by **Horrendous**, NP at 09/03/21 2107
Electronically signed by ██ **Relentless** ██, MD at 09/16/21 0840

A chest X-ray clearly showed the **pneumomediastinum** (as also noted on the previous page). When Rob was moved to the ICU at **9:05 PM** (21:05), **VELETRI** (more on that later) was added to the **remdesivir assault**. As shown here, the Nurse Practitioner in the ED said Rob was "at high risk for needing intubation" while he was stabilizing on Oxygen alone (as shown on the next page)—making it clear that "intubation" was their plan for Rob from the moment he arrived. Why were they forcing the Covid protocol on a patient who was already improving on oxygen alone?

Sk████
MR████
Adm████2021, D/C: 10/13/2021
████████ DOB: ████████, Sex: M

Printed by ██████████ at 10/26/21 2:44 PM

Exhibit 4–Rob's Vital Signs the Evening of His Arrival (Evening of 9/3/21)

09/03/2021 - ED to Hosp-Admission (Discharged) in ███████████ Intensive Care Unit (continued)

Flowsheets (group 10 of 32) (continued)

Hand Off - Professional

Row Name	09/03/21 2053	09/03/21 2054	09/04/21 0700	09/04/21 1900	09/04/21 2009
Reviewed and	Given	—	Given	—	Given
Reviewed and	—	Received	—	Received	—

Row Name	09/05/21 0720	09/05/21 1635	09/06/21 0729	09/06/21 1848	09/06/21 2247
Reviewed and	Given	Given	Given	Given	Given

Row Name	09/10/21 0700	09/11/21 0700	09/11/21 1917	09/13/21 1025	09/13/21 1802
Reviewed and	—	—	Given	—	Given
Reviewed and	Received	Received	—	Received	

Row Name	09/15/21 0700	09/15/21 1835	09/17/21 ██		
Reviewed and	Given	Given	—		
Reviewed and	—	—	Rec		

Row Name	09/19/21 0700	09/23/21 1910	09/24 ██		
Reviewed and	Given	—			
Reviewed and	—	Received	Receiv		

Row Name	09/25/21 1858	10/04/21 0645	10/04/2 ██		
Reviewed and	Given	Given	Given		
Reviewed and	—	—	—		

Row Name	10/09/21 0701				
Reviewed and	Given				

As shown below, Rob's **SpO2** (Serum Pressure O2)—the percent of oxygen-carrying hemoglobin in the blood—was **95%** to **98%** on supplemental oxygen **within hours of his arrival**, yet the hospital staff **immediately** began debilitating Rob with **remdesivir** and other **off-label drugs** while **pushing him to agree to intubation and ventilation.** Why were they doing this to Rob?

Hemodynamics

Row Name	09/03/21 2115	09/03/21 2130	09/03/21 2200	09/03/21 2300	09/04/21 0000
Weight	76 kg (167 lb 8.8 oz)	—	—	—	—
Method of weight	Bed scale	—	—	—	—
Pulse	—	—	96	91	87
BP	—	145/67	135/91	—	—
BP Mean (MAP) (device)	—	97 MMHG	108 MMHG	—	—
Shock Index	—	—	0.71	—	—
Resp	—	—	(!) 32	29	(!) 36
SpO2	—	—	95 %	98 %	96 %
Temp	98.4 °F (36.9 °C)	—	—	—	98.1 °F (36.7 °C)

Skiba, Robert
MRN: 2000087384, DOB: ████████, Sex: M
Adm: 9/3/2021, D/C: 10/13/2021

Printed by ██████ at 10/26/21 2:48 PM

Exhibit 5–Rob's Vital Signs the Next Morning (Morning of 9/4/21 at 1:00-9:00 AM)

09/03/2021 - ED to Hosp-Admission (Discharged) in ▮▮▮▮▮▮ Intensive Care Unit (continued)

Flowsheets (group 10 of 32) (continued)

Temp src	Oral	—	—	—	Oral
Daily weight change in kg	76 kg	—	—	—	—

Row Name	09/04/21 0001	09/04/21 0100	09/04/21 0200	09/04/21 0300	09/04/21 0400
Weight	—	—	—	—	76 kg (167 lb 8.8 oz)
Method of weight	—	—	—	—	Bed scale
Pulse	88	83	82	87	73
BP	144/84	130/84	121/86	141/92	116/70
BP Mean (MAP) (device)	108 MMHG	103 MMHG	100 MMHG	112 MMHG	88 MMHG
Shock Index	0.61	0.64	0.68	0.62	0.63
Resp	—	(!) 36	(!) 47	(!) 33	(!) 44
⇨ SpO2	—	92 %	95 %	96 %	92 %
Daily weight change in kg	—	—	—	—	0 kg

Row Name	09/04/21 0500	09/04/21 0600	09/04/21 0700	09/04/21 0800	09/04/21 0900
Pulse	69	72	72	78	82
BP	121/72	127/73	134/83	132/88	145/98
BP Mean (MAP) (device)	92 MMHG	96 MMHG	104 MMHG	106 MMHG	117 MMHG
Shock Index	0.57	0.57	0.54	0.59	0.57
Resp	(!) 46	(!) 38	(!) 41	(!) 32	(!) 39
⇨ SpO2	95 %	94 %	91 %	93 %	94 %
SPO2 Monitoring	—	—	—	Continuous central	—
Temp	—	—	—	97.1 °F (36.2 °C)	—
Temp src	—	—	—	Temp...	
Glasgow Coma Scale Best Eye Response	—	—	—		
Glasgow Coma Scale Best Verbal Response	—	—	—		
Glasgow Coma Scale Best Motor Response	—	—	—		
Glasgow Coma Scale Score	—	—	—		

Row Name	09/04/21 1000	09/04/21 1100	09/04/2...		
Pulse	78	75	84		
BP	150/93	140/87	159/98		
BP Mean (MAP) (device)	115 MMHG	108 MMHG	122 MMH...		
Shock Index	0.52	0.54	0.53		
Resp	(!) 35	(!) 35	(!) 35		(!) 38

*Rob's **blood oxygen level** remained **in the low to mid-90s** from 1:00 AM to 9:00 AM on 9/4/21, the day after his arrival. **Continued O₂** and **no drugs other than antibiotics** (for pneumonia) **and steroids** (for inflammation) would likely have allowed Rob to go home on supplemental oxygen within days. Unfortunately, getting Rob stabilized so he could be discharged to recover at home on O₂ was not in the plan.*

Skiba, Robert
MRN: 2000087384, DOB: ▮▮▮▮▮ , Sex: M
Adm: 9/3/2021, D/C: 10/13/2021

Printed by ▮▮▮▮▮ at 10/26/21 2:48 PM

09/03/2021 - ED to Hosp-Admission (Discharged) in ▮▮▮▮▮▮▮ Intensive Care Unit (continued)

Consults (continued)

Consults by ▮Torture▮, MD at 9/4/2021 0947

Author: ▮Torture▮, MD	Service: Infectious Disease	Author Type: Physician
Filed: 09/04/21 1959	Date of Service: 09/04/21 0947	Creation Time: 09/04/21 0947
Status: Signed	Editor: ▮Torture▮, MD (Physician)	

Error, Duplicate

Electronically signed by ▮Torture▮, MD at 09/04/21 1959

Consults by ▮Torture▮, MD at 9/4/2021 1442

Author: ▮Torture▮, MD	Service: Infectious Disease	Author Type: Physician
Filed: 09/04/21 1452	Date of Service: 09/04/21 1442	Creation Time: 09/04/21 1442
Status: Addendum	Editor: ▮Torture▮, MD (Physician)	

Infectious Disease Consult Note

Name:　　Robert Skiva　　　　　　Date:　　9/4/▮▮
MR#:　　2000087384　　　　　　DO▮
Room #:　C297/C29701　　　　　　Age▮
Admit Date: 9/3/2021　　　　　　Adm▮

Acct #:

Consult requested by: ▮Horrendous▮, NP
Reason for Consult: COVID 19 infection complica▮▮

Past History:

History of present illness:
　　Chief Complaint
　　Patient presents with
　　• Covid Like Symptoms
　　　pt reports congestion, cough and shortness ▮
　　　PTA. pt was 71% on room air at triage

The blatant and bolded "He has not been vaccinated" note helped make Rob a target who needed to be made an example of. Since when has someone's vaccination status been an issue in how the patient is to be treated? Also, why would they be giving Rob VELETRI—which should **NEVER** be given to a patient who is already short of breath because it may cause **SERIOUS** side effects that include "**severe shortness of breath, gasping for breath, and anxiety**"—instead of budesonide which, as noted in Appendix F, was known to reduce the relative risk of requiring urgent care or hospitalization by 90%?

History of Present Illness: Robert Skiva is a 52 y.o. ▮▮▮ who presents to the emergency department with complaints of shortness of breath and cough with clear sputum production. Symptoms began 2 weeks ago. However shortness of breath has been more obvious in the last 1 week. Cough is productive of clear sputum. **_He has not been vaccinated._** He reports being at a conference on August 26th where he may have been exposed to the virus. He was treated in the outpatient setting with azithromycin and ivermectin and steroid but without improvement in his symptoms. He presented to the ED where he was hypoxic with a saturation of 71% on room air the time of arrival. He had a chest x-ray done and a CT angiogram which revealed bilateral pulmonary opacities. He was started on supplemental oxygen, IV antibiotic and antiviral therapy and it was felt that he will benefit from admission to the hospital for further care.

The patient is seen in the ICU and is currently on OptiFlow 55 L/98%
D-dimer was elevated to 9.35, down to 4.39 today
LDH 1532
Ferritin 4834 yesterday, down to 3782
He was started on Veletri, Remdesivir

	Skiba, Robert
	MRN: 2000087384, DOB: ▮▮▮▮, Sex: M
	Adm: 9/3/2021, D/C: 10/13/2021

Printed by ▮▮▮▮ at 10/26/21 2:44 PM

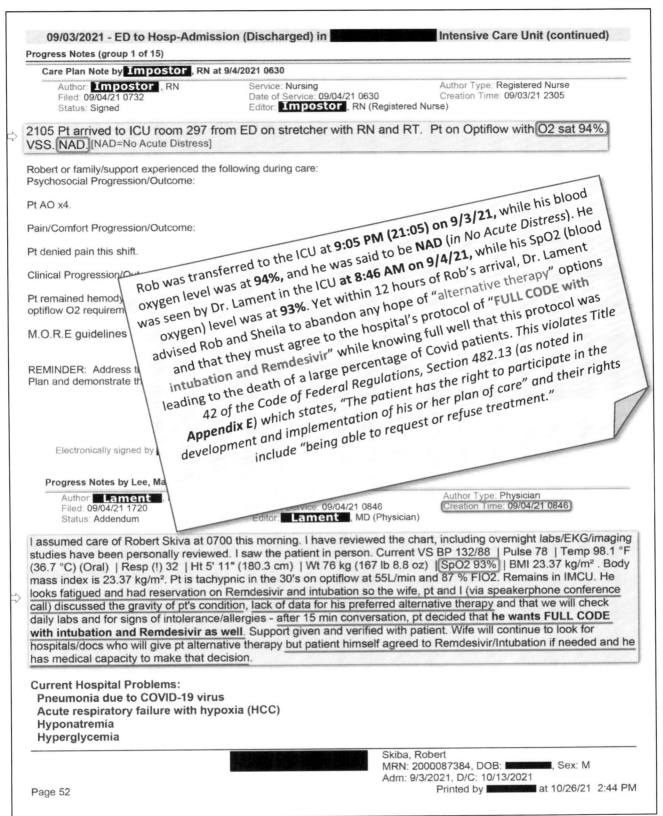

| 09/03/2021 - ED to Hosp-Admission (Discharged) in ███████ Intensive Care Unit (continued) |

Progress Notes (group 1 of 15)

Care Plan Note by **Impostor**, RN at 9/4/2021 0630

Author: **Impostor**, RN	Service: Nursing	Author Type: Registered Nurse
Filed: 09/04/21 0732	Date of Service: 09/04/21 0630	Creation Time: 09/03/21 2305
Status: Signed	Editor: **Impostor**, RN (Registered Nurse)	

2105 Pt arrived to ICU room 297 from ED on stretcher with RN and RT. Pt on Optiflow with O2 sat 94%. VSS. NAD. [NAD=No Acute Distress]

Robert or family/support experienced the following during care:
Psychosocial Progression/Outcome:

Pt AO x4.

Pain/Comfort Progression/Outcome:

Pt denied pain this shift.

Clinical Progression/Out...

Pt remained hemod...
optiflow O2 requirem...

M.O.R.E guidelines...

REMINDER: Address t...
Plan and demonstrate th...

Electronically signed by...

Rob was transferred to the ICU at 9:05 PM (21:05) on 9/3/21, while his blood oxygen level was at 94%, and he was said to be NAD (in No Acute Distress). He was seen by Dr. Lament in the ICU at 8:46 AM on 9/4/21, while his SpO2 (blood oxygen) level was at 93%. Yet within 12 hours of Rob's arrival, Dr. Lament advised Rob and Sheila to abandon any hope of "alternative therapy" options and that they must agree to the hospital's protocol of "FULL CODE with intubation and Remdesivir" while knowing full well that this protocol was leading to the death of a large percentage of Covid patients. This violates Title 42 of the Code of Federal Regulations, Section 482.13 (as noted in Appendix E) which states, "The patient has the right to participate in the development and implementation of his or her plan of care" and their rights include "being able to request or refuse treatment."

Progress Notes by Lee, Ma...

Author **Lament**,		Author Type: Physician
Filed: 09/04/21 1720	Service: 09/04/21 0846	Creation Time: 09/04/21 0846
Status: Addendum	Editor: **Lament**, MD (Physician)	

I assumed care of Robert Skiva at 0700 this morning. I have reviewed the chart, including overnight labs/EKG/imaging studies have been personally reviewed. I saw the patient in person. Current VS BP 132/88 | Pulse 78 | Temp 98.1 °F (36.7 °C) (Oral) | Resp (!) 32 | Ht 5' 11" (180.3 cm) | Wt 76 kg (167 lb 8.8 oz) | SpO2 93% | BMI 23.37 kg/m². Body mass index is 23.37 kg/m². Pt is tachypnic in the 30's on optiflow at 55L/min and 87 % FIO2. Remains in IMCU. He looks fatigued and had reservation on Remdesivir and intubation so the wife, pt and I (via speakerphone conference call) discussed the gravity of pt's condition, lack of data for his preferred alternative therapy and that we will check daily labs and for signs of intolerance/allergies - after 15 min conversation, pt decided that **he wants FULL CODE with intubation and Remdesivir as well**. Support given and verified with patient. Wife will continue to look for hospitals/docs who will give pt alternative therapy but patient himself agreed to Remdesivir/Intubation if needed and he has medical capacity to make that decision.

Current Hospital Problems:
Pneumonia due to COVID-19 virus
Acute respiratory failure with hypoxia (HCC)
Hyponatremia
Hyperglycemia

Skiba, Robert
MRN: 2000087384, DOB: ████, Sex: M
Adm: 9/3/2021, D/C: 10/13/2021
Page 52   Printed by ████ at 10/26/21 2:44 PM

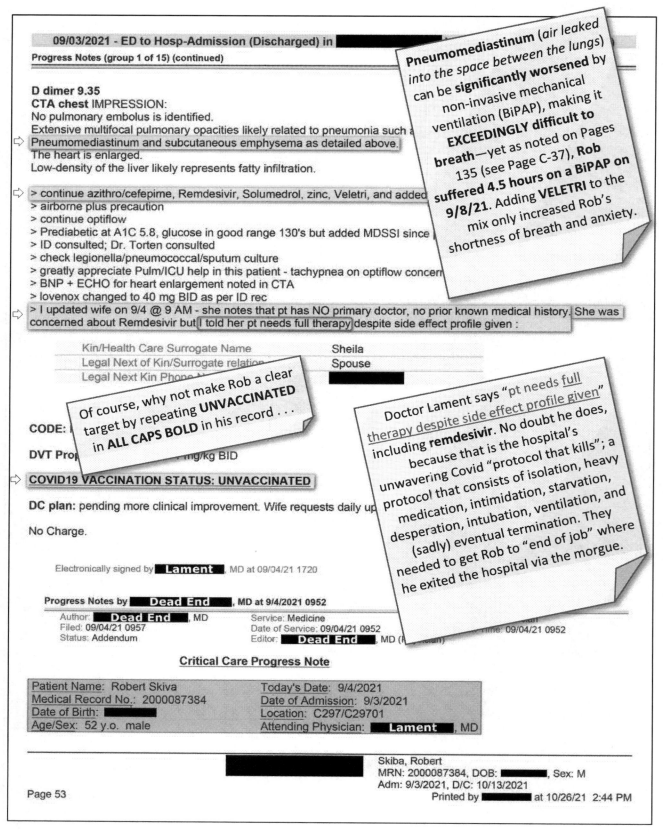

09/03/2021 - ED to Hosp-Admission (Discharged) in ▓▓▓▓

Progress Notes (group 1 of 15) (continued)

D dimer 9.35
CTA chest IMPRESSION:
No pulmonary embolus is identified.
Extensive multifocal pulmonary opacities likely related to pneumonia such a▓
Pneumomediastinum and subcutaneous emphysema as detailed above.
The heart is enlarged.
Low-density of the liver likely represents fatty infiltration.

> continue azithro/cefepime, Remdesivir, Solumedrol, zinc, Veletri, and added▓
> airborne plus precaution
> continue optiflow
> Prediabetic at A1C 5.8, glucose in good range 130's but added MDSSI since ▓
> ID consulted; Dr. Torten consulted
> check legionella/pneumococcal/sputum culture
> greatly appreciate Pulm/ICU help in this patient - tachypnea on optiflow concern▓
> BNP + ECHO for heart enlargement noted in CTA
> lovenox changed to 40 mg BID as per ID rec
> I updated wife on 9/4 @ 9 AM - she notes that pt has NO primary doctor, no prior known medical history. She was concerned about Remdesivir but I told her pt needs full therapy despite side effect profile given :

Kin/Health Care Surrogate Name	Sheila
Legal Next of Kin/Surrogate relation▓	Spouse
Legal Next Kin Phone ▓	▓▓▓▓

CODE: ▓

DVT Pro▓ ▓ ▓g/kg BID

COVID19 VACCINATION STATUS: UNVACCINATED

DC plan: pending more clinical improvement. Wife requests daily up▓

No Charge.

Electronically signed by **Lament**, MD at 09/04/21 1720

Progress Notes by **Dead End**, MD at 9/4/2021 0952

Author: **Dead End**, MD	Service: Medicine
Filed: 09/04/21 0957	Date of Service: 09/04/21 0952
Status: Addendum	Editor: **Dead End**, MD (▓▓▓)

Critical Care Progress Note

Patient Name: Robert Skiva	Today's Date: 9/4/2021
Medical Record No.: 2000087384	Date of Admission: 9/3/2021
Date of Birth: ▓▓	Location: C297/C29701
Age/Sex: 52 y.o. male	Attending Physician: **Lament**, MD

▓▓▓▓ Skiba, Robert
MRN: 2000087384, DOB: ▓▓, Sex: M
Adm: 9/3/2021, D/C: 10/13/2021

Page 53

Printed by ▓▓▓▓ at 10/26/21 2:44 PM

Handwritten-style annotation notes:

*Pneumomediastinum (air leaked into the space between the lungs) can be **significantly worsened** by non-invasive mechanical ventilation (BiPAP), making it **EXCEEDINGLY difficult to breath**—yet as noted on Pages 135 (see Page C-37), **Rob suffered 4.5 hours on a BiPAP on 9/8/21**. Adding **VELETRI** to the mix only increased Rob's shortness of breath and anxiety.*

*Of course, why not make Rob a clear target by repeating **UNVACCINATED** in **ALL CAPS BOLD** in his record . . .*

*Doctor Lament says "pt needs <u>full therapy despite side effect profile given</u>" including **remdesivir**. No doubt he does, because that is the hospital's unwavering Covid "protocol that kills"; a protocol that consists of isolation, heavy medication, intimidation, starvation, desperation, intubation, ventilation, and (sadly) eventual termination. They needed to get Rob to "end of job" where he exited the hospital via the morgue.*

Exhibit 9– Rob Wishes to **Not** Be Placed on a Ventilator or Be Intubated (9:52 AM on 9/4/21)

Progress Notes (group 1 of 15) (continued)

Chief complaint: COVID-19

Subjective:

⇨ Overnight events reviewed. Patient wishes to not be placed on ventilator or intubated in emergency. Has increased work of breathing and hypoxia

Ventilator/Blood Gas
Current Ventilator Settings:

Oxygen Therapy O2
Device: high-flow
oxygen device;high-
flow nasal cannula
(09/04/21 0831)

Last Arterial Blood Gas:
POC ABG Results
Lab Results
Component
POC

Oxygen
Concentr
88 (09/04
Oxygen Th
Flow (L/mi
(09/04/21 0

Current Facility-Administered Medications

Medication	Route	Fre
• epoprostenol (arginine)	Continuous Nebulization	CC US

Current Facility-Administered Medications

Medication	Route	Freque
• azithromycin	IV PIGGYBACK	EVERY HOURS
• cefepime	SLOW IV PUSH	EVERY HOURS
• enoxaparin	SUBCUTANEOU S	EVERY 1 HOURS
• famotidine	ORAL	AT BEDTIM

at
09/03/2
1 2153

Skiba, Robert
MRN: 2000087384, DOB: ████████, Sex: M
Adm: 9/3/2021, D/C: 10/13/2021

Printed by ████████ at 10/26/21 2:44 PM

Despite being continually badgered and pressured, Rob made it clear <u>the morning after his arrival at the hospital</u> that he "wishes to not be placed on ventilator or intubated." This note directly contradicts Dr. Lament's statement on Page 52 of the hospital records (see Page C-7 above) where she alleged "he wants FULL CODE with intubation."

The multiple "Orders" extracted from Pages 1001 to 1018 (see Page C-53) show how four doctors flip-flopped Rob's status from **FULL** to **Limited** resuscitation from September 4, 2021 (the morning after his admission) to September 8, 2021 (the day he was intubated) due to their <u>persistent insistence</u> that he to consent to "elective intubation," followed by Rob's consistently reminding them (we counted a total of 17 times in the records) that he **DID NOT agree** to being intubated and placed on a ventilator.

In a text message Rob sent a friend (Bonnie) at 10:11 AM on September 5, 2021 (which appears in Chapter 4), he said, "**In ICU where doctors all disagree with me. Feeling hopeless and afraid.**" Rob had every right to participate in the design of his plan of care and be totally free of any form of harassment by the doctors. What Rob endured is deplorable and totally inexcusable.

Exhibit 10-Second Dose of Remdesivir & Blood Oxygen Level at 93% (Morning of 9/4/21)

Progress Notes (group 1 of 15) (continued)

• insulin lispro	SUBCUTANEOUS	EVERY 6 HOURS	
• l.acid,para-b.bifidum-s.therm	ORAL	DAILY	
• methylprednisoLONE sodium PF	IV PUSH	EVERY 12 HOURS	
• montelukast	ORAL	AT BEDTIME	10 mg at 09/03/21 2154
• remdesivir (Veklury) IVPB	IV PIGGYBACK	EVERY 24 HOURS	100 mg at 09/04/21 0841
And			
• NORMAL SALINE	INTRAVENOUS	EVERY 24 HOURS	
• sodium chloride	SALINE LOCK	24 HOURS STOP	10 mL at 09/04/21 0854
• zinc sulfate	ORAL/FEEDING TUBE	TWICE DAILY	220 mg at 09/04/21 0844

Vital Signs
Current:
Temp: 97.1 °F (36.2 °C)   Pulse: 78   Resp: (I) 32   BP: 132/88   SpO2: 93 %   Weight: 76 kg (167 lb 8.8 oz)
   Body mass index is 23.37 kg/m².
Ranges:
Systolic (24hrs), Avg:135 , Min:116 , Max:155
Diastolic (24hrs), Avg:83, Min:67, Max:92

Temp Avg: 97.9 °F (36.6 °C)
Pulse Avg: 86.6 Min: 69 Max:
Resp Avg: 32.6 Min: 16 Max:
SpO2 Avg: 93.8 % Min: 71 %

Intake/Output Summary (Last 24 hou
Last data filed at 9/4/2021 0030
                Gross per 24 hour
Intake   661.87 ml
Output   500 ml
Net   **161.87 ml**

No data found.

The morning after Rob's arrival at the hospital, as shown above, they documented that Rob had been given **a second dose of remdesivir** at 8:41 AM, yet Rob and Sheila had made it clear that they **did not** want him to receive this medication. Regrettably, Rob was given 8 vials during six doses of this poison (two were "double doses"). As noted earlier on Page C-7, this violates Title 42 of the Code of Federal Regulations, Section 482.13 (as noted in **Appendix E**) which states, "The patient has the right to participate in the development and implementation of his or her plan of care," and their rights include "being able to request or refuse treatment."

Skiba, Robert
MRN: 2000087384, DOB: ▇▇▇▇▇, Sex: M
Adm: 9/3/2021, D/C: 10/13/2021
Printed by ▇▇▇▇▇ at 10/26/21 2:44 PM

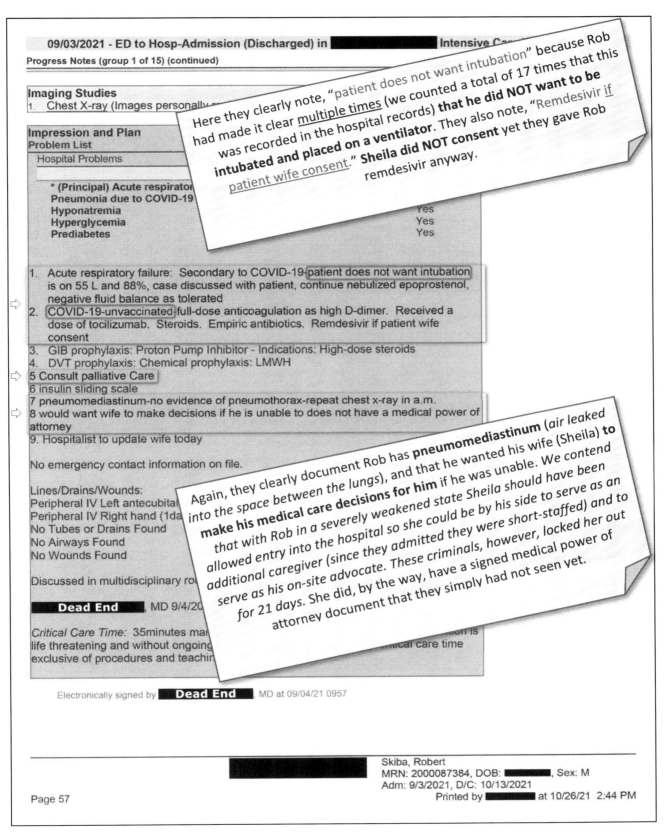

09/03/2021 - ED to Hosp-Admission (Discharged) in ▓▓▓▓▓▓▓▓ Intensive Ca▓▓▓
Progress Notes (group 1 of 15) (continued)

Imaging Studies
1. Chest X-ray (Images personally ▓▓

Impression and Plan
Problem List

Hospital Problems

* (Principal) Acute respirator▓
Pneumonia due to COVID-19
Hyponatremia   Yes
Hyperglycemia   Yes
Prediabetes   Yes

1. Acute respiratory failure: Secondary to COVID-19-patient does not want intubation
   is on 55 L and 88%, case discussed with patient, continue nebulized epoprostenol,
   negative fluid balance as tolerated
2. COVID-19-unvaccinated-full-dose anticoagulation as high D-dimer. Received a
   dose of tocilizumab. Steroids. Empiric antibiotics. Remdesivir if patient wife
   consent
3. GIB prophylaxis: Proton Pump Inhibitor - Indications: High-dose steroids
4. DVT prophylaxis: Chemical prophylaxis: LMWH
5 Consult palliative Care
6 insulin sliding scale
7 pneumomediastinum-no evidence of pneumothorax-repeat chest x-ray in a.m.
8 would want wife to make decisions if he is unable to does not have a medical power of
attorney
9. Hospitalist to update wife today

No emergency contact information on file.

Lines/Drains/Wounds:
Peripheral IV Left antecubital
Peripheral IV Right hand (1da
No Tubes or Drains Found
No Airways Found
No Wounds Found

Discussed in multidisciplinary ro▓

▓▓▓ **Dead End** ▓▓, MD 9/4/20▓

Critical Care Time: 35minutes ma▓
life threatening and without ongoing ▓▓▓▓▓▓▓▓▓ ▓▓▓ is
exclusive of procedures and teachir▓ ▓▓cal care time

Electronically signed by ▓▓ **Dead End** ▓▓, MD at 09/04/21 0957

Skiba, Robert
MRN: 2000087384, DOB: ▓▓▓▓▓▓, Sex: M
Adm: 9/3/2021, D/C: 10/13/2021
Printed by ▓▓▓▓▓ at 10/26/21 2:44 PM

Page 57

Here they clearly note, "patient does not want intubation" because Rob
had made it clear <u>multiple times</u> (we counted a total of 17 times that this
was recorded in the hospital records) **that he did NOT want to be
intubated and placed on a ventilator.** They also note, "Remdesivir <u>if</u>
<u>patient wife consent.</u>" **Sheila did NOT consent** yet they gave Rob
remdesivir anyway.

Again, they clearly document Rob has **pneumomediastinum** (air leaked
into the space between the lungs), and that he wanted his wife (Sheila) **to
make his medical care decisions for him** if he was unable. We contend
that with Rob in a severely weakened state Sheila should have been
allowed entry into the hospital so she could be by his side to serve as an
additional caregiver (since they admitted they were short-staffed) and to
serve as his on-site advocate. These criminals, however, locked her out
for 21 days. She did, by the way, have a signed medical power of
attorney document that they simply had not seen yet.

Exhibit 12–Planning 5-day Course of Remdesivir, Other Drugs (Afternoon of 9/4/21)

09/03/2021 - ED to Hosp-Admission (Discharged) in ▓▓▓▓▓▓▓ **Intensive Care Unit (continued)**

Consults (continued)

Problem List

Hospital Problems

	POA
* (Principal) Acute respiratory failure with hypoxia (HCC)	Y
Pneumonia due to COVID-19 virus	
Hyponatremia	
Hyperglycemia	
Prediabetes	

> *Note the plan for a "5-day course" of **remdesivir** and **off-label use** of **nitazoxanide** (an antiparasitic clinical trial drug that would have required informed consent, which was not provided by Rob) and **colchicine** (a drug that treats gout symptoms). **Nausea** and **diarrhea** are common side-effects of both, and these drugs later had to be discontinued because <u>that's exactly what they caused</u>. Why assault Rob with these destructive drugs that further weakened him when he was already being malnourished?*

Plan:

1. For his community-acquired p▓▓▓▓▓
cefepime and azithromycin are a▓▓▓▓▓
Azithromycin will also provide ant▓▓▓▓▓

2. Agree with current dose of Solu▓▓▓▓▓ ▓▓▓▓continue with Singulair.

3. Check vitamin-D levels and add ▓▓▓▓in-C, D and zinc.

4. The patient meets criteria for use of Remdesivir, plan a 5 day course unless gets intubated.

5. With his increased inflammatory markers and respiratory failure, the patient meets criteria for tocilizumab, which was given last night, *although his oxygen requirements are still very high, his inflammatory markers have improved.*

6. Recommend to decrease Lovenox to 40 mg every 12 hours moderate dose since he does not have any pulmonary embolus on his CT angiogram.

7. Management of severe sepsis and respiratory failure per Critical Care Team.

9. Will give off-label Nitazoxanide and colchicine to target as anti-inflammatory and interference with the gamma interferon pathway.

10. The patient is out of the window to benefit from convalescent plasma as this late out he likely has his own IgG. I will check COVID IgG and if it is negative will reconsider.

Patient has been encouraged to self prone and use the incentive spirometer.

Further recommendations will depend on his progress and trending labs▓▓▓▓▓

Thank you for this consultation, will continue to fo▓▓▓

Seen in the ICU

> *Once you have developed **IgG antibodies to COVID-19** (see the "he likely has his own IgG" note), you are usually no longer contagious. So, **why lock Sheila out of the hospital for 21 days** vs. allowing her to assist Rob as his on-site advocate and extra caregiver?*

Torture, MD 9/4/2021 14:42

Skiba, Robert
MRN: 2000087384, DOB: ▓▓▓▓▓, Sex: M
Adm: 9/3/2021, D/C: 10/13/2021

Page 31

Printed by ▓▓▓▓▓ at 10/26/21 2:44 PM

C-12

Exhibit 13–Rob's Vital Signs the Afternoon of 9/4/21 (3:00-7:00 PM)

09/03/2021 - ED to Hosp-Admission (Discharged) in ▮▮▮▮▮▮ Intensive Care Unit (continued)

Flowsheets (group 10 of 32) (continued)

Row Name					
SpO2	93 %	96 %	95 %	95 %	92 %
SPO2 Monitoring	—	Continuous central	—	—	—
Temp	—	98 °F (36.7 °C)	—	—	—
Temp src	—	Temporal Artery	—	—	—
Glasgow Coma Scale Best Eye Response	—	4 - (E4) spontaneous	—		
Glasgow Coma Scale Best Verbal Response	—	5 - (V5) oriented	—	—	—
Glasgow Coma Scale Best Motor Response	—	6 - (M6) obeys commands	—	—	—
Glasgow Coma Scale Score	—	15	—	—	—

Row Name	09/04/21 1500	09/04/21 1600	09/04/21 1700	09/04/21 1800	09/04/21 1900
Pulse	71	75	76	71	69
BP	146/82	138/82	121/56	109/61	110/60
BP Mean (MAP) (device)	111 MMHG	101 MMHG	80 MMHG	80 MMHG	78 MMHG
Shock Index	0.49	0.54	0.63	0.65	0.63
Resp	(!) 44	(!) 39	(!) 35	(!) 34	(!) 32
⇨ SpO2	98 %	95 %	98 %	98 %	98 %
SPO2 Monitoring	—	Continuous central	—	—	—
Temp	—	97 °F (36.1 °C)	—	—	—
Temp src	—	Temporal Artery	—	—	—
Glasgow Coma Scale Best Eye Response	—	4 - (E4) spontaneous	—		
Glasgow Coma Scale Best Verbal Response	—				
Glasgow Coma Scale Best Motor Response	—				
Glasgow Coma Scale Score					

Row Name					0000
Pulse					70
BP				—	129/63
BP Mean (MAP) (device)	1		106 MMHG	—	88 MMHG
Shock Index	0.5	0.61	0.55	—	0.54
Resp	(!) 36	(!) 38	(!) 31	(!) 41	(!) 38
SpO2	98 %	96 %	98 %	95 %	98 %
Temp	97.6 °F (36.4 °C)	—	—	—	98.1 °F (36.7 °C)
Temp src	Oral	—	—	—	Oral

As shown above, Rob's blood oxygen levels continued to improve throughout the afternoon of 9/4/21. **A conservative approach** of oxygen, antibiotics, steroids, and budesonide—in addition to adequate fluids and nutrition which he was NOT provided—could have stabilized Rob for a rapid discharge to recover at home. Sadly, that's not part of "the protocol that kills" and would not have been of financial benefit to the hospital and the doctors. So, instead, they gave him injurious drugs and therapies that eventually that led to Rob's death.

Skiba, Robert
MRN: 2000087384, DOB: ▮▮▮▮▮▮, Sex: M
Adm: 9/3/2021, D/C: 10/13/2021

Printed by ▮▮▮▮▮▮ at 10/26/21 2:48 PM

Exhibit 14–Rob's Vital Signs the Early Morning of 9/5/21 (1:00-8:00 AM)

Flowsheets (group 10 of 32) (continued)

Row Name	09/05/21 0100	09/05/21 0200	09/05/21 0300	09/05/21 0328	09/05/21 0400
Weight	—	—	—	73.4 kg (161 lb 13.1 oz)	—
Method of weight	—	—	—	Bed scale	—
Pulse	66	—	67	—	62
BP	134/62	118/58	100/81	—	107/64
BP Mean (MAP) (device)	89 MMHG	84 MMHG	86 MMHG	—	80 MMHG
Shock Index	0.49	0.55	0.67	—	0.58
Resp	(!) 42	(!) 42	(!) 31	—	(!) 37
SpO2	100 %	—	97 %	—	95 %
Temp	—	—	—	—	97.6 °F (36.4 °C)
Temp src	—	—	—	—	Oral
Daily weight change in kg	—	—	—	-2.6 kg -IB at 09/05/21 0330	—

Row Name	09/05/21 0500	09/05/21 0600	09/05/21 0700	09/05/21 0712	09/05/21 0800
Pulse	(!) 59	62	70	64	63
BP	116/67	122/57	—	113/67	125/71
BP Mean (MAP) (device)	87 MMHG	82 MMHG	—	86 MMHG	93 MMHG
Shock Index	0.51	0.51	—	0.57	0.5
Resp	(!) 34	(!) 35	28	(!) 33	19
SpO2	98 %	95 %	93 %	96 %	—
SPO2 Monitoring	—	—	—	—	Continuous central
Temp	—	—	—	—	98 °F (36.7 °C)
Temp src	—	—	—	—	Temporal
Glasgow Coma Scale Best Eye Response	—	—	—	—	
Glasgow Coma Scale Best Verbal Response	—	—	—	—	
Glasgow Coma Scale Best Motor Response	—	—	—	—	
Glasgow Coma Scale Score	—				
RASS Score	—				0 Alert and calm
Ramsay Scale Score	—			—	2 - awake: patient cooperative, oriented and tranquil

Rob's SpO2 (blood oxygen) level **improved even more** the morning of 9/5/21, and yet as noted on the next page Dr. Dead End **continues to push remdesivir** and **expresses his dismay** that Sheila "has refused remdesivir" and "has refused elective intubation." Why are they even talking about intubation at this point?

Skiba, Robert
MRN: 2000087384, DOB: ▮▮▮▮, Sex: M
Adm: 9/3/2021, D/C: 10/13/2021
Printed by ▮▮▮▮ at 10/26/21 2:48 PM

Page 3008

Exhibit 15–Staff Frustrated by Sheila's Refusal of Remdesivir and Intubation (9/5/21)

09/03/2021 - ED to Hosp-Admission (Discharged) in ▓▓▓▓▓▓▓▓▓▓ **Intensive Care Unit (continued)**

Progress Notes (group 1 of 15) (continued)

2130 Spoke with pt's wife. Pt's wife states, " We don't want him to have Remdesivir. He was railroaded today and was given it. Please do not give this to him anymore." Pt's wife informed that I would let the day shift RN aware that pt is not to get Remdesivir. Wife also requested to know all medications that the patient was receiving. Pt's wife also requested to have an increase in Vit D dosage as well as wanting to have pt to be given Vit C. Pt's wife informed that she would need to speak with the doctor who is providing care to the patient. Pt's wife verbalized understanding. Pt's wife also stated, "We do not want him to be intubated but if he stops breathing it is ok but just to intubate him because his oxygen levels are low and someone thinks its a good idea we do not want him intubated." Pt's wife informed that I would communicate this information to the night on call provider.

2140 spoke with night on call provider regarding conversation that I had with pt's wife.

M.O.R.E guidelines implemented appropriately.

REMINDER: Address the patient/family progress this shift (including the ab____
Plan and demonstrate the compassionate care given.

You can clearly see how frustrated the staff are at Sheila's continued insistence that Rob NOT be given remdesivir, and the NOT be intubated and placed on a ventilator. Sadly, she had to continue to conduct her fight for Rob by phone because she was shut out by an unwritten policy for 21 days.

Electronically signed by **Impostor**, RN at 09/0▓

Progress Notes by **Malicious**, RN at 9/5/2021 090▓

Author: **Malicious**, RN	Service: Nursing	Author Type: Registered Nurse
Filed: 09/05/21 0912	Date of Service: 09/05/21 0909	Creation Time: 09/05/21 0909
Status: Signed	Editor: **Malicious**, RN (Registered Nurse)	

Pt's wife spoke with him and **Dr Dead End** on phone speaker and refused remdesivir. She stated that she will speak with hospital administrator regarding the medications she would like him to be treated with.

Electronically signed by **Malicious**, RN at 09/05/21 0912

Progress Notes by **Dead End**, MD at 9/5/2021 0931

Author: **Dead End**, MD	Service: Medicine	Author T▓
Filed: 09/05/21 0936	Date of Service: 09/05/21 0931	▓
Status: Signed	Editor: **Dead End** ▓	

Critical Care Pro▓

Unfortunately, by his 5th day (on 9/8/21) they had their way after starving Rob into submission (no family was allowed in to help feed him) and bombarding him with harmful drugs and therapies that brought him to a point of desperation where he could no longer breathe for himself as noted in the pages that follow.

Patient Name: Robert Skiva
Medical Record No.: 2000087384
Date of Birth: ▓▓▓▓▓▓
Age/Sex: 52 y.o. male

Chief complaint: COVID-19

Subjective:

Overnight events reviewed. Patient's wife was upset with us. Thinks we are trying to harm patient. She has refused remdesivir. She has refused elective intubation, she has advised her husband to not proceed with intubation if necessary. She would want resuscitative measures done

▓▓▓▓▓▓▓▓
Skiba, Robert
MRN: 2000087384, DOB: ▓▓▓▓▓▓, Sex: M
Adm: 9/3/2021, D/C: 10/13/2021

Exhibit 16–Patient Does NOT Want Intubation, Refusing Remdesivir (9/5/21)

09/03/2021 - ED to Hosp-Admission (Discharge...

Progress Notes (group 1 of 15) (continued...

"Patient does not want intubation" is noted (note 1), *"unvaccinated"* is listed, *"Patient and family are refusing remdesivir"* is stated, **ivermectin** and **hydroxychloroquine** are said to be not approved or indicated (note 2), and Dr. Dead End is threatening that Rob will die without *"elective intubation"* and he turned the family's **directives** into **"wishes,"** admitting, *"I have also notified the ICU charge nurse of the patient's wishes."* He also noted that Rob wanted his **"wife to make decisions if he is unable"** (note 8), yet that request was blatantly ignored. The *"does not have a medical power of attorney"* (note 8) statement is patently false, and *"No emergency contact information on file"* makes no sense as Sheila is listed as the surrogate on the record on Page 53 of the records (see Page C-8).

Imaging Studies
1. Chest X-ray (Images pe...

Impression and Plan
Problem List

Hospital Problems

* (Principal) Acute respirato...
Pneumonia due to COVID-19
Hyponatremia
Hyperglycemia
Prediabetes

Yes
Yes

1. Acute respiratory failure: Secondary to COVID-19-patient does not want intubation is on 55 L and 88%, at this point if patient does not wish for intubation if needed Will transfer to floor. To utilize ICU beds for patient and may need elective intubation
2. COVID-19-unvaccinated-full-dose anticoagulation as high D-dimer. Received a dose of tocilizumab. Steroids. Empiric antibiotics. Patient and family are refusing remdesivir. They have been counseled that this is the only approved antiviral.. They have requested ivermectin, vitamin C, vitamin D IV, hydroxychloroquine. I have offered oral vitamin-C. None of the other medications are approved or indicated
3 unfortunately at some point he may code., I hope that he makes improvement. Can continue steroids and anticoagulation and empiric antibiotics
4 given the limited resource is available in the intensive care unit Will triaged the patient up stairs is they do not want intubation if necessary to prolonged and save his life. I have advised patient and his family that he may die without elective intubation, and they understand those risks. I have asked the nurse to contact the house supervisor. I have also notified the ICU charge nurse of the patient's wishes

3. GIB prophylaxis: Proton Pump Inhibitor - Indications: High-dose steroids
4. DVT prophylaxis: Chemical prophylaxis: LMWH
5 Consult palliative Care
6 insulin sliding scale
7 pneumomediastinum-no evidence of pneumothorax-x-ray improved
8 would want wife to make decisions if he is unable to does not have a medical power of attorney
9. Long conversation with patient and his wife

No emergency contact information on file.

Lines/Drains/Wounds:
Peripheral IV Left antecubital (2days)
Peripheral IV Right hand (2days)
No Tubes or Drains Found
No Airways Found
No Wounds Found

Exhibit 17–Lengthy Discussion with Rob About Intubation & Remdesivir (9/5/21)

09/03/2021 - ED to Hosp-Admission (Discharged) in ▮▮▮▮▮▮ Intensive ▮▮▮▮▮▮ ▮ed)

Progress Notes (group 1 of 15) (continued)

Psychosocial Progression/Outcome:
Pt is alert, oriented. Vitals stable.Plan of care dis▮▮

Pain/Comfort Progression/Outcome:
Breathing better today than yesterday. On 40L▮

Clinical Progression/Outcome:
Vitals stable. Tolerating PO liquids. Poor appetit▮

Electronically signed by **Malicious**, RN at 09/0▮

Progress Notes by ▮▮▮ **Jackedup** ▮▮ at 9/5/▮

Author: ▮▮ **Jackedup** ▮▮ Service▮
Filed: 09/05/21 1648 Date o▮
Status: Signed Editor: ▮

Pastoral Care Vi▮

Name: Robert Skiba Date: ▮
MR#: 2000087384 DOB: ▮
Room #: C297/C29701 Age/Sex▮
Admit Date: 9/3/2021 Admitting▮
:

Acct #:

Source of referral: Staff
Visited with: Spouse;Children;Extended Family

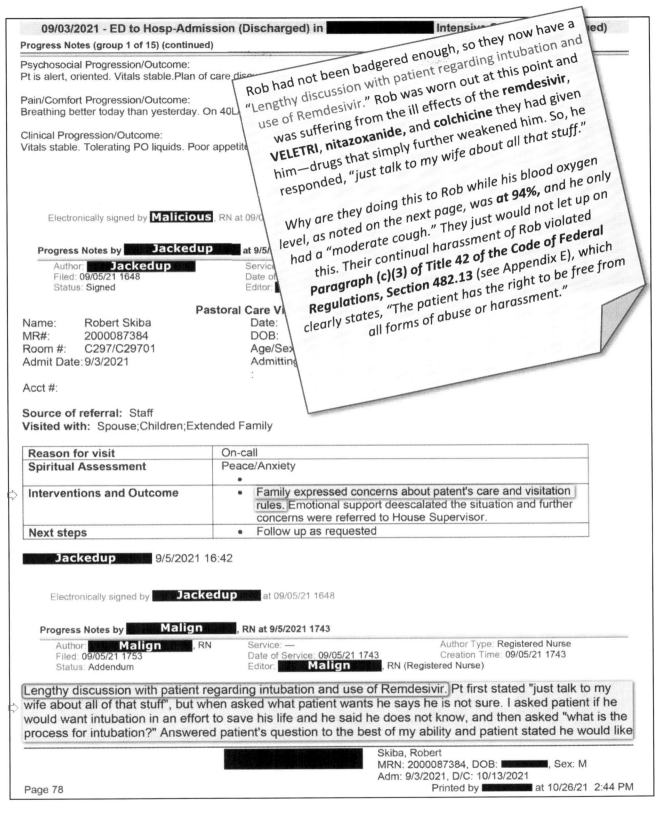

Rob had not been badgered enough, so they now have a "Lengthy discussion with patient regarding intubation and use of Remdesivir." Rob was worn out at this point and was suffering from the ill effects of the **remdesivir**, **VELETRI**, **nitazoxanide**, and **colchicine** they had given him—drugs that simply further weakened him. So, he responded, "*just talk to my wife about all that stuff.*"

Why are they doing this to Rob while his blood oxygen level, as noted on the next page, was **at 94%**, and he only had a "*moderate cough*." They just would not let up on this. Their continual harassment of Rob violated **Paragraph (c)(3) of Title 42 of the Code of Federal Regulations, Section 482.13** (see Appendix E), which clearly states, "*The patient has the right to be free from all forms of abuse or harassment.*"

Reason for visit	On-call
Spiritual Assessment	Peace/Anxiety
	•
Interventions and Outcome	• Family expressed concerns about patent's care and visitation rules. Emotional support deescalated the situation and further concerns were referred to House Supervisor.
Next steps	• Follow up as requested

▮▮ **Jackedup** ▮ 9/5/2021 16:42

Electronically signed by ▮▮ **Jackedup** ▮ at 09/05/21 1648

Progress Notes by ▮▮▮ **Malign** ▮▮, RN at 9/5/2021 1743

Author: ▮▮ **Malign** ▮, RN Service: — Author Type: Registered Nurse
Filed: 09/05/21 1753 Date of Service: 09/05/21 1743 Creation Time: 09/05/21 1743
Status: Addendum Editor: ▮▮ **Malign** ▮, RN (Registered Nurse)

Lengthy discussion with patient regarding intubation and use of Remdesivir. Pt first stated "just talk to my wife about all of that stuff", but when asked what patient wants he says he is not sure. I asked patient if he would want intubation in an effort to save his life and he said he does not know, and then asked "what is the process for intubation?" Answered patient's question to the best of my ability and patient stated he would like

▮▮▮▮▮▮ Skiba, Robert
MRN: 2000087384, DOB: ▮▮▮, Sex: M
Adm: 9/3/2021, D/C: 10/13/2021

Exhibit 18–Continuing to Wear Rob Down about Intubation (9/5/21)

09/03/2021 - ED to Hosp-Admission (Discharged) in ▓▓▓▓▓▓▓▓ Intensive Care Unit (continued)

Progress Notes (group 1 of 15) (continued)

to think about it and said "would I have to go back downstairs?". Informed him he would need to be in the ICU. Patient stated "I am getting a lot of different information from a lot of people and I just don't know". Expressed empathy and understanding for pt's situation. Explained to patient he is on a high volume of oxygen and is breathing at a fast rate and patient asked "what should I do right now to help myself?" Explained to patient the need for rest and deep breathing and to use call light if he feels short of breath. Pt expressed understanding and very appreciative of discussion. O2 94% on 40L/96% Optiflow, RR 30, lying in bed with moderate cough at this time.

Electronically signed by ▓▓▓ **Malign** ▓▓▓ , RN at 09/05/21 1753

Progress Notes by ▓▓ **Felonious** ▓▓ , RN at 9/5/2021 2115
Author: ▓▓ **Felonious** ▓▓ , RN   Service: Nursing
Filed: 09/06/21 0622   Date of Ser▓▓▓
Status: Signed

Lab called and notified ▓▓▓
obtains

Electronically signed by ▓▓ **F**▓▓

Progress Notes by ▓▓▓ **Felon**▓▓
Author: ▓▓ **Felonious** ▓▓ , ▓
Filed: 09/05/21 2316
Status: Signed

As noted below, Rob's **DNR** (Do Not Resuscitate) **status** is brought to his attention (again) and he reiterates "**I want to avoid Intubation**," which must have been a real frustration for the doctors and staff. Sadly, they are working to wear Rob down at a time when he is weaker than when he arrived two days prior because of the barrage of unnecessary and harmful drugs that were forced on him and a lack of adequate nutrition— which is apparently in the script they follow for all their unvaccinated COVID-19 patients.

1930: pt' wife called and to g▓▓ ▓▓▓▓dated pt's condition and vitals with wife. Pt is resting comfortably at this time.

2240: When checked with pt about limited DNR status, pt states," I want to avoid Intubation, but open to discuss more." Explained to pt best of my ability. Pt is made aware that RN will notify On call MD to discuss with pt. **Dr. Heartless** is paged and made aware.

Electronically signed by ▓▓ **Felonious** ▓▓ , RN at 09/05/21 2316

Progress Notes by ▓▓ **Heartless** ▓▓ , MD at 9/5/2021 2340
Author: ▓▓ **Heartless** ▓▓ , MD   Service: Hospitalist   Author Type: Physician
Filed: 09/05/21 2345   Date of Service: 09/05/21 2340   Creation Time: 09/05/21 2340
Status: Signed   Editor: ▓▓ **Heartless** ▓▓ , MD (Physician)

Hospitalist X-cover Note

Called by nurse because pt told nurse that he wants to avoid intubation but is open to discussing it some more. However, when nurse went to ask him if he wants to discuss it tonight, pt told nurse that he would prefer to talk with doctors again in the morning - does not want to revisit this discussion tonight.

Will defer to dayshift doctors to discuss code status/intubation with patient in morning.

▓▓ **Heartless** ▓▓ , MD

Electronically signed by ▓▓ **Heartless** ▓▓ , MD at 09/05/21 2345

▓▓▓▓▓▓▓▓▓▓▓   Skiba, Robert
                              MRN: 2000087384, DOB: ▓▓▓▓ , Sex: M
                              Adm: 9/3/2021, D/C: 10/13/2021
Page 79   Printed by ▓▓▓▓ at 10/26/21 2:44 PM

C-18

Exhibit 19–Rob's Vital Signs the Evening of 9/5/21 (5:07 PM) to 9/6/21 (9:30 PM)

CPN Comprehensive Flowsheet

Row Name	09/05/21 1707	09/05/21 1911	09/05/21 2330	09/06/21 0318	09/06/21 0731
Temp	97.4 °F (36.3 °C)	97.6 °F (36.4 °C)	98.3 °F (36.8 °C)	97.5 °F (36.4 °C)	98 °F (36.7 °C)
Temp src	Temporal Artery	Temporal Artery	Temporal Artery	Temporal Artery	—
Orthostatic Position	Semi-Fowlers	Supine	Supine	Supine	Supine
BP	154/93	158/90	154/100	155/99	(!) 169/88
Pulse	65	66	74	66	73
Resp	20	20	19	20	18
					MH (t) at 09/06/21
SpO2	95 %	91 %	94 %	94 %	(!) 89 %
Weight	—	—	—	76.1 kg (167 lb 12.3 oz)	—
BP Cuff Location	Right Upper Arm	Left Upper Arm	Left Upper Arm	Left Upper Arm	Right Upper Arm
Pulse Source (Device)	SpO2	—	—	—	
SPO2 Monitoring	Spot check	—	—		
Safety (WDL)	WDL	WDL			
Purposeful Rounding	Within defined limit	Within defin			
General Activity	Awake;In bed	—			in bed
					(r) MH (t) at 09/06/21 0732

Row Name	09/06/21 1151	09/06/21 1542		09/06/21 1958	09/06/21 2130
Temp	97.2 °F (36.2 °C)	97.6 °F (36.4		97.2 °F (36.2 °C)	—
Temp src	—	—	—	Temporal Artery	—
Orthostatic Position	Supine	Supine	—	Supine	Supine
BP	157/97	155/94	—	154/100	(!) 160/103
Pulse	76	76	—	81	75
Resp	18	(!) 32	—	19	—
SpO2	93 %	93 %	—	93 %	92 %

*Rob's SpO2 (blood oxygen) level **remained good** (in the low to mid 90s) with respirations generally 20 or below the evening of 9/5/21 through the evening of 9/6/21. So, why the **constant badgering** about "limited DNR status" and the need for "elective intubation"?*

Skiba, Robert
MRN: 2000087384, DOB: ▮▮▮▮▮, Sex: M
Adm: 9/3/2021, D/C: 10/13/2021
Printed by ▮▮▮▮▮ at 10/26/21 2:46 PM

09/03/2021 - ED to Hosp-Admission (Discharged) in ▮▮▮▮▮▮▮ Intensive Care Unit (continued)

Progress Notes (group 1 of 15) (continued)

		0253	PT	13.4	09/03/2021
ALKPHOS	85	09/06/2021			1709
		0253	INR	1.02	09/03/2021
AST	78 (H)	09/06/2021			1709
		0253			
ALT	84.0 (H)	09/06/2021			
		0253			
TBILI	0.9	09/06/2021			
		0253			

Imaging Studies
1. Chest X-ray (Images personally reviewed): Diffuse bilateral ground-glass opacities

Impression and Plan
Problem List

Hospital Problems

	POA
* (Principal) Acute respiratory failure with hypoxia (HCC)	Yes
Pneumonia due to COVID-19 virus	Yes
Hyponatremia	Yes
Hyperglycemia	Yes
Prediabetes	Yes

1. Acute respiratory failure: continue optiflo. Encourage self proning, deep breathing exercises.
2. COVID-19: s/p remdesivir X 1 dose, tocilizumab 1 dose. Continue empiric abx, solu medrol, zinc, vit D.
3. Hyperglycemia 2/2 steroids: insulin sliding scale.
4. Pneumomediastinum: no evidence of pneumothorax-x-ray improved
5. GIB prophylaxis: Proton Pump Inhibitor - Indications: High-dose steroids
6. DVT prophylaxis: Chemical prophylaxis: LMWH
7. Pt does not wish to be intubated and refusing standard treatment. Consult palliative Care

No emergency contact information on file.

Lines/Drains/Wounds:
Peripheral IV Left antecubital (3days)
Peripheral IV Right hand (3days)
No Tubes or Drains Found
No Airways Found
No Wounds Found

Discussed in multidisciplinary rounds today.

▮▮▮ **Yoyo** ▮, PA 9/6/2021

PA Yoyo notes "Pt does not wish to be intubated and refusing standard treatment." As you can see, they are dead set on Rob begin **intubated** and for him to follow their "standard treatment" protocol of **remdesivir** and being placed on a **ventilator** (you know, *"the protocol that kills"*).

Electronically signed by ▮▮▮ **Yoyo** ▮, PA at 09/06/21 0957

Skiba, Robert
MRN: 2000087384, DOB: ▮▮▮▮, Sex: M
Adm: 9/3/2021, D/C: 10/13/2021
Printed by ▮▮▮▮ at 10/26/21 2:44 PM

Page 84

Exhibit 21–Not a Candidate for BiPAP & Continues to Refuse Intubation (9/6/21)

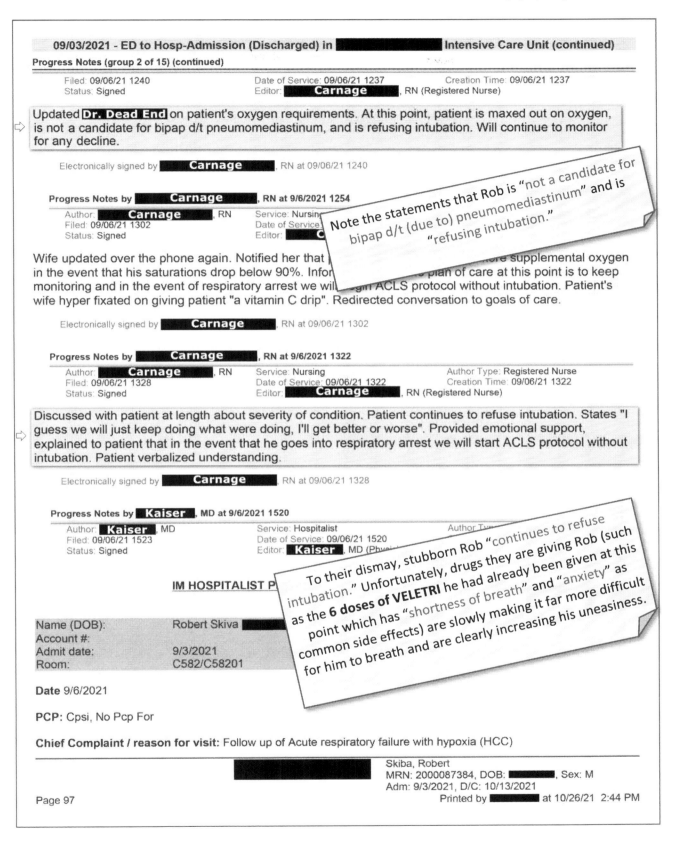

09/03/2021 - ED to Hosp-Admission (Discharged) in ▓▓▓▓▓▓▓▓▓▓ Intensive Care Unit (continued)

Progress Notes (group 2 of 15) (continued)

Filed: 09/06/21 1240	Date of Service: 09/06/21 1237	Creation Time: 09/06/21 1237
Status: Signed	Editor: ▓▓▓ **Carnage** ▓▓, RN (Registered Nurse)	

Updated **Dr. Dead End** on patient's oxygen requirements. At this point, patient is maxed out on oxygen, is not a candidate for bipap d/t pneumomediastinum, and is refusing intubation. Will continue to monitor for any decline.

Electronically signed by ▓▓▓ **Carnage** ▓▓, RN at 09/06/21 1240

Progress Notes by ▓▓▓ **Carnage** ▓▓, RN at 9/6/2021 1254

Author: ▓▓ **Carnage** ▓, RN	Service: Nursing	
Filed: 09/06/21 1302	Date of Service	
Status: Signed	Editor: ▓ **C**	

Note the statements that Rob is "not a candidate for bipap d/t (due to) pneumomediastinum" and is "refusing intubation."

Wife updated over the phone again. Notified her that ▓▓▓▓▓▓▓▓▓▓▓▓▓ ore supplemental oxygen in the event that his saturations drop below 90%. Infor▓▓▓▓▓▓▓▓▓ plan of care at this point is to keep monitoring and in the event of respiratory arrest we wil▓▓▓▓ ACLS protocol without intubation. Patient's wife hyper fixated on giving patient "a vitamin C drip". Redirected conversation to goals of care.

Electronically signed by ▓▓▓ **Carnage** ▓▓, RN at 09/06/21 1302

Progress Notes by ▓▓▓ **Carnage** ▓▓, RN at 9/6/2021 1322

Author: ▓▓ **Carnage** ▓, RN	Service: Nursing	Author Type: Registered Nurse
Filed: 09/06/21 1328	Date of Service: 09/06/21 1322	Creation Time: 09/06/21 1322
Status: Signed	Editor: ▓▓ **Carnage** ▓▓, RN (Registered Nurse)	

Discussed with patient at length about severity of condition. Patient continues to refuse intubation. States "I guess we will just keep doing what were doing, I'll get better or worse". Provided emotional support, explained to patient that in the event that he goes into respiratory arrest we will start ACLS protocol without intubation. Patient verbalized understanding.

Electronically signed by ▓▓▓ **Carnage** ▓▓, RN at 09/06/21 1328

Progress Notes by ▓ **Kaiser** ▓, MD at 9/6/2021 1520

Author ▓ **Kaiser** ▓, MD	Service: Hospitalist	Author T▓▓▓
Filed: 09/06/21 1523	Date of Service: 09/06/21 1520	
Status: Signed	Editor: ▓▓ **Kaiser** ▓, MD (Phys▓▓	

IM HOSPITALIST P▓▓

*To their dismay, stubborn Rob "continues to refuse intubation." Unfortunately, drugs they are giving Rob (such as the **6 doses of VELETRI** he had already been given at this point which has "shortness of breath" and "anxiety" as common side effects) are slowly making it far more difficult for him to breath and are clearly increasing his uneasiness.*

Name (DOB):	Robert Skiva ▓▓▓▓
Account #:	
Admit date:	9/3/2021
Room:	C582/C58201

Date 9/6/2021

PCP: Cpsi, No Pcp For

Chief Complaint / reason for visit: Follow up of Acute respiratory failure with hypoxia (HCC)

▓▓▓▓▓▓▓ Skiba, Robert
MRN: 2000087384, DOB: ▓▓▓▓, Sex: M
Adm: 9/3/2021, D/C: 10/13/2021

Printed by ▓▓▓▓ at 10/26/21 2:44 PM

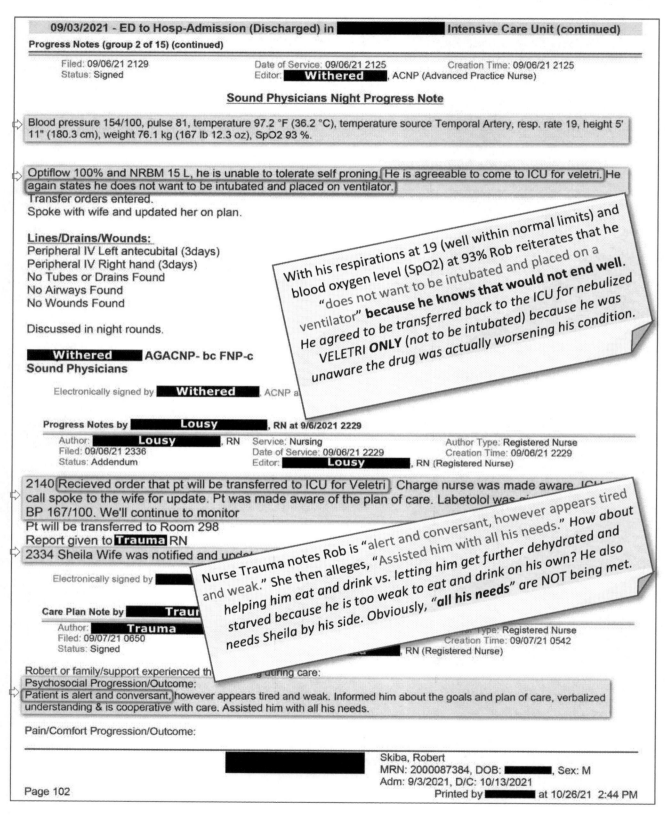

09/03/2021 - ED to Hosp-Admission (Discharged) in ▮▮▮▮▮ Intensive Care Unit (continued)

Progress Notes (group 2 of 15) (continued)

Filed: 09/06/21 2129   Date of Service: 09/06/21 2125   Creation Time: 09/06/21 2125
Status: Signed   Editor: ▮▮ **Withered** ▮▮, ACNP (Advanced Practice Nurse)

Sound Physicians Night Progress Note

⇨ Blood pressure 154/100, pulse 81, temperature 97.2 °F (36.2 °C), temperature source Temporal Artery, resp. rate 19, height 5' 11" (180.3 cm), weight 76.1 kg (167 lb 12.3 oz), SpO2 93 %.

⇨ Optiflow 100% and NRBM 15 L, he is unable to tolerate self proning. He is agreeable to come to ICU for veletri. He again states he does not want to be intubated and placed on ventilator.
Transfer orders entered.
Spoke with wife and updated her on plan.

Lines/Drains/Wounds:
Peripheral IV Left antecubital (3days)
Peripheral IV Right hand (3days)
No Tubes or Drains Found
No Airways Found
No Wounds Found

Discussed in night rounds.

▮▮ **Withered** ▮▮ AGACNP- bc FNP-c
Sound Physicians

Electronically signed by ▮▮ **Withered** ▮▮, ACNP a▮▮

Progress Notes by ▮▮ **Lousy** ▮▮, RN at 9/6/2021 2229

Author: ▮▮ **Lousy** ▮▮, RN   Service: Nursing   Author Type: Registered Nurse
Filed: 09/06/21 2336   Date of Service: 09/06/21 2229   Creation Time: 09/06/21 2229
Status: Addendum   Editor: ▮▮ **Lousy** ▮▮, RN (Registered Nurse)

2140 Recieved order that pt will be transferred to ICU for Veletri. Charge nurse was made aware. ICU call spoke to the wife for update. Pt was made aware of the plan of care. Labetolol was ▮▮▮
BP 167/100. We'll continue to monitor
Pt will be transferred to Room 298
Report given to Trauma RN
2334 Sheila Wife was notified and upd▮▮

Electronically signed by ▮▮▮

Care Plan Note by ▮▮ Trau▮▮

Author: ▮▮ **Trauma** ▮▮   ▮▮ Type: Registered Nurse
Filed: 09/07/21 0650   Creation Time: 09/07/21 0542
Status: Signed   ▮▮, RN (Registered Nurse)

Robert or family/support experienced th▮▮▮ during care:
Psychosocial Progression/Outcome:
Patient is alert and conversant, however appears tired and weak. Informed him about the goals and plan of care, verbalized understanding & is cooperative with care. Assisted him with all his needs.

Pain/Comfort Progression/Outcome:

Skiba, Robert
MRN: 2000087384, DOB: ▮▮, Sex: M
Adm: 9/3/2021, D/C: 10/13/2021

Page 102   Printed by ▮▮ at 10/26/21 2:44 PM

Annotation (top): With his respirations at 19 (well within normal limits) and blood oxygen level (SpO2) at 93% Rob reiterates that he "does not want to be intubated and placed on a ventilator" **because he knows that would not end well**. He agreed to be transferred back to the ICU for nebulized VELETRI **ONLY** (not to be intubated) because he was unaware the drug was actually worsening his condition.

Annotation (bottom): Nurse Trauma notes Rob is "alert and conversant, however appears tired and weak." She then alleges, "Assisted him with all his needs." How about helping him eat and drink vs. letting him get further dehydrated and starved because he is too weak to eat and drink on his own? He also needs Sheila by his side. Obviously, **"all his needs"** are NOT being met.

Exhibit 23–Rob's Vital Signs the Early Morning of 9/7/21 (1:30 AM to 8:30 AM)

SPO2 Monitoring	—	Continuous bedside	—	—
Temp	—	98.2 °F (36.8 °C)	—	
Temp src	—	Temporal Artery	—	
Daily weight change in kg	—	2.1 kg	—	
Humalog	2 Units	—	—	—

> Rob's vitals the early morning of 9/7/21 show that Rob was doing relatively well with his blood oxygen levels at **91% to 96%**.

Row Name	09/07/21 0130	09/07/21 0200	09/07/21 0230	09/07/21 0300	09/07/21 0326
Pulse	74	72	80	76	—
BP	155/91	155/91	158/95	154/89	—
BP Mean (MAP) (device)	117 MMHG	118 MMHG	120 MMHG	114 MMHG	—
Shock Index	0.48	0.46	0.51	0.49	—
Resp	25	28	26	17	—
⇨ SpO2	94 %	93 %	93 %	96 %	—
Humalog	—	—	—	—	2 Units

Row Name	09/07/21 0330	09/07/21 0400	09/07/21 0430	09/07/21 0500	09/07/21 0530
Pulse	75	80	79	63	71
BP	157/88	(!) 166/109	156/95	159/87	157/94
BP Mean (MAP) (device)	116 MMHG	132 MMHG	119 MMHG	115 MMHG	119 MMHG
Shock Index	0.48	0.48	0.51	0.4	0.45
Resp	23	(!) 31	30	(!) 33	21
⇨ SpO2	96 %	93 %	95 %	96 %	96 %
Temp	—	98.6 °F (37 °C)	—	—	—
Temp src	—	Temporal Artery	—	—	—

Row Name	09/07/21 0600	09/07/21 0700	09/07/21 0756	09/07/21 0800	09/07/21 0830
Pulse	62	70	72	87	65
BP	(!) 167/95	147/87	159/93	(!) 178/102	(!) 161/90
BP Mean (MAP) (device)	124 MMHG	111 MMHG	120 MMHG	130 MMHG	120 MMHG
Shock Index	0.37	0.48	0.45	0.49	0.4
Resp	27	26	26	(!) 35	24
⇨ SpO2	95 %	96 %	96 %	91 %	95 %
SPO2 Monitoring	—	—	—	Continuous central	—
Temp	—	—	—	97.5 °F (36.4 °C)	—
Temp src	—	—	—	Temporal Artery	—

Exhibit 24–Rob's Vital Signs Continued the Morning of 9/7/21 (9:00 AM to 1:00 PM)

09/03/2021 - ED to Hosp-Admission (Discharged) in ▮▮▮▮▮▮▮ Intensive Care Unit (continued)

Flowsheets (group 10 of 32) (continued)

Row Name	09/07/21 0900	09/07/21 0930	09/07/21 1000	09/07/21 1130	09/07/21 1200
Pulse	72	63	61	60	75
BP	(!) 167/94	148/91	147/82	153/80	
BP Mean (MAP) (device)	124 MMHG	114 MMHG	109 MMHG		
Shock Index	0.43	0.43	0.		
Resp	23	25	30	28	27
SpO2	96 %	96 %	95 %	95 %	96 %
SPO2 Monitoring	—	—	—	—	Continuous central
Temp	—	—	—	—	97.7 °F (36.5 °C)

Rob's blood oxygen level remained between 92% to 97% throughout the day on 9/7/21.

Row Name	09/07/21 1300	09/07/21 1400	09/07/21 1430	09/07/21 1500	09/07/21 1530
Pulse	68	72	72	—	69
BP	153/83	(!) 170/94	(!) 167/99	—	(!) 162/101
BP Mean (MAP) (device)	111 MMHG	126 MMHG	128 MMHG	128 MMHG	127 MMHG
Shock Index	0.44	0.42	0.43	—	0.43
Resp	16	22	25	26	26
SpO2	95 %	92 %	93 %	94 %	93 %
SPO2 Monitoring	—	—	—	—	Continuous central

Row Name	09/07/21 1630	09/07/21 1730	09/07/21 1800	09/07/21 1900	09/07/21 2000
Pulse	72	68	66	75	85
BP	159/98	155/91	(!) 164/90	(!) 183/97	134/76
BP Mean (MAP) (device)	123 MMHG	118 MMHG	120 MMHG	133 MMHG	99 MMHG
Shock Index	0.45	0.44	0.4	0.41	0.63
Resp	25	23	26	27	28
SpO2	93 %	93 %	95 %	93 %	93 %
SPO2 Monitoring	Continuous central	—	—	—	—
Temp	97.7 °F (36.5 °C)	—	—	—	98.4 °F (36.9 °C)
Temp src	Temporal Artery	—	—	—	Temporal Artery

Row Name	09/07/21 2100	09/07/21 2200	09/07/21 2300	09/08/21 0000	09/08/21 0100
Pulse	86	92	96	90	80
BP	125/64	132/73	154/86	147/88	142/82
BP Mean (MAP) (device)	88 MMHG	97 MMHG	114 MMHG	111 MMHG	106 MMHG
Shock Index	0.69	0.7	0.62	0.61	0.56
Resp	27	27	(!) 31	25	26
SpO2	97 %	92 %	92 %	92 %	96 %
SPO2 Monitoring	—	—	—	Continuous	—

Skiba, Robert
MRN: 2000087384, DOB: ▮▮▮▮▮, Sex: M
Adm: 9/3/2021, D/C: 10/13/2021

Printed by ▮▮▮▮▮ at 10/26/21 2:48 PM

ADMISSION ACKNOWLEDGEMENTS AND GENERAL CONSENT FOR TREATMENT
** SCROLL TO BOTTOM TO COMPLETE THE SIGNATURE ON THIS FORM **

1. **General consent.** I understand that my health condition requires inpatient or outpatient admission. I consent to and authorize testing, treatment and health care at this facility ("Facility"), a **Covid Coven Hospital** Facility, by facility nurses, employees, and others as ordered by my physician and his/her consultants, associates, and assistants, or as directed pursuant to standing medical orders or protocols. I understand that it may be necessary for representatives of outside health care companies to assist in my care. I also understand that persons in professional training programs may be among the persons who provide care to me. I understand that in connection with my treatment, photos or videos may be taken. Any tissue or body parts removed from my body may be retained or disposed of by the Facility at its sole discretion.

2. **Independent physicians.** I acknowledge that the physicians taking part in my care or providing a professional service to me do not work for the Facility and that the Facility is not responsible for their judgment or conduct. They practice independently and are not employees or agents of the Facility. The exception to this is that some physicians may be medical residents in a graduate medical education program of the Facility under the supervision of more experienced physicians. In addition to my attending physician, other physicians who may take part in my care may include radiologists, pathologists, anesthesiologists, hospitalists, neonatologists, cardiologists, emergency physicians, psychiatrists, and other specialists. The physician and professional services are not covered by the **CCH** Financial Assistance Policy.

3. **No guarantee.** I acknowledge that no guarantees or warranties have been made to me with the respect to treatment or services to be provided at this Facility. I understand that all supplies, medical devices and other goods provided or billed to me by the Facility are provided by the Facility on an "AS IS" basis, and the Facility disclaims any expressed or implied warranties with respect to them. With respect to specific supplies and devices, manufacturers ' warranties may apply, and I may request manufacturer 's warranty information concerning such supplies and/or devices.

4. **My valuables:** I understand that the Facility does not assume responsibility for personal property I keep with me during my treatment/Facility stay. I understand that unnecessary items should be sent home and that a safe is available for my valuables.

5. **Assignment of benefits:** I hereby irrevocably assign to the Facility and any practitioner providing care and treatment to me, any and all benefits and all interest and rights (including causes of action and the right to enforce payment) under any insurance policies, benefit plans, indemnity plans, prepaid health plans, third-party liability policies, or from any other payer providing benefits on my behalf, for and to the extent of the services and goods provided to me during this admission. Under this assignment, the Facility shall have an independent, non-exclusive right to appeal or pursue any denied or delayed claims on behalf of the insured or beneficiary. This assignment is not and shall not be construed as an obligation of the Facility and/or Facility-based physician to pursue such interest and rights. In signing this form, I (as the patient or patient's agent) am directing any applicable health insurer, health benefit plan, indemnity plan, reinsurer, third-party liability insurer or other payer providing benefits on my behalf to pay the Facility and/or Facility-based physicians directly for the services and goods the Facility and/or Facility-based physicians provide to me.

6. **Financial agreement:** I hereby promise to pay the Facility its full billed charges for all services and goods provided to me. I understand that the Facility, as a courtesy to me, may bill my insurance company, health benefit plan, or other non-governmental payer concerning the services and goods provided by the Facility to me but that the Facility is under no obligation to do so. Except as prohibited by law or by written agreement of the Facility, I agree to pay for any charges not covered and covered charges not paid in full by any applicable insurance and/or health benefit plan including charges payable as co-insurance, deductibles, and non-covered benefits due to policy and/or plan limitations, exclusions, and/or failure to comply with insurance and/or plan requirements. I further understand that the Facility, by mutual agreement with me or a person and/or entity making payments on my behalf, may agree to accept a discounted amount of its charges in full payment of the charges; however, to the extent the Facility has not agreed to accept less than the charges, I agree to be responsible for payment of the full amount of the charges less any amounts already paid by me or on my behalf. If I am entitled to benefits under a governmental plan, such as Medicare or Medicaid, I further understand the Facility may bill such plan and may accept as payment in full a discounted payment for the services and goods provided to me. **CCH** Financial Assistance Policy may be available if Facility eligibility criteria are met. An estimate of the anticipated charges is available upon request. I understand that estimates may vary significantly from the final charges because of a variety of factors such as the course of my treatment, intensity of care, physician practices, and the necessity of providing additional services and goods.I hereby consent to credit bureau inquiries and to receiving auto-dialed/artificial or pre-recorded [...] or text messages to my cellular telephone and to any telephone number provided during my registration process. I [...] attempts could be performed by from **Covid Coven Hospital** or its affiliates/agents including, with [...] [...], independent contractors or collection agents.

7. **Medicaid patients only:** I understand that the services or go[...] [...] covered under the Texas Medical Assistance Program as being reasonable and n[...] [...] the Texas Department of Human Services or its health insuring agent determines the me[...] [...] request and receive. I also understand that I am responsible for payment of the services or goods [...] are determined not to be reasonable and medically necessary for my care. If I am a Medicaid Star patie[...] [...].

8. **Communicable disease testing.** I acknowledge that Texas law provides if any health care worker is exposed to my blood or other bodily fluid, the Facility may perform tests, without my consent, on my blood or other bodily fluid to look for the presence of hepatitis B and C and HIV. I understand that such testing is needed to protect those who will be caring for me while I am a patient at the Facility. I understand that the results of tests taken under these circumstances are confidential and do not become a part of my Facility patient record.

9. **Obstetrics patients only:** This *Admission Acknowledgement and General Consent for Treatment* also applies to any child(ren) born to me during this hospitalization.

10. **OPTION TO RECEIVE INFORMATION AS TEXT MESSAGES:** As indicated below, I make the following election regarding whether to receive information about my care from the Facility and/or my physician in the form of a text message.

  ◉ I elect to receive information about my care, including information the privacy of which is protected under federal and state law, from the Facility and/or my physician in the form of a text message.

  ○ I elect NOT to receive information about my care, including information the privacy of which is protected under federal and state law, from the Facility and/or my physician in the form of a text message.

Page 1 of 2-page General Consent for Treatment form "signed" on the next page.

If the person signing this form is not the patient, please give full name, phone number and address:

Name:

Phone Number:

Address:

Relationship: ➪ spouse

Acknowledgement: I, the undersigned, c_____ its terms.

Signature captured with Topaz 1x5 by Robert Skiba

Skiba,Robert   09/07/21 1:07 PM

Witness Admission Specialist [Redacted Name]

Covid Coven Hospital
Admission Acknowledgements
And General Consent for Treatment
998543135 (Rev. 05/19) Page 1 of 1

Four days after Rob's admission (why wait this long?) a hospital "Admission Specialist" signed "**Verbal**" on the *General Consent* form shown above and, as shown in the signature blocks below, on two other forms. These forms were "signed" at 1:07, 1:08, and 1:09 PM—and by entering "**spouse**" they implied Sheila had given her verbal consent (which she had not) at a time when they were ignoring her directives because (as they admit) Rob was alert, aware, and fully capable of making his own decisions. Rob was fully capable of signing these and any other consent forms they needed. They should have obtained **Rob's signature** on these and other clearly "missing" consents for treatment, yet these three basic consent forms are the ONLY ones filed in the hospital records. Why did they not ask Rob to sign these forms, and why did they wait until four days after Rob's admission? **See Appendix I – Falsification of Hospital Consent Forms** for more on this troubling discovery.

Signatu____

PROTECTED HEALTH INFORMATION, T____ ___ TO PATIENTS, ADVANCE DIRECTIVES

Acknowledgement:
I, the undersigned, certify that I have read and fully understand the information in this Protected Health Information, Third Party Payer Notice to Patients, Advance Directives. I understand that if I need to change any information I have provided on this form, I will notify a facility staff member promptly.

Tap Once To Sign

Signature captured at 9/7/2021 01:08 PM

Skiba,Robert

➪ spouse

Relationship to patient

Signature Block Only (Not Full Form)

CONSENT FOR HEALTH INFORMATION EXCHANGE

Acknowledgment:
I, the undersigned, certify that I have read and fully understand the information in this Consent for Health Information Exchange form. I understand that if I need to change any information I have provided on this form, I will notify a staff member promptly.

Signature of patient or authorized representative

Signature captured at 9/7/2021 01:09 PM

Skiba,Robert

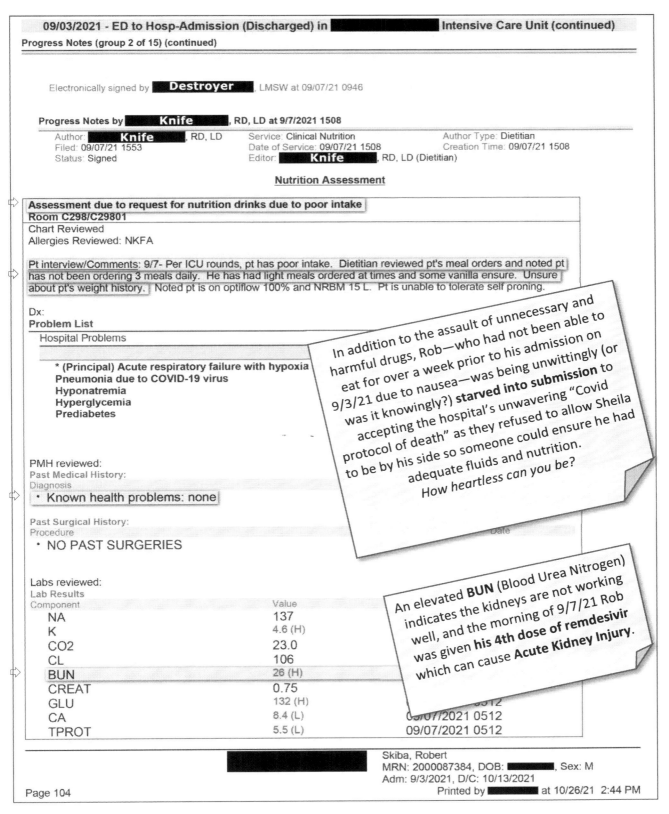

09/03/2021 - ED to Hosp-Admission (Discharged) in ⬛⬛⬛⬛ Intensive Care Unit (continued)

Progress Notes (group 2 of 15) (continued)

Electronically signed by ⬛ **Destroyer** ⬛, LMSW at 09/07/21 0946

Progress Notes by ⬛ **Knife** ⬛, RD, LD at 9/7/2021 1508

Author: ⬛ **Knife** ⬛, RD, LD	Service: Clinical Nutrition	Author Type: Dietitian
Filed: 09/07/21 1553	Date of Service: 09/07/21 1508	Creation Time: 09/07/21 1508
Status: Signed	Editor: ⬛ **Knife** ⬛, RD, LD (Dietitian)	

Nutrition Assessment

Assessment due to request for nutrition drinks due to poor intake
Room C298/C29801
Chart Reviewed
Allergies Reviewed: NKFA

Pt interview/Comments: 9/7- Per ICU rounds, pt has poor intake. Dietitian reviewed pt's meal orders and noted pt has not been ordering 3 meals daily. He has had light meals ordered at times and some vanilla ensure. Unsure about pt's weight history. Noted pt is on optiflow 100% and NRBM 15 L. Pt is unable to tolerate self proning.

Dx:
Problem List

Hospital Problems

* **(Principal)** Acute respiratory failure with hypoxia
* Pneumonia due to COVID-19 virus
* Hyponatremia
* Hyperglycemia
* Prediabetes

*In addition to the assault of unnecessary and harmful drugs, Rob—who had not been able to eat for over a week prior to his admission on 9/3/21 due to nausea—was being unwittingly (or was it knowingly?) **starved into submission** to accepting the hospital's unwavering "Covid protocol of death" as they refused to allow Sheila to be by his side so someone could ensure he had adequate fluids and nutrition. How heartless can you be?*

PMH reviewed:
Past Medical History:
Diagnosis
• Known health problems: none

Past Surgical History:
Procedure
• NO PAST SURGERIES

Labs reviewed:
Lab Results

Component	Value	
NA	137	
K	4.6 (H)	
CO2	23.0	
CL	106	
BUN	26 (H)	
CREAT	0.75	
GLU	132 (H)	
CA	8.4 (L)	09/07/2021 0512
TPROT	5.5 (L)	09/07/2021 0512

*An elevated **BUN** (Blood Urea Nitrogen) indicates the kidneys are not working well, and the morning of 9/7/21 Rob was given **his 4th dose of remdesivir** which can cause **Acute Kidney Injury**.*

Skiba, Robert
MRN: 2000087384, DOB: ⬛⬛⬛, Sex: M
Adm: 9/3/2021, D/C: 10/13/2021

Page 104   Printed by ⬛⬛ at 10/26/21 2:44 PM

C-27

Exhibit 28–Malnutrition Weakens Rob, Making Him More Compliant (9/7/21)

09/03/2021 - ED to Hosp-Admission (Discharged) in ▮▮▮▮▮▮ **Intensive C▮▮▮▮▮▮tinued)**

Progress Notes (group 2 of 15) (continued)

ALB   2.5 (L)
GLOB
ALKPHOS
AST
ALT
TBILI

Meds reviewed: vitamin C 500mg BID, zithromax, m▮
pepcid, Medium dose correctional insulin, flora Q, lab▮
and to go through 9/13/21, electrolyte replacements p▮

Height: 5' 11" (180.3 cm)
Weight:
9/6/21- 75.5 kg (166 lb 7.2 oz) bed scale
9/4/21- 76 kg (167 lb 8.8 oz) bed scale
Admission Weight [09/03/21 1658] stated
Weight   **77.1 kg (170 lb)**

Body mass index is 23.21 kg/m².   (Classification: WNL)
IBW: 166 lbs ± 10%

Current Diet order/Regimen: regular

Nursing Flowsheets Reviewed. Noted:
    GI fxn: Last noted BM type 7 on 9/6
    Oral: none
    Skin/physical appearance: Total Braden 18 noted.
    Edema: none
    Dietary intake/appetite: poor < 50%
Pulse 77, BP 171/99, MAP 123

Diagnosis

Nutrition Dx: Inadequate oral intake related to decreased appetite with Covid 19 pneumonia as evidenced by
documentation and pt not ordering much at meals or skipping meals. .

Intervention
Nutrition Prescription:
Est. Kcal Needs: 2000-2200 kcals/day
Est. Protein Needs: 95-105g protein/day
Est. Fluid Needs: 2000-2200ml fluid/day

Nutrition Interventions: Meals and Snacks: General/healthf▮
Specific foods/beverages or groups:
    Per RD, send vanilla ensure enlive on all trays.   Order plac▮

RECOMMENDATIONS:
1. Continue regular diet and encourage meals/nutrition dri▮
2. Weigh pt daily
3. Vit/Mineral supplementation with COVID-19:
    *Continue minimum Vitamin D 50mcg (2000 Internati▮

Page 105

▮▮▮▮▮▮087384, DOB: ▮▮▮▮▮, Sex: M
Adm: 9/3/2021, D/C: 10/13/2021
Printed by ▮▮▮▮▮ at 10/26/21 2:44 PM

Rob was being **starved into submission** due to a lack of adequate food and water because Sheila was shut out of the hospital, and no one on staff would help Rob eat or drink between breaths. Rob's admission weight (as shown here) was **170 lbs.**, yet in a later record (not included) on the morning of September 9, 2021 (less than six full days after his admission), they recorded his weight as **160 lbs.**, thus Rob lost **10 pounds in less than six days** in the hospital. Of course, his "Dietary intake" was poor, and he was "skipping meals" because he needed someone to help him eat and drink!

Rob desperately needed Sheila by his side to aid him in taking in adequate food and water. Yet this criminal enterprise kept Sheila out for 21 days because they did not want her interfering with their plans for Rob—and they knew a starved and weakened patient would, in time, become "compliant" with their Covid "death protocol."

Nice of them to **send vanilla Ensure Enlive on all trays** while no one ensured that Rob was even able to drink this only 350-calorie "meal replacement beverage." Rob texted Sheila at 7:30 PM on September 5, 2021, over 48 hours after his arrival at the hospital, **"No food."** He then texted, **"No strength, no hope left."**

How can these criminals sleep at night knowing they are allowing their patients to starve?

Exhibit 29–In "No Acute Distress" Just Over 24 Hours Prior to Intubation (9/7/21 at 3:25 PM)

Progress Notes (group 2 of 15) (continued)

Last data filed at 9/7/2021 1525

	Gross per 24 hour
Intake	818.08 ml
Output	1820 ml
Net	**-1001.92 ml**

Physical Exam:

⇨ general - awake, no acute distress
Neuro - alert and oriented x 3. Speech fluent. Moving all limbs independently
head,eyes,ears,nose, and throat - moist mucous membranes, oropharynx clear
cv - regular rate and rhythm
pulm - rhonchi bilaterally
gi/abdomen - soft, non tender, non distended

RADIOLOGY/LABORATORY:

Labs
Lab Results

Component	Value	
NA	137	
K	4.6 (H)	
CO2	23.0	
CL	106	
BUN	26 (H)	
CREAT	0.75	
GLU	132 (H)	09/07/2021 0512
CA	8.4 (L)	09/07/2021 0512
TPROT	5.5 (L)	09/07/2021 0512
ALB	2.5 (L)	09/07/2021 0512
ALKPHOS	109	09/07/2021 0512
AST	102 (H)	09/07/2021 0512
ALT	120.0 (H)	09/07/2021 0512
TBILI	1.0	09/07/2021 0512

Component	Value	Date/Time
TROPONIN	0.048 (H)	09/03/2021 1709
DIMERQ	17.05 (H)	09/07/2021 0512
BNP	25	09/04/2021 0539

Lab Results

Component	Value	Date/Time
PT	13.4	09/03/2021 1709
INR	1.02	09/03/2021 1709

*Note that the **Physical Exam** shows Rob is awake and in "no acute distress" with his "speech fluent." However, Rob continued to decline due to a lack of adequate water and food and the onslaught of harmful medications such as **remdesivir** (which he had 4 doses of by now) and **VELETRI** (which he had been given 5 nebulized treatments of by now).*

***Remdesivir** is known to be able to cause **Acute Kidney Injury** (which was the secondary cause of death noted on Rob's death certificate). **VELETRI** (as noted earlier on Page C-6) should **NEVER** be given to a patient who is already short of breath because it may cause **SERIOUS** side effects that include "**severe shortness of breath, gasping for breath, and anxiety.**"*

Skiba, Robert
MRN: 2000087384, DOB: ▉▉▉▉▉, Sex: M
Adm: 9/3/2021, D/C: 10/13/2021

Page 114

Printed by ▉▉▉▉▉ at 10/26/21 2:44 PM

09/03/2021 - ED to Hosp-Admission (Discharged) in ████████ Intensive Care Unit (continued)

Progress Notes (group 2 of 15) (continued)

Acct #:

Source of referral: Family
Visited with: Spouse (Sheila)

Reason for visit	Family Support
Spiritual Assessment	Peace/Anxiety • Chaplain received call to reach out to spouse • She named distress around him not having personal touch, human connection ⇨ She asked if chaplain could enter covid room to remind him of the love that surrounds him and offer prayer and support • I let her know that i would discuss this with supervisor since our protocol has not included going to covid rooms- • She says video calls agitate him and she would prefer a minute of a real person and not a screen
Intervention	• Called spouse and listened to her request without making promises, other than to ask and clarify
Next steps	⇨ Will follow up tomorrow to tell her what our department's policy is on entering covid rooms

Joker

Electronically sig... ...07/21 1724

Care Plan Note by 16
Author: **Strife** ...ice: Nursing
Filed: 09/07/21 18... ...of Service: 09/07/21 1816
Status: Signed ... **Strife**, RN (Register...

Robert or family/support ... ...ring care:
Psychosocial Progression ...
Calm and fatigued. Receiv... ...dated.

Pain/Comfort Progression/Outcome:
Denies any pain.

Clinical Progression/Outcome:
⇨ Weak and fatigued. Oriented x4, MAE, follows commands. On Optiflow 93%, 60L with NRB mask. Spo2 >92%. Exertional
⇨ dyspnea. Poor apatite, refused lunch and breakfast. Encouraged to drink ensure for dinner. Safety maintained.

REMINDER: Address the patient/family progress this shift (including the abo... ...
Plan and demonstrate the compassionate care given.

Electronically signed by **Strife**

(handwritten note overlay:) Sheila could not even get a hospital Chaplain to visit Rob to offer him prayer and support. What a total waste of a department! And once again, it is noted here that Rob has a **poor appetite**. They neither notice nor care that he is wasting away—or was it their intention to starve him so he would "submit" to "the protocol"? Locking Sheila out was a totally inexcusable, criminal act.

(note overlay:) Despite the continued neglect and abuse, Rob's SpO2 (blood oxygen level) **remains above 90%**. Sadly, in just 24 hours, Rob will be weakened to the point where they can force him to be drugged, intubated, and placed on a ventilator, which has been their clearly orchestrated plan all along.

(note overlay:) The "Poor apatite [sic]..." note makes it even more clear that Rob's absolute lack of nutrition (essential to keeping up his strength) is being **totally ignored**. Of course, Rob is "Weak and fatigued" because they are unwittingly or wittingly starving him into submission. They know full well that a "weakened" patient would be a "compliant" patient who will not have the strength to resist succumbing to "the protocol."

Exhibit 31–Patient Has Not Been Ordering Meals, Unsure About Weight History (9/7/21)

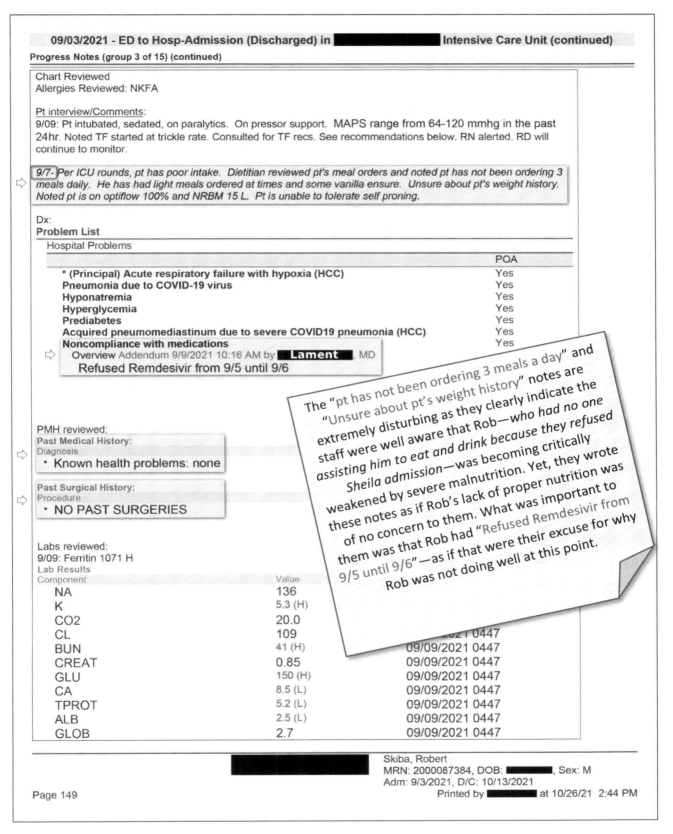

09/03/2021 - ED to Hosp-Admission (Discharged) in ███████████ **Intensive Care Unit (continued)**
Progress Notes (group 3 of 15) (continued)

Chart Reviewed
Allergies Reviewed: NKFA

Pt interview/Comments:
9/09: Pt intubated, sedated, on paralytics. On pressor support. MAPS range from 64-120 mmhg in the past 24hr. Noted TF started at trickle rate. Consulted for TF recs. See recommendations below. RN alerted. RD will continue to monitor.

9/7- Per ICU rounds, pt has poor intake. Dietitian reviewed pt's meal orders and noted pt has not been ordering 3 meals daily. He has had light meals ordered at times and some vanilla ensure. Unsure about pt's weight history. Noted pt is on optiflow 100% and NRBM 15 L. Pt is unable to tolerate self proning.

Dx:
Problem List

Hospital Problems

	POA
* (Principal) Acute respiratory failure with hypoxia (HCC)	Yes
Pneumonia due to COVID-19 virus	Yes
Hyponatremia	Yes
Hyperglycemia	Yes
Prediabetes	Yes
Acquired pneumomediastinum due to severe COVID19 pneumonia (HCC)	Yes
Noncompliance with medications	Yes

⇨ Overview Addendum 9/9/2021 10:16 AM by ███ **Lament** ███, MD
Refused Remdesivir from 9/5 until 9/6

The "pt has not been ordering 3 meals a day" and "Unsure about pt's weight history" notes are extremely disturbing as they clearly indicate the staff were well aware that Rob—who had no one assisting him to eat and drink because they refused Sheila admission—was becoming critically weakened by severe malnutrition. Yet, they wrote these notes as if Rob's lack of proper nutrition was of no concern to them. What was important to them was that Rob had "Refused Remdesivir from 9/5 until 9/6"—as if that were their excuse for why Rob was not doing well at this point.

PMH reviewed:
Past Medical History:
Diagnosis
· Known health problems: none

Past Surgical History:
Procedure
· NO PAST SURGERIES

Labs reviewed:
9/09: Ferritin 1071 H
Lab Results

Component	Value	
NA	136	
K	5.3 (H)	
CO2	20.0	
CL	109	
BUN	41 (H)	...21 0447
CREAT	0.85	09/09/2021 0447
GLU	150 (H)	09/09/2021 0447
CA	8.5 (L)	09/09/2021 0447
TPROT	5.2 (L)	09/09/2021 0447
ALB	2.5 (L)	09/09/2021 0447
GLOB	2.7	09/09/2021 0447

Skiba, Robert
MRN: 2000087384, DOB: ████████, Sex: M
Adm: 9/3/2021, D/C: 10/13/2021

Page 149

Printed by ████████ at 10/26/21 2:44 PM

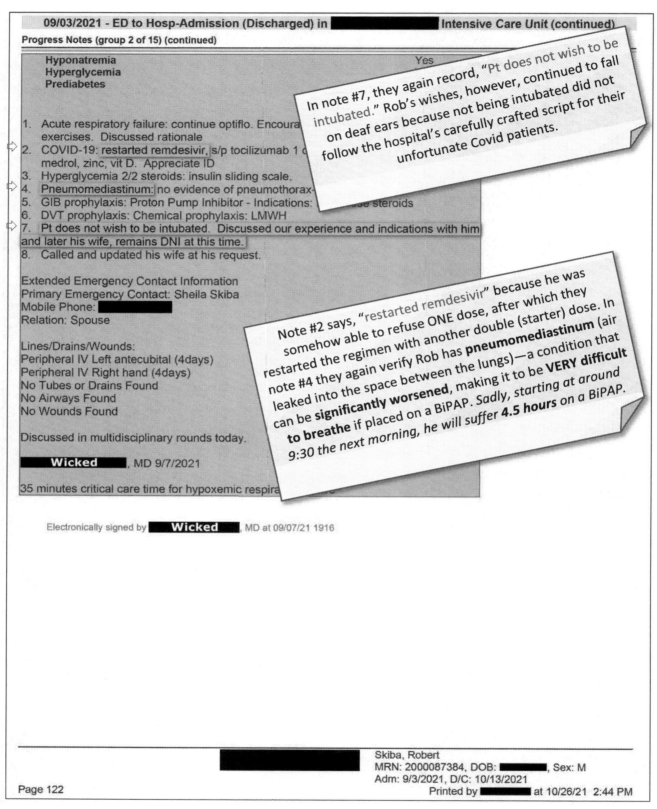

09/03/2021 - ED to Hosp-Admission (Discharged) in [REDACTED] **Intensive Care Unit (continued)**

Progress Notes (group 2 of 15) (continued)

Hyponatremia   Yes
Hyperglycemia
Prediabetes

1. Acute respiratory failure: continue optiflo. Encoura[ge]
   exercises. Discussed rationale
2. COVID-19: restarted remdesivir, s/p tocilizumab 1 [REDACTED]
   medrol, zinc, vit D. Appreciate ID
3. Hyperglycemia 2/2 steroids: insulin sliding scale.
4. Pneumomediastinum: no evidence of pneumothorax-[REDACTED]
5. GIB prophylaxis: Proton Pump Inhibitor - Indications: [REDACTED] se steroids
6. DVT prophylaxis: Chemical prophylaxis: LMWH
7. Pt does not wish to be intubated. Discussed our experience and indications with him
   and later his wife, remains DNI at this time.
8. Called and updated his wife at his request.

Extended Emergency Contact Information
Primary Emergency Contact: Sheila Skiba
Mobile Phone: [REDACTED]
Relation: Spouse

Lines/Drains/Wounds:
Peripheral IV Left antecubital (4days)
Peripheral IV Right hand (4days)
No Tubes or Drains Found
No Airways Found
No Wounds Found

Discussed in multidisciplinary rounds today.

Wicked [REDACTED], MD 9/7/2021

35 minutes critical care time for hypoxemic respira[tory]

Electronically signed by [REDACTED] **Wicked** [REDACTED], MD at 09/07/21 1916

In note #7, they again record, "Pt does not wish to be intubated." Rob's wishes, however, continued to fall on deaf ears because not being intubated did not follow the hospital's carefully crafted script for their unfortunate Covid patients.

*Note #2 says, "restarted remdesivir" because he was somehow able to refuse ONE dose, after which they restarted the regimen with another double (starter) dose. In note #4 they again verify Rob has **pneumomediastinum** (air leaked into the space between the lungs)—a condition that can be **significantly worsened**, making it to be **VERY difficult to breathe** if placed on a BiPAP. Sadly, starting at around 9:30 the next morning, he will suffer **4.5 hours** on a BiPAP.*

Skiba, Robert
MRN: 2000087384, DOB: [REDACTED], Sex: M
Adm: 9/3/2021, D/C: 10/13/2021

Page 122   Printed by [REDACTED] at 10/26/21 2:44 PM

09/03/2021 - ED to Hosp-Admission (Discharged) in ▓▓▓▓▓▓▓▓▓▓ d)

Orders (group 6 of 28)

SMALL VOLUME NEBULIZER, CONTINUOUS

Electronically signed by: **Blea** ▓
Ordering user: **Bleak**, RT
Authorized by: **Relentless**
Frequency: Routine CONTINUOUS
Quantity: 1

Discontinued by: **Bleak**, RT

Adult High Flow Oxygen [1136632927

Electronically signed by: **Ogre**
Mode: Ordering in Verbal w/Read-back
mode
Ordering
Ordering user: **Chaos**, RT
Authorized by: **Ogre**, MD
Frequency: Routine CONTINUOUS 09/03/
Quantity: 1

Discontinued by: **Senseless**, R

METERED DOSE INHALER [1136632930] (D

Electronically signed by: **Pointless**, RT
Ordering user: **Pointless**, RT 09/06/21 1
Authorized by: **Killer**, MD
Frequency: Routine DAILY 09/07/21 0900 - Unt
Quantity: 1

Discontinued by: **Harmful**, RRT 09

On this **"Orders"** record you can see that at **9:40 AM** on **9/8/21**, Dr. Wicked entered a **"FULL RESUSCITATION"** order as they were placing Rob on a **BiPAP**, a positive pressure therapy that forced air into his lungs and, as noted on the pages that follow, caused **barotrauma**—the rupturing of the air sacks (the alveoli) in Rob's lungs. This order removed the formerly active **DNI** (Do Not Intubate) order that was entered because Rob had continually insisted that he **DID NOT want** to be intubated. This gave Dr. Wicked the authority to have Rob intubated and placed on a ventilator if the BiPAP caused the devastation of Rob's lungs they fully expected it would. **NOTE:** Page C-53 shows how four doctors flip-flopped Rob's status to **FULL,** then back to **Limited,** then back to **FULL** resuscitation **five times** over a four-day period due to their persistent insistence that he consent to "elective intubation."

▓▓▓▓▓▓ed by: **Pointless**, RT (auto-released) 9/8/2021

9:00 AM

▓▓▓ [THERAPY COMPLETED]

FULL RESUSCITATION [1136632932] (Discontinued)

Electronically signed by: **Wicked**, MD on 09/08/21 0940
Ordering user: **Wicked**, MD 09/08/21 0940
Authorized by: **Wicked**, MD
Frequency: Routine Continuous 09/08/21 0942 - Until Specified
Quantity: 1
Instance released by: **Wicked**, MD (auto-released)
9/8/2021 9:40 AM

Ordering provider: **Wicked**, MD
Ordering mode: Standard
Class: Normal
Code status: Full Code

Status: **Discontinued**

Discontinued by: Interface, Adtinv 10/14/21 0304 [Pt Discharge]

enoxaparin (Lovenox) syringe [1136632935] (Discontinued)

Electronically signed by: **Wicked**, MD on 09/08/21 0947
Ordering user: **Wicked**, MD 09/08/21 0947
Authorized by: **Wicked**, MD
Frequency: Routine EVERY 12 HOURS 09/08/21 2100 - 09/17/21 0852
Discontinued by: **Wicked**, MD 09/17/21 0852
Acknowledged: **Rabid**, RN 09/08/21
Admin instructions: Administer by deep SubQ injection to the left or right anterolateral or left or right posterolateral abdominal wall. Wait to administer at least 2 hours after epidural catheter removal.
Package: 60505-0792-0
Modified from: enoxaparin (Lovenox) syringe

Ordering provider: **Wicked**, MD
Ordering mode: Standard
Class: ePrescribe

Status: **Discontinued**

BiPAP / CPAP [1136632937] (Discontinued)

Electronically signed by: **Wicked**, MD on 09/08/21 1508
Mode: Ordering in Verbal w/Read-back (Co-Sign REQUIRED) mode
Ordering user: **Grief**, RT 09/08/21 1017
Authorized by: **Wicked**, MD
Frequency: Routine CONTINUOUS 09/08/21 1019 - Until Specified
Quantity: 1

Communicated by: **Grief**, RT

Ordering provider: **Wicked**, MD
Ordering mode: Verbal w/Read-back (Co-Sign REQUIRED)
Class: Normal
Instance released by: **Grief**, RT (auto-released) 9/8/2021 10:17 AM

Status: **Discontinued**

Skiba, Robert
MRN: 2000087384, DOB: ▓▓▓▓▓▓, Sex: M
Adm: 9/3/2021, D/C: 10/13/2021

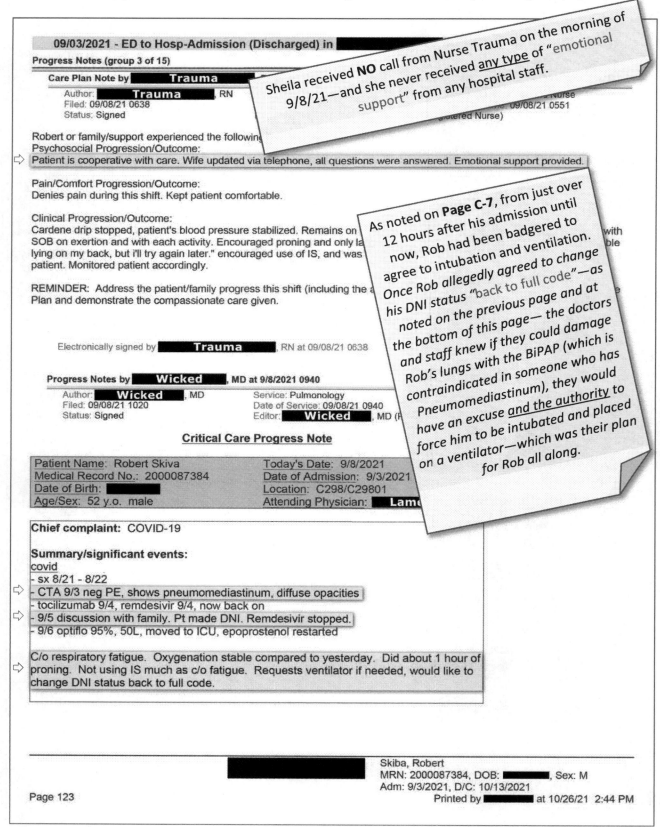

09/03/2021 - ED to Hosp-Admission (Discharged) in

Progress Notes (group 3 of 15)

Care Plan Note by ▮▮▮▮ **Trauma**

Author: ▮▮▮▮ **Trauma** ▮▮▮▮, RN
Filed: 09/08/21 0638
Status: Signed

*Sheila received **NO** call from Nurse Trauma on the morning of 9/8/21—and she never received any type of "emotional support" from any hospital staff.*

Robert or family/support experienced the following
Psychosocial Progression/Outcome:
⇨ Patient is cooperative with care. Wife updated via telephone, all questions were answered. Emotional support provided.

Pain/Comfort Progression/Outcome:
Denies pain during this shift. Kept patient comfortable.

Clinical Progression/Outcome:
Cardene drip stopped, patient's blood pressure stabilized. Remains on ▮▮▮ with SOB on exertion and with each activity. Encouraged proning and only la▮▮▮ lying on my back, but i'll try again later." encouraged use of IS, and was ▮▮▮ble patient. Monitored patient accordingly.

REMINDER: Address the patient/family progress this shift (including the ▮▮
Plan and demonstrate the compassionate care given.

Electronically signed by ▮▮▮▮ **Trauma** ▮▮▮▮, RN at 09/08/21 0638

Progress Notes by ▮▮▮▮ **Wicked** ▮▮▮▮, MD at 9/8/2021 0940

Author: ▮▮▮ **Wicked** ▮▮▮, MD   Service: Pulmonology
Filed: 09/08/21 1020   Date of Service: 09/08/21 0940
Status: Signed   Editor: ▮▮▮ **Wicked** ▮▮▮, MD (P

*As noted on **Page C-7**, from just over 12 hours after his admission until now, Rob had been badgered to agree to intubation and ventilation. Once Rob allegedly agreed to change his DNI status "back to full code"—as noted on the previous page and at the bottom of this page— the doctors and staff knew if they could damage Rob's lungs with the BiPAP (which is contraindicated in someone who has Pneumomediastinum), they would have an excuse and the authority to force him to be intubated and placed on a ventilator—which was their plan for Rob all along.*

Critical Care Progress Note

Patient Name: Robert Skiva	Today's Date: 9/8/2021
Medical Record No.: 2000087384	Date of Admission: 9/3/2021
Date of Birth: ▮▮▮	Location: C298/C29801
Age/Sex: 52 y.o. male	Attending Physician: ▮▮▮ **Lam**

Chief complaint: COVID-19

Summary/significant events:
covid
- sx 8/21 - 8/22
⇨ - CTA 9/3 neg PE, shows pneumomediastinum, diffuse opacities
- tocilizumab 9/4, remdesivir 9/4, now back on
⇨ - 9/5 discussion with family. Pt made DNI. Remdesivir stopped.
- 9/6 optiflo 95%, 50L, moved to ICU, epoprostenol restarted

⇨ C/o respiratory fatigue. Oxygenation stable compared to yesterday. Did about 1 hour of proning. Not using IS much as c/o fatigue. Requests ventilator if needed, would like to change DNI status back to full code.

Skiba, Robert
MRN: 2000087384, DOB: ▮▮▮, Sex: M
Adm: 9/3/2021, D/C: 10/13/2021
Printed by ▮▮▮ at 10/26/21 2:44 PM

Page 123

09/03/2021 - ED to Hosp-Admission (Discharged) in ▮▮▮▮ ▮▮▮▮ ued)
Progress Notes (group 3 of 15) (continued)

CA	
TPROT	
ALB	2
ALKPHOS	12
AST	106
ALT	130.0
TBILI	1.1

Imaging Studies
1. No new studies

Impression and Plan
Problem List
Hospital Problems

* (Principal) Acute respirator▮
Pneumonia due to COVID-19
Hyponatremia
Hyperglycemia
Prediabetes

The excessive oxygen concentrations Rob was subjected to during his first five days at the hospital (see the chart at the top of Page C-54), resulted in **atelectasis** (a condition where alveoli in a lung or a part of a lung deflate, causing a partial or complete collapsed lung) as shown in **Note 1**. This condition causes shortness of breath and painful breathing. Thus, they placed Rob on a BiPAP to "see if it helps atelectasis." In the same note, you'll see "Monitor for barotrauma given already with pneumomediastinum," which was written at **10:20 AM**, about an hour after Rob was started on 4.5 hours on a BiPAP. This shows Dr. Wicked (who wrote this note) knew full well that with **pneumomediastinum** (listed in **Note 4**), there was a significant risk that the BiPAP **would cause barotrauma**—the rupturing of the alveoli (the air sacs of the lungs). The "Repeat CXR [Chest X-ray] this afternoon to **monitor** barotrauma" note on Page 141 of the hospital records (see Page C-44) makes it clear that 4.5 hours on the BiPAP **DID** rupture the alveoli of Rob's lungs with the BiPAP. We contend that the injury (the **barotrauma**) directly led to Rob ending up being intubated and placed on a ventilator.

⇨ 1. Acute respiratory failure: continu▮ ▮▮▮▮ ▮ncourage self proning, deep breathing exercises. Trial of BiPAP given c/o fatigue and see if helps atelectasis. Monitor for barotrauma given already with pneumomediastinum
2. COVID-19: restarted remdesivir, s/p tocilizumab 1 dose. Continue empiric abx, solumedrol, zinc, vit D. Appreciate ID. Inflammatory markers improving, plan to wean steroids soon
3. Hyperglycemia 2/2 steroids: insulin sliding scale.
⇨ 4. Pneumomediastinum: no evidence of pneumothorax-x-ray improved
5. GIB prophylaxis: Proton Pump Inhibitor - Indications: High-dose steroids
6. DVT prophylaxis: Chemical prophylaxis: LMWH
7. Removed DNI from his code status per his request.
8. Called and updated his wife via phone at his request.

Extended Emergency Contact Information
Primary Emergency Contact: Sheila Skiba
Mobile Phone: ▮▮▮▮▮▮▮
Relation: Spouse

Lines/Drains/Wounds:
Peripheral IV Left antecubital (5days)
Peripheral IV Right wrist (1days)

Skiba, Robert
MRN: 2000087384, DOB: ▮▮▮▮▮, Sex: M
Adm: 9/3/2021, D/C: 10/13/2021

Printed by ▮▮▮▮▮ at 10/26/21 2:44 PM

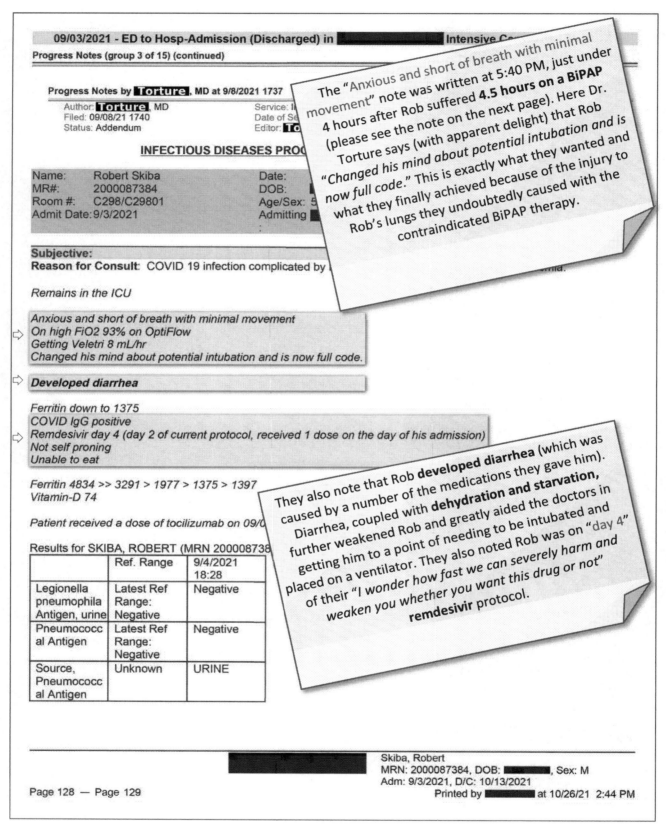

09/03/2021 - ED to Hosp-Admission (Discharged) in ▇▇▇▇▇▇▇▇ **Intensive C**▇▇▇

Progress Notes (group 3 of 15) (continued)

Progress Notes by **Torture**, MD at 9/8/2021 1737

Author: **Torture**, MD   Service: I▇▇
Filed: 09/08/21 1740   Date of Se▇▇
Status: Addendum   Editor: **To**▇▇

INFECTIOUS DISEASES PRO▇▇

Name:	Robert Skiba	Date:	
MR#:	2000087384	DOB:	
Room #:	C298/C29801	Age/Sex:	5▇
Admit Date:	9/3/2021	Admitting	

Subjective:
Reason for Consult: COVID 19 infection complicated by ▇▇▇▇▇▇▇▇ ▇▇▇▇▇▇▇▇ ▇▇ia.

Remains in the ICU

⇨ Anxious and short of breath with minimal movement
On high FiO2 93% on OptiFlow
Getting Veletri 8 mL/hr
Changed his mind about potential intubation and is now full code.

⇨ **Developed diarrhea**

⇨ Ferritin down to 1375
COVID IgG positive
Remdesivir day 4 (day 2 of current protocol, received 1 dose on the day of his admission)
Not self proning
Unable to eat

Ferritin 4834 >> 3291 > 1977 > 1375 > 1397
Vitamin-D 74

Patient received a dose of tocilizumab on 09/0▇

Results for SKIBA, ROBERT (MRN 200008738▇

	Ref. Range	9/4/2021 18:28
Legionella pneumophila Antigen, urine	Latest Ref Range: Negative	Negative
Pneumococcal Antigen	Latest Ref Range: Negative	Negative
Source, Pneumococcal Antigen	Unknown	URINE

The "Anxious and short of breath with minimal movement" note was written at 5:40 PM, just under 4 hours after Rob suffered **4.5 hours on a BiPAP** (please see the note on the next page). Here Dr. Torture says (with apparent delight) that Rob "*Changed his mind about potential intubation and is now full code.*" This is exactly what they wanted and what they finally achieved because of the injury to Rob's lungs they undoubtedly caused with the contraindicated BiPAP therapy.

They also note that Rob **developed diarrhea** (which was caused by a number of the medications they gave him). Diarrhea, coupled with **dehydration and starvation,** further weakened Rob and greatly aided the doctors in getting him to a point of needing to be intubated and placed on a ventilator. They also noted Rob was on "day 4" of their "*I wonder how fast we can severely harm and weaken you whether you want this drug or not*" **remdesivir** protocol.

Skiba, Robert
MRN: 2000087384, DOB: ▇▇▇▇▇▇, Sex: M
Adm: 9/3/2021, D/C: 10/13/2021
Printed by ▇▇▇▇▇▇ at 10/26/21 2:44 PM

Page 128 — Page 129

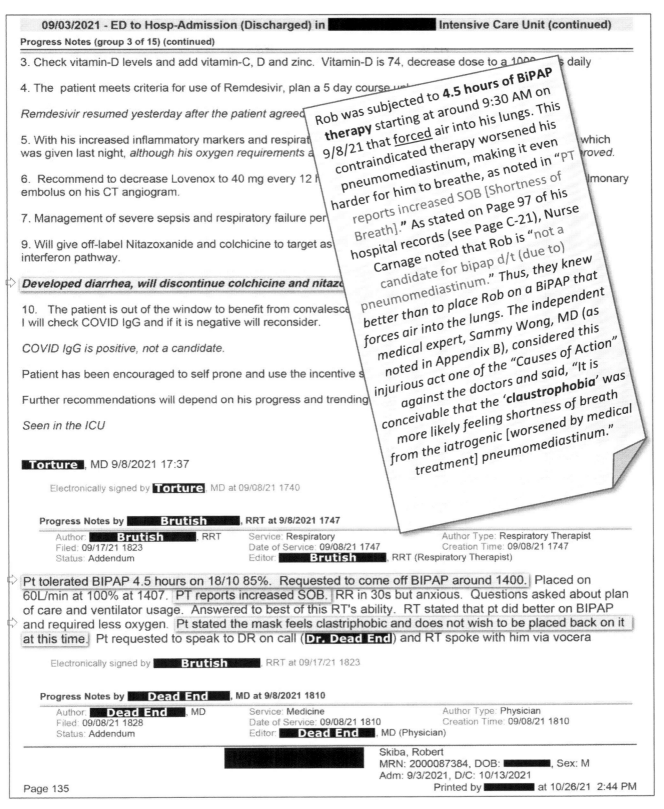

09/03/2021 - ED to Hosp-Admission (Discharged) in ▮▮▮▮▮▮▮▮▮ Intensive Care Unit (continued)

Progress Notes (group 3 of 15) (continued)

3. Check vitamin-D levels and add vitamin-C, D and zinc. Vitamin-D is 74, decrease dose to a 1000 ▮▮▮▮s daily

4. The patient meets criteria for use of Remdesivir, plan a 5 day course ▮▮▮

Remdesivir resumed yesterday after the patient agreed ▮▮▮

5. With his increased inflammatory markers and respirat▮▮▮ ▮▮▮ which was given last night, *although his oxygen requirements a* ▮▮▮ *roved.*

6. Recommend to decrease Lovenox to 40 mg every 12 ▮ ▮▮▮ lmonary embolus on his CT angiogram.

7. Management of severe sepsis and respiratory failure per ▮▮▮

9. Will give off-label Nitazoxanide and colchicine to target as▮▮▮ interferon pathway.

⇨ ***Developed diarrhea, will discontinue colchicine and nitaz▮▮▮***

10. The patient is out of the window to benefit from convalesc▮▮▮ I will check COVID IgG and if it is negative will reconsider.

COVID IgG is positive, not a candidate.

Patient has been encouraged to self prone and use the incentive s▮▮▮

Further recommendations will depend on his progress and trending▮▮▮

Seen in the ICU

▮**Torture**▮, MD 9/8/2021 17:37

Electronically signed by **Torture**▮, MD at 09/08/21 1740

Progress Notes by ▮▮**Brutish**▮▮, RRT at 9/8/2021 1747

Author: ▮▮**Brutish**▮▮, RRT	Service: Respiratory	Author Type: Respiratory Therapist
Filed: 09/17/21 1823	Date of Service: 09/08/21 1747	Creation Time: 09/08/21 1747
Status: Addendum	Editor: ▮▮**Brutish**▮▮, RRT (Respiratory Therapist)	

⇨ Pt tolerated BIPAP 4.5 hours on 18/10 85%. Requested to come off BIPAP around 1400. Placed on 60L/min at 100% at 1407. PT reports increased SOB. RR in 30s but anxious. Questions asked about plan of care and ventilator usage. Answered to best of this RT's ability. RT stated that pt did better on BIPAP
⇨ and required less oxygen. Pt stated the mask feels clastriphobic and does not wish to be placed back on it at this time. Pt requested to speak to DR on call (**Dr. Dead End**) and RT spoke with him via vocera

Electronically signed by ▮▮**Brutish**▮▮, RRT at 09/17/21 1823

Progress Notes by ▮**Dead End**▮, MD at 9/8/2021 1810

Author: ▮**Dead End**▮, MD	Service: Medicine	Author Type: Physician
Filed: 09/08/21 1828	Date of Service: 09/08/21 1810	Creation Time: 09/08/21 1810
Status: Addendum	Editor: ▮**Dead End**▮, MD (Physician)	

Skiba, Robert
MRN: 2000087384, DOB: ▮▮▮▮, Sex: M
Adm: 9/3/2021, D/C: 10/13/2021

Page 135

Printed by ▮▮▮▮ at 10/26/21 2:44 PM

Rob was subjected to **4.5 hours of BiPAP therapy** starting at around 9:30 AM on 9/8/21 that <u>forced</u> air into his lungs. This contraindicated therapy worsened his pneumomediastinum, making it even harder for him to breathe, as noted in "PT reports increased SOB [Shortness of Breath]." As stated on Page 97 of his hospital records (see Page C-21), Nurse Carnage noted that Rob is "not a candidate for bipap d/t (due to) pneumomediastinum." Thus, they knew better than to place Rob on a BiPAP that forces air into the lungs. The independent medical expert, Sammy Wong, MD (as noted in Appendix B), considered this injurious act one of the "Causes of Action" against the doctors and said, "It is conceivable that the '**claustrophobia**' was more likely feeling shortness of breath from the iatrogenic [worsened by medical treatment] pneumomediastinum."

Exhibit 38–Rob's Vital Signs Early to Mid-Afternoon of 9/8/21 (2:00 AM to 3:00 PM)

Flowsheets (group 10 of 32) (continued)

Row Name	09/08/21				0600
Temp	—				
Temp src	—				
Pulse	88				
BP	129/80				
BP Mean (MAP) (device)	99 MMHG			110 MMHG	
Shock Index	0.68			0.6	0.59
Resp	22		23	25	29
⇨ SpO2	92 %	(!) 88 %	95 %	94 %	93 %
Temp	—	—	98.4 °F (36.9 °C)	—	—
Temp src	—	—	Temporal Artery	—	—

> Rob was placed on a BiPAP from **around 9:30 AM (0930) to 2:00 PM (1400)**, which caused **barotrauma** (the rupturing of the alveoli)—leading to his SpO2 (blood oxygen level) dropping to 89% at 12:00 PM (1200). Once off the BiPAP at 2:00 PM (1400) he breathed more normally (22 respirations/min.), *yet the damage was already done.*

Row Name	09/08/21 0700	09/08/21 0800	09/08/21 0900	09/08/21 1000	09/08/21 1100
Pulse	80	83	87	78	82
BP	(!) 161/99	(!) 161/96	148/93	134/95	—
BP Mean (MAP) (device)	123 MMHG	123 MMHG	116 MMHG	111 MMHG	—
Shock Index	0.5	0.52	0.59	0.58	—
Resp	25	26	28	28	26
⇨ SpO2	95 %	91 %	92 %	94 %	92 %
Temp	—	98.7 °F (37.1 °C)	—	—	—
Temp src	—	Temporal Artery	—	—	—
Humalog	—	—	—	2 Units	—

Row Name	09/08/21 1200	09/08/21 1300	09/08/21 1400	09/08/21 1456	09/08/21 1500
Pulse	79	87	92	—	100
BP	121/75	155/94	159/100	—	148/100
BP Mean (MAP) (device)	92 MMHG	125 MMHG	124 MMHG	—	139 MMHG
Shock Index	0.65	0.56	0.58	—	0.68
Resp	(!) 33	28	22	—	27
⇨ SpO2	(!) 89 %	92 %	92 %	—	—
Temp	98.6 °F (37 °C)	—	—	—	—
Temp src	Temporal Artery	—	—	—	—
Humalog	—	—	—	—	—

> On Page 136 of the records (see Page C-37) Dr. Dead End alleges that Rob was "borderline" and "will need intubation" at 1400 (2:00 PM). Yet, Rob's respirations were only 22 (intubation criteria is generally > 30 breaths/minute) and his SpO2 (blood oxygen level) was at 92% (within the NIH's acceptable target range). Obviously, Dr. Dead End was dead set on getting Rob intubated no matter what.

Skiba, Robert
MRN: 2000087384, DOB: ▉▉▉, Sex: M
Adm: 9/3/2021, D/C: 10/13/2021

Printed by ▉▉▉ at 10/26/21 2:48 PM

Exhibit 39–Rob's Vital Signs Before and After Intubation (Afternoon & Evening of 9/8/21)

09/03/2021 - ED to Hosp-Admission (Discharged) in ██████			Intensive Care Unit (continued)	

Flowsheets (group 10 of 32) (continued)

INTUBATED

Row Name	09/08/21 1600	09/08/21 1700	09/08/21 1900	09/08/21 1930	09/08/21 2000
Pulse	(!) 108	100	93	96	86
BP	147/96	156/91	115/74	100/66	96/66
BP Mean (MAP) (device)	129 MMHG	133 MMHG	91 MMHG	79 MMHG	76 MMHG
Shock Index	0.73	0.64	0.81	0.96	0.9
Resp	(!) 34	(!) 36	24	23	26
SpO2	91 %	(!) 88 %	95 %	93 %	(!) 87 %
SPO2 Monitoring	—	—		—	Continuous central
Glasgow Coma Scale Best Eye Response	—			—	1 - (E1) none
Glasgow Coma Scale Best Verbal Response					1 - (V1) none
Glasgow Coma Scale Best Motor Response					4 - (M4) withdraws from pain
Glasgow Coma Scale Score					6
Pain Management Interventions					not indicated
RASS Score	—				-3 Moderate sedation, movement or eye opening. No eye contact

> As noted earlier, the BiPAP caused **barotrauma** and **likely forced more air between Rob's lungs**— making it nearly impossible for him to breathe adequately on his own. This gave the doctors **the excuse they had been waiting for** to force their sedation, intubation, and ventilation protocol on Rob at 6:43 PM (18:43). Once on the ventilator, Rob's blood oxygen level soon dropped to **below 90%** for a period of time.

Row Name	09/08/21 2015	09/08/21 2030	09/08/21 2045	09/08/21 2100	09/08/21 2115
Pulse	93	92	91	88	91
BP	90/63	90/60	94/62	94/63	(!) 89/65
BP Mean (MAP) (device)	72 MMHG	71 MMHG	72 MMHG	74 MMHG	73 MMHG
Shock Index	1.03	1.02	0.97	0.94	1.02
Resp	22	23	23	22	20
SpO2	(!) 88 %	(!) 88 %	(!) 88 %	(!) 87 %	(!) 89 %

Row Name	09/08/21 2130	09/08/21 2145	09/08/21 2200	09/08/21 2215	09/08/21 2221
Pulse	89	91	93	91	—
BP	92/62	91/60	90/59	90/53	—
BP Mean (MAP) (device)	72 MMHG	69 MMHG	70 MMHG	65 MMHG	—
Shock Index	0.97	1	1.03	1.01	—
Resp	24 -KC at 09/08/21 2205	25 -KC at 09/08/21 2205	24 -KC at 09/08/21 2205	19 -KC at 09/08/21 2234	—
SpO2	(!) 89 %	(!) 87 %	(!) 89 %	(!) 89 %	—
Humalog	—	—	—	—	2 Units

Skiba, Robert
MRN: 2000087384, DOB: ██████, Sex: M
Adm: 9/3/2021, D/C: 10/13/2021
Printed by ██████ at 10/26/21 2:48 PM

09/03/2021 - ED to Hosp-Admission (Discharged) in ███████████ Intensive Care Unit (continued)

Flowsheets (group 19 of 32) (continued)

		bedside sitting, hygiene;L Diversional activity	bedside sitting, hygiene;L		
ID Band Verification					—
Precautions					—
Device/Implant					—
Isolation Precautions		air pre mai			—
Cognitive/Perceptual/Neuro (WDL)		Exce Excep		Exception/WDL Except 09/08/21 2256	—
⇨ Ramsay Scale Score		2 - awake: patient cooperative, oriented and tranquil 09/08/21 1315	2 - awake: patient cooperative, oriented and tranquil 09/08/21 1748	—	—
⇨ Level of Consciousness		alert 09/08/21 1315	alert 09/08/21 1748	sedated 09/08/21 2256	—
⇨ Arousal Level		spontaneous / aware 09/08/21 1315	spontaneous / aware 09/08/21 1748	pain 09/08/21 2256	—
⇨ Orientation		oriented x 4 09/08/21 1315	oriented x 4 09/08/21 1748	Unable to evaluate (see comments) 09/08/21 2256	—
⇨ Speech		clear 09/08/21 1315	clear 09/08/21 1748	intubated 09/08/21 2256	—
Glasgow Coma Scale Best Eye Response		4 - (E4) spontaneous 09/08/21 1315	4 - (E4) spontaneous 09/08/21 1748	—	—
Glasgow Coma Scale Best Verbal Response		5 - (V5) oriented 09/08/21 1315	5 - (V5) oriented 09/08/21 1748	—	—
Glasgow Coma Scale Best Motor Response		6 - (M6) obeys commands 09/08/21 1315	6 - (M6) obeys commands 09/08/21 1748	—	—
Glasgow Coma Scale Score		15 09/08/21 1315	15 09/08/21 1748	—	—
Feature 1: Acute Onset or Fluctuating Course		—	—	09/08/21 2256	—
Hand Grip, Left		strong 09/08/21 1315	strong 09/08/21 1748	other (see comments) 09/08/21 2256	—
Hand Grip, Right		strong 09/08/21 1315	strong 09/08/21 1748	other (see comments) 09/08/21 2256	—
Dorsiflexion, Left		strong 09/08/21 1315	strong 09/08/21 1748	—	—
Dorsiflexion, Right		strong 09/08/21 1315	strong 09/08/21 1748	—	—

Sammy Wong, MD, our medical expert witness, noted in his **Interim Analysis** on Page B-2 of Appendix B (based on this page): "At 5:48 PM, the nurse noted that the patient was 'alert, awake, cooperative, oriented (x4) and tranquil' and that his 'speech was clear.'" However, less than 60 minutes later, at 6:43 PM, Rob was coerced into being sedated, intubated, and placed on a ventilator by Dr. Dead End soon after he had said (as noted on the next page) that Rob was only in "mild respiratory distress." Why, then, was Rob pressured to be intubated and placed on a ventilator?

Skiba, Robert
MRN: 2000087384, DOB: ████████, Sex: M
Adm: 9/3/2021, D/C: 10/13/2021
Printed by ██████████ at 10/26/21 2:48 PM

Exhibit 41–From Mild Respiratory Distress to Intubation & Ventilation (Afternoon of 9/8/21)

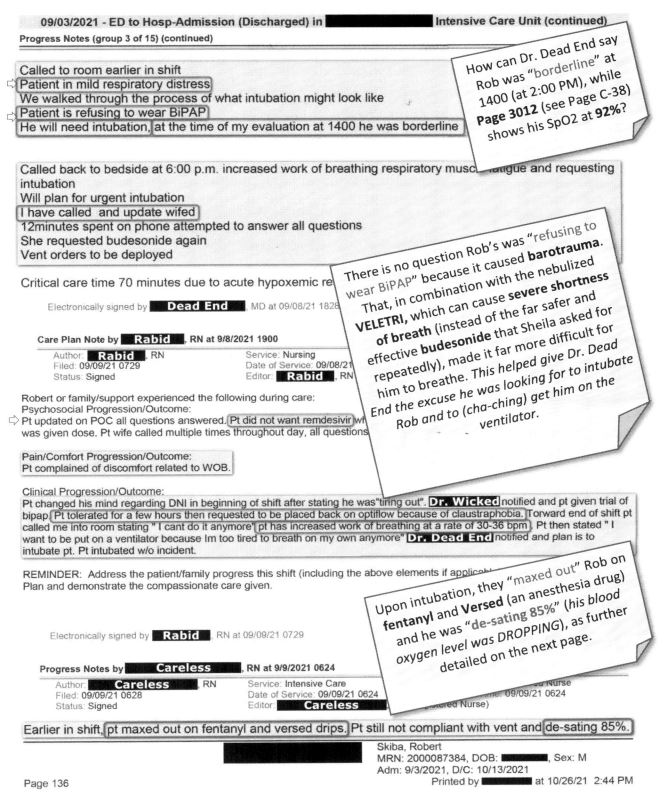

09/03/2021 - ED to Hosp-Admission (Discharged) in ███████████ **Intensive Care Unit (continued)**

Progress Notes (group 3 of 15) (continued)

Called to room earlier in shift
Patient in mild respiratory distress
We walked through the process of what intubation might look like
Patient is refusing to wear BiPAP
He will need intubation, at the time of my evaluation at 1400 he was borderline

> How can Dr. Dead End say Rob was "borderline" at 1400 (at 2:00 PM), while **Page 3012** (see Page C-38) shows his SpO2 at **92%**?

Called back to bedside at 6:00 p.m. increased work of breathing respiratory musc~~fatigue~~ and requesting intubation
Will plan for urgent intubation
I have called and update wifed
12minutes spent on phone attempted to answer all questions
She requested budesonide again
Vent orders to be deployed

Critical care time 70 minutes due to acute hypoxemic re~~

Electronically signed by ███ **Dead End** ███, MD at 09/08/21 1828

> There is no question Rob's was "refusing to wear BiPAP" because it caused **barotrauma**. That, in combination with the nebulized **VELETRI**, which can cause **severe shortness of breath** (instead of the far safer and effective **budesonide** that Sheila asked for repeatedly), made it far more difficult for him to breathe. This helped give Dr. Dead End the excuse he was looking for to intubate Rob and to (cha-ching) get him on the ventilator.

Care Plan Note by ███ **Rabid** ███, RN at 9/8/2021 1900

Author: ███ **Rabid** ███, RN	Service: Nursing
Filed: 09/09/21 0729	Date of Service: 09/08/21
Status: Signed	Editor: ███ **Rabid** ███, RN

Robert or family/support experienced the following during care:
Psychosocial Progression/Outcome:
Pt updated on POC all questions answered. Pt did not want remdesivir w~~ was given dose. Pt wife called multiple times throughout day, all questions

Pain/Comfort Progression/Outcome:
Pt complained of discomfort related to WOB.

Clinical Progression/Outcome:
Pt changed his mind regarding DNI in beginning of shift after stating he was"tiring out". **Dr. Wicked** notified and pt given trial of bipap. Pt tolerated for a few hours then requested to be placed back on optiflow because of claustraphobia. Toward end of shift pt called me into room stating " I cant do it anymore" pt has increased work of breathing at a rate of 30-36 bpm. Pt then stated " I want to be put on a ventilator because Im too tired to breath on my own anymore" **Dr. Dead End** notified and plan is to intubate pt. Pt intubated w/o incident.

REMINDER: Address the patient/family progress this shift (including the above elements if applic~~
Plan and demonstrate the compassionate care given.

> Upon intubation, they "maxed out" Rob on fentanyl and **Versed** (an anesthesia drug) and he was "de-sating 85%" (his blood oxygen level was DROPPING), as further detailed on the next page.

Electronically signed by ███ **Rabid** ███, RN at 09/09/21 0729

Progress Notes by ████ **Careless** ████, RN at 9/9/2021 0624

Author: ███ **Careless** ███, RN	Service: Intensive Care
Filed: 09/09/21 0628	Date of Service: 09/09/21 0624
Status: Signed	Editor: ███ **Careless** ███

Earlier in shift, pt maxed out on fentanyl and versed drips. Pt still not compliant with vent and de-sating 85%.

Skiba, Robert
MRN: 2000087384, DOB: ███████, Sex: M
Adm: 9/3/2021, D/C: 10/13/2021

Exhibit 42–Blood Oxygen Level Drops to 81% After Intubation (Evening of 9/8/21)

Flowsheets (group 10 of 32) (continued)

Row Name	09/08/21 2230	09/08/21 2245	09/08/21 2300	09/08/21 2315	09/08/21 2330
Pulse	89	88	88	90	93
⇒ BP	(!) 88/58	(!) 89/59	96/70	103/64	96/62
Shock Index	1.01	0.99	0.92	0.87	0.97
Resp	22	24	25	29	24
⇒ SpO2	(!) 86 %	(!) 89 %	(!) 82 %	91 %	(!) 81 %
Temp	—	96.8 °F (36 °C)	—	—	—

Row Name	09/08/21 2345	09/09/21 0000	09/09/21 0015	09/09/21 0030	09/09/21 0045
Pulse	84	86	85	85	84
BP	98/65	95/62	95/61	99/62	97/60
BP Mean (MAP) (device)	76 MMHG	73 MMHG	73 MMHG	75 MMHG	74 MMHG
Shock Index	0.86	0.91	0.89	0.86	0.87
Resp	22	22	22	22	
⇒ SpO2	96 %	96 %	96 %		
SPO2 Monitoring	—				
Glasgow Coma Scale Best Eye Response					
Glasgow Coma Scale Best Verbal Response					
Glasgow Coma Scale Best Motor Response					
Glasgow Coma Scale Score					
Pain Management Interventions				—	—
RASS Score	—	-5 Unarousable, no response to voice or physical stimulation	—	—	—

Row Name	09/09/21 0100	09/09/21 0115	09/09/21 0130	09/09/2▮ ▮	09/09/21 0200
Weight	—	—	72.8 kg (160 lb ▮ ▮z)		—
Method of weight	—				—
Pulse	8▮				79
⇒					(!) 88/55
B					67 MMHG
S				0.84	0.9
Re			22	22	22
⇒ SpO		96 %	96 %	96 %	98 %

Rob was placed on the ventilator at 6:43 PM [18:43], yet less than 4 hours later (at 23:30 as noted above), he was **struggling with blood oxygen levels as low as 81%**. Thus, he was doing far better **PRIOR** to being intubated. It took over five hours, until 11:45 PM [23:45], to get Rob's blood oxygen level *above 90%* where it had generally been prior to being placed on a ventilator. As further evidence of the harm being done to Rob by being placed on a ventilator see the **SOFA Score Assessment** at the end of this appendix.

At **11:30 PM** on **9/9/21**, Rob's blood pressure dropped to **88/58** as he was going into **septic shock**. That caused them to add **Levophed**, a brand name norepinephrine bitartrate vasopressor used for patients in septic shock to increase systemic blood pressure and coronary artery blood flow, as noted in the "Okay to add levophed" note on the next page.

Skiba, Robert
MRN: 2000087384, DOB: ▮▮▮▮, Sex: M
Adm: 9/3/2021, D/C: 10/13/2021

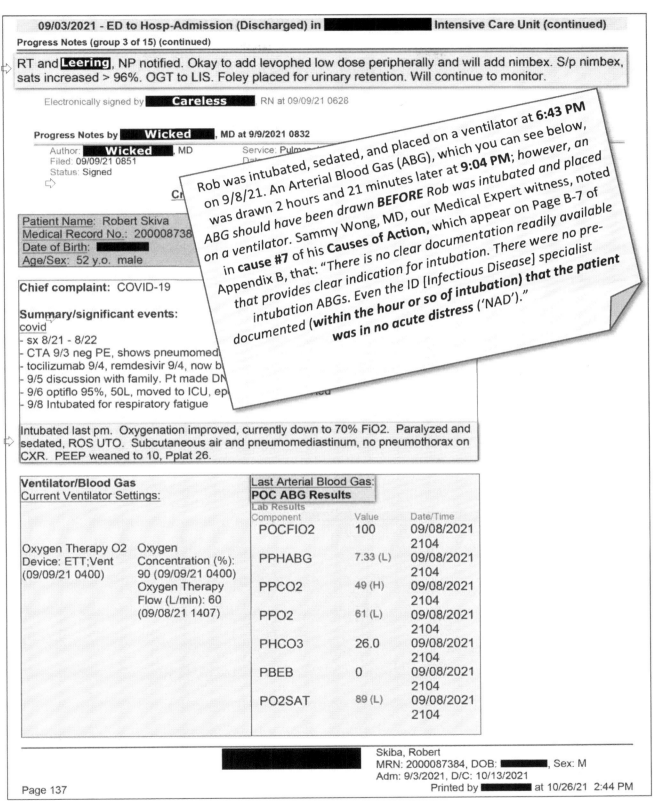

	09/03/2021 - ED to Hosp-Admission (Discharged) in ▮▮▮▮▮▮▮ Intensive Care Unit (continued)

Progress Notes (group 3 of 15) (continued)

RT and **Leering**, NP notified. Okay to add levophed low dose peripherally and will add nimbex. S/p nimbex, sats increased > 96%. OGT to LIS. Foley placed for urinary retention. Will continue to monitor.

Electronically signed by ▮▮▮ **Careless** ▮▮▮, RN at 09/09/21 0628

Progress Notes by ▮▮▮ **Wicked** ▮▮▮, MD at 9/9/2021 0832

Author: ▮▮▮ **Wicked** ▮▮▮, MD   Service: Pulmo▮▮
Filed: 09/09/21 0851   Da▮▮
Status: Signed

Cr▮▮

Patient Name: Robert Skiva
Medical Record No.: 200008738
Date of Birth: ▮▮▮▮▮▮
Age/Sex: 52 y.o. male

Chief complaint: COVID-19

Summary/significant events:
covid
- sx 8/21 - 8/22
- CTA 9/3 neg PE, shows pneumomed▮
- tocilizumab 9/4, remdesivir 9/4, now b▮
- 9/5 discussion with family. Pt made DN▮
- 9/6 optiflo 95%, 50L, moved to ICU, ep▮
- 9/8 Intubated for respiratory fatigue

Intubated last pm. Oxygenation improved, currently down to 70% FiO2. Paralyzed and sedated, ROS UTO. Subcutaneous air and pneumomediastinum, no pneumothorax on CXR. PEEP weaned to 10, Pplat 26.

Rob was intubated, sedated, and placed on a ventilator at **6:43 PM** on 9/8/21. An Arterial Blood Gas (ABG), which you can see below, was drawn 2 hours and 21 minutes later at **9:04 PM**; however, an ABG should have been drawn **BEFORE** Rob was intubated and placed on a ventilator. Sammy Wong, MD, our Medical Expert witness, noted in **cause #7** of his **Causes of Action**, which appear on Page B-7 of Appendix B, that: "There is no clear documentation readily available that provides clear indication for intubation. There were no pre-intubation ABGs. Even the ID [Infectious Disease] specialist documented **(within the hour or so of intubation) that the patient was in no acute distress ('NAD')."**

Ventilator/Blood Gas
Current Ventilator Settings:

Oxygen Therapy O2
Device: ETT;Vent
(09/09/21 0400)

Oxygen
Concentration (%):
90 (09/09/21 0400)
Oxygen Therapy
Flow (L/min): 60
(09/08/21 1407)

Last Arterial Blood Gas:
POC ABG Results

Lab Results Component	Value	Date/Time
POCFIO2	100	09/08/2021 2104
PPHABG	7.33 (L)	09/08/2021 2104
PPCO2	49 (H)	09/08/2021 2104
PPO2	61 (L)	09/08/2021 2104
PHCO3	26.0	09/08/2021 2104
PBEB	0	09/08/2021 2104
PO2SAT	89 (L)	09/08/2021 2104

▮▮▮▮▮   Skiba, Robert
MRN: 2000087384, DOB: ▮▮▮▮, Sex: M
Adm: 9/3/2021, D/C: 10/13/2021

Printed by ▮▮▮▮ at 10/26/21 2:44 PM

Exhibit 44–Admission BiPAP Caused Barotrauma (Morning of 9/9/21)

09/03/2021 - ED to Hosp-Admission (Discharged) in ████████ Intensive Care Unit (continued)

Progress Notes (group 3 of 15) (continued)

CO2	20.0	09/09/2021 0447	HCT	47.8	09/09/2021 0447
CL	109	09/09/2021 0447	PLT	233	09/0█
BUN	41 (H)	09/09/2021 0447			
CREAT	0.85				
GLU	150 (H)				
CA	8.5 (L)				
TPROT	5.2 (L)				
ALB	2.5 (L)				
ALKPHOS	117				
AST	67 (H)				
ALT	112.0 (H)				
TBILI	1.0				

As noted on Page 104 of the records (see Page C-27), on the morning of 9/7/21 Rob was given his **4th dose** of **remdesivir**, and that afternoon he had an elevated **BUN** (Blood Urea Nitrogen) of **26**, which indicated his kidneys were not working well. Rob then had his **5th dose** of Remdesivir on the morning of 9/8/21. By the morning of 9/9/21, his BUN had risen to **41** (more than double the normal range). At 6:43 PM on 9/8/21 (the moment Rob was fully sedated and intubated), Sheila's Medical Power of Attorney took full effect. Although they knew full well Sheila had consistently said, "NO" to Remdesivir—as noted below, Remdesivir was being **"restarted per ID [the Infectious Disease doctor]."** Despite Sheila's directives, at 9:45 AM on 9/9/21, Rob was given his **6th dose** of this toxic drug.

Imaging Studies
1. CXR personally reviewed

The "Repeat CXR [Chest X-ray] this afternoon to monitor barotrauma" note confirms that the 4.5 hours Rob was placed on the positive pressure BiPAP not only worsened his Pneumomediastinum but it also created **barotrauma**, a well-recognized and potentially life-threatening complication of mechanical ventilation where the alveoli (the air sacs of the lungs).

Impression and Plan
Problem List

Hospital Problems

* (Principal) Acute respiratory failur█
Pneumonia due to COVID-19 virus
Hyponatremia   Yes
Hyperglycemia   Yes
Prediabetes   Yes

1. Acute respiratory failure: Intubated. Repeat CXR this afternoon to monitor barotrauma. Lung protective strategy, current Pplat good at 26. Lower PEEP strategy given pneumomediastinum. Once FiO2 down to about 60% will try weaning off paralytics then epoprostenol.
2. COVID-19: restarted remdesivir per ID. S/p tocilizumab 1 dose, continue empiric abx, zinc, vit D. Appreciate Dr. Torten's assistance. Inflammatory markers continue to improve, wean steroids
3. Hyperglycemia 2/2 steroids: insulin sliding scale.
4. Starting tube feeds
5. GIB prophylaxis: pepcid
6. DVT prophylaxis: Chemical prophylaxis: LMWH

Skiba, Robert
MRN: 2000087384, DOB: ████████, Sex: M
Adm: 9/3/2021, D/C: 10/13/2021

Printed by ████ at 10/26/21 2:44 PM

Exhibit 45–Now Intubated Will Extend Remdesivir to 10 Days (Afternoon of 9/9/21)

09/03/2021 - ED to Hosp-Admission (Discharged) in ███████ Intensive Care Unit (continued)

Progress Notes (group 3 of 15) (continued)

Toxic Granulation	Present
Differential Type	Manual
Neutrophil #	16.68 (H)
Neutrophil %	97.0

RADIOLOGY: I have personally reviewed all available imaging studies

Assessment and Plan:

ACTIVE PROBLEMS:
Problem List
Hospital Problems

	POA
* (Principal) Acute respiratory failure with hypoxia (HCC)	Yes
Pneumonia due to COVID-19 virus	Yes
Hyponatremia	Yes
Hyperglycemia	Yes
Prediabetes	Yes
Acquired pneumomediastinum due to severe COVID19 pneumonia (HCC)	Yes
Noncompliance with medications	Yes

Overview Addendum 9/9/2021 10:16 AM by **Lament**, MD
⇨ Refused Remdesivir from 9/5 until 9/6

PLAN:

1. For his community-acquired pneumonia with cefepime and azithromycin are adequa Azithromycin will also provide anti-inflamma

Now he is intubated will get a sputum cult

2. Agree with current dose of Solu-Medrol 62.

3. Check vitamin-D levels and add vitamin-C, D...crease dose to a 1000 units daily

4. The patient meets criteria for use of Remdesi...plan a 5 day course unless gets intubated.

Remdesivir resumed yesterday after the patient agreed to get it
⇨ *Now that he is intubated will extend Remdesivir to 10 days*
Renal function is normal, LFTs are improving.

5. With his increased inflammatory markers and respiratory failure, the patient meets criteria for tocilizumab, which was given last night, *although his oxygen requirements are still very high, his inflammatory markers have improved.*

6. Recommend to decrease Lovenox to 40 mg every 12 hours moderate dose since he does not have any pulmonary embolus on his CT angiogram.

Torture, MD 9/9/2021 15:16

Electronically signed by **Torture**, MD at 09/09/21 1519

As you can see, they make special note of the fact that Rob "Refused Remdesivir from 9/5 until 9/6" as if that was a major cause of his decline and eventual intubation. They seem to almost gleefully state: "Now that he is intubated (that is, now that we finally succeeded) will extend Remdesivir to 10 days." Can you hear someone shouting, "Goal!"?

Skiba, Robert
MRN: 2000087384, DOB: ███, Sex: M
Adm: 9/3/2021, D/C: 10/13/2021

Printed by ███ at 10/26/21 2:44 PM

09/03/2021 - ED to Hosp-Admission (Discharged) in ▮▮▮▮▮ Intensive Care Unit (continued)

Progress Notes (group 3 of 15) (continued)

A/P:
  Acute respiratory failure with hypoxia (HCC)
DUE TO
  SEVERE Pneumonia due to COVID-19 virus
WITH
  Acquired pneumomediastinum due to severe COVID19 pneumonia (HCC)
COMPLICATED BY
  Noncompliance with medications
> Continue cefepime, azithromycin, flora Q, vitamin C, vitamin D, zinc, Solu-Medrol 40 mg q 12 hrs, Veletri at 8 ml/hr neb, remdesivir resumed 9/6 evening
> ID stopped colchicine and nitazoxanide and gave him Questran and Lomotil due to diarrhea.
> refused Remdesivir from 9/5-9/6, refused BiPAP, pt changed his mind on these issues and received Remdesivir 9/6 evening onwards until he got intubated for progressive respiratory failure 9/8 evening.
> Wife refused Remdesivir again, removed from MAR.
> Continue IV azithromycin as well as cefepime, trend inflammatory markers.
> greatly appreciate ID/ICU teams

Hyponatremia
> resolved. SIADH from the pneumon...

Hyperkalemia
> K 5.3, improved after insulin/glucose...

Hyperglycemia
FROM
  Prediabetes
> A1c of 5.8, continue LDSSI

Code Status: FULL

DVT prophylaxis: lovenox

COVID19 VACCINATION STATUS: Unvaccinated

DC Plan: intubated last night. Critically ill. Anticipate at least 5 more days in hospital

Anticipated Date of Discharge (retired): (not recorded)
Discharge Disposition: (not recorded)
Facility Name: (not recorded)

Surrogate decision maker:

Legal Next of Kin/Health Care Surrog...
Legal Next of Kin/Surrogate relation: ...
Legal Next Kin Phone Number: ▮▮▮

▮▮▮ Lament ▮▮▮, MD

Electronically signed by ▮▮ Lament ▮▮, ...

*Here Dr. Lament implies that Rob's condition was "COMPLICATED BY Noncompliance with medications." Really? The one drug Rob and Sheila refused was **remdesivir**, yet that drug was forced upon Rob without his consent. We contend <u>what complicated Rob's condition</u> was his starvation, the harmful drugs he was placed on, and the contraindicated BiPAP therapy. They apparently believed food and water were not at all essential to Rob's being able to heal, while remdesivir was absolutely essential.*

Here Dr. Lament says, "Anticipate at least 5 more days in hospital." Unfortunately, the damage had already been done to the point they were never able to get Rob off the ventilator <u>that they should never have placed him on</u>—and Rob spent another 33 days on the ventilator until they had damaged his lungs with high pressures and high oxygen levels to the point he could no longer survive.

Skiba, Robert
MRN: 2000087384, DOB: ▮▮▮▮, Sex: M
Adm: 9/3/2021, D/C: 10/13/2021
Printed by ▮▮▮▮ at 10/26/21 2:44 PM

Page 170 — Page 171

09/03/2021 - ED to Hosp-Admission (Discharged) in ██████████ **Intensive Care Unit (continued)**

Progress Notes (group 4 of 15) (continued)

Care Plan Note by ██Outlaw██, RN at 9/12/2021 0510

Author: ██Outlaw██, RN	Service: —	Author Type: Registered Nurse
Filed: 09/12/21 0801	Date of Service: 09/12/21 0510	Creation Time: 09/12/21 0757
Status: Signed	Editor: ██Outlaw██, RN (Registered Nurse)	

Robert or family/support experienced the following during care:
Psychosocial Progression/Outcome:
Sedated and paralyzed with Versed and Nimbex drips. GCS 3, TOF 2/4.

Pain/Comfort Progression/Outcome:

⇨ Fetanyl drip to address pain.

Clinical Progression/Outcome:
Tried weaning Fio2 as per RT, now down to 90%, saturating >95%. Titrated paralytics and sedation accordingly. Discontinued restraints. Observed airborne plus precautions at all times. VSS. Wife called for updates, answered all questions. Provided patient a conducive environment for rest.

REMINDER: Address the patient/family progress this shift (including the above elements if applicable) to individualize the Care Plan and demonstrate the compassionate care given.

Electronically signed by ██Outlaw██, RN at 09/12/21 0801

Progress Notes by ██Obliterate██, M

Author: ██Obliterate██, MD
Filed: 09/12/21 1217
Status: Signed

IM HOSPITALIST

Name (DOB):	Robert Skiba (██)
Account #:	
Admit date:	9/3/2021
Room:	C298/C29801

Date 9/12/2021

PCP: ██ **Jaded** ██

Chief Complaint / reason for visit: Follow up of
Chief Complaint
Patient presents with
• Covid Like Symptoms
  pt reports congestion, cough and shortness of breath x 2 weeks PTA. pt was 71% on room air at triage

Subjective:
⇨ Patient seen and observed through his ICU glass door
He is intubated and sedated

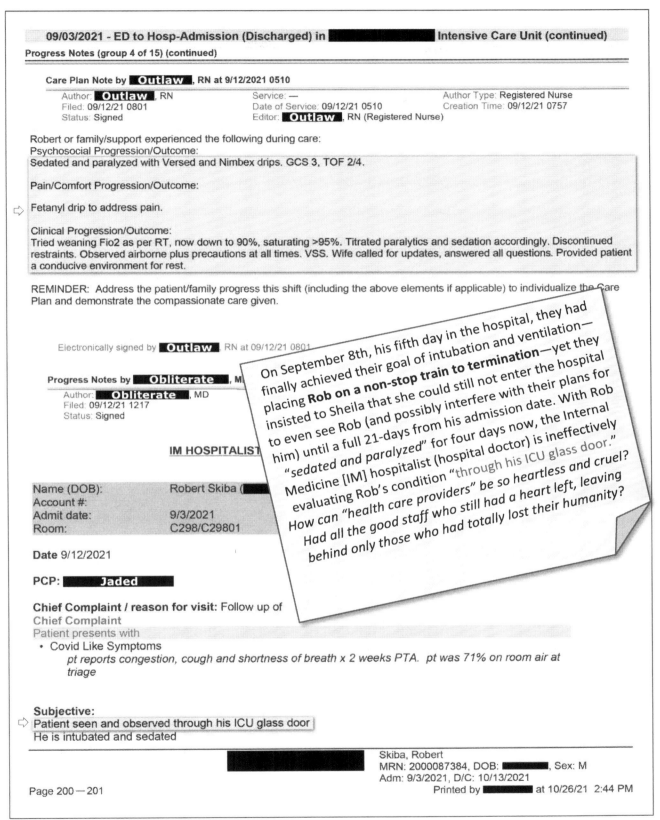

On September 8th, his fifth day in the hospital, they had finally achieved their goal of intubation and ventilation—yet they insisted to Sheila that she could still not enter the hospital placing **Rob on a non-stop train to termination**—yet they insisted to Sheila that she could still not enter the hospital to even see Rob (and possibly interfere with their plans for him) until a full 21-days from his admission date. With Rob "sedated and paralyzed" for four days now, the Internal Medicine [IM] hospitalist (hospital doctor) is ineffectively evaluating Rob's condition "through his ICU glass door." How can "health care providers" be so heartless and cruel? Had all the good staff who still had a heart left, leaving behind only those who had totally lost their humanity?

	Skiba, Robert
	MRN: 2000087384, DOB: ██████, Sex: M
	Adm: 9/3/2021, D/C: 10/13/2021
Page 200 — 201	Printed by ██████ at 10/26/21 2:44 PM

Exhibit 48–Did Not Tolerate Weaning Well, Had to Increase FiO2 to 100% (9/14/21)

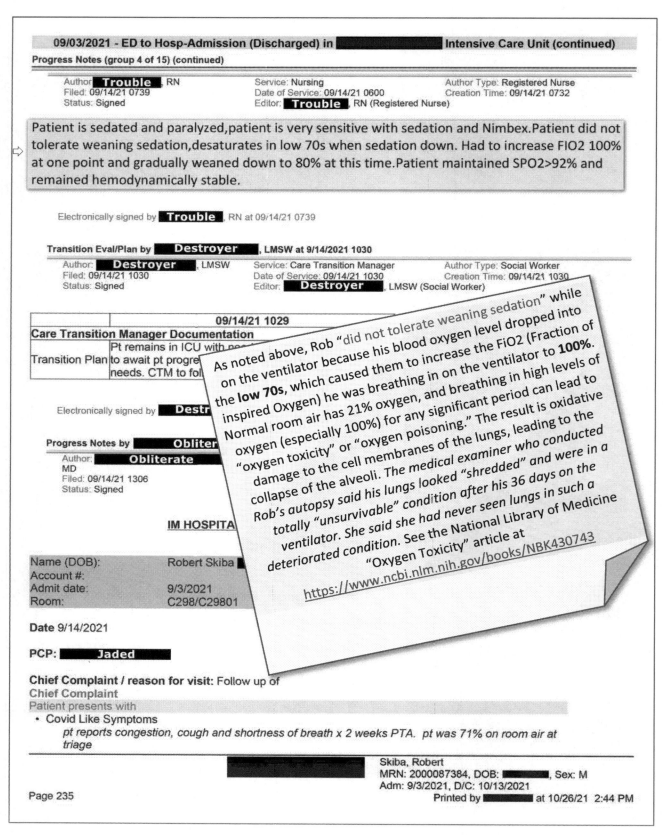

09/03/2021 - ED to Hosp-Admission (Discharged) in ▆▆▆▆▆ Intensive Care Unit (continued)

Progress Notes (group 4 of 15) (continued)

Author ▆**Trouble**▆, RN	Service: Nursing	Author Type: Registered Nurse
Filed: 09/14/21 0739	Date of Service: 09/14/21 0600	Creation Time: 09/14/21 0732
Status: Signed	Editor: ▆**Trouble**▆, RN (Registered Nurse)	

Patient is sedated and paralyzed,patient is very sensitive with sedation and Nimbex.Patient did not tolerate weaning sedation,desaturates in low 70s when sedation down. Had to increase FIO2 100% at one point and gradually weaned down to 80% at this time.Patient maintained SPO2>92% and remained hemodynamically stable.

Electronically signed by ▆**Trouble**▆, RN at 09/14/21 0739

Transition Eval/Plan by ▆**Destroyer**▆, LMSW at 9/14/2021 1030

Author: ▆**Destroyer**▆, LMSW	Service: Care Transition Manager	Author Type: Social Worker
Filed: 09/14/21 1030	Date of Service: 09/14/21 1030	Creation Time: 09/14/21 1030
Status: Signed	Editor: ▆**Destroyer**▆, LMSW (Social Worker)	

09/14/21 1029

Care Transition Manager Documentation	
Transition Plan	Pt remains in ICU with ▆▆▆ to await pt progre▆▆ needs. CTM to fol▆▆

Electronically signed by ▆**Destr**▆

Progress Notes by ▆▆▆ **Obliter**▆

Author: ▆ **Obliterate** ▆
MD
Filed: 09/14/21 1306
Status: Signed

IM HOSPITA▆

Name (DOB): Robert Skiba ▆
Account #:
Admit date: 9/3/2021
Room: C298/C29801

Date 9/14/2021

PCP: ▆ **Jaded** ▆

Chief Complaint / reason for visit: Follow up of
Chief Complaint
Patient presents with
- Covid Like Symptoms
  pt reports congestion, cough and shortness of breath x 2 weeks PTA. pt was 71% on room air at triage

Skiba, Robert
MRN: 2000087384, DOB: ▆▆▆, Sex: M
Adm: 9/3/2021, D/C: 10/13/2021
Printed by ▆▆▆ at 10/26/21 2:44 PM

Page 235

As noted above, Rob "did not tolerate weaning sedation" while on the ventilator because his blood oxygen level dropped into the **low 70s**, which caused them to increase the FiO2 (Fraction of inspired Oxygen) he was breathing in on the ventilator to **100%.** Normal room air has 21% oxygen, and breathing in high levels of oxygen (especially 100%) for any significant period can lead to "oxygen toxicity" or "oxygen poisoning." The result is oxidative damage to the cell membranes of the lungs, leading to the collapse of the alveoli. The medical examiner who conducted Rob's autopsy said his lungs looked "shredded" and were in a totally "unsurvivable" condition after his 36 days on the ventilator. She said she had never seen lungs in such a deteriorated condition. See the National Library of Medicine "Oxygen Toxicity" article at
https://www.ncbi.nlm.nih.gov/books/NBK430743

Exhibit 49–Liver Function Test Going Up—Likely Due to Medications (9/14/21)

Progress Notes (group 4 of 15) (continued)

⇨ *Renal function is normal, **LFTs going up now, likely related to medications.***

5. With his increased inflammatory markers and respiratory failure, the patient meets criteria for tocilizumab, which was givent, *although his oxygen requirements are still very high, his inflammatory markers have improved.*

6. Recommend to decrease Lovenox to 40 mg every 12 hours moderate dose since he does not have any pulmonary embolus on his CT angiogram.

7. Management of severe sepsis and respiratory failure per Critical Care Team.

9. Will give off-label Nitazoxanide and colchicine to target as anti-inflammatory and interference with ~~interferon~~ pathway.

Developed diarrhea, will discontinue colchicine and nitazoxanide

10. The patient is out of the window to ~~~ I will check COVID IgG and if it is negativ~~~

COVID IgG is positive, not a candidate.

Patient has been encouraged to self prone ~~~

Further recommendations will depend on his ~~~

Seen in the ICU

> With the massive amounts of powerful and harmful drugs Rob was being bombarded with (remdesivir, VELETRI, fentanyl, propofol, morphine, Tylenol, Nimbex, nitazoxanide, colchicine, etc.), it is no surprise that by 9/14/21 he was suffering from **liver damage**, which they admit in their "**LFTs [Liver Function Tests] going up now, likely related to medications**" statement. How is this atrocity considered "health care"?

███Torture███, MD 9/14/2021 15:54

Electronically signed by ███Torture███, MD at 09/14/21 1556

Care Plan Note by ███Trouble███, RN at 9/15/2021 0428

Author ███Trouble███, RN	Service: Nursing	Author Type: Registered Nurse
Filed: 09/15/21 0439	Date of Service: 09/15/21 0428	Creation Time: 09/15/21 0428
Status: Signed	Editor: ███Trouble███, RN (Registered Nurse)	

⇨ Patient is sedated and paralyzed,Patient desaturates at times.still needing nimbex,not tolerating weaning Nimbex.Patient is also on fentanyl drip ,versed,and on veletri @8ml/hr.

Electronically signed by ███Trouble███, RN at 09/15/21 0439

Progress Notes by ███Wicked███, MD at 9/15/2021 1127

Author: ███Wicked███, MD	Service: Pulmonology	Author Type: Physician
Filed: 09/15/21 1332	Date of Service: 09/15/21 1127	Creation Time: 09/15/21 1127
Status: Signed	Editor: ███Wicked███, MD (Physician)	

Critical Care Progress Note

Patient Name: Robert Skiva	Today's Date: 9/15/2021
Medical Record No.: 2000087384	Date of Admission: 9/3/2021
Date of Birth: ████	Location: C298/C29801

Skiba, Robert
MRN: 2000087384, DOB: ███████, Sex: M
Adm: 9/3/2021, D/C: 10/13/2021

Printed by ████████ at 10/26/21 2:44 PM

Exhibit 50–Drugs Damage Liver While Doctors Wait for 8X Upper Limit (Morning of 9/15/21)

09/03/2021 - ED to Hosp-Admission (Discharged) in ███████████ Intensive Care Unit (continued)

Progress Notes (group 4 of 15) (continued)

		0436	PT		13.4	09/03/2021
ALKPHOS	55	09/15/2021				1709
		0436	INR		1.02	09/03/2021
AST	90 (H)	09/15/2021				1709
		0436				
ALT	404.0 (H)	09/15/2021				
		0436				
TBILI	1.1	09/15/2021				
		0436				

Imaging Studies
1. CXR personally reviewed, overall █████

Impression and Plan
Problem List

Hospital Problems

* (Principal) Acute respiratory failure █████
Pneumonia due to COVID-19 virus ... Yes
Hyponatremia ... Yes
Hyperglycemia ... Yes
Prediabetes ... Yes
Acquired pneumomediastinum due to severe COVID19 pneumonia ... Yes
(HCC)
Noncompliance with medications ... Yes
    Overview Addendum 9/9/2021 10:16 AM by ██Lament██, MD
    Refused Remdesivir from 9/5 until 9/6

1. Acute respiratory failure: Intubated. CXR no pneumothorax. Continue lung protective strategy, current Pplat good at 31. Close monitoring given pneumomediastinum. FiO2 currently at 60%, continue try weaning off paralytics again once back to 60%. Plan to then wean epoprostenol and PEEP.
2. COVID-19: restarted remdesivir once patient agreed, d/w Mrs. Skiba 9/10 am, she declines further remdesivir given length of time since diagnosis and her concern for his renal function, d/c'd from MAR. S/p tocilizumab 1 dose, continue empiric abx, zinc, vit D, vit C. Appreciate Dr. ██Torture██ assistance. Inflammatory markers overall improved, weaning steroids
3. LFTs up. Monitor. Cefepime most likely culprit though not for sure, seems to be flattening, still under 8x upper limit normal.
4. Hyperglycemia 2/2 steroids: insulin sliding scale.
5. Continue tube feeds.
6. GIB prophylaxis: pepcid
7. DVT prophylaxis: Chemical prophylaxis: LMWH
8. D/w RN, RT
9. Updated Mrs. Skiba via phone

Extended Emergency Contact Information
Primary Emergency Contact: Sheila Skiba
Mobile Phone: ██████

██████████ , DOB: ██████ , Sex: M
██████ 9/3/2021, D/C: 10/13/2021

Printed by ██████ at 10/26/21 2:44 PM

They again note, "Noncompliance with medications." As noted on **Page C-45**, the one drug Rob and Sheila refused was **Remdesivir**, yet that drug was forced upon Rob without his consent. The "d/w Mrs. Skiba 9/10 am" means they "**discussed with**" Sheila. . . and then they **FINALLY** agreed to stop giving Rob this destructive drug.

Note #3 states, "LFTs up. Monitor. Cefepime [an antibiotic] most likely culprit.... still under 8x upper limit normal." They reiterate that the LFTs (Liver Function Tests) are up (which indicates inflammation or damage to cells in the liver), yet they are perfectly fine as long as they are <u>under 8x the upper limit normal</u>. Why wait for LFTs to be **8x normal**?

09/03/2021 - ED to Hosp-Admission (Discharged) in ████████████ Intensive Care Unit (continued)

Progress Notes (group 5 of 15)

Progress Notes by **Torture**, MD at 9/15/2021 1704

Author: **Torture**, MD	Service: Infectious Disease	Author Type: Physician
Filed: 09/15/21 1707	Date of Service: 09/15/21 1704	Creation Time: 09/15/21 1704
Status: Addendum	Editor: **Torture**, MD (Physician)	

INFECTIOUS DISEASES PROGRESS NOTE

Name:	Robert Skiba	Date:
MR#:	2000087384	DOB:
Room #:	C298/C29801	Age/Sex:
Admit Date:	9/3/2021	Admitting

Subjective:
Reason for Consult: COVID 19 infection complicated

Remains in the ICU

⇨ Sedated on propofol
Paralytics being tapered off

> Finally, on 9/15/21, the hospital recognized Sheila's Medical Power of Attorney, and in unquestionable frustration, Dr. Torture notes, "Remdesivir discontinued as per wife's wishes." That is a small consolation to a wife who has been shut out of the hospital and will remain shut out for a full 21 days from her husband's 9/3/21 date of admission.

⇨ **Due to increasing LFTs Tylenol discontinued, will also change cefepime to Zosyn since GPT increased to 404**

FiO2 down to 60% and remains there.
Subcutaneous emphysema stable
Ferritin down to 800 >> 733
LFTs increased but less than 10 times the upper limit of normal.

> Again, they note "increasing LFTs," which indicates further liver damage caused by needless and harmful medications.

⇨ Remdesivir discontinued as per wife's wishes

Diarrhea better after stopping colchicine and Nitazoxanide, ~~Lomotil.~~

COVID IgG positive
⇨ *Remdesivir day 5 (day 2 of current protocol, received 1 dose on the day of his admission)*
Not self proning
Unable to eat

Ferritin 4834 >> 3291 > 1977 > 1375 > 1397 >> 902 >>> 1890
Vitamin-D 74

Patient received a dose of tocilizumab on 09/04

> It is interesting that they note that a fully sedated and paralyzed patient is "Unable to eat."

Results for SKIBA, ROBERT (MRN 2000087384) as of 9/6/2021

	Ref. Range	9/4/2021 18:28
Legionella pneumophila Antigen, urine	Latest Ref Range: Negative	Negative
Pneumococcal Antigen	Latest Ref Range: Negative	Negative
Source, Pneumococc	Unknown	URINE

Skiba, Robert
MRN: 2000087384, DOB: ████████, Sex: M
Adm: 9/3/2021, D/C: 10/13/2021

Printed by ████████ at 10/26/21 2:44 PM

09/03/2021 - ED to Hosp-Admission (Discharged) in ███████████ Intensive Care Unit (continued)

Progress Notes (group 11 of 15) (continued)

⇨ Refused Remdesivir from 9/5 until 9/6

A/P:
Acute respiratory failure with hypoxia (HCC)
DUE TO
SEVERE Pneumonia due to COVID-19 virus
WITH
Acquired pneumomediastinum due to severe COVID19 pneumonia (HCC)
Septic shock-
> Continue zosyn, azithromycin, flora Q, vitamin C, vitamin D
⇨ Continue Solu-Medrol , remdesivir received x6 doses-refused to complete 10 doses
> ID stopped colchicine and nitazoxanide and gave him Questran and Lomotil due to diarrhea.
⇨ Remains on Baracitinib; veletri
> trend inflammatory markers.
> Appreciate ID/ICU teams
-off rotaprone
- new fevers; concern for super impose bacterial infection
- started on vanc and cefepime
NOW ON LEVOPHED AND LOW-DOSE DOPAMINE
Blood cultures concerning for Gram-negative ba[...]

Septic shock
Likely due to Gram-negative bacteremia
Remains on pressor support
Continue on cefepime

Klebsiella bacteremia
Patient on cefepime
Await culture results

⇨ **elevated LFTs**
Liver ultrasound Hepatic steatosis. 2
. Minimal pericholecystic edema of indeterminate etiology, the gallbladder is otherwise unremarkable in appearance
Was likely due to COVID

Candidemia
Continue on Mycamine

Hyponatremia
resolved. SIADH from the pneumonia

Hyperkalemia
improved after insulin/glucose
Monitor

Hyperglycemia
> A1c of 5.8, continue ISS

An ultrasound indicates Rob is now suffering from "**Hepatic steatosis,**" which may be due to iatrogenic hepatic injury (injury to the liver directly caused by the drugs being ordered by the doctors). They also noted that Rob received **a total of 6 doses of remdesivir** and that he "**refused to complete 10 doses**"—which went totally against their lethal protocol.

Skiba, Robert
MRN: 2000087384, DOB: ████████, Sex: M
Adm: 9/3/2021, D/C: 10/13/2021

Page 646

Printed by ████████ at 10/26/21 2:44 PM

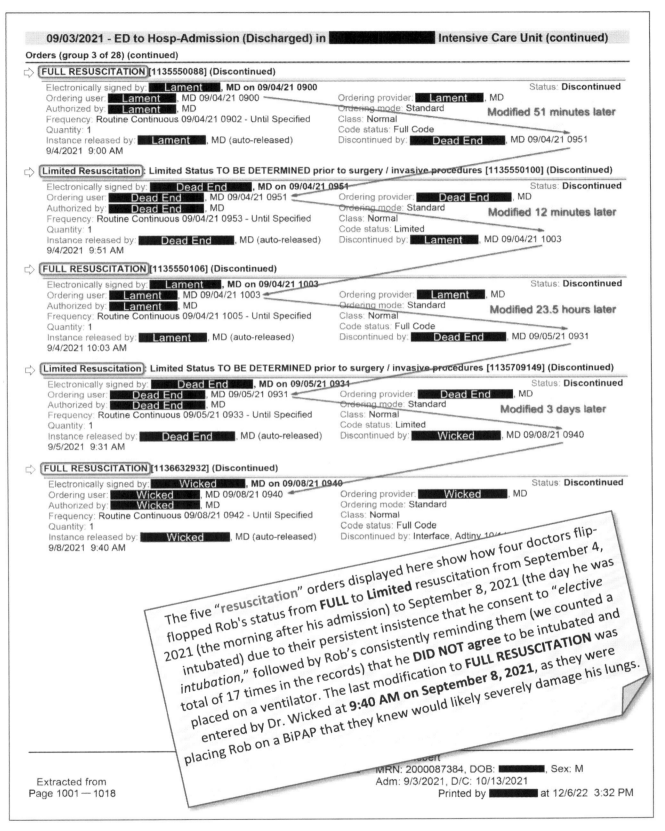

09/03/2021 - ED to Hosp-Admission (Discharged) in ▓▓▓▓▓▓▓▓ Intensive Care Unit (continued)

Orders (group 3 of 28) (continued)

FULL RESUSCITATION [1135550088] (Discontinued)

Electronically signed by: ▓ Lament ▓, **MD on 09/04/21 0900**   Status: **Discontinued**
Ordering user: ▓ Lament ▓, MD 09/04/21 0900   Ordering provider: ▓ Lament ▓, MD
Authorized by: ▓ Lament ▓, MD   Ordering mode: Standard   *Modified 51 minutes later*
Frequency: Routine Continuous 09/04/21 0902 - Until Specified   Class: Normal
Quantity: 1   Code status: Full Code
Instance released by: ▓ Lament ▓, MD (auto-released)   Discontinued by: ▓ Dead End ▓, MD 09/04/21 0951
9/4/2021 9:00 AM

Limited Resuscitation : Limited Status TO BE DETERMINED prior to surgery / invasive procedures [1135550100] (Discontinued)

Electronically signed by: ▓ Dead End ▓, **MD on 09/04/21 0951**   Status: **Discontinued**
Ordering user: ▓ Dead End ▓, MD 09/04/21 0951   Ordering provider: ▓ Dead End ▓, MD
Authorized by: ▓ Dead End ▓, MD   Ordering mode: Standard   *Modified 12 minutes later*
Frequency: Routine Continuous 09/04/21 0953 - Until Specified   Class: Normal
Quantity: 1   Code status: Limited
Instance released by: ▓ Dead End ▓, MD (auto-released)   Discontinued by: ▓ Lament ▓, MD 09/04/21 1003
9/4/2021 9:51 AM

FULL RESUSCITATION [1135550106] (Discontinued)

Electronically signed by: ▓ Lament ▓, **MD on 09/04/21 1003**   Status: **Discontinued**
Ordering user: ▓ Lament ▓, MD 09/04/21 1003   Ordering provider: ▓ Lament ▓, MD
Authorized by: ▓ Lament ▓, MD   Ordering mode: Standard   *Modified 23.5 hours later*
Frequency: Routine Continuous 09/04/21 1005 - Until Specified   Class: Normal
Quantity: 1   Code status: Full Code
Instance released by: ▓ Lament ▓, MD (auto-released)   Discontinued by: ▓ Dead End ▓, MD 09/05/21 0931
9/4/2021 10:03 AM

Limited Resuscitation : Limited Status TO BE DETERMINED prior to surgery / invasive procedures [1135709149] (Discontinued)

Electronically signed by: ▓ Dead End ▓, **MD on 09/05/21 0931**   Status: **Discontinued**
Ordering user: ▓ Dead End ▓, MD 09/05/21 0931   Ordering provider: ▓ Dead End ▓, MD
Authorized by: ▓ Dead End ▓, MD   Ordering mode: Standard   *Modified 3 days later*
Frequency: Routine Continuous 09/05/21 0933 - Until Specified   Class: Normal
Quantity: 1   Code status: Limited
Instance released by: ▓ Dead End ▓, MD (auto-released)   Discontinued by: ▓ Wicked ▓, MD 09/08/21 0940
9/5/2021 9:31 AM

FULL RESUSCITATION [1136632932] (Discontinued)

Electronically signed by: ▓ Wicked ▓, **MD on 09/08/21 0940**   Status: **Discontinued**
Ordering user: ▓ Wicked ▓, MD 09/08/21 0940   Ordering provider: ▓ Wicked ▓, MD
Authorized by: ▓ Wicked ▓, MD   Ordering mode: Standard
Frequency: Routine Continuous 09/08/21 0942 - Until Specified   Class: Normal
Quantity: 1   Code status: Full Code
Instance released by: ▓ Wicked ▓, MD (auto-released)   Discontinued by: Interface, Adtiny ▓▓
9/8/2021 9:40 AM

The five "resuscitation" orders displayed here show how four doctors flip-flopped Rob's status from **FULL** to **Limited** resuscitation from September 4, 2021 (the morning after his admission) to September 8, 2021 (the day he was intubated) due to their persistent insistence that he consent to "*elective intubation*," followed by Rob's consistently reminding them (we counted a total of 17 times in the records) that he **DID NOT agree** to be intubated and placed on a ventilator. The last modification to **FULL RESUSCITATION** was entered by Dr. Wicked at **9:40 AM on September 8, 2021**, as they were placing Rob on a BiPAP that they knew would likely severely damage his lungs.

▓▓▓ ▓bert
MRN: 2000087384, DOB: ▓▓▓▓, Sex: M
Adm: 9/3/2021, D/C: 10/13/2021
Printed by ▓▓▓▓ at 12/6/22 3:32 PM

Extracted from
Page 1001 — 1018

Exhibit 54–Excessively High O2 Levels on Optiflow (High-Flow Nasal Cannula) and Ventilator

These charts show the **excessively high levels of oxygen** Rob was subjected to <u>before</u> and <u>after</u> being placed on a ventilator. *Levels **above 60% for over 24 hours** can create pulmonary toxicity, extensive damage to the alveoli, and **atelectasis** (where alveoli in a lung or a part of a lung deflate, causing a partially or completely collapsed lung), resulting in shortness of breath and painful breathing.* As noted on **Page 127** of the hospital records (see Page C-35 in this Appendix), Rob was diagnosed with **atelectasis** on September 8, 2021, the day he was placed on a ventilator. The **atelectasis** followed by **barotrauma** caused by 4.5 hours of BiPAP therapy (see Pages C-37 and C-38) resulted in Rob's ending up on a ventilator against his will.

Optiflow High-Flow Nasal Cannula Oxygen Concentration Settings (High & Low)

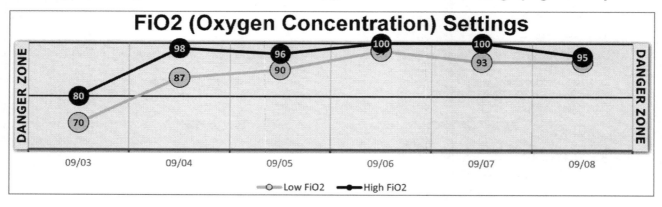

Ventilator Oxygen Concentration and PEEP Settings (High & Low)

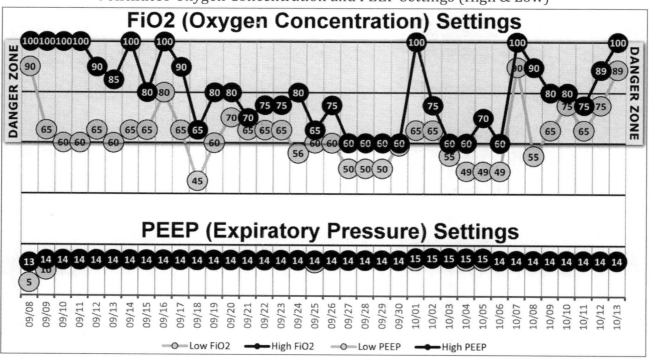

The assault of high concentrations of oxygen (above 60%) continued on the ventilator. This further damaged Rob's lungs to the extent that the medical examiner who conducted Rob's private autopsy said his lungs looked "shredded," were "unsurvivable," and did not look human. The continuously high PEEP (Positive End-Expiratory Pressure), pressure applied by the ventilator at the end of each breath (high = above 5 cm H_2O) placed added stress on Rob's fragile lungs. *Removing Rob from the ventilator required a PEEP setting of 8 cm H_2O or lower, yet they kept it at 14 to 15 cm H_2O for the entire 35 days Rob was on the ventilator.*

Exhibit 55–Weights Recorded in Hospital Records (9/3/21 to 10/13/21)

Below is a chart showing each of the daily weights recorded in Rob's hospital records. A massive daily change in weight indicates that their beds, especially the RotoProne bed, generally displayed inaccurate weights.

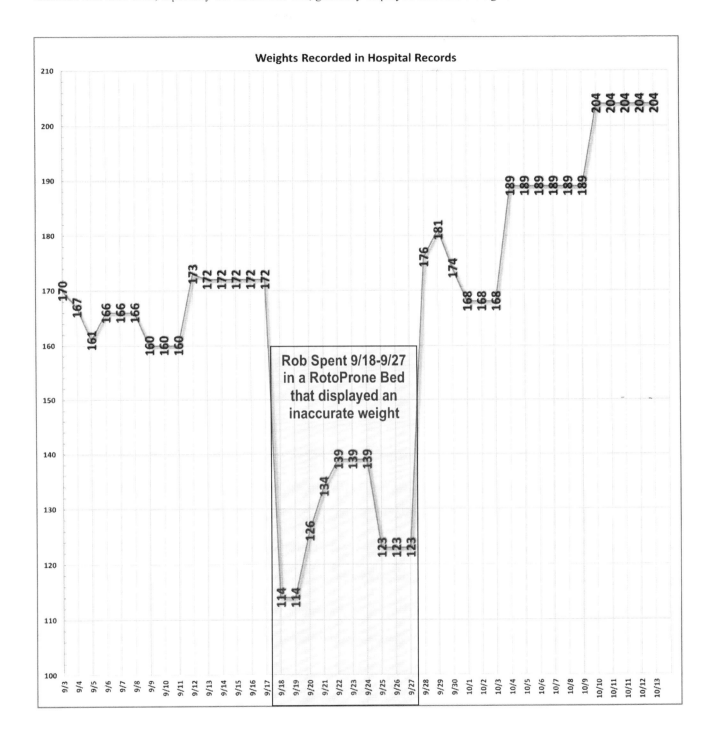

SOFA Score Assessment

Based on the Hospital Records, Pages 4584-4590

(NOTE: Pages 4584-4590 of the records are not included in the book as exhibits.)

The **SOFA** (Sequential Organ Failure Assessment) Score is used to track a patient's status and forecast the likelihood of mortality while in an ICU. It is based on calculations of both the number and the severity of organ dysfunctions in six organ systems: respiratory, cardiovascular, hepatic (liver), renal (kidneys) and neurological systems along with coagulation (blood clotting).

- Rob's post-admission SOFA Score **remained at a 4** (which equates to about a 7% mortality rate), yet it **jumped up to a 10** (a 40-50% mortality rate) the evening of 9/8/21 *right after he was intubated and placed on a ventilator.*

- Around 12 hours after intubation and ventilation **his SOFA Score peaked at 14** (a 50-60% mortality rate).

- His SOFA Score then settled down and remained **in the range of 7 to 9** (a 15-20% mortality rate) until 10/1/21 when it **popped up to 10 to 13** (a 40-60% mortality rate) for three days. Rob's SOFA Score then settled back down to the **7-9 range** (a 15-20% mortality rate) until 10/11/21.

- Then, on 10/11/21 something obviously changed, as his SOFA Score **jumped up to 15** (which equates to a greater than 80% mortality rate). The Score then continued to climb (never falling below 15) until 10/13/21, they day Rob died, when it **reached 19** (a greater than 90% mortality rate).

Postulation

- **Considering his early score of only 4** (which is about a 7% mortality rate) **followed by a massive rise up to 10** (a 40-50% mortality rate) <u>the very evening he was intubated</u> it is apparent that *Rob's likelihood of survival **vastly decreased** the moment he was intubated and placed on a ventilator.*

- **Something significant must have occurred/changed on 10/11/21** that caused Rob's SOFA Score—a Score that for over 30 days (other than a 3-day period from 10/1 to 10/4) had been in the 7-9 range (an only 15-20% mortality rate)—to **jump up to 15** (a greater than 80% mortality rate) after which it **continued to climb up to 19** (a greater than 90% mortality rate) on 10/13/21.

Appendix D – Hospitals' Incentive Payments for COVID-19

NOVEMBER 17, 2021
Hospitals' Incentive Payments for COVID-19

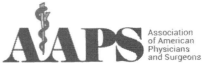

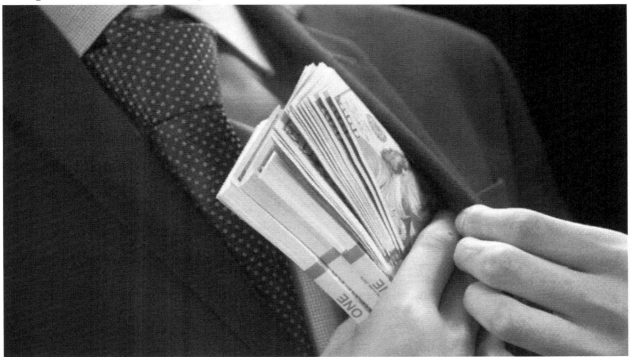

By Elizabeth Lee Vliet, M.D. and Ali Shultz, J.D.

Source: https://aapsonline.org/bidens-bounty-on-your-life-hospitals-incentive-payments-for-covid-19

Upon admission to a once-trusted hospital, American patients with COVID-19 become virtual prisoners, subjected to a rigid treatment protocol with roots in Ezekiel Emanuel's "Complete Lives System" for rationing medical care in those over age 50. They have a shockingly high mortality rate. How and why is this happening, and what can be done about it?

As exposed in audio recordings, hospital executives in Arizona admitted meeting several times a week to *lower* standards of care, with coordinated restrictions on visitation rights. Most COVID-19 patients' families are deliberately kept in the dark about what is really being done to their loved ones.

The combination that enables this tragic and avoidable loss of hundreds of thousands of lives includes (1) The CARES Act, which provides hospitals with bonus incentive payments for all things related to COVID-19 (testing, diagnosing, admitting to hospital, use of remdesivir and ventilators, reporting COVID-19 deaths, and vaccinations) and (2) waivers of customary and long-standing patient rights by the Centers for Medicare and Medicaid Services (CMS).

In 2020, the Texas Hospital Association submitted requests for waivers to CMS. According to Texas attorney Jerri Ward, *"CMS has granted 'waivers' of federal law regarding patient rights.*

Specifically, CMS purports to allow hospitals to <u>violate the rights of patients</u> or their surrogates about medical record access, to have patient visitation, and to be free from seclusion." She notes that *"rights do not come from the hospital or CMS and cannot be waived, as that is the antithesis of a 'right.' The purported waivers are meant to isolate and gain total control over the patient and to deny patient and patient's decision-maker the ability to exercise informed consent."*

Creating a "National Pandemic Emergency" provided justification for such sweeping actions that override individual physician medical decision-making and patients' rights. The CARES Act provides incentives for hospitals to use treatments dictated solely by the federal government under the auspices of the NIH. These "bounties" must be paid back if not "earned" by making the COVID-19 diagnosis and following the COVID-19 protocol.

The hospital payments include:
- A "free" *required* PCR test in the Emergency Room or upon admission for every patient, with government-paid fee to hospital.
- Added bonus payment for each positive COVID-19 diagnosis.
- Another bonus for a COVID-19 admission to the hospital.
- A 20 percent "boost" bonus payment from Medicare on the *entire hospital bill* for use of remdesivir instead of medicines such as Ivermectin.
- Another and larger bonus payment to the hospital if a COVID-19 patient is mechanically ventilated.
- More money to the hospital if cause of death is listed as COVID-19, even if patient did not die directly of COVID-19.
- A COVID-19 diagnosis also provides extra payments to coroners.

CMS implemented "value-based" payment programs that track data such as how many workers at a healthcare facility receive a COVID-19 vaccine. Now we see why many hospitals implemented COVID-19 vaccine mandates. They are paid more.

Outside hospitals, physician MIPS quality metrics link doctors' income to performance-based pay for treating patients with COVID-19 EUA drugs. Failure to report information to CMS can cost the physician 4% of reimbursement.

Because of obfuscation with medical coding and legal jargon, we cannot be certain of the actual amount each hospital receives per COVID-19 patient. But Attorney Thomas Renz and CMS whistleblowers have calculated a total payment of at least $100,000 per patient.

What does this mean for your health and safety as a patient in the hospital?

There are deaths from the government directed COVID treatments. For remdesivir, studies show that 71–75 percent of patients suffer an adverse effect, and the drug often had to be stopped after five to ten days because of these effects, such as kidney and liver damage, and death. Remdesivir trials during the 2018 West African Ebola outbreak had to be discontinued because *death rate exceeded 50%.* Yet, in 2020, Anthony Fauci directed that remdesivir was to be the drug hospitals use to treat COVID-19, even when the COVID clinical trials of remdesivir showed similar adverse effects.

In ventilated patients, the death toll is staggering. A National Library of Medicine January 2021 report of 69 studies involving more than 57,000 patients concluded that fatality rates were 45 percent in COVID-19 patients receiving invasive mechanical ventilation, increasing to 84 percent in older patients. Renz announced at a Truth for Health Foundation Press Conference that CMS data showed that in Texas hospitals, 84.9% percent of all patients died after more than 96 hours on a ventilator.

Then there are deaths from restrictions on effective treatments for hospitalized patients. Renz and a team of data analysts have estimated that more than 800,000 deaths in America's hospitals, in COVID-19 and other patients, have been caused by approaches restricting fluids, nutrition, antibiotics, effective antivirals, anti-inflammatories, and therapeutic doses of anti-coagulants.

We now see government-dictated medical care at its worst in our history since the federal government *mandated* these ineffective and dangerous treatments for COVID-19, and then *created financial incentives* for hospitals and doctors to use only those "approved" (and paid for) approaches.

Our formerly trusted medical community of hospitals and hospital-employed medical staff have effectively become "bounty hunters" for *your* life. Patients need to now take unprecedented steps to *avoid* going into the hospital for COVID-19.

Patients need to take active steps to plan before getting sick to use early home-based treatment of COVID-19 that can help you *save* your life.

Appendix E – Title 42 of the Code of Federal Regulations, Section 482.13

[**NOTE 1:** The **Centers for Medicare & Medicaid Services (CMS)**—which is referred to in the article above—has developed "Conditions of Participation" and "Conditions for Coverage" that all health care organizations must meet to begin and continue participating in the Medicare and Medicaid programs. The hospital Rob Skiba was admitted to was required to but did not comply with the following key regulations that are part of Title 42 of the Code of Federal Regulations which you can read at https://www.ecfr.gov/current/title-42]

PART 482 - CONDITIONS OF PARTICIPATION FOR HOSPITALS Section 482.13 - Condition of participation: Patient's rights of Title 42 of the Code of Federal Regulations clearly state the following (among other things).

[**NOTE 2:** The highlighted requirements are those we believe the hospital clearly violated (underlines are ours).]

(a) Standard: Notice of rights.
(1) A hospital must inform each patient, or when appropriate, the patient's representative (as allowed under State law), of the patient's rights, in advance of furnishing or discontinuing patient care whenever possible.
(2) The hospital must establish a process for prompt resolution of patient grievances and must inform each patient whom to contact to file a grievance.
(b) Standard: Exercise of rights.
(1) The patient has the right to participate in the development and implementation of his or her plan of care.
(2) The patient or his or her representative (as allowed under State law) has the right to make informed decisions regarding his or her care. The patient's rights include being informed of his or her health status, being involved in care planning and treatment, and being able to request or refuse treatment. This right must not be construed as a mechanism to demand the provision of treatment or services deemed medically unnecessary or inappropriate.
(3) The patient has the right to formulate advance directives and to have hospital staff and practitioners who provide care in the hospital comply with these directives.
(c) Standard: Privacy and safety.
(1) The patient has the right to personal privacy.
(2) The patient has the right to receive care in a safe setting.
(3) The patient has the right to be free from all forms of abuse or harassment.
(h) Standard: Patient visitation rights. A hospital must have written policies and procedures regarding the visitation rights of patients, including those setting forth any clinically necessary or reasonable restriction or limitation that the hospital may need to place on such rights and the reasons for the clinical restriction or limitation. A hospital must meet the following requirements:
(1) Inform each patient (or support person, where appropriate) of his or her visitation rights, including any clinical restriction or limitation on

such rights, when he or she is informed of his or her other rights under this section.

(2) Inform each patient (or support person, where appropriate) of the right, subject to his or her consent, to receive the visitors whom he or she designates, including, but not limited to, a spouse, a domestic partner (including a same-sex domestic partner), another family member, or a friend, and his or her right to withdraw or deny such consent at any time.

(3) Not restrict, limit, or otherwise deny visitation privileges on the basis of race, color, national origin, religion, sex, gender identity, sexual orientation, or disability.

(4) Ensure that all visitors enjoy full and equal visitation privileges consistent with patient preferences.

Appendix F – University of Oxford Study–Budesonide Reduces Covid-19 Recovery Time

FEBRUARY 9, 2021

Common asthma treatment reduces need for hospitalisation in COVID-19 patients, study suggests

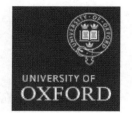

Early treatment with a medication commonly used to treat asthma appears to significantly reduce the need for urgent care and hospitalisation in people with COVID-19, researchers at the University of Oxford have found.

The STOIC study found that inhaled budesonide given to patients with COVID-19 within seven days of the onset of symptoms also reduced recovery time. Budesonide is a corticosteroid used in the long-term management of asthma and chronic obstructive pulmonary disease (COPD).

Findings from the phase 2 randomised study, which was supported by the NIHR Oxford Biomedical Research Centre (BRC), were published on the medRxiv pre-print server.

The findings from 146 people – of whom half took 800 micrograms of the medication twice a day and half were on usual care – suggests that inhaled budesonide reduced the relative risk of requiring urgent care or hospitalisation by 90% in the 28-day study period. Participants allocated the budesonide inhaler also had a quicker resolution of fever, symptoms, and fewer persistent symptoms after 28 days.

Professor Mona Bafadhel of the University's Nuffield Department of Medicine, who led the trial, said: 'There have been important breakthroughs in hospitalised COVID-19 patients, but equally important is treating early disease to prevent clinical deterioration and the need for urgent care and hospitalisation, especially to the billions of people worldwide who have limited access to hospital care.'

Common asthma treatment reduces need for hospitalisation in covid-19. University of Oxford. (n.d.). From https://www.ox.ac.uk/news/2021-02-09-common-asthma-treatment-reduces-need-hospitalisation-covid-19-patients-study

Appendix G – Questionable Drugs & Dosages Given Between 9/8/21 and 9/10/21

Drug Name	Amount Given	Date	Time	Ordered By
September 7, 2021				
epoprostenol (arginine) VELETRI 1 mg/50 mL	8 mL/hr	9/7/2021	4:30 AM	Dr. Dead End
labetalol solution	10 mg	9/7/2021	8:07 AM	Horrendous, NP
enoxaparin Lovenox syringe	80 mg	9/7/2021	8:08 AM	Dr. Dead End
nitazoxanide (Alinia) tablet	500 mg	9/7/2021	8:08 AM	Dr. Torture
remdesivir (Veklury) 100 mg	100 mg	9/7/2021	8:22 AM	Dr. Torture
epoprostenol (arginine) VELETRI 1 mg/50 mL	8 mL/hr	9/7/2021	10:35 AM	Dr. Dead End
labetalol solution	20 mg	9/7/2021	3:00 PM	Dr. Wicked
enalaprilat (Vasotec IV) solution	1.25 mg	9/7/2021	3:42 PM	Dr. Wicked
epoprostenol (arginine) VELETRI 1 mg/50 mL	8 mL/hr	9/7/2021	5:24 PM	Dr. Dead End
niCardipine (Cardene) drip infusion	2 mg/hr	9/7/2021	7:32 PM	Dr. Wicked
niCardipine (Cardene) drip infusion	3 mg/hr	9/7/2021	9:02 PM	Dr. Wicked
enoxaparin Lovenox syringe	80 mg	9/7/2021	9:06 PM	Dr. Dead End
nitazoxanide (Alinia) tablet	500 mg	9/7/2021	9:06 PM	Dr. Torture
niCardipine (Cardene) drip infusion	5 mg/hr	9/7/2021	10:10 PM	Dr. Wicked
epoprostenol (arginine) VELETRI 1 mg/50 mL	8 mL/hr	9/7/2021	11:26 PM	Dr. Dead End
September 8, 2021				
enoxaparin Lovenox syringe	80 mg	9/8/2021	8:33 AM	Dr. Dead End
remdesivir (Veklury) 100 mg	100 mg	9/8/2021	9:01 AM	Dr. Torture
epoprostenol (arginine) VELETRI 1 mg/50 mL	8 mL/hr	9/8/2021	5:01 AM	Dr. Dead End
nitazoxanide (Alinia) tablet	500 mg	9/8/2021	8:31 AM	Dr. Torture
epoprostenol (arginine) VELETRI 1 mg/50 mL	8 mL/hr	9/8/2021	9:25 AM	Dr. Dead End
epoprostenol (arginine) VELETRI 1 mg/50 mL	8 mL/hr	9/8/2021	5:14 PM	Dr. Dead End
ROB WAS INTUBATED AT 6:43 PM				
midazolam / Versed solution	5 mg	9/8/2021	6:43 PM	Dr. Dead End
succinylcholine (Anectine) solution	100 mg	9/8/2021	6:46 PM	Dr. Dead End
etomidate (Amidate) solution	20 mg	9/8/2021	6:46 PM	Dr. Dead End
midazolam in NS 1 mg/mL (Versed) solution	5 mg/hr	9/8/2021	6:52 PM	Dr. Wicked
fentanyl in NS PF drip infusion 10 mcg/mL	50 mcg/hr 5 mL/hr	9/8/2021	6:54 PM	Dr. Wicked
fentanyl in NS PF drip infusion 10 mcg/mL	75 mcg/hr 7.5 mL/hr	9/8/2021	7:07 PM	Dr. Wicked

midazolam in NS 1 mg/mL (Versed) solution	7.5 mg/hr	9/8/2021	7:07 PM	Dr. Wicked
fentanyl in NS PF drip infusion 10 mcg/mL	150 mcg/hr 15 mL/hr	9/8/2021	7:10 PM	Dr. Wicked
midazolam in NS 1 mg/mL (Versed) solution	10 mg/hr	9/8/2021	7:10 PM	Dr. Wicked
fentanyl in NS PF drip infusion 10 mcg/mL	175 mcg/hr 17.5 mL/hr	9/8/2021	7:40 PM	Dr. Wicked
fentanyl in NS PF drip infusion 10 mcg/mL	200 mcg/hr 20 mL/hr	9/8/2021	7:45 PM	Dr. Wicked
midazolam in NS 1 mg/mL (Versed) solution	12 mg/hr	9/8/2021	8:04 PM	Dr. Wicked
fentanyl in NS PF drip infusion 10 mcg/mL	225 mcg/hr 22.5 mL/hr	9/8/2021	8:07 PM	Dr. Wicked
enoxaparin Lovenox syringe	40 mg	9/8/2021	9:28 PM	Dr. Wicked
midazolam in NS 1 mg/mL (Versed) solution	12 mg/hr	9/8/2021	10:00 PM	Dr. Wicked
fentanyl in NS PF drip infusion 10 mcg/mL	250 mcg/hr 25 mL/hr	9/8/2021	10:12 PM	Dr. Wicked
norepinephrine (Levophed) drip infusion	0.01 mcg/kg/min 1.42 mL/hr	9/8/2021	10:12 PM	Rabid, NP
norepinephrine (Levophed) drip infusion	0.03 mcg/kg/min 4.25 mL/hr	9/8/2021	10:16 PM	Rabid, NP
fentanyl in NS PF drip infusion 10 mcg/mL	250 mcg/hr 25 mL/hr	9/8/2021	11:00 PM	Dr. Wicked
norepinephrine (Levophed) drip infusion	0.03 mcg/kg/min 4.25 mL/hr	9/8/2021	11:00 PM	Rabid, NP
epoprostenol (arginine) VELETRI 1 mg/50 mL	8 mL/hr	9/8/2021	11:14 PM	Dr. Dead End
cisatracurium / Nimbex drip infusion	3 mcg/kg/min 13.59 mL/hr	9/8/2021	11:30 PM	Rabid, NP
September 9, 2021				
cisatracurium / Nimbex drip infusion	3 mcg/kg/min 13.59 mL/hr	9/9/2021	12:00 AM	Rabid, NP
fentanyl in NS PF drip infusion 10 mcg/mL	250 mcg/hr 25 mL/hr	9/9/2021	12:00 AM	Dr. Wicked
midazolam in NS 1 mg/mL (Versed) solution	12 mg/hr	9/9/2021	12:00 AM	Dr. Wicked
norepinephrine (Levophed) drip infusion	0.03 mcg/kg/min 4.25 mL/hr	9/9/2021	12:00 AM	Rabid, NP
cisatracurium / Nimbex drip infusion	2.5 mcg/kg/min 11.33 mL/hr	9/9/2021	12:17 AM	Rabid, NP
midazolam in NS 1 mg/mL (Versed) solution	12 mg/hr	9/9/2021	12:17 AM	Dr. Wicked
cisatracurium / Nimbex drip infusion	2.5 mcg/kg/min 11.33 mL/hr	9/9/2021	1:00 AM	Rabid, NP
fentanyl in NS PF drip infusion 10 mcg/mL	250 mcg/hr 25 mL/hr	9/9/2021	1:00 AM	Dr. Wicked
midazolam in NS 1 mg/mL (Versed) solution	12 mg/hr	9/9/2021	1:00 AM	Dr. Wicked
norepinephrine (Levophed) drip infusion	0.03 mcg/kg/min 4.25 mL/hr	9/9/2021	1:00 AM	Rabid, NP

Medication	Rate/Dose	Date	Time	Provider
cisatracurium / Nimbex drip infusion	2.5 mcg/kg/min 11.33 mL/hr	9/9/2021	2:00 AM	Rabid, NP
fentanyl in NS PF drip infusion 10 mcg/mL	250 mcg/hr 25 mL/hr	9/9/2021	2:00 AM	Dr. Wicked
midazolam in NS 1 mg/mL (Versed) solution	12 mg/hr	9/9/2021	2:00 AM	Dr. Wicked
norepinephrine (Levophed) drip infusion	0.03 mcg/kg/min 4.25 mL/hr	9/9/2021	2:00 AM	Rabid, NP
cisatracurium / Nimbex drip infusion	2.5 mcg/kg/min 11.33 mL/hr	9/9/2021	3:00 AM	Rabid, NP
fentanyl in NS PF drip infusion 10 mcg/mL	250 mcg/hr 25 mL/hr	9/9/2021	3:00 AM	Dr. Wicked
midazolam in NS 1 mg/mL (Versed) solution	12 mg/hr	9/9/2021	3:00 AM	Dr. Wicked
norepinephrine (Levophed) drip infusion	0.03 mcg/kg/min 4.25 mL/hr	9/9/2021	3:00 AM	Rabid, NP
midazolam in NS 1 mg/mL (Versed) solution	12 mg/hr	9/9/2021	4:00 AM	Dr. Wicked
norepinephrine (Levophed) drip infusion	0.03 mcg/kg/min 4.25 mL/hr	9/9/2021	4:00 AM	Rabid, NP
cisatracurium / Nimbex drip infusion	2.5 mcg/kg/min 11.33 mL/hr	9/9/2021	4:00 AM	Rabid, NP
fentanyl in NS PF drip infusion 10 mcg/mL	250 mcg/hr 25 mL/hr	9/9/2021	4:00 AM	Dr. Wicked
fentanyl in NS PF drip infusion 10 mcg/mL	250 mcg/hr 25 mL/hr	9/9/2021	4:27 AM	Dr. Wicked
epoprostenol (arginine) VELETRI 1 mg/50 mL	8 mL/hr	9/9/2021	4:38 AM	Dr. Dead End
cisatracurium / Nimbex drip infusion	2.5 mcg/kg/min 11.33 mL/hr	9/9/2021	6:00 AM	Rabid, NP
fentanyl in NS PF drip infusion 10 mcg/mL	250 mcg/hr 25 mL/hr	9/9/2021	6:00 AM	Dr. Wicked
midazolam in NS 1 mg/mL (Versed) solution	12 mg/hr	9/9/2021	6:00 AM	Dr. Wicked
norepinephrine (Levophed) drip infusion	0.03 mcg/kg/min 4.25 mL/hr	9/9/2021	6:00 AM	Rabid, NP
norepinephrine (Levophed) drip infusion	0.04 mcg/kg/min 5.66 mL/hr	9/9/2021	7:52 AM	Rabid, NP
albumin 25% Solution	12.5g 100 mL/hr 30 min	9/9/2021	9:26 AM	Dr. Wicked
midazolam in NS 1 mg/mL (Versed) solution	12 mg/hr	9/9/2021	9:27 AM	Dr. Wicked
enoxaparin Lovenox syringe	40 mg	9/9/2021	9:28 AM	Dr. Wicked
fentanyl in NS PF drip infusion 10 mcg/mL	225 mcg/hr 22.5 mL/hr	9/9/2021	9:34 AM	Dr. Wicked
midazolam in NS 1 mg/mL (Versed) solution	11 mg/hr	9/9/2021	9:34 AM	Dr. Wicked
remdesivir (Veklury) 100 mg	100 mg	9/9/2021	9:46 AM	Dr. Torture
epoprostenol (arginine) VELETRI 1 mg/50 mL	8 mL/hr	9/9/2021	10:07 AM	Dr. Dead End
norepinephrine (Levophed) drip infusion	0.02 mcg/kg/min 2.83 mL/hr	9/9/2021	10:12 AM	Rabid, NP

fentanyl in NS PF drip infusion 10 mcg/mL	200 mcg/hr 20 mL/hr	9/9/2021	11:03 AM	Dr. Wicked
ketamine (Ketalar) sedation drip infusion	40 mcg/kg/min 41.33 mL/hr	9/9/2021	12:32 PM	Dr. Wicked
norepinephrine (Levophed) drip infusion	0.03 mcg/kg/min 4.25 mL/hr	9/9/2021	1:16 PM	Rabid, NP
albumin 25% Solution	12.5g 100 mL/hr 30 min	9/9/2021	1:17 PM	Dr. Wicked
midazolam in NS 1 mg/mL (Versed) solution	11 mg/hr	9/9/2021	1:39 PM	Dr. Wicked
norepinephrine (Levophed) drip infusion	0.02 mcg/kg/min 2.83 mL/hr	9/9/2021	2:04 PM	Rabid, NP
cisatracurium / Nimbex drip infusion	2.5 mcg/kg/min 11.33 mL/hr	9/9/2021	2:13 PM	Rabid, NP
epoprostenol (arginine) VELETRI 1 mg/50 mL	8 mL/hr	9/9/2021	3:55 PM	Dr. Dead End
norepinephrine (Levophed) drip infusion	0.01 mcg/kg/min 1.42 mL/hr	9/9/2021	4:17 PM	Rabid, NP
fentanyl in NS PF drip infusion 10 mcg/mL	175 mcg/hr 17.5 mL/hr	9/9/2021	4:19 PM	Dr. Wicked
albumin 25% Solution	12.5g 100 mL/hr 30 min	9/9/2021	7:37 PM	Dr. Wicked
enoxaparin Lovenox syringe	40 mg	9/9/2021	7:38 PM	Dr. Wicked
epoprostenol (arginine) VELETRI 1 mg/50 mL	8 mL/hr	9/9/2021	10:32 PM	Dr. Dead End
ketamine (Ketalar) sedation drip infusion	40 mcg/kg/min 41.33 mL/hr	9/9/2021	11:45 PM	Dr. Wicked
September 10, 2021				
albumin 25% Solution	25g 200 mL/hr 30 min	9/10/2021	12:03 AM	Dr. Wicked
epoprostenol (arginine) VELETRI 1 mg/50 mL	8 mL/hr	9/10/2021	4:57 AM	Dr. Dead End
midazolam in NS 1 mg/mL (Versed) solution	11 mg/hr	9/10/2021	4:58 AM	Dr. Wicked
albumin 25% Solution	12.5g 100 mL/hr 30 min	9/10/2021	4:59 AM	Dr. Wicked
albumin 25% Solution	12.5g 100 mL/hr 30 min	9/10/2021	7:30 AM	Dr. Wicked
enoxaparin Lovenox syringe	40 mg	9/10/2021	7:32 AM	Dr. Wicked
fentanyl in NS PF drip infusion 10 mcg/mL	150 mcg/hr 15 mL/hr	9/10/2021	8:54 AM	Dr. Wicked
epoprostenol (arginine) VELETRI 1 mg/50 mL	8 mL/hr	9/10/2021	11:11 AM	Dr. Dead End
furosemide (Lasix) Injection	20 mg	9/10/2021	12:04 PM	Dr. Wicked
ketamine (Ketalar) sedation drip infusion	40 mcg/kg/min 41.33 mL/hr	9/10/2021	2:50 PM	Dr. Wicked
midazolam in NS 1 mg/mL (Versed) solution	11 mg/hr	9/10/2021	2:55 PM	Dr. Wicked
albumin 25% Solution	25g 200 mL/hr 30 minutes	9/10/2021	5:26 PM	Dr. Wicked
epoprostenol (arginine) VELETRI 1 mg/50 mL	8 mL/hr	9/10/2021	5:39 PM	Dr. Dead End

cisatracurium / Nimbex drip infusion	2.5 mcg/kg/min 11.33 mL/hr	9/10/2021	6:06 PM	Rabid, NP
fentanyl in NS PF drip infusion 10 mcg/mL	150 mcg/hr 15 mL/hr	9/10/2021	6:06 PM	Dr. Wicked
midazolam in NS 1 mg/mL (Versed) solution	11 mg/hr	9/10/2021	6:06 PM	Dr. Wicked
enoxaparin Lovenox syringe	40 mg	9/10/2021	9:01 PM	Dr. Wicked
midazolam in NS 1 mg/mL (Versed) solution	11 mg/hr	9/10/2021	10:24 PM	Dr. Wicked
epoprostenol (arginine) VELETRI 1 mg/50 mL	8 mL/hr	9/10/2021	11:44 PM	Dr. Dead End

Appendix H - Darkness Exposed by a Respiratory Therapist

[Sheila's comments: *At the start of our conversation, the RT asked me what hospital Rob had died in. His demeanor slightly changed when I told him the hospital's name, but I did not initially know why. As you will read below, I later learned he was a close friend of one of Rob's primary physicians. Thus, he held back on being totally candid with me regarding the harm caused to Rob at Covid Coven Hospital of Plano, Texas.]*

Sheila: I'm trying to figure out exactly what happened to Rob and looking for closure. He died a year ago, and I've reviewed his hospital records. The first question I would like to ask you is, if somebody has something called pneumomediastinum, would they ever be put on a BiPAP? I'm asking because a nurse said he wasn't a candidate for it.

RT: It depends. *It's not the normal recommended thing—no, it's not.* But you got to understand that with COVID affecting their lungs and issues of this sort and breathing problems, you kind of get caught in what we call a Catch-22. Sometimes you have to do things you really are not particularly wanting to do. Sometimes you don't have a lot of choices.

[Sheila's comments: *In a war zone, in a field hospital, you may not "have a lot of choices" when trying to save a life with limited resources. However, in a modern American hospital, many choices are available. Thus, I put this comment on the back burner to think about later.]*

Sheila: "My husband and I vowed to each other NO vent and NO remdesivir. He knew the ventilator was a death sentence. I have X-rays and ventilation settings, and his vitals. I believe he was intubated against his will and certainly against my will because he had put in his chart DNI. (Do Not Intubate). I was locked out for 21 days, and they had already damaged him by the time I could get in there.

RT: *I want to apologize because the worst thing medicine ever did was lock the families out of the hospital. Not just you. But for him, too. Anytime you have oxygen greater than 60% for long periods of time, you can get what's called "nitrogen wash out" in the lungs to where it makes the lungs where they stick together, okay? There's a lubricant in the lungs all the time, and if this washes out, and of course, 100% O_2 for a long period of time will do it faster. And then, the lungs will have a tendency to stick together, and it makes it harder to ventilate them. And it makes it harder for them to breathe, as well.* Unfortunately, depending on what his oxygen levels were in his blood, you don't have a choice but to give him 100% O_2. I would have to see what his blood gas values were before intubation."

[Sheila's comments: *The high levels of oxygen Rob was subjected to while on the ventilator were making it even more difficult for them to wean him from the ventilator.]*

Sheila: Well, the doctors did not do a blood gas before intubating him, nor did they do any X-rays before intubation. They had over four hours available after he came off the BiPAP to do X-rays and an arterial blood gas, but they did not do them.

RT: I'll be honest with you; I mean, if you tell me something that I know is wrong, I'll tell you it's wrong.

Sheila: Okay, well, that's what I'm wanting. I want the brutal truth. So, here's a fact. Rob texted me early in his stay that there was *no food*.

RT: *Well, I don't really understand that unless they were giving him something IV-wise.* COVID was one of these things. And to be honest with you, I'm more than pissed off about COVID. We were lied to so much in the beginning. And things changed so much every day. *And so, it was mismanaged greatly in a lot of ways. But it was all coming from CDC and NIH.*

Sheila: Did anybody survive the ventilator?

RT: In the first six months of COVID, the majority of people that went on a ventilator passed away. *There was a problem with ventilation.* And with COVID, the lungs got hit so hard. And it's very difficult to try to ventilate someone; the stiffer the lungs got, the worse they became.

RT: *When you could get a patient in sync with the ventilator, and they're comfortable with it, and they were relaxed, and they worked with the machine, that would be a miracle.* However, sometimes people freak out because they feel like they're breathing through a small straw, and they panic. Then we have to start the whole process over again, adding a bunch of sedatives and paralytics. And you start fighting the machine, the machine can hurt you, okay, because the machine is gonna win that battle. And so, to avoid that, <u>sometimes</u> you have to paralyze the patients. I know that in COVID, there were a lot of people that were paralyzed, but we do our best.

*[**Sheila's comments:** He admitted they did not <u>always</u> have to paralyze a patient. So, now I wanted to know why Rob had to be paralyzed. I believe the reason was that he did not want to be on the ventilator in the first place, which led to him "fighting" the ventilator.]*

RT: But now, you're dealing with a serious illness. His lungs would have gotten that ground-glass look to them. The resulting Acute Respiratory Distress Syndrome (ARDS) creates horrible oxygenation issues. The lungs get very stiff, they get inflamed, and it causes a spiral where the patient is deteriorating. The trick is always trying to stop the decline because if you don't stop the decline, they die.

*[**Sheila's comments:** All of that may be true. However, Rob's doctor said he was improving, and I had spoken to Rob earlier in the day before he was placed on the ventilator. He also thought he was improving. But, then, the ventilator as the "only option" suddenly appeared.]*

RT: *Sometimes doctors get in too big of a hurry. Sometimes, you just need to leave the patient alone, just on that plateau. And I've always hated when they had that "one size fits all" approach where everybody gets X, Y, or Z when they are put on a ventilator. That's not the way it works.* I mean, everybody's different. And hopefully, you get the right settings that work for you.

Sheila: Is it normal for a doctor not to tell the spouse that he removed her husband's DNI (Do Not Intubate) order?

RT: *It's not normal. They should have told you.* But, I mean, I have actually had patients change their minds, and I've seen that myself, where someone didn't want to be intubated, and then they changed their mind and decided they did. But you do need to inform the families about these situations when they occur because the *family should be on the same page. And Rob had a DNI before, right? But they do need to be notified if it's removed, yes.*

Sheila: Rob acquired barotrauma after the BiPAP. What's with that?

RT: *If his lungs were sticking by this time, and his alveoli were not opening as they should, and the pressure built up and kind of tore the alveoli, then you could get some barotrauma from that.*

Sheila: Rob was reported to have felt claustrophobic with the BiPAP.

RT: Oh, well, when they're on a BiPAP, they put that mask on you. And some just don't do well with a mask. And they use soft restraints, which makes them feel claustrophobic. And then, depending on the skill of the therapist, and things of this sort, getting the flows adjusted right so they didn't feel like they are starving for air, which is another problem called air hunger. That's because they don't feel as if the air is coming to them fast enough, and then they start fighting and bucking everything. And the difference between being in an acidic state versus an alkaline state is that oxygen releases much easier in an alkaline state. Oxygen can get bound and doesn't release very well. But now you can have a critical acidosis where the acidic state is really, really bad. But I've never seen that kill anybody. But you do have to address alkalosis, on the other hand, for it will kill you.

Sheila: It seems like our medical system today has been hijacked.

RT: *We were hijacked, all right! And it's put a very bitter taste in a lot of people's mouths. And I know a lot of people that have just walked away and said they had had enough. What's happening now with the medical system is political.*

Sheila: Do you think that there is a difference between the treatment of vaccinated or unvaccinated patients?

RT: No, there wasn't a difference in treatment. *Because a lot of us,* **we** *didn't want the damn vaccination. Because you got to understand that's a lie too. It's not a vaccination, right?* But when I grew up and went to school, we had vaccinations. We had smallpox, polio, and all this stuff we took as kids. We never got any of those illnesses because that's what a vaccine does. Right? *This new thing? This was not a vaccine because it doesn't prevent you from getting COVID. It doesn't prevent you from spreading it. And I don't even know for sure what the hell it does. If you really want to know the truth. Well, the new vaccine kills you very quickly. We don't have any clue what the long-term effects you're gonna have. I took the vaccine back when I was working in the hospital because I still needed to work. But if I had not been working, there's no way in hell I would have taken it. To this day, I wouldn't have taken it because they don't know enough about it.*

Sheila: The doctor who insisted that he was put on a ventilator was Dr. Dead End. That was his name, but Dr. Wicked was the one who . . .

RT: Dr. Wicked?

Sheila: Yes, do you know him?

RT: Yes, he is a good friend.

Sheila: That's interesting. Oh, he's a good friend? Well, that's good to know.

*[**Sheila's comments:** From this point on, I knew he could not give me his unbiased opinion. However, I still hoped he could shed some light on what really happened to Rob.]*

RT: I worked with him during his "baby time" at another hospital. I'll never forget the day that I had to put him on a ventilator during a teaching session because the chief of service over there made all of the doctors experience the ventilator firsthand. What I would do to them is say, "Okay, give me the orders that you think you deserve or think you need. I'll give you the pressures and everything exactly the way you tell me, according to what you think." And I would look at them and let them do this, and then I would look at them and say, "Is this okay? How's the flow of oxygen coming now?" But Dr. Wicked is a really nice man.

Sheila: Dr. Wicked was the doctor who called me the day of intubation, saying Rob was getting better and all his lab tests were improving. Of course, all that good news came after he had already removed Rob's DNI without telling me. He already had a plan of action and a planned outcome, which makes me feel he had a quota to fill, as ventilators can't just sit vacant if they're being rented.

RT: I would trust what Dr. Wicked had to say.

Sheila: Dr. Wicked initially told me all Rob needed was rest, oxygen, time, and nutrition. So, at that time, I trusted him fully.

RT: I was wondering if Covid Coven Hospital in Plano, Texas, was where Dr. Wicked was working. Yes, I knew he was in Plano, but I wasn't exactly sure where he was working. Rob's first blood gas shows his pH is high. And that's an alkalotic state. So that's not good. I don't like alkalosis. Because what happens in the blood is oxygen is transferred through the body through the red blood cells. When you have an alkalotic state, what happens is oxygen is bound to the red hemoglobin, and it doesn't release. And so, if this were his first blood gas, then the first thing I would have done to him right away, I would purposely let his CO_2 come up, okay? *In other words, I would have underventilated him to allow his CO_2 to rise, which would have put him in a mild acidotic state because when you're acidotic, oxygen is released very easily.* You've got to understand that the brain controls everything. The one thing is oxygen; the body screams for oxygen, and there's not a single part of your body that doesn't need oxygen. And unfortunately, when you start decreasing the amount of oxygen the body has, the brain starts turning systems off. The first thing it does is it goes to the skin. Your skin starts getting blue, and if that's not enough, your gut is the next most important thing it starts turning off. And so, your bowels do not work like they should. Then it shuts down the kidneys. So it's one domino effect after the other when you have a severe oxygenation issue, and then you end up in a multi-system problem.

Sheila: But when he went into the hospital, they put him on Optiflow, which immediately increased his blood oxygen level to 98%.

RT: In the records, I see his PO_2 was 62. That's the oxygen level in the blood recorded on this blood gas, which is low but not too low.

Sheila: So when a person is put on a ventilator, all these oxygen numbers should improve, correct? But that's not what happened. *He was better off **before** they intubated him, and after that, he began to deteriorate. Why would they risk damaging his lungs by using the positive pressure of a BiPAP?*

RT: *My guess is they probably didn't adjust it [the BiPAP] right.*

Sheila: Rob had pneumomediastinum, and I was told he wasn't a candidate for the BiPAP. So I don't know why they would put him on it for 4.5 hours."

RT: *With the pneumomediastinum, you normally don't put anybody on a BiPAP with that positive pressure. You don't want that pressure, positive pressure; **it can make that worse**.* If Dr. Wicked was willing to do it, and if he was kind of stuck between a rock and a hard place knowing him the way I know him, we would have had a long discussion about it if I had been there.

Sheila: Rob was like a prisoner of war. They were treating him worse than a prisoner of war.

RT: I could tell you personally that many of them would reach out and grab my hand.

Sheila: Yeah, they drugged him and tortured him with threats of the ventilator and then forced it on him. *You wouldn't treat a dog like this.*

RT: *Oh, trust me, I agree. I actually made this comment one time. I said, "I could go out on the street, pick up stray dogs or cats, bring them into this building, and do what you make me do all day to the patients, and it wouldn't be allowed. It would be called inhumane, and I would be thrown into jail." Don't get me started. I cried with the patients many times.* I couldn't tell you how many funerals I've attended through the years. You try your best. You have to distance yourself to some degree from the patients, but there are always some patients who managed to get under my defensive mechanisms, and I got too emotionally involved in their lives. The biggest thing I'm looking for when it comes to the vent *is I want to see notes that the doctors wrote on the vent or BiPAP and then **blood gases**. Because that's how I determine whether they were doing what they were supposed to do even on the BiPAP. The hospitals always are short of respiratory therapists. It's been an ongoing problem, and it boiled down to hospitals being corporate and a money-mongering machine.* Respiratory therapists go into their jobs knowing they're not going to be able to get to everybody who needs them. *Some patients will fall through the cracks. And you spend your day putting out fires and praying nobody dies.*

Sheila: Why is the health care system ailing like this?

RT: *Basically, they don't care. Health care is no longer health care. For the past almost 20 years now, health care has been taken over by corporate America. It used to be that health care was run by healthcare people. It is not anymore. To them, you're nothing but a part moving down the assembly line. It is all about the almighty dollar.*

Sheila: Well, the thing is, if you try to do anything about it, you're going to get censored. You can't speak out publicly. My husband was censored two months before he was hospitalized and kicked off Facebook for what he said. My husband was a truth seeker and a truther. The truth must be told. We need to be on the offense and stand up for what's right and stop these hospital killings.

RT: As I look further at the records, here on September 8th, there are notes that his pneumomediastinum was getting better. That's a good thing.

Sheila: Right. Exactly. And then what happened? The protocol is what happened. Oh yeah, they also weren't feeding him. *Rob texted me that there was no food and no water.*

RT: They didn't have any tube feedings on him. I am surprised. He didn't have a feeding tube down his nose?

Sheila: Nope. I asked Dr. Wicked the morning of September 8th before Rob was placed on a ventilator. But he would not agree to TPN (Total Parenteral Nutrition), where nutrients and calories are provided via an IV, because he believed it presented too much of an infection risk. *He said he would consider putting in a nasogastric feeding tube first, yet he already had plans for*

If Rob had the strength to make a meal order, he was not strong enough to feed himself. Rob had already lost about 15 pounds by September 8th. My husband was tiring out due to a lack of nutrition and not having family by his side, yet Dr. Wicked said he thought he was just anxious.

RT: Here, we are in an acidotic state. They hypoventilated him. I'm not surprised because I know Dr. Wicked. That would have been the first thing I did. Dr. Wicked was the only one who could fix it. And I see his kidneys took a bit of a hit.

Sheila: Well, they gave him a drug called **remdesivir**, which is known to shut the kidneys down and cause acute kidney injury. We both refused it, but he still got a total of 800 mg with six doses against our will.

RT: Okay. Every single medication you take, even over-the-counter stuff, affects your kidneys and your liver—every single drug.

Sheila: My husband was like a boy scout. He never took a drug in his life. He was clean. He did not smoke or drink.

RT: Here, it says he requested the ventilator if needed.

Sheila: These are the hospital records. Who's to say my husband *really* said that? I have my husband's texts which say something totally different. I don't believe the hospital records. It's not true. *They had been trying to get him to be intubated and on a ventilator since day one. My husband texted, "If they intubate me, I'm dead." That's what he said. He also said, "They're trying everything they can to intubate me."* I can show you two pictures of the text messages. I told him to stay strong because they were using fear tactics. *He said, "I'm dead if they do," because he knew being on a ventilator would be a death sentence. My husband was in the military like you were, and he would rather have died at home than be put on a ventilator because he knew it was a one-way ticket to a miserable death.*

RT: *But see, that's the thing that irritates me about this. It wasn't necessary. Now in the very first initial days of early 2020 and February, and March, when the main cases first started hitting the hospital. Shit, they would not let us even touch them. We stood there and watched people die. They would not let us touch them. And we're looking at each other like, "What the hell is going on." I mean, we were all in total shock.* But it's our job to try to save people, yeah.

Sheila: So, the hospital became a morgue.

RT: *As a hospital employee, you are not programmed to see that.* You are programmed to help. I've worked around COVID, of course. I had those two "stupid shots" that I wished I never got. I did it to keep my job.

Sheila: Rob's records on September 8th said he was breathing at a rate of 36 breaths a minute. At the same time, a nurse noted in the records that he was "alert, awake, cooperative, oriented, and tranquil." *Would it be possible for someone breathing this rapidly, at 36 breaths per minute, to say anything?*

RT: *No. Not at all.*

Sheila: Well, isn't that interesting, because in his records, they quoted my husband to have been able to say the afternoon of September 8th, "*I want to be put on a ventilator because I'm too tired to breathe on my own anymore.*" That's a total of eighteen words and twenty-three syllables he was supposed to have been able to say while breathing in and out over twice per second. So he was either NOT breathing that rapidly and not in trouble, or he did NOT make that statement.

Do you have any other thoughts on VELETRI? I'm asking because the morning after his arrival, they put him on **VELETRI**. Have you heard of it? I've talked to other critical care doctors, and they are bewildered at the use of it for Covid. It was not part of the "standard protocol." It's typically used for pulmonary hypertension, which he did not have, and it's considered a "high-risk drug." So I don't know why they would give that to him. It wasn't a normal COVID drug.

*[**Sheila's comments:** Rob was assaulted with VELETRI from the morning after his admission to the ICU. Sammy Wong, MD, our medical expert witness, said using this medication subjected Rob to "unnecessary risks" and helped lead to his death.]*

RT: *The only thing I really know about it [VELETRI], and I've never used it, was a patient would have to be weaned from it very carefully and slowly because if you tried to take them off too fast, you could have this horrible rebound. And if you have a big swing in the pressure like that, I call it "scrambled eggs." The brain just goes "poof." So, you have to be really careful with that particular family of drugs when you're using it because it has to be weaned very slowly. It's not something you can just turn off.*

Sheila: But they **did** suddenly turn it off in Rob's case.

RT: They would have slowly turned it down, lowering the dosage slowly over the eight hours. And so, what they're doing is they're decreasing it, they're watching their blood pressure, and as long as they don't get a spike in blood pressure, they can turn it off once they get to a certain level. *But you won't take it from a max dose to off, right? Right, because if you do, their brain is going to scramble.*

*[**Sheila's comments:** His comment deeply disturbed me because Rob had received his first nebulized dose of VELETRI on September 4, 2021, at 3:25 AM. They then continued to administer this drug <u>every 6 hours</u> for a total of six doses until he was booted out of the ICU and sent to a regular hospital room by Dr. Dead end at 5:05 PM on September 5th because Rob refused to be placed on a ventilator. The drug was not restarted until <u>over 38 hours later</u> on September 6th at 11:35 PM when Rob was returned to the ICU. Thus, Dr. Dead End had abruptly withdrawn Rob from this risky drug, knowing doing so could cause him severe and irreparable harm.]*

Sheila: I hope this didn't happen to Rob's brain. My husband had never done any drugs. His body was clean until the hospital got ahold of him. Then, he was placed on fentanyl, Versed, ketamine, propofol, and more. I mean, how could a patient survive all this?

RT: I don't know. I'm not sure what to do. If they had to increase the sedations, that's telling me that he was fighting the ventilator more. *But when you fight against that machine, the machine is gonna win. And the problem is that it [fighting the ventilator] causes damage to the lungs.* If you take an average eight-year-old child, if I took their lungs out and started pulling them apart, I could carpet a tennis court. So, if you can get that much lung material from an eight-year-old, what do you think adults have? And all these little, tiny layers in all of these little, tiny air sacs, and you've got all the blood vessels wrapping around because the oxygen goes into these little air sacs, and it has to get out of the air sacs into the blood vessel. And if these air sacs are closed, if it's full of goop, oxygen cannot get in it to get into the bloodstream.

Sheila: What about the use of a surfactant? Could that have been beneficial?

RT: *I wanted the surfactant one time so bad I couldn't stand it.* They give it to babies. And they go, "If we gave you surfactant, and for this one patient, there would be no surfactant left in the information was a shock to me; I don't know if it is verifiable. *Once the nitrogen in the surfactant gets washed out of the lungs, you're in trouble.* This happens at a high FiO2 level. You have to be really, really careful not to allow the lungs to collapse; that's true because the minute the alveoli close, they stick to themselves. And that's where that PEEP comes in. That keeps the alveoli from closing. But if you take someone coughing really hard, yeah, they're gonna close off the alveoli because they cough the surfactant all out. And then they stick together, and then when they try to open up again, they tear, and then you get all the cytokine releases, you get all kinds of other mediators and things that break loose and create problems for you as well, and the shedding of that tissue begins. *That's probably why they paralyzed him because of the barotrauma. I can't promise that was what it was, but I'd be willing to bet.*

Sheila: The barotrauma was something Rob got **not** from coughing because his coughing had subsided according to several reports—one of them made by Dr. Wicked on the 7th of September, the day before the intubation. *The barotrauma happened due to the BiPAP because Dr. Wicked told me after he was intubated that all the doctors knew Rob had barotrauma before intubation. Why wasn't I told? Because they had purposely harmed him with the BiPAP to get the incentive money from being placed on the ventilator. Do you think there is a conflict of interest when the government gives incentive money to hospitals?*

RT: *There was a lot of conflict of interest where that was concerned.* Well, it's like the testing for Covid lines they had, for instance, right? I had a lady call me who wanted to know about how to get tested. And I told her, I said, you know, so all you got to do is call the hospital if you want to get tested, and they'll put you on the list, and you just drive down here, and they swab you, and you go on. Well, she just said, "Okay." So she went home, called, and signed up to be tested. But then she decided not to come in. *Three days later, she got a letter that she was positive for Covid, and she never went in for the test. This scenario happened a lot. The issue is that the truth will never come out. Because if it did, it would make a REVOLUTION. Oh, yeah. It would make January 6 look like a damn picnic.*

Sheila: Literally, it was a setup.

RT: *There would not be a sitting senator or congressman, or anybody in any federal building, that would not be jerked out on the street and thrown into the damn jail if the truth was really told. At some point in time, the American public needs to know. Because I'm sorry, they don't care anything about you, me, or anyone else!* They don't. Why is it we haven't cured the common cold, or anything else for that matter, with the billions and billions of dollars spent? They don't want to cure it. They wouldn't have a business anymore if they cured it. Because if you cure it, you don't have it anymore, right?

Sheila: Can you tell me any more about incentivized medicine?

RT: *The issue was it was $13,000 for every COVID-positive admission, $33,000 If they were intubated, and so forth. In fact, the hospitals were laying people off, okay? Full-time employees were being laid off because they were using contract people, right? Then, so they didn't have to pay the contract people <u>the government</u> paid them. So, they were getting free labor paid for by the government. Don't ask me why. I haven't a clue. Our tax-paying dollars at work.*

Sheila: Can you explain further how Rob's lungs got shredded? I am asking because I have proof that they were from his autopsy report.

RT: *The stiffness of the lungs and the fact that he was on such a high level of oxygen for so long made the surfactant and the nitrogen wash out. And him coughing as vigorously as he was and* *lowering the PEEP, causing his alveoli to collapse, and when they raise the PEEP again, then they're going to tear when they open back up. This will worsen barotrauma and increase inflammation. That's the shredding. Well, you're gonna have damage. That's what the pneumomediastinum was—damaged lungs.*

Sheila: Everyone else who looked at the same records voiced their findings differently. They believed the ventilator hastened his death.

RT: I believe Dr. Wicked did everything right.

Sheila: Yeah, a nurse on the 9th told me he had deteriorated significantly.

RT: Yeah, and I'm looking here on the 9th. And they had weaned back down to 70% FiO2 [oxygen concentration] at 11:48 AM, and then, they got down to 65% by 3:30. And then boom! At 8:00 PM, the oxygen concentration goes up to 85%, then back to 100%, and then stays at 100%.

Sheila: How long can you stay at 100% oxygen?

RT: As long as you have to.

Sheila: *Every time I called, he was on 100% oxygen. So, I started writing them down; according to their records, he was between 70% and 100% oxygen concentration, like, every day.*

RT: *And that's not an uncommon thing. Nor was killing patients uncommon, either.*

Sheila: Dr. Wicked told me a dog could live on 65% oxygen for a week, but we're talking about 35 days here on the ventilator cranked up to 100% a lot of the time.

RT: So, I'm sorry, I don't have a magic bullet.

Sheila: Can you tell me about the blood cultures they took? They came back negative, but they gave him tons of drugs for infections he didn't have.

RT: The blood cultures are outside my field of expertise. Well, strictly when I'm looking at vent settings, I haven't found anything wrong with the way Dr. Wicked was manipulating this vent up to this point. So on September 13th, he took a hell of a dive at 9:00 at night. His respiratory rate went all the way to 44. And his saturation [blood oxygen level] went in the 40s.

Sheila: Did his brain survive that one?

RT: Oh, well, he lost a few cells, I can tell you that.

Sheila: So, if he could have survived at that moment, what would his life have been like?

RT: The doctors were probably thinking, "What the HELL Just happened?" And some have a bad habit of doing a review of what took place during the night or the day, and they don't get a full report. Back on the 12th and the 13th, we're back down to 60% FiO2 again, right? That's better. And then, at midnight, it went back to 85% and then back to 100%

Sheila: Wouldn't that mean a night nurse was doing something weird?

RT: It does seem strange because, on the 13th and the 14th, he was back down to 60% FiO2 (oxygen concentration) on the 13th. Then at midnight, he tanked, and we're back at 100% oxygen. The same thing happened on the 14th.

Sheila: I think I figured it out; see, the night nurse was turning Rob all by himself, causing him trauma. And his vitals were showing it. And what did the nurse do after he injured Rob? He drugged him some more because he was taught to chase problems with drugs instead of avoiding them.

RT: So, when did they trach him?

Sheila: I discussed this with the doctor on September 27th, but he did not have a trach yet.

RT: Normally, we don't like to go more than 21 days with a tube down someone's throat without traching him."

Sheila: Rob had 35 days of an endotracheal tube down his raw and damaged throat.

RT: *Here, Look, I found three days where Rob was not fighting the ventilator, and it might have been possible to wean him. September 12-14.*

Sheila: Except for the night nurse who had been sabotaging Rob's chances by risking his wellbeing, turning him by himself, and "getting him all riled up." What about the fact that there was no arterial blood gas test before he was placed on the ventilator?

RT: Well, the thing I taught Dr. Wicked about blood gases was that he didn't need to take blood gases every two to three damn hours on these people, right? It's downright painful. And you don't need a blood gas every morning and every damn evening unless you're making a change, a big change, or you have an alteration in the patient's status.

Sheila: Why is it painful?

RT: It's sticking a needle into the artery, okay. In other words, wherever you can feel your pulse. On your arm or groin, in places where you can feel your pulse, right?

Sheila: And do they usually do an arterial blood gas before putting somebody on a ventilator?

RT: *Generally, you do it right before placing someone on a ventilator. **The blood gas readings are what determine the need.** It's why you're having to be intubated, because of the arterial blood gas deteriorating so badly. And then you'll do another blood gas once you've got them all situated on the ventilator after 30 minutes to an hour to see that your settings are appropriate for them. But some doctors were the world's worst about doing blood gases.*

Sheila: *Dr. Wicked did not take a blood gas just before intubating Rob, even though he told me that he would not intubate Rob unless he were 100% sure he would die without the ventilator. It seems to me that for a doctor to be 100% sure a patient would die without the ventilator, he would have to take a blood gas. And on top of that, he would have to let the wife in to see her husband if he thought the patient was in critical condition and might die without being placed on a ventilator. Neither a blood gas nor calling me to allow me to see Rob was done! Would you say trying to wean someone off drugs and get them safely off the ventilator is like jumping from a 120-mile-per-hour train?*

RT: *Yes. So, it is nearly impossible. Those who survive the ventilator are rare.* I got into this job because my wife died young, leaving me with two small children, and I needed a stable job. So, I became a respiratory therapist and strove to become the best in my field because I cared about my patients. I was told by a doctor friend, "If you find yourself in trouble, you don't want the smartest doctor. You want the one with the heart," because if you could get the doctor with the heart, they would keep digging for answers. They'll keep pushing until they get what needs to be done to save your life. ***The smart one might not give a shit.*** *That's true in every walk of life.*

I look at patients as this is someone's husband, wife, daughter, son, and parent. They're human beings, for God's sake. But you'd be amazed how many people just don't care.

Sheila: *I agree with you 100%. Some of Rob's doctors never went into his room to examine him but simply looked at him through the glass door. They then had the nerve to record things like, "patient has coarse breath sounds." How could a doctor hear breath sounds through the glass door?*

RT: *I am not surprised. Some doctors are just pulling a paycheck, and they just don't care. They're buying their time and gliding through Covid. Dr. Wicked is very good at only going to a ventilator when you have to. And back in the day, I asked him a question. One time, I said, when do you start thinking about extubating the patient? And he goes, well, it depends. And I said, <u>NO, you should think about that.</u> <u>You need to think about needing to put an end to it.</u> It makes sense that **before** you put them on a ventilator, you need to be thinking about how the hell am I gonna get them off?"*

Sheila*: I agree with you. That's what I've been asking. But you have to consider that they have incentives dangling in front of them. I was always asking, "What's your exit plan," or "What's your Discharge Plan," yet none of the doctors ever had one. That's the thing. When there's a conflict of interest, they just let the incentive money keep piling up. They get dollar signs in their eyes. The truth is that if you fail to plan, then you're planning to fail. In this case, they failed big time because my husband is now dead.*

RT: Were you ever able to ask your husband if he changed his DNI?

Sheila: No, because apparently Dr. Wicked never told Rob that he [the doctor] had removed it. Rob would have told me on the phone when we spoke that morning on September 8th if he had agreed to have the doctor remove it. Dr. Wicked had every opportunity to tell me he had removed it when I spoke with him that morning, right after I talked to Rob. This whole scenario was suspicious, and I smell a rat. Have you heard of any benefits of using budesonide?

RT: I don't know anything about it. I stay far away from stuff like that.

Sheila: Why?

RT: Well, it's just that you can fall into the trap of a quick fix with a pill or a shot, and it doesn't work. It lasts for a short period of time. I'm old school; I want something that's going to move it and keep it moving in the right direction. I'm looking through Rob's X-rays, and here on September 21st, there might have been a landmark—a point of no return for Rob.

Sheila: I asked Dr. Wicked on October 11th what the chances were of Rob surviving. His response was that if I had asked him a few days earlier, he would have given him a 50/50 chance. However, since the "we don't know what happened" <u>event day,</u> which was on October 9th, he believed Rob would not survive. At that point, my whole family should have been invited into the ICU to say our goodbyes. So, when did Dr. Wicked or Dr. Liar plan on telling me?

RT: So Dr. Wicked never told you anything about a specific event that changed Rob's chances of survival?

Sheila: I still don't know what he was referring to, and he claimed he did not know what happened.

RT: I see here on October 2nd, as I'm looking at his X-rays, that there was possibly another day that something terrible happened. I believe this was probably another possible point of no return. I'm sorry I wasn't much help to you. Dr. Wicked would have only gone to the ventilator if he had no choice. I know Dr. Wicked very well. He's a good man.

Sheila: So, do the doctors get incentive money at all?

RT: The doctors don't get a thing.

Sheila: So the incentives are all for the hospital, then. I felt Rob was discriminated against because he wasn't vaccinated. I don't know for sure, but UNVACCINATED was in his records in large bold, underlined letters. So, I want to know how many people in that hospital with COVID died that were not vaccinated versus how many people who died were vaccinated.

RT: I don't know. From my personal experience, I never saw any staff treat a patient differently, whether they had been vaccinated or not vaccinated.

Sheila: *A pharmacist friend told me his doctor friends at a different hospital in Dallas told him they didn't put anybody on the ventilator that had the vaccine. I have a problem with that. I was hoping there would be some public statistics that would say one way or the other.*

RT: *It's not that you probably can't get that data, but they're gonna make you jump through hoops to get it because they don't want that information made public. It's just like the heart problems that some, especially the young ones, have after taking COVID vaccines, right? They don't want the public to know.*

Sheila: I also want to know how many patients died on the ventilator at Covid Coven Hospital of Plano, Texas. Dr. Wicked told me that 45% died and 55% survived. I wonder where he got those numbers. So, there's nothing you could have or would have done differently?

RT: I don't see anything from a respiratory standpoint I would have done differently. *However, if I had a family member who was adamant and did <u>not</u> want their loved one on a vent, and I knew that the patient also did not want to be on a vent, then circumstances changed, and that patient told me differently, "I now want to be put on the vent," trust me I would have made damn sure when I charted that it stood out where God and everybody could see that he <u>really</u> wanted it. Everybody would be able to see it.*

Sheila: Isn't there a consent form a patient must sign to be placed on a ventilator?

RT: Actually, no. There's a consent form for all kinds of surgeries, but you don't have to sign a consent form to be put on the ventilator because so many times, you don't have anyone there to sign a consent form to put someone on the vent.

Sheila: That is a lame excuse. The DNI was taken off before the BiPAP, and there was plenty of time for Dr. Wicked to have Rob sign an "informed consent" form identifying that he was aware of the risks of the BiPAP before the damage of the BiPAP was done. The same is true of the ventilator. Besides, patients who might be considered progressively hypoxic, like they said my husband was right before he was intubated, might not understand what they're requesting or doing. A patient with no advocate could easily be persuaded to do something they would not usually agree to. The hospital and doctors had financial incentives that could fog their judgment if given a full reign of power. My husband never signed a consent form for the BiPAP or ventilator, nor did I.

RT: There were so many things that were going on at that time. They were short-staffed. The limited staff was getting so many things from the CDC and NIH. Literally, they tell you one thing in the morning, and two hours later, they just threw every damn thing they told you in the trash and would give you something else. Then by 1:00 PM, they would have done away with that and changed it again. We walked around like, "Okay, well, which damn way is it?"

[**Sheila's comments:** *Regardless, everyone has a conscience which, if ignored, makes it easy to become an accomplice in a criminal act. I say, "Be present. Pay attention. Take note of what is really going on. If you are NOT willing to say NO to senseless guidelines or harmful actions being taken by others, you are then, by default, saying YES, it is okay. You cannot just stand there and watch people die, as standing by and doing nothing makes you complicit, and you might as well have pulled the trigger yourself.*]

RT: *All of us were doing everything we could to* **avoid** *putting someone on the ventilator. That was the last thing we wanted.* We were pulling out the high flows [high flow nasal cannula oxygen like Rob was initially on]. God only knows how much money we spent on high flows because that's not something we normally keep. We would usually keep two or three, but we then used 100 a day and sometimes 200 or 300. So we were, you know, renting equipment like crazy. And initially, we didn't even use BiPAP because we were afraid of spreading COVID more because you don't have a sealed system. So initially, we wouldn't put anybody on the BiPAP. And then we got away from that because it was like, "the high flows not doing it, they've got to have some help," and because they were just fatigued. And so, then we started using the BiPAP. And even to this day, most of us are still hesitant to put them on a vent unless we have to. But luckily, recently, it hasn't been as severe, and most of them going in now are surviving it. *But in the early stages, it was bad. I mean, it was just that it was a madhouse everywhere, and we didn't have a hint of what we were doing because we couldn't get any straight answers from everybody. And all of us were going home just sick to death because we felt so useless.*

LEGAL COUNSEL STATEMENT

Members of the jury, even though the respiratory therapist was (and still is) a good friend of Dr. Wicked's, he shared some invaluable insights. Rather than interpret them, we have called out a few highlights for your review and consideration:

- Placing someone suffering from pneumomediastinum on a BiPAP is *"not the normal recommended thing"* because *"With the pneumomediastinum, you don't put anybody on a BiPAP with that positive pressure. You don't want that pressure, positive pressure; it can make that worse."*
- It *"would be a miracle"* to *"get a patient in sync with the ventilator."* Whenever patients ended up *"fighting"* the ventilator (as Rob did), they had to *"start the whole process over again, adding a bunch of sedatives and paralytics."* He also said, *"But when you fight against that machine, the machine is gonna win. And the problem is that it [fighting the ventilator] causes damage to the lungs."*
- Unfortunately, anyone who cannot get *"in sync with the ventilator"* ends up on a one-way trip to the morgue—which is what happened to Rob. *We contend that Rob should not have been placed on a ventilator and that conservative drugs and therapies could have saved his life.*
- With regards to placing patients on a ventilator, he said, *"Sometimes doctors get in too big of a hurry."* He also confirmed that he *"always hated when they had that 'one size fits all' approach where everybody gets X, Y, or Z when they are put on a ventilator. That's not the way it works."*
- When asked whether it was normal for Dr. Wicked to have **not** advised her that he had removed Rob's (Do Not Intubate) order the morning of September 8, 2021, he admitted, *"It's not normal. They should have told you."*
- He admitted the BiPAP could cause barotrauma, saying about Rob, *"If his lungs were sticking by this time, and his alveoli were not opening as they should, and the pressure built up and kind of tore the alveoli, then you could get some barotrauma from that."* He went on to say, *"My guess is they probably didn't adjust it [the BiPAP] right,"* and noted, *"That's probably why they paralyzed him because of the barotrauma. I can't promise that was what it was, but I'd be willing to bet."*
- When Sheila asked if Rob could have said the phrase, *"I want to be put on a ventilator because I'm too tired to breathe on my own anymore,"* as a nurse alleged in the hospital records while Rob was supposedly breathing at a rate of 36 breaths per minute (breathing in and out over two times per second) he confirmed, *"No. Not at all."*

H-13

- Regarding VELETRI, which Rob was abruptly withdrawn from upon being ejected from the ICU by Dr. Dead End (because Rob refused to agree to be intubated and placed on a ventilator), he confirmed a rapid withdrawal was hazardous to patients because "*their brain is going to scramble.*"
- Regarding Rob's being subjected to long periods of breathing in up to 100% oxygen, he said, "*And that's not an uncommon thing. Nor was killing patients uncommon, either.*" He also noted that subjecting patients to oxygen levels of greater than 60% can cause a rapid loss of the surfactant in the lungs, making it even harder for patients to breathe. *You can see the excessive levels of oxygen Rob was subjected to each day in the charts on Page C-54 in Appendix C.*
- When Sheila asked about the benefits of a surfactant, which Sheila had asked Dr. Liar for on September 23, 2021, but was denied, he said, "*I wanted the surfactant one time so bad I couldn't stand it.*" He then noted, "*The stiffness of the lungs and the fact that he was on such a high level of oxygen for so long made the surfactant and the nitrogen wash out. Once the nitrogen in the surfactant gets washed out of the lungs, you're in trouble.*"
- When Sheila noted that the Medical Examiner who did Rob's autopsy said his lungs appeared "*shredded*," he admitted the high PEEP and oxygen settings Rob was on "*will worsen barotrauma and increase inflammation. That's the shredding. Well, you're gonna have damage.*"
- When Sheila asked if an Arterial Blood Gas (ABG) should have been drawn BEFORE placing Rob on the ventilator to verify he urgently needed to be intubated, he noted, "*You do it right before placing someone on a ventilator, generally. The blood gas readings are what determine the need. It's why you're having to be intubated, because of the arterial blood gas deteriorating so badly.*"
- When asked whether attempting to get someone off all the drugs and safely weaning them from a ventilator was like jumping from a 120-mile-per-hour train, he admitted, "*Yes. So, it is nearly impossible. Those who survive the ventilator are rare.*"
- Regarding doctors sometimes not caring about their patients and not having a clear "exit strategy" or "discharge plan" for those on ventilators, he recalled a conversation he had with Dr. Wicked when he knew him in his early days, saying, "*One time, I said, 'When do you start thinking about extubating the patient?' Dr. Wicked said, 'Well, it depends.'* He admonished Dr. Wicked, "*'NO, you should think about that. You need to think about needing to put an end to it.' It makes sense that before you put them on a ventilator, you need to be thinking about how the hell am I gonna get them off?*"
- Finally, when Sheila asked him if the medical system had been hijacked, he said, "*We were hijacked, all right! And it's put a very bitter taste in a lot of people's mouths. And I know a lot of people that have just walked away and said they had had enough. What's happening now with the medical system is political.*" He also confirmed, "*I actually made this comment one time. I said, 'I could go out on the street, pick up stray dogs or cats, bring them into this building, and do what you make me do all day to the patients, and it wouldn't be allowed. It would be called inhumane, and I would be thrown into jail.' Don't get me started. I cried with the patients many times.*" He then said, "*Basically, they don't care. Health care is no longer health care. For the past almost 20 years now, health care has been taken over by corporate America. It used to be that health care was run by healthcare people. It is not anymore. To them, you're nothing but a part moving down the assembly line. It is all about the almighty dollar.*" He also noted, "*The issue was it was $13,000 for every COVID-positive admission, $33,000 if they were intubated, and so forth.*"

Thus, although he did not wish to disparage the decisions his friend, Dr. Wicked, made, he clearly admitted that there were cases of gross negligence, willful misconduct, and conscious indifference that led to needless injuries and deaths—and confirmed that the medical establishment had been hijacked by an incentivized protocol that was causing needless deaths.

Erich Fromm said, "*Greed is a bottomless pit which exhausts the person in an endless effort to satisfy the need without ever reaching satisfaction.*"

When specific pharmaceuticals and therapies become incentivized, hospitals and the physicians who practice there become predatory, and patients become their prey. The word of God says, "*The **love** of money is the root of all evil.*" Andrew Weil said, "*Fear and greed are potent motivators.*" Unfortunately, when fear, greed, and financial incentives are combined, they form a powerful force that can lead to unspeakable evils.

Appendix I – Falsification of Hospital Consent Forms

Transcript of Dec 22, 2022, Meeting at Covid Coven Hospital

Sheila: My husband was hospitalized last year [in 2021] from September 3rd through October 13th. A year later, while going through his medical records, I came across consent forms that he *supposedly* signed, yet *that's not a signature*. So, I want you to look at these because where it says "Witness," it says "Admission Specialist," followed by your name. Each of these forms [some of which were rather lengthy and would have taken time to read] was "signed" within a minute of each other, which I find rather strange. Your name was listed as the witness on each of these documents on September 7, 2021, and Rob was admitted on September 3rd.

Specialist: And so, these are not his signature?

*[**Sheila's comments:** When she saw the alleged "signatures" on the form, she knew the word she had written on the forms was in her handwriting. Even then, she innocently asked, "And so, these are not his signature?" while knowing it was not.]*

Sheila: He was admitted on September 3rd. These were all "*signed*" on September 7th within one minute of each other while he was coherent and calling us, and that is not his signature.

Jeremiah: I have pictures of his signatures I can show you. No, this is not his signature.

Sheila: Here's his driver's license. There's his signature right there.

Specialist: Are you Mrs. Skiba?

Sheila: Yes, I am Sheila. And the confusing part is that one of the forms says, "*If the person signing this form is not the patient, please give full name, phone number, and address.* Yet no name, phone number, or address was entered. Then, someone typed "*spouse*" in the "Relationship" field, and I wasn't here to sign it because I wasn't allowed into the hospital. I was forbidden to come in. So, on September 7, 2021, at 1:07 PM, it makes no sense for someone to type in "*spouse*" as the signing party because I was not even allowed in at that time. Since your name is here as the witness, do you remember this?

[Sheila's comments: At this point, the Admission Specialist's supervisor, who was listening in on our conversation in the background, stepped forward and interrupted.]

Supervisor: I am the supervisor. So, what I can do is I can go back and listen to an audio recording of that encounter to see what happened in this situation.

[Sheila's comments: As you will discover from the emails exchanged with the hospital below, they could not locate any recordings of a call with me.]

Sheila: Oh, I would love that.

Supervisor: So, he was here in the hospital on this day?

Sheila: Yes, he was, and all three "signatures" on these forms look the same. They were all "signed" within a minute of each other. I wasn't allowed in due to the hospital's 21-day isolation policy. My husband was calling and texting me on this day. I know for sure that's not *his* signature. We've had it forensically tested, and it is not his signature. Rob should have had something to sign like the Consent for Treatment form when he first got here.

Supervisor: Can I compare your signature here?

Sheila: It's on my driver's license, here.

Supervisor: Do you mind if I make a copy so we can compare these?

Sheila: Not at all.

Jeremiah: [Directing his question to the Specialist] Why would they put your name here? I'm just curious.

Specialist: Because I may have registered him

[Sheila's comments: She now suggests that the "signature" on the consent forms might be hers].

Sheila: They admitted him to ICU. And then they got mad at him because he wouldn't do what they wanted him to do [to agree to be intubated and placed on a ventilator]. So, they then put him on the fifth floor two days later, on September 5th. And then they tricked him into going back down to ICU [to get nebulized VELETRI, which they told him he needed].

Specialist: Okay, so if I was working in admissions on that day, then this says "*Verbal.*"

[Sheila's comments: Apparently, she recognizes her handwriting. With her name typed on the form as the witness (which we have redacted, as shown on Page C-26 in Appendix C), she was undoubtedly "working in admissions on that day."]

Sheila: So how does that work?

Supervisor: So, that would mean I would have to find a recording of it [since it was a "verbal" vs. written/signed consent].

Sheila: Okay. And can I get a copy of that recording as a witness?

Supervisor: I'm gonna have to listen to it. Do you have time to wait so I can investigate?

Sheila: Yes, sure. That is what we are trying to uncover.

Sheila: So, I'm just curious. It says "Verbal" while my husband was calling me and texting me, yet why wouldn't you just have him sign it?

Supervisor: *Maybe he was incoherent.* Maybe there was a doctor in the room?

[Sheila's comments: On September 7, 2021, when Rob was fully conscious and coherent, even with my Medical Power of Attorney, I could not legally sign any "consents" for his treatment. My right to "consent" to treatments for Rob only became effective, by law, on the evening of September 8, 2021, after he was fully sedated and unconscious when they placed him on a ventilator against our will. Then again, if he were deemed incoherent on September 7, 2021, they would NOT have had the authority to remove his DNI (Do Not Intubate) order nor to place him on a ventilator without my permission. So, none of this made any sense.]

Sheila: I have the phone log between his phone and my phone. *He **was** coherent because we talked that day and the morning of September 8th.*

Supervisor: Sometimes there is a nurse in the room, or sometimes we have to call the patient if we can't get to him in person.

Sheila: Okay. And if he was incoherent, I had Medical Power of Attorney. They knew I had Medical Power of Attorney, so I would have had to have been notified *immediately* if he had become incoherent.

Supervisor: Okay, so yeah, let me do my investigation and see what I can find on my recordings.

Sheila: It's confusing to me because there were many drugs given to him that were trial drugs. When my dad had a heart attack at Disneyland, he was taken to the hospital. When they asked my son Jeremiah to sign the consent, he said, "I don't feel comfortable doing that." So they had to wake my dad up to sign the consent form. So in this hospital, if somebody is doing a procedure like a BiPAP, where there's a significant risk because he had pneumomediastinum, would he have to sign a consent for that?

Supervisor: Not that I'm aware of. But that is over my head. That is on the clinical end.

Sheila: Another reason why this is so important to me is that my husband was strong enough to put a DNI [Do Not Intubate] in his record in his chart on the 5th of September, okay? We talked for 15 minutes that night. Then, three days later, on September 8th, we spoke at 9:00 AM, yet later that day, they intubated him, and I wasn't told they had removed his DNI.

Supervisor: So, we're . . . well, the question is, in what documentation does it say do not intubate?

Sheila: Oh, it was in the hospital records. On September 5th, he had them document the DNI. It's all over if you look at the first 100 pages. It's in there 17 times, okay. But he had them put it in his records because they kept coming to his room and harassing him about being intubated. And he said No. I'm just gonna put it in my records so they leave me alone.

Supervisor: Yeah. So there are multiple things that are going on in your situation. We are just the registration, okay? There's very little that I can do about that. What I can do is I will work on my investigation to figure out where these "signatures" [the "verbal" consent] came from.

Sheila: So, do you keep audio records? Do you always record if there's a witness to a verbal consent?

and try to find it. But what I'm going to do is, I'm going to go ahead and send you to our *patient advocate.* Since there are so many concerns, let me get her contact information because she's on campus now.

*[**Sheila's comments:** Sadly, over a year after Rob's death, I was NOW being told that they DO have people working at Covid Coven Hospital of Plano, Texas, who are supposed to serve as patient advocates. Why did the hospital administration not advise me they had patient advocates on staff when I asked to speak with an ombudsman on September 17, 2021? I explained that I was looking for someone who acted as a liaison between patients or their families and hospital staff to help resolve complaints and concerns. I was told that the hospital had **no one** in that role. Instead, they directed me to Risk Management, whose role was to protect the hospital from potential backlashes from patients or their families. Thus, five days later, I had to hire my own patient advocate.]*

Specialist: You're correct. There should be a name, a phone number, and an address on the form [since it was supposedly a "verbal" consent from someone]. *There is a whole procedure. And I missed out on that one. Sorry.*

Sheila: That is your handwriting?

Specialist: Yes

Sheila: This IS your handwriting. Oh, you recognize it?

Supervisor: Yeah.

*[**Sheila's comments:** The Administration Specialist and her supervisor finally admitted that the "signature" (or the handwritten word "Verbal") on the consent forms was written by the Specialist. Clearly, she had not followed the hospital's documented procedures for obtaining verbal consent. In addition, I knew she had not spoken with me. Furthermore, since she wrote in "spouse" as the party giving the consent, it was apparent she had NOT spoken with Rob. Thus, it appeared (unless they could find a recording of a conversation with one of us to the contrary—which they did not— the "consent" had been fraudulently fabricated.]*

Sheila: Oh, well, that's good to know.

Specialist: First, I was, like, thinking it says "*V*" something. But . . then . . . when she said . . . I was because . . . I cover multiple departments [stuttering as she realized she might now be in serious trouble].

Sheila: So, what? Would you have had to be in the room with my husband to get *his* verbal consent, or would you have called his room?

Specialist: It just depends on the situation.

Sheila: But this is when he was getting better. So what actually happened?

Specialist: I don't remember.

Supervisor: I'm going to go and look for the recording, and I'm going to get you the phone number for the patient advocate. She's on campus; if I can, I will have her come down and see you. [At this point, the Supervisor walked away to attempt to locate the audio recording of the verbal consent.]

Specialist: That just says "Verbal." I missed out on that. And I normally don't work with inpatients. So, I missed out on that, entering your name and stuff. So yeah . . . because we're not used to doing it every day, sometimes you can miss out on it. So, it is my fault; I should have put it there.

Sheila: So, someone called you and said to get a set of consent forms signed?

Specialist: So, I get a list of patients that I go and see inside their rooms. So, we registered them by going into their rooms.

Sheila: Like an ICU room?

Specialist: Yes, sometimes, if we can get to the room. If we can't, we call the patient's room, and then we get all that over the phone,

Sheila: And then it will be recorded? If you have a recording, then that's fine. As long as there is a recording of him saying "Yes."

Specialist: If there is a recording, then that should be fine. If not, then I don't know . . . we'll see. I don't remember, hahaha. Yeah . . . sometimes we have technical difficulties. Sometimes things are not working. The machines are not working.

*[**Sheila's comments:** I found it implausible that they would happen to have had "technical difficulties" that day. What I did find plausible, and what I did believe likely, was that I was being lied to about what really happened.]*

Sheila: I want to *hear* my husband giving someone verbal consent because there's nothing in his records with his signature. The "General Consent for Treatment" form is the most important. The question is, did he agree to this because he was a real stickler for reading everything?

Specialist: Since it says "Verbal," I did it over the phone. I would have kind of briefly told him what this is, like general consent for treatment that we can see you at the hospital today and all that stuff. And he probably said, "Okay." So I just wrote in "*Verbal.*"

Sheila: On September 7, 2021, he was in the ICU. That day, we talked for 15 minutes. I have a phone log of all of our calls.

Specialist: What happens, I call the room, and if they're able to pick up and talk to me, then that's when I get all the verbal consents over the phone.

Sheila: And you probably were not going in the room when there was a Covid patient.

Specialist: No.

Sheila: Well, he was diagnosed with Covid, but he actually had organized pneumonia, which is different from Covid.

Specialist: Sometimes, if I'm not able to reach the patient, then I call the spouse; I don't know if I called you that day. Probably not, because we need consent from the patient anyway. The second option is the spouse. *So, did I call you?*

Sheila: He came in on September 3rd. I got a call on either Friday or Saturday, and I'm pretty sure it was admissions. I was asked if I had Medical Power of Attorney, and I said, "Yes."

Specialist: We also notate it on our hard [handwritten] notes. So, if I registered him, I would have said, "Patient . . . registered patient . . . Verbal consents done" in my notes. So, I should have that noted as well. I think my supervisor is gonna check on that.

Sheila: I am so thankful that you were here.

Specialist: I'm glad I'm here too. Because I only work three days a week because I work part-time. So now we know, like, yea, "Verbal" . . . Now I know that I covered that day.

Supervisor: [Upon returning after checking for the recording] Okay, so it's gonna take me some time to try to find that recording since it was last year. But I did try to contact the patient message with your phone number so she can give you a call. The best that I can give you right now is that I will continue my investigation to see if I can find that recording.

Sheila: I know it might take time because I don't know how many people you've had to do this with. But if you could find the recording, it would give me a lot of peace. I don't see anything in the record that shows that he agreed to anything.

Supervisor: Right. Which is why I want you to continue with the patient advocate because she can get a lot more done than I can. So, I left her your phone number in my message.

Sheila: She is not a Social Worker?

Supervisor: No. she's the hospital's patient advocate.

Sheila: Okay. So you don't have an ombudsman anymore, right?

Supervisor: That term does not sound familiar. She knows how to pull all those strings and whatever to get the information you're after. You can still talk to her to give her the full story because so much of what you asked about is clinical.

Sheila: At least we know it says "*Verbal*" in the signature box.

Specialist: Yes. So, thank you. Good luck to you.

Supervisor: Thank you. And hopefully, we can get the recording.

Sheila: It would help me feel better. Thank you.

Below are copies of written communications between the hospital and Sheila as a follow-on to the December 22, 2022, face-to-face meeting.

December 27, 2022

Dear Ms. Skiba:

Thank you for contacting us with your concerns regarding your concerns regarding your husband's hospital stay September 3, 2021, through October 13, 2021. Covid Coven Hospital of Plano, Texas, strives to provide excellent care and service, and we regret that you were not satisfied with some aspects of your hospital experience.

I am forwarding these concerns to the appropriate departments for review and response. While it may take us some time to review the concerns, we will respond within 30 days from the date we received the complaint by January 20, 2023.

We appreciate the opportunity to review our services. In the meantime, should you have any questions, please feel free to contact our Patient Advocate office at Phone Number.

Sincerely,
Redacted Signature
Patient Advocate's Name
Covid Coven Hospital of Plano, Texas

January 19, 2023—Second Letter from Hospital to Sheila

[**Bolded** text by us to highlight their admission that no recording of the alleged verbal consent was located.]

January 19, 2023

Dear Mrs. Skiba:

On January 19, 2023, we completed our investigation of your concerns regarding your husband, Robert's care during his hospital stay of September 3, 2021 through October 13, 2021. Please accept our deepest condolences on his passing and for your loss. Covid Coven Hospital of Plano, Texas, strives to provide excellent care and service, and we hope that you will accept our sincere apology that you were not satisfied with some aspects of his hospital experience.

On December 22, 2022, we learned of your concerns when you came to the hospital and spoke to staff at the main registration. The Patient Advocate contacted you via telephone to follow up. To investigate your concerns, the Director of Patient Access Services (admissions), and the Manager of Request of Information Department (ROI) reviewed the documentation created in their department and spoke with their staff; the ICU Nurse Manager reviewed Mr. Skiba's medical record and spoke with staff who provided his care; and the Director of Information Systems/Information Technology provided additional information. Below I have listed your concerns followed by the outcome of our investigation.

1. Mr. Skiba was brought to the hospital emergency department (ED) by you. You were not able to remain with him in the ED at the time due to his COVID diagnosis. You obtained copies of his medical record and were upset that his consent forms were not with the copies when you requested them; however, you did obtain them subsequently. You came to the hospital on December 22, 2022, and tracked down the person who is designated as the witness on the consents and were told that the consents were all obtained as "verbal" and that there is a voice recording giving verbal consent on these forms. You would like to hear your husband's voice giving verbal consent for treatment.

The Director of Patient Access Services (PAS) investigated the obtaining of consents and found the following documentation:

09/06/2021 11:13 am: Inpatient Registration attempted to obtain consents. Notes indicated "Pt in isolation, called the room to get verbal consents, no answer."

09/07/2021 1:09 pm: Inpatient Registration notes indicate "Pt in isolation, tried to call the room, no answer/ called to get verbal consents from spouse."

The Patient Access Services Representative indicated verbal consent was given by you as Mr. Skiba's spouse. During the initial conversation between you and the PAS supervisor on December 22, 2022, she informed you that the consents were obtained verbally from you on September 7, 2021, due to Mr. Skiba's very serious condition and inability to consent for himself. She recalls that you acknowledged that you could have verbally consented but did not remember due to so many doctors and others discussing his care with you at the time. **We did find that there was no trace recording made of the conversation and that the consents were not fully completed with your full name, phone number and address as they should have been.** When this was discovered, the staff member involved was re-educated on the importance of completing the forms. In addition, department wide reminders and reeducation has also been conducted. We apologize that this occurred.

2. You asked why the admission consent forms were not included in the medical records that you requested and received. You feel that there is some sort of cover up.

The Manager of the Release of Information Department (ROI) verified and confirmed that a copy of all medical records were printed and sent to you on December 6, 2022. The documents included all admission consents referenced above.

3. On the day of Mr. Skiba's passing, October 13, 2021, you asked the ICU Nurse Manager for the official cause of death. She told you that she did not know and advised you to look for information in Mr. Skiba's MyChart. When you attempted to do so you found that the MyChart had been deactivated. You are requesting immediate reactivation of the MyChart and feel that you are entitled to access as next of kin and POA.

The ROI Department's process is to disable the MyChart account of a deceased patient shortly after the death of the patient. After the account is disabled, the next of kin must request a copy of the medical record from the Department. We apologize that was not explained to you at the time.

The ICU Nurse Manager was not the primary nurse, but as the department leader she was present at the time of Mr. Skiba's death and when you arrived to offer support if needed. She does not recall the conversation about cause of death but explains that as a nurse she is not authorized to discern or declare an official cause of death. She believes she would have referred you to either MyChart or to Medical Records, ROI to obtain that information.

4. You stated that your POA was never honored when Mr. Skiba passed and you were denied information on the day he died.

Based on the information in the medical record, you were provided information that was available to the staff. According to Mr. Skiba's medical record you spoke with the nurse via telephone on October 13, 2021 at 5:46 am and received a status update of your husband's current condition and plan of care. At 8:44 am you are noted to be at the bedside during a visit by the Nephrologist. The Nephrologist documented that following this visit he had a long discussion with you in the conference room regarding his recommendation that Continuous Renal Replacement Therapy (CRRT) be initiated, including a discussion on the risks and benefits of the treatment and that your questions were answered. At 4:50 pm CRRT was initiated; however, Mr. Skiba's oxygen concentration immediately decreased despite 100% oxygen support. Resuscitation efforts were immediately initiated but unsuccessful. The time of death was 5:11 pm. The Care Transitions Manager attempted to call your phone while physicians and staff were attempting resuscitation but the call went to voicemail. Shortly thereafter you arrived at Mr. Skiba's bedside. Staff offered support however you declined and asked staff to leave you alone with patient. Staff complied with your wishes. At shift change you remained at the bedside with a group of family/friends and requested the staff to continue to leave you and your support group alone with Mr. Skiba. You and the group left the hospital shortly after 8:30 pm with Mr. Skiba's belongings and personal effects.

It is certainly understandable that you are continuing to grieve your husband's death. We regret any stress you may have experienced due to your dissatisfaction over some aspects of Mr. Skiba's hospital experience and hope his letter has given you some assurance that your concerns were addressed.

In closing, I again wish to extend our sincere sympathy to you and your family. It is our hope that you will have confidence in the care you can expect to receive here, or any Covid Coven Hospital facility, if you or your family should need future health care services. If you have any further questions, feel free to contact the patient advocate at Covid Coven Hospital of Plano, Texas.

Sincerely,
Redacted Signature
Patient Advocate's Name
Covid Coven Hospital of Plano, Texas

January 25, 2023—Email from Sheila to Hospital

Emailed January 25, 2023
Dear Patient Advocate's Name :

Thank you so much for your mailed response concerning the investigation about the three consent documents in my husband's hospital record. It cleared up a lot of things for me. But, I do have a few more questions.

You stated that the Director of Patient Access Services (PAS), the Manager of Request of Information Department (ROI), and the Director of Information Systems (IS)/Information Technology (IT) were involved in the outcome of this investigation. Please share this email with the directors above.

It was my understanding that the investigation would include you looking for my husband's voice-recorded audio consent, which led to "*Verbal*" written on all three of his consent forms (Admission and Consent, PHI, and HIE). All three were signed the same ("*Verbal*"), and it was not his signature. I was told by Supervisor's Name that it is your practice to record all "Verbal" consents obtained.

You stated that your findings are: *Inpatient Registration attempted to obtain consents. Notes indicated "Pt in isolation, called the room to get verbal consents, no answer."* Are you stating in this response letter that consent was given by me? If so, I would like to see the evidence of your findings: Please provide a copy of:
1. your call log
2. what number you called from
3. what number you called
4. the duration of your call
5. the time of your call.

The witness, Specialist's Name, spoke to me (and my son) in person at Covid Coven Hospital of Plano, Texas on December 22, 2022. We inquired whom she spoke with and asked her if she signed the three documents.

Her response was initially that she did not remember. She later said, "Yes," she admitted to signing them and acknowledged that the word in the signature box on all three was the word "*Verbal*." She also said, "We also notate on our hard notes. So if I registered him, I would have said patient, registered patient verbal consents done. So I should have that noted as well."

If you could, also provide us with a copy of Specialist's Name's hard notes, which should confirm who she communicated with concerning these three consent forms. This information is critical for me and my son as we continue to heal from our tragic loss.

ALSO, PLEASE SEE ATTACHMENT OF PHI FORM.

Specialist's Name was the witness again. We would like to know whom did she speak with? What day and what time did this occur? Who answered these questions for her? They are not correct. This form is confusing to us because the button reflects that "The patient" is filling the form, and also reflects "spouse."

As you can understand, this is inconsistent and confusing to us. We need answers.
Your quick and speedy response will help me in my healing process.

Sincerely,
Sheila Skiba

February 1, 2021—Certified Letter from Sheila to Hospital

[Below is an updated version of the email that Sheila sent to the hospital patient advocate on January 25, 2021. This slightly modified edition was sent to the hospital via Certified Mail to ensure prompt attention to the issue.]

Covid Coven Hospital of Plano, Texas
Dear Patient Advocate's Name :

Thank you so much for your mailed response concerning the investigation of the three consent documents for Robert Skiba. Your response raises a few more questions.

You stated that the Director of Patient Access Services (PAS), the Manager of Request of Information Department (ROI), and the Director of Information Systems (IS)/Information Technology (IT) were involved in conducting an investigation of how the consent forms were completed for my husband's hospitalization.

As you know, my son and I came to the hospital on December 22, 2022, to meet with Specialist's Name to ask who gave her the consent for the three forms she wrote "*Verbal*" on. At that time, Supervisor's Name told us it was your practice to record all "*Verbal*" consents. She then agreed to launch an investigation to search for my husband's recorded audio consent that led to Specialist's Name writing "*Verbal*" on all three consent forms.

She launched the investigation because Specialist's Name could not recall whom she spoke with and even asked me, "*Did I call you?*" I told her, "*I do not remember getting a call from you nor do I remember your name.*"

In truth, the only call I remember receiving from anyone in hospital administration was one where I was asked if I had a Medical POA, and I responded that I did.

Your letter to me stated that you were not able to find any trace of a recording, which I find very disconcerting. In addition, your reprimand of Specialist's Name has not aided me in getting closure on how these forms were completed.

In addition, the attached PHI form that Specialist's Name filled out (and wrote "*Verbal*" on) contains responses that do not match those I would have given her if she had spoken with me. This clearly indicates I was not the person who provided the answers for this form.

Also, you alleged that I did not remember giving verbal consent. If I had provided verbal consent (a) the answers on the PHI form would match the answers I would have given, and (b) I would have definitely recalled someone taking the time to read each of the three lengthy consent forms that ended up logged, one minute apart, in your system, and (c) I would have definitely asked a number of questions about the consent forms during the call.

Thus, I am writing you to request that you conduct a follow-up investigation and provide me with answers to these important questions:
1. Who specifically told you they spoke with me and received my verbal consent?
2. What evidence do they have that they spoke with me? Please provide:
   a. The date and time of the phone call.
   b. The phone number they called.
   c. The phone number they placed the call from.
   d. The duration of the call.

Your prompt reply will be greatly appreciated and will aid my son and me with our healing process.

Sincerely,

ADMISSION ACKNOWLEDGEMENTS AND GENERAL CONSENT FOR TREATMENT
** SCROLL TO BOTTOM TO COMPLETE THE SIGNATURE ON THIS FORM **

1. **General consent.** I understand that my health condition requires inpatient or outpatient admission. I consent to and authorize testing, treatment and health care at this facility ("Facility"), a **Covid Coven Hospital** Facility, by facility nurses, employees, and others as ordered by my physician and his/her consultants, associates, and assistants, or as directed pursuant to standing medical orders or protocols. I understand that it may be necessary for representatives of outside health care companies to assist in my care. I also understand that persons in professional training programs may be among the persons who provide care to me. I understand that in connection with my treatment, photos or videos may be taken. Any tissue or body parts removed from my body may be retained or disposed of by the Facility at its sole discretion.

2. **Independent physicians.** I acknowledge that the physicians taking part in my care or providing a professional service to me do not work for the Facility and that the Facility is not responsible for their judgment or conduct. They practice independently and are not employees or agents of the Facility. The exception to this is that some physicians may be medical residents in a graduate medical education program of the Facility under the supervision of more experienced physicians. In addition to my attending physician, other physicians who may take part in my care may include radiologists, pathologists, anesthesiologists, hospitalists, neonatologists, cardiologists, emergency physicians, psychiatrists, and other specialists. The physician and professional services are not covered by the **CCH** Financial Assistance Policy.

3. **No guarantee.** I acknowledge that no guarantees or warranties have been made to me with the respect to treatment or services to be provided at this Facility. I understand that all supplies, medical devices and other goods provided or billed to me by the Facility are provided by the Facility on an "AS IS" basis, and the Facility disclaims any expressed or implied warranties with respect to them. With respect to specific supplies and devices, manufacturers' warranties may apply, and I may request manufacturer's warranty information concerning such supplies and/or devices.

4. **My valuables:** I understand that the Facility does not assume responsibility for personal property I keep with me during my treatment/Facility stay. I understand that unnecessary items should be sent home and that a safe is available for my valuables.

5. **Assignment of benefits:** I hereby irrevocably assign to the Facility and any practitioner providing care and treatment to me, any and all benefits and all interest and rights (including causes of action and the right to enforce payment) under any insurance policies, benefit plans, indemnity plans, prepaid health plans, third-party liability policies, or from any other payer providing benefits on my behalf, for and to the extent of the services and goods provided to me during this admission. Under this assignment, the Facility shall have an independent, non-exclusive right to appeal or pursue any denied or delayed claims on behalf of the insured or beneficiary. This assignment is not and shall not be construed as an obligation of the Facility and/or Facility-based physician to pursue such interest and rights. In signing this form, I (as the patient or patient's agent) am directing any applicable health insurer, health benefit plan, indemnity plan, reinsurer, third-party liability insurer or other payer providing benefits on my behalf to pay the Facility and/or Facility-based physicians directly for the services and goods the Facility and/or Facility-based physicians provide to me.

6. **Financial agreement:** I hereby promise to pay the Facility its full billed charges for all services and goods provided to me. I understand that the Facility, as a courtesy to me, may bill my insurance company, health benefit plan, or other non-governmental payer concerning the services and goods provided by the Facility to me but that the Facility is under no obligation to do so. Except as prohibited by law or by written agreement of the Facility, I agree to pay for any charges not covered and covered charges not paid in full by any applicable insurance and/or health benefit plan including charges payable as co-insurance, deductibles, and non-covered benefits due to policy and/or plan limitations, exclusions, and/or failure to comply with insurance and/or plan requirements. I further understand that the Facility, by mutual agreement with me or a person and/or entity making payments on my behalf, may agree to accept a discounted amount of its charges in full payment of the charges; however, to the extent the Facility has not agreed to accept less than the charges, I agree to be responsible for payment of the full amount of the charges less any amounts already paid by me or on my behalf. If I am entitled to benefits under a governmental plan, such as Medicare or Medicaid, I further understand the Facility may bill such plan and may accept as payment in full a discounted payment for the services and goods provided to me. **CCH** Financial Assistance Policy may be available if Facility eligibility criteria are met. An estimate of the anticipated charges is available upon request. I understand that estimates may vary significantly from the final charges because of a variety of factors such as the course of my treatment, intensity of care, physician practices, and the necessity of ~~providing~~ additional services and goods. I hereby consent to credit bureau inquiries and to receiving auto-dialed/artificial or pre-recorded ~~...~~ or text messages to my cellular telephone and to any telephone number provided during my registration process. I ~~...~~ attempts could be performed by from **Covid Coven Hospital** or its affiliates/agents including, ~~without~~ ~~...~~ ~~...parties,~~ independent contractors or collection agents.

7. **Medicaid patients only:** I understand that the services or ~~...~~ ~~...~~ ~~...~~ be covered under the Texas Medical Assistance Program as being reasonable and ~~...~~ ~~...~~ that the Texas Department of Human Services or its health insuring agent determines the ~~...~~ ~~...~~ quest and receive. I also understand that I am responsible for payment of the services or goods ~~...~~ ~~...~~ are determined not to be reasonable and medically necessary for my care. If I am a Medicaid Star patie~~...~~ ~~...~~ pay.

8. **Communicable di~~...~~ se testing.** I acknowledge that Texas law provides if any health care worker is exposed to my blood or other bodily fluid, the Facility may perform tests, without my consent, on my blood or other bodily fluid to look for the presence of hepatitis B and C and HIV. I understand that such testing is needed to protect those who will be caring for me while I am a patient at the Facility. I understand that the results of tests taken under these circumstances are confidential and do not become a part of my Facility patient record.

9. **Obstetrics patients only:** This *Admission Acknowledgement and General Consent for Treatment* also applies to any child(ren) born to me during this hospitalization.

10. **OPTION TO RECEIVE INFORMATION AS TEXT MESSAGES:** As indicated below, I make the following election regarding whether to receive information about my care from the Facility and/or my physician in the form of a text message.

    ⦿ I elect to receive information about my care, including information the privacy of which is protected under federal and state law, from the Facility and/or my physician in the form of a text message.

    ○ I elect NOT to receive information about my care, including information the privacy of which is protected under federal and state law, from the Facility and/or my physician in the form of a text message.

Page 1 of 2-page General Consent for Treatment form "signed" on the next page.

If the person signing this form is not the patient, please give full name, phone number and address:

Name:

Phone Number:

Address:

Relationship: ⇨ spouse

Acknowledgement: I, the undersigned, ⬚ ⬚ ⬚ ⬚ ⬚ ⬚ ⬚ ⬚ ⬚ ⬚ ⬚ by
its terms.

⇨ *[signature]*

Signature captured with Topaz 1x5 by Robert Skiba

Skiba, Robert   09/07/21 1:07 PM

Witness Admission Specialist Redacted Name

Covid Coven Hospital
**Admission Acknowledgements
And General Consent for Treatment**
998543135 (Rev. 05/19) Page 1 of 1

Four days after Rob's admission (why wait this long?) a hospital "Admission Specialist" signed **"Verbal"** on the *General Consent* form shown above and, as shown in the signature blocks below, on two other forms. These forms were "signed" at 1:07, 1:08, and 1:09 PM—and by entering **"spouse"** they implied Sheila had given her verbal consent (which she had not) at a time when they were ignoring her directives because (as they admit) Rob was alert, aware, and fully capable of making his own decisions. Rob was fully capable of signing these and any other consent forms they needed. They should have obtained **Rob's signature** on these and other clearly "missing" consents for treatment, yet these three basic consent forms are the ONLY ones filed in the hospital records. Why did they not ask Rob to sign these forms, and why did they wait until four days after Rob's admission? See **Appendix I – Falsification of Hospital Consent Forms** for more on this troubling discovery.

Signatu⬚

PROTECTED HEALTH INFORMATION, T⬚ ⬚E TO PATIENTS, ADVANCE DIRECTIVES

Acknowledgement:
I, the undersigned, certify that I have read and fully understand the information in this Protected Health Information, Third Party Payer Notice to Patients, Advance Directives. I understand that if I need to change any information I have provided on this form, I will notify a facility staff member promptly.

Tap Once To Sign

⇨ *[signature]*

Signature captured at 9/7/2021 01:08 PM

Skiba, Robert

⇨ spouse

Relationship to patient

Signature Block Only (Not Full Form)

CONSENT FOR HEALTH INFORMATION EXCHANGE

Acknowledgment:
I, the undersigned, certify that I have read and fully understand the information in this Consent for Health Information Exchange form. I understand that if I need to change any information I have provided on this form, I will notify a staff member promptly.

Signature of patient or authorized representative

⇨ *[signature]*

Signature captured at 9/7/2021 01:09 PM

Skiba, Robert

February 6, 2023—Final Letter from Hospital to Sheila

February 6, 2023

Dear Mrs. Skiba:

On January 19, 2023, we provided you with the outcome of our investigation of your concerns regarding your late husband, Robert Skiba's hospital stay of September 3, 2021 until his passing on October 13, 2021. After receiving our letter you followed up with an e-mail on January 25, 2023 in which you requested additional information.

Below is a list of the additional information you requested, followed by our response.

1. You asked for evidence of our findings including a copy of the recorded audio consent with your voice.

As noted in our previous letter the staff member who took the consent mistakenly did not record any of the registrations she did that day in violation of hospital procedure. As mentioned in our January 19th letter, the staff member involved was re-educated on the importance of completing the forms. In addition, department wide reminders and reeducation has also been conducted. We apologize that this occurred.

2. You requested a copy of our call log.

We do not keep a call log. All calls are supposed to be saved by the recording. However, as previously discussed, a mistake was made and we failed to record the call.

3. You asked which number we called from.

To the best of our knowledge the phone numbers that would have been utilized to call from would have been Phone Number 1 or Phone Number 2. However, we are unable to verify this.

4. You asked what number we called.

Staff utilizes the emergency contact as listed in the Medical Record to make such calls. The following was the information in the medical record that the staff member would have referred to:
Emergency Contact 1
Sheila Skiba (Spouse)
Phone Number (M)

5. You asked for the duration of the call.

We do not have that information as the call was not properly documented as discussed previously.
6. You asked for the time of the call.

According to the documentation provided by the staff member, the call would have taken place between 1:00-1:09 pm on September 7, 2021. The staff member noted in the medical record:

9/7/2021 13:09:45 "Patient in isolation, tried to call the room.
No answer/called to get verbal consents from spouse."

7. You asked for a copy of Specialist's Name's hard notes.

Enclosed is a copy of the hard notes. For your convenience I have highlighted Specialist's Name's entry. The "hard note" is part of the electronic record kept of the patient encounter but is not technically a part of the medical record.

8. Specialist's Name was the witness on the PHI form you sent. You asked who she spoke-with, the day and time

The registration employees failed to follow the hospital process and incorrectly completed this form. She indicated the patient was the individual answering the questions and should have written instead that it was the person with patient, filled in the name of the spouse and address on the last page, and legibly written "verbal" in the signature box. We do not have any of the other information you requested on this issue because as we explained above the employee mistakenly did not record the conversation.

We again sincerely apologize that we did not follow our process for appropriate documentation of this consent and want to assure you that we have taken this matter very seriously and that coaching and corrective action has taken place with the employee.

We are very sorry that our failure to properly document consent continues to trouble you as you grieve the loss of your husband. If you have any further questions, feel free to contact the patient advocate at Phone Number.

Sincerely,
Redacted Signature
Patient Advocate's Name
Covid Coven Hospital of Plano, Texas

Rob Skiba—the Man Behind the Story

Robert A. Skiba II (Rob Skiba) was a beloved husband, father, son, brother, and friend. His heart's desire was to see people redeemed, set free, and made whole.

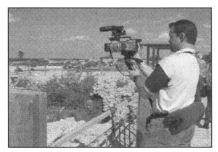

From a young age, Rob's dream was to become a filmmaker. His dream became a reality when a world missions organization hired him to create short films for missionaries in foreign countries to help publicize and promote their work.

As his colleague within the same organization, I produced printed materials supporting the films and further describing each mission's objectives and positive impact.

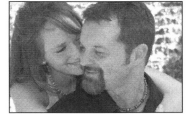

We wished to use our skills to advance God's kingdom, and we formed a strong team. We tied the knot on 7/7/07 (three 7s) and enjoyed 14 wonderful years of marriage (two 7s). Rob was more than what I had prayed for. He was my best friend, and being his wife was such a blessing and gift that I often had to pinch myself.

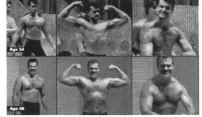

As a former Eagle Scout and Army helicopter pilot in the U.S. Army Reserve, Rob was devoted to maintaining his health and taking care of his body. Comparing his photographs in his twenties to those he took more recently reveals that he had a lifelong goal of remaining physically fit.

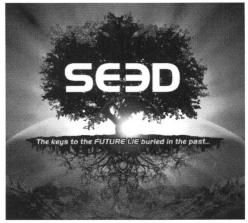

Soon after our wedding, we felt compelled to take a leap of faith to pursue Rob's lifelong dream of creating a television series titled SEED, which you can learn more about at https://seedtheseries.com.

Rob also investigated ancient history, and after recording his findings, he published his first book, Babylon Rising, which describes the impact of pre-flood giants/Nephilim. In his second book, Archon Invasion, he delved into transhumanism and genetic manipulation.

Due to the immense interest in Rob's discoveries, he became a sought-after speaker, and we soon found ourselves traveling the world to share his findings. Rob also launched a YouTube channel at https://www.youtube.com/robskiba.

In 2013, he established a "Virtual House Church" on the Internet to make it easier for people from around the world to study the scriptures together. You can learn more at http://virtualhousechurch.com.

As a result of Rob's insightful books, videos, and conference presentations, numerous individuals sent him emails and letters expressing gratitude for their newfound or restored faith. It was a fruitful season, and we relished every moment of it!

Rob's *"truth radar"* was always on, and in 2020, after researching the disconcerting response to the COVID-19 pandemic with its attendant travel restrictions, lockdowns, experimental mRNA "vaccines," and banned versus approved treatments, he began sounding the alarm. As was his nature, Rob had no problem delving deeply into a nefarious and troubling subject and was not afraid to share his findings with anyone willing to listen.

Most importantly, Rob devoted his life to helping others find Yeshua (Jesus) through Internet interviews, creating hundreds of YouTube videos, and designing websites that shed light on the darkness and revealed the truth. His tragic and needless death is a loss felt by many who appreciated his insightful teachings. Moreover, when Rob died at the hands of *"the protocol that kills,"* it completely shattered the lives of his family—and especially impacted mine.

My son, Jeremiah Skiba, and I are committed to continuing Rob's research and preserving his voice to uphold his legacy of uncovering and revealing the truth. Jeremiah launched his own YouTube news channel titled "Skiba News Nation," which can be viewed at https://youtube.com/skibanewsnation. Jeremiah's weekly broadcast, which airs every Friday at 4:44 PM Central, covers a wide range of historical and contemporary topics and frequently features engaging guests.

Jeremiah also authored his own book, <u>Never Got To Say Goodbye</u>, which provides a more in-depth look at who Rob Skiba truly was as a father and as a man.

Rob's legacy endures in the hearts of those who loved him and his teachings. Although he is greatly missed, his impact lives on in the countless lives he touched and those he led to Yeshua during his time on Earth. I believe he is alive now and forever with Yeshua and enjoying fellowshipping with many historical greats he regarded as his heroes.

To see the teachings of the man behind the story, visit the following websites:
- https://robschannel.com
- https://seedtheseries.com
- http://virtualhousechurch.com
- https://babylonrisingbooks.com
- https://ephraimawakening.com

You might also enjoy these YouTube channels:
- https://www.youtube.com/robskiba
- https://youtube.com/skibanewsnation

Sheila Skiba

Made in the USA
Columbia, SC
13 April 2024